硬膜下血肿
——过去、现在与未来的临床管理

Subdural Hematoma:
Past to Present to Future Management

原著 Mehmet Turgut・Ali Akhaddar
Walter A. Hall・Ahmet T. Turgut

主译 刘伟明 吴 量

主审 高国一

北京大学医学出版社

YINGMO XIA XUEZHONG——GUOQU、XIANZAI YU WEILAI DE LINCHUANG GUANLI

图书在版编目（CIP）数据

硬膜下血肿：过去、现在与未来的临床管理 /（土）穆罕默德·图尔古特（Mehmet Turgut）等原著；刘伟明，吴量主译 . -- 北京：北京大学医学出版社，2025. 8. -- ISBN 978-7-5659-3464-3

I . R651.1

中国国家版本馆 CIP 数据核字第 2025YA8814 号

北京市版权局著作权合同登记号：图字：01-2025-2232

First published in English under the title
Subdural Hematoma: Past to Present to Future Management
edited by Mehmet Turgut, Ali Akhaddar, Walter A. Hall and Ahmet T. Turgut
Copyright © Mehmet Turgut, Ali Akhaddar, Walter A. Hall and Ahmet T. Turgut, 2021
This edition has been translated and published under licence from
Springer Nature Switzerland AG.

Simplified Chinese translation Copyright © 2025 by Peking University Medical Press.
All Rights Reserved.

硬膜下血肿——过去、现在与未来的临床管理

主　　译：	刘伟明　吴　量
出版发行：	北京大学医学出版社
地　　址：	（100191）北京市海淀区学院路 38 号　北京大学医学部院内
电　　话：	发行部 010-82802230；图书邮购 010-82802495
网　　址：	http://www.pumpress.com.cn
E-mail：	booksale@bjmu.edu.cn
印　　刷：	北京金康利印刷有限公司
经　　销：	新华书店
责任编辑：	高　瑾　　责任校对：靳新强　　责任印制：李　啸
开　　本：	889 mm×1194 mm　1/16　印张：19.75　字数：600 千字
版　　次：	2025 年 8 月第 1 版　2025 年 8 月第 1 次印刷
书　　号：	ISBN 978-7-5659-3464-3
定　　价：	185.00 元

版权所有，违者必究
（凡属质量问题请与本社发行部联系退换）

译者名单

主译

刘伟明　首都医科大学附属北京天坛医院神经外科
吴　量　首都医科大学附属北京天坛医院神经外科

主审

高国一　首都医科大学附属北京天坛医院神经外科

译者（按姓氏笔画排序）

马永杰　首都医科大学北京宣武医院神经外科
王李傲　首都医科大学附属北京天坛医院神经外科
石　禹　首都医科大学附属北京天坛医院神经外科
田润发　首都医科大学附属北京天坛医院神经外科
朱炳城　首都医科大学附属北京天坛医院神经外科
汤　劼　首都医科大学北京宣武医院神经外科
李　姝　首都医科大学附属北京天坛医院麻醉科
李云飞　首都医科大学附属北京天坛医院神经外科
李锦平　首都医科大学附属北京朝阳医院神经外科
张　烁　首都医科大学附属北京天坛医院神经外科
陈思畅　首都医科大学北京宣武医院神经外科
欧云尉　首都医科大学附属北京天坛医院神经外科
郭　鹏　首都医科大学附属北京朝阳医院神经外科
郭旭飞　首都医科大学附属北京天坛医院神经外科

小说月报

译者序

慢性硬膜下血肿是神经外科临床实践中的常见病、多发病，其发病率在我国各级医院均占有相当比重。然而，长期以来，国内对于这一疾病的系统认知、规范化诊疗路径以及基于高级别循证医学证据的共识性标准，仍存在显著不足。译者前期进行的全国性问卷调查清晰地揭示了这一现状：广大神经外科医师普遍反映，现有的专业书籍对该病的阐述相对匮乏且滞后，导致临床实践中对疾病的认识深度不一，治疗方式多依赖个人经验，疗效亦参差不齐。这种状况，无疑对提升我国慢性硬膜下血肿的整体诊疗水平构成了挑战。

值此背景下，我们怀着极大的热忱，将 Mehmet Turgut 教授、Ali Akhaddar 教授、Walter A. Hall 教授以及 Ahmet T. Turgut 教授共同编著的《硬膜下血肿：过去、现在与未来的临床管理》引入中国。本书的出版恰逢其时，其价值不言而喻。

本书堪称一部关于慢性硬膜下血肿的集大成之作。它对该病的全貌进行了系统而深入的梳理与总结，内容涵盖病因学、危险因素、病理生理机制、解剖病理特征、流行病学规律、临床表现、影像学诊断精髓、多样化的治疗策略、术后并发症管理以及预后评估等各个核心临床环节。尤为可贵的是，全书贯穿了循证医学的理念，提供了大量基于高等级证据的诊疗要点，为临床决策提供了坚实的科学依据。更难能可贵的是，作者们并未止步于现状，还前瞻性地探讨了该病未来的研究方向与潜在的治疗创新领域，为读者打开了通往学科前沿的视野。

本书的四位主编均是享誉国际的顶尖学者，他们在神经外科、放射学及相关交叉领域拥有深厚的学术造诣和丰富的临床经验。Mehmet Turgut 教授在发育神经科学、儿童神经外科及中枢神经系统感染等领域建树卓著；Ali Akhaddar 教授在中枢神经系统感染、脊柱外科及医学史方面成果斐然，其著作已有中文译本惠及中国读者；Walter A. Hall 教授在脑肿瘤创新治疗模式（如术中磁共振导航手术）方面是公认的权威；Ahmet T. Turgut 教授则在肿瘤影像诊断与介入领域贡献突出。他们汇聚各自专长，确保了本书内容的权威性、前沿性和全面性。

我们深信，本书中文版的推出，将有效填补国内在该疾病领域系统性、高质量专业参考书的空白。它不仅是各级神经外科医师、神经内科医师、放射科医师、急诊科医师及相关专业研究生、规培生不可或缺的知识资源，更能为临床实践提供清晰的指引，有力推动我国慢性硬膜下血肿诊疗的规范化、标准化进程，最终惠及广大患者。

本书的翻译工作凝聚了多位专家的心血，感谢各位译者在专业术语审定和内容校对上付出的努力。同时，特别感谢出版社编辑团队的严谨把关，确保了译稿的质量。

我们衷心希望，这部凝聚了国际顶尖专家智慧结晶的著作，能够成为国内同仁案头常备的实用指南，助力大家深化对这一"熟悉又陌生"的常见疾病的理解，提升诊疗水平。

谨为序。

刘伟明　吴　量
2025 年 6 月

प्रास्ताविक

原著序

本书及时全面地介绍了神经外科常见但却被严重忽视的疾病之一——硬膜下血肿（SDH）。慢性硬膜下血肿（CSDH）或如 Virchow 创造的"内出血性硬脑膜炎"一词（1857 年），是 SDH 的慢性变异型，其发病率与我们人类的寿命成正比。本书系统性介绍了 SDH 的诱发因素及其多样的临床表现。

虽然动静脉畸形和动脉瘤相对罕见，但其相关书籍却很多；SDH 在现实生活中更为普遍，但对 SDH 进行深入分析的书籍却很少。同时，SDH 通常是许多神经外科医生在过去、现在和未来第一次主刀的手术。

在大多数情况下，通过一个小手术就可以让 SDH 患者获得快速恢复。然而，SDH 也可能发展成为不断恶性循环的血肿，无论临床医生进行何种治疗尝试，患者最终结局都将恶化且无法挽回。尤其是对 CSDH 患者的治疗，较差的预后常常会令临床医生们感到沮丧。

虽然很少有人会自称为治疗"CSDH"的外科医生，但我们不都治疗过此类患者吗？作为合格的治疗"CSDH"的外科医生，我们的义务就是不断提高自身的知识和水平。改善 SDH 患者的命运可能会很容易，临床医生会因患者的"奇迹"康复而感到自豪。有时尽管我们尽了最大的努力，但还是无法帮助到患者，这可能是无法逃脱的命运，但我们仍有责任尽一切努力来提高治愈患者的概率。用严谨科学和真诚的态度治疗患者是我们应尽的责任。

Turgut、Akhaddar、Turgut 和 Hall 的研究成果为本书提供了基础。他们的著作将成为年轻医生的行医标准，同时也提醒所有人在最重要的方面不断提高专业水平。

Arya Nabavi，MD，PhD，MaHM，IFAAN
神经外科教授
神经外科主任
北施塔特医院
德国 汉诺威

原著前言

硬膜下血肿（SDH）是一种需要谨慎对待的疾病，尽管它是外科实践中最常见的疾病，也是神经外科住院医师培训中最先教授的外科手术，但其标准治疗方式仍未统一。由于人类预期寿命的延长和广泛的抗血栓治疗，这种临床疾病的发病率在世界范围内逐渐增加。受其病因和患病个体因素的影响，SDH 主要表现为急性、亚急性和慢性 3 种形式。SDH 发生发展的病理生理学可以通过其在颅顶或椎管中的位置来解释。在 SDH 中观察到的各种组织病理学变化，可因血肿的形成时间不同而异，特定的易感风险因素也可导致 SDH 的发生。

SDH 的临床表现与其颅内位置有关，其临床表现会随发病时的年龄不同而有所差异。在颅内 SDH 中，可能会出现常规临床表现如癫痫发作，或不寻常的表现形式如精神障碍。脊髓压迫综合征通常发生在受影响的脊髓区域。当出现神经系统症状时应采取影像学检查，检查方法包括计算机断层成像或磁共振成像，以确定出血的位置和原因。细致的临床病史采集也可以发现 SDH 的潜在病因，如曾接受腰椎穿刺或脑脊液分流手术，进行电疗，以及存在潜在的血液病或自发性颅内低压。在一些情况下，可确定与 SDH 相关的特定颅内异常病变，如动静脉畸形和蛛网膜囊肿。头部创伤和与运动相关的损伤也可能导致 SDH 的发展，甚至老年人的轻微创伤也可能导致 SDH。

SDH 的主要治疗方式是外科手术治疗，手术治疗通常涉及多种麻醉技术，以便能够安全地清除血肿。新的手术方式，如内镜引流和脑膜中动脉栓塞，已成功地应用于 SDH 的治疗。药物治疗可能包括使用皮质类固醇和氨甲环酸治疗。尽管治疗方法不断进步，但 SDH 的术后并发症仍可能导致疾病复发。对于患有 SDH 的老年人群，术后进行专业的康复治疗是必需的，且预后和临床结局往往受治疗过程的影响。从医疗法律的角度来看，除了错误诊断和延误治疗外，还应始终牢记各种失职行为，如漏诊婴儿摇晃综合征，这些都可能会使 SDH 患者的治疗变得复杂。

Aydın，Turkey	Mehmet Turgut
Marrakech，Morocco	Ali Akhaddar
Syracuse，NY，USA	Walter A. Hall
Ankara，Turkey	Ahmet T. Turgut

目　录

第 1 章　急性、亚急性及慢性硬膜下血肿综述 ····· 1
第 2 章　颅内急性及亚急性硬膜下血肿 ·········· 16
第 3 章　颅内硬膜下血肿研究发展史 ············ 21
第 4 章　慢性硬膜下血肿：病理生理学 ·········· 27
第 5 章　慢性硬膜下血肿的实验模型 ············ 34
第 6 章　颅腔形态对慢性硬膜下血肿好发部位的
　　　　 影响 ································ 42
第 7 章　慢性硬膜下血肿的解剖病理学和组织
　　　　 病理学变化 ·························· 46
第 8 章　慢性硬膜下血肿的流行病学和诱发
　　　　 因素 ································ 56
第 9 章　慢性硬膜下血肿的主要临床表现 ········ 61
第 10 章　慢性硬膜下血肿与癫痫 ················ 67
第 11 章　伴精神障碍的慢性硬膜下血肿 ·········· 75
第 12 章　小儿慢性硬膜下血肿 ·················· 80
第 13 章　慢性硬膜下血肿的影像学表现 ·········· 89
第 14 章　机化的慢性硬膜下血肿 ··············· 102
第 15 章　钙化或骨化的硬膜下血肿 ············· 110
第 16 章　颅脑创伤性硬膜下积液后的慢性硬膜下
　　　　 血肿 ······························· 117
第 17 章　继发于脑脊液分流术和神经外科内镜
　　　　 手术的硬膜下出血 ··················· 124
第 18 章　腰椎穿刺及椎管内麻醉后慢性硬膜下
　　　　 血肿 ······························· 128
第 19 章　低颅内压 ··························· 136
第 20 章　电休克疗法后的慢性硬膜下血肿：
　　　　 一种罕见但严重的并发症 ············· 144
第 21 章　血液病导致的慢性硬膜下血肿 ········· 148
第 22 章　合并颅内血管畸形的急性和慢性硬膜下
　　　　 血肿 ······························· 156
第 23 章　慢性硬膜下血肿与颅内蛛网膜囊肿 ···· 161
第 24 章　慢性硬膜下血肿的罕见颅内部位 ······ 167
第 25 章　运动性头部损伤相关慢性硬膜下
　　　　 血肿 ······························· 172
第 26 章　慢性硬膜下血肿的神经影像学鉴别诊断
　　　　（影像学层面）······················ 184
第 27 章　慢性硬膜下血肿的非手术治疗 ········· 194
第 28 章　慢性硬膜下血肿的麻醉治疗 ··········· 202
第 29 章　慢性硬膜下血肿的外科治疗 ··········· 221
第 30 章　神经内镜在慢性硬膜下血肿手术
　　　　 治疗中的作用 ······················· 228
第 31 章　脑膜中动脉栓塞治疗慢性硬膜下
　　　　 血肿 ······························· 231
第 32 章　慢性硬膜下血肿围手术期管理 ········· 236
第 33 章　颅内慢性硬膜下血肿术后并发症 ······ 246
第 34 章　慢性硬膜下血肿的术后处理及随访
　　　　 策略 ······························· 258
第 35 章　慢性硬膜下血肿的皮质类固醇治疗 ···· 267
第 36 章　慢性硬膜下血肿复发的处理 ··········· 273
第 37 章　老年慢性硬膜下血肿的康复治疗 ······ 284
第 38 章　慢性硬膜下血肿的转归和预后 ········· 288
第 39 章　硬膜下血肿的法医学问题 ············· 293
第 40 章　脊柱硬膜下血肿 ····················· 299
结语 ··· 304

第1章 急性、亚急性及慢性硬膜下血肿综述

Ali Akhaddar

译者：刘伟明

1.1 引言

硬膜下血肿（SDH）是由于血液在硬脑膜和蛛网膜之间积聚而形成的。硬膜包括保护颅腔脑组织的硬脑膜以及保护椎管内脊髓和神经根的硬脊膜。一般情况下，硬膜下间隙桥静脉的破裂是大多数SDH发生的原因。导致桥静脉破裂的最常见因素是创伤，其他因素包括医源性并发症以及使用抗凝、抗血小板治疗等。

SDH在神经外科是一种常见且被较多研究的疾病，其特点包括血肿位置不同、临床表现多样、神经影像表现各异，以及对大脑的重要功能区域产生不同的影响。为了简化SDH的分类，依据血肿的形状范围以及进展时间分为三类：

- "第一类"颅脑急性/亚急性SDH
- "第二类"颅脑慢性SDH
- "第三类"脊髓SDH

本书将尽可能探究不同类型SDH之间的联系。急性和亚急性SDH的区别以及亚急性和慢性SDH的区别并不典型，主要是通过发生发展时间及神经影像特征进行区别。

颅脑SDH对年轻人和老年人均会产生影响。年轻患者典型表现为继发于高能损伤的急性创伤性SDH，而老年患者则更易出现慢性SDH，其主要与微小颅脑创伤伴/不伴诱因如脑萎缩、饮酒、凝血功能障碍等有关。颅脑急性SDH通常会严重影响生活，慢性SDH如果得到规范治疗预后相对较好。

截至目前文献报道中，脊髓SDH患者数量少于260例，与颅脑SDH相比不常见[61]。

对于颅脑和脊髓SDH，本章将会讨论血肿的发展时间以及不同类型SDH的潜在联系。

1.2 颅脑急性及亚急性硬膜下血肿

急性及亚急性SDH一般与严重颅脑创伤有关，桥静脉破裂、脑挫裂伤以及皮质血管断裂也可能导致其发生，而且多达1/3伴有急性SDH的颅脑损伤患者可能合并严重的多发伤[24, 40]。这些血肿同样与其他的颅脑损伤如脑震荡、脑内血肿、脑水肿、弥散性轴索损伤以及硬膜外血肿有关。一些急性或亚急性SDH患者可能没有颅脑创伤史，但是可能有出血性疾病（接受抗凝治疗或者患凝血性疾病）以及肿瘤、血管畸形等非少见潜在病因[13, 16, 27, 32, 41, 58]，甚至少数病例曾接受过颅脑或脊柱手术[10, 12, 52, 62, 64]。

症状可能继发于颅底压迫、脑实质损伤、脑水肿以及中线偏移。额叶和颞叶是最常见的发生部位。然而，部分急性或亚急性SDH可能位于大脑半球间、小脑幕或者颅后窝[19]。SDH可能会有多种临床表现，如意识改变、癫痫发作、神经功能缺失以及累及心脏呼吸等全身性疾病。

在急诊情况下，计算机断层成像（CT）因其更普遍、更快以及更便宜的优点被认为是颅脑创伤患者的最佳首选检查。经典颅脑SDH的CT表现为边缘向内凹陷的轴外新月形肿块，通常伴有脑水肿、占位效应以及中线偏移，若出现严重的临床症状可能伴随脑挫裂伤、脑实质内部血肿、钩回疝、基底池消失以及对侧颞角扩张。急性和亚急性出血之间的区别一般是不明确的，大多数急性血肿（少于3天）是高密度的，亚急性血肿（3天至2周）与脑实质相比是等密度或者混杂密度的（图1.1和1.2）。一些SDH类型不能通过CT平扫与硬膜外血肿鉴别，甚至有时二者并存[4]。当某血管区域怀疑病变时，及时进行血管造影CT或血管磁共振造影（MRA）（较少见的脑血管造影）能够帮助定位以及诊断病因[13, 18, 58]。其他检查同样有效，如

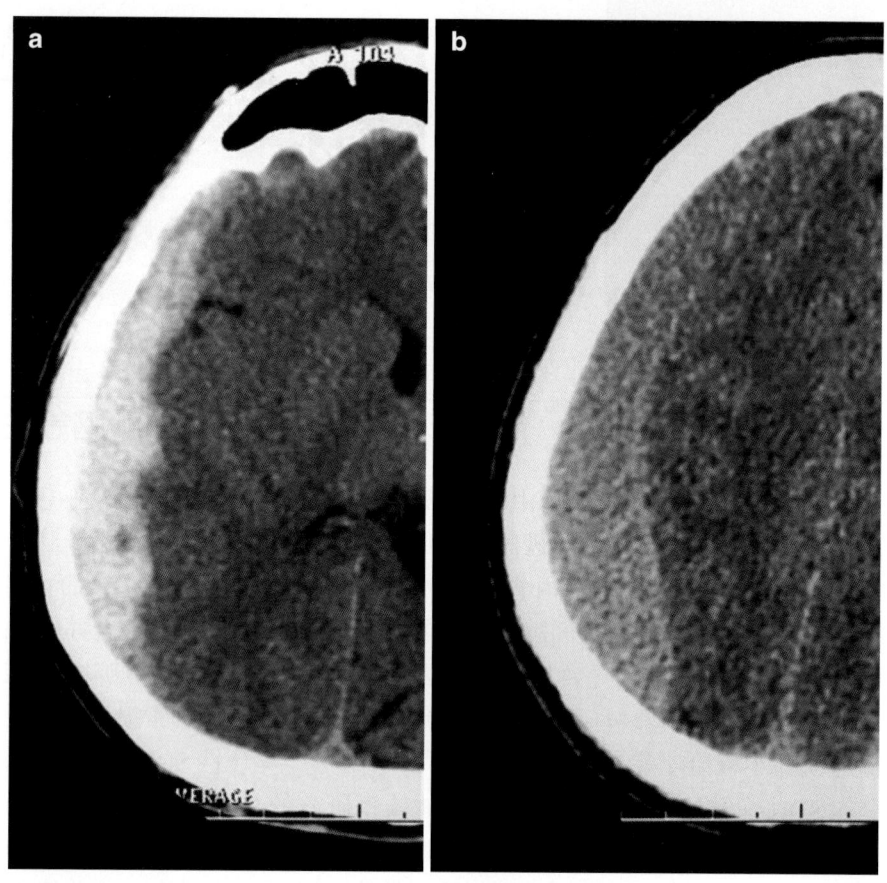

图 1.1 急性（a）和亚急性（b）硬膜下血肿 CT 扫描表现

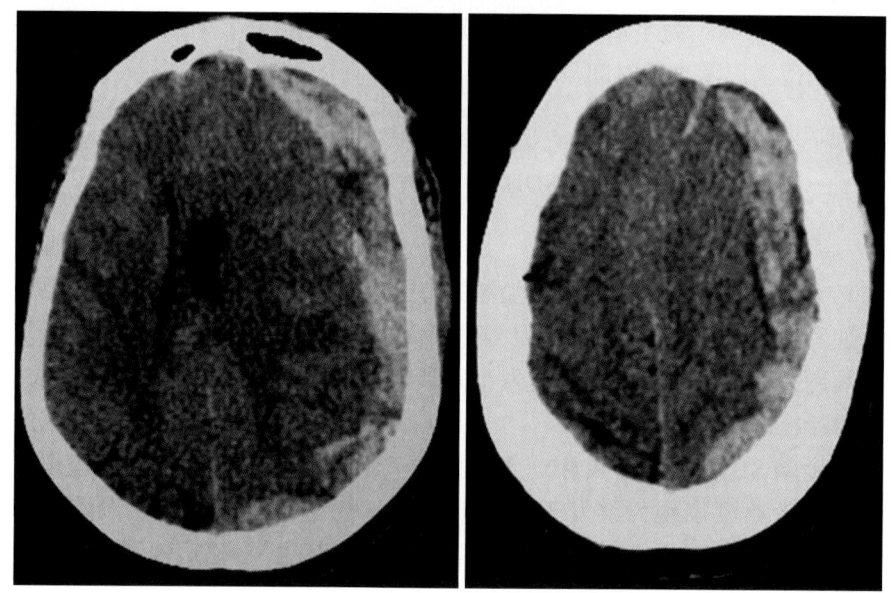

图 1.2 头颅轴位 CT 扫描：使用抗凝治疗的患者出现了自发性（非创伤性）左侧急性硬膜下出血

相关实验室检查能够用来判断隐匿性凝血功能障碍或血液病。

绝大多数急性 SDH 患者需要神经重症监护[19, 36]。当可能需要手术治疗时，神经外科医生应该考虑潜在的出血风险、患者的一般状况和相关的凝血功能障碍。急性或亚急性 SDH 的治疗需根据血肿大小、增长速度及潜在的颅脑损伤程度决定。一些小血肿（成人血肿厚度小于 10 mm，儿童血肿厚度小于 5 mm）可能会自行吸收，可以保守治疗[28, 76]。其他血肿类型尤其是亚急性和液化性的血肿类型，可以钻孔引流治疗。然而，由于血凝块的长期存在，体积较大或有临床症状的急性 SDH 需要行开颅术清除血肿并控制出血（图 1.3）[19]，必要时行去骨瓣减压术[40, 60]。术后并发症包括颅内高压、脑肿

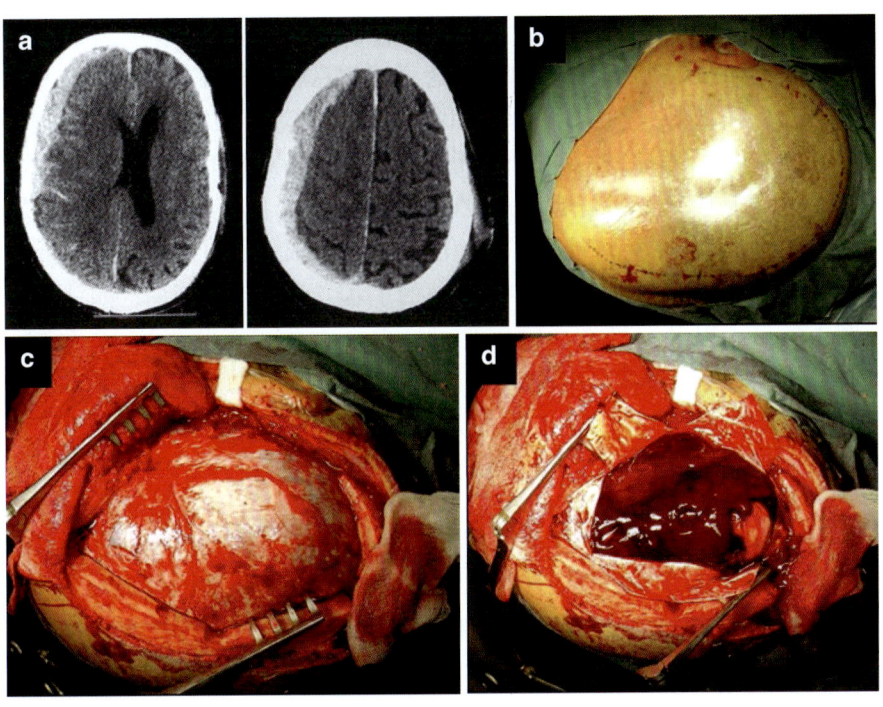

图1.3 轴向CT扫描：右侧外伤后急性硬膜下血肿（a）。头部切口标记（问号形状）（b）。去除额顶颞骨瓣后的手术视图（c）。十字形打开硬脑膜后，清除硬膜下的急性血肿（血凝块）（d）

胀、新发颅内出血、硬膜下血肿复发、感染、癫痫发作以及心肺功能紊乱。因此，术后联合多学科的重症监护是必需的[36, 70]。

急性SDH预后通常较慢性SDH以及硬膜外血肿更差。急性硬膜下血肿的原发性脑损伤类型可能是影响预后的最重要因素[22, 33, 70]，积极的医疗干预以及及时的手术减压能够提高患者术后初始的神经功能状态[33, 40]。（颅脑急性及亚急性SDH相关内容，详情查阅本书第2章）

1.3 慢性硬膜下血肿

慢性硬膜下血肿是指积聚在硬脑膜下的陈旧性血肿块（时间大于3周），由于年龄增长导致的脑萎缩及硬膜下间隙增宽，慢性SDH在老年人中更常见。这种硬膜下血肿发生率大约是每10万名老年人中有80～120人患病[11, 65]。然而，这项数据预计从2020年到2040年将会大幅增加，到2030年慢性SDH将会成为美国成年人中最常见的神经外科疾病[11, 59]。

颅内慢性SDH有多种可能病因（颅脑损伤、肿瘤、血管畸形、颅高压及其他）以及危险因素（慢性酒精中毒、癫痫发作、脑脊液分流、颅脑/脊柱手术、凝血功能障碍、男性及其他）。然而，其病理生理学机制尚未明确[5, 11, 34, 38, 59]。3个世纪以前，慢性SDH被看作是一种卒中[75]。2个世纪前，该病被认为是一种炎症[63, 69, 75]。然后，在20世纪早期，创伤被看作是其病因（连接大脑皮质和硬脑膜的桥静脉创伤性撕裂）[63, 71]。此后，渗透压和液体弥散等各种更进一步的假说被提出。一些研究人员同样发现凝血和纤溶系统在慢性SDH中同样十分活跃，因此提出了可能涉及更多复杂因素的病因猜想，包括血管生成、炎症、反复微小出血、渗出以及局部凝血功能障碍[21, 25]。

另外，一些危险因素也被视为与颅内慢性SDH有关。大量研究人员最新提出"颅骨形态"（对称或不对称）在慢性SDH的定位和发展中起着重要作用（详情查阅本书第6章）[5]。

通常，慢性SDH的临床发展被分为三个独立阶段：初始的创伤事件（通常微小或者没有被注意到）、延迟阶段以及真正的临床症状阶段。因此，慢性SDH患者通常是无症状的或者有非常轻微的症状如头痛、意识模糊、语言困难、恶心、呕吐、眩晕、乏力、进行性精神退化、步态异常、四肢无力或失禁。患者也可能表现为各种程度的偏瘫、癫痫发作甚至昏迷等急性和严重症状[6-7]。

颅脑慢性SDH通常可通过CT扫描诊断。这种血肿的典型表现为沿着颅脑凸面的新月状脑周液体积聚。这种血肿绝大多数是低密度的，然而同样可以看到等密度、混杂密度或者非均匀密度病变

（图 1.4a～d）。慢性 SDH 通常发生在单侧并有明显占位效应和中线偏移；然而一些患者可能发生在双侧、大脑半球之间，但是很少发生在后颅窝或与颅底相邻。虽然罕见，一些血肿可能出现机化、钙化甚至骨化（图 1.4e，f）[73]，辅以增强 CT 甚至更佳的 MR 检查能够提供重要的影像学特征来判断血肿的准确形状以及可能的潜在病因（如肿瘤、血管畸形、炎症病变、感染等）（图 1.5、1.6 以及 1.7）[15]。同时，相关实验室检查有助于探究有无隐匿性凝血疾病或血液疾病。由于慢性 SDH 临床表现多样以及潜在的微小神经影像表现，该病的临床诊断比较困难（详情查阅本书第 26 章）。因此，当高度怀疑患者出现慢性 SDH 时需要进行严格的临床治疗管理，并警惕其潜在并发症。

尽管部分患者可以选择非手术治疗（图 1.8 和 1.9）（详情查阅本书第 27 章），但对于有症状的患者来说外科闭式引流仍是必需的治疗方式。这种外科治疗方式在很大程度上降低了慢性 SDH 的复发可能性，缩短出院时间，减少术后并发症并降低死亡率。多种成熟的手术方式被广泛使用，如钻孔术（图 1.10）（两孔、单个大孔或环形孔）、床旁颅骨钻孔术以及伴/不伴硬膜下闭式引流的开颅术（图 1.11）。全世界范围内已经实施了多种其他外科手术，但是目前结果有限，患者预后尚不明确[66]。已经报道的手术技术列举如下：中空螺钉、硬膜下腹腔分流、可植入于硬膜下用于反复穿刺/抽吸血肿

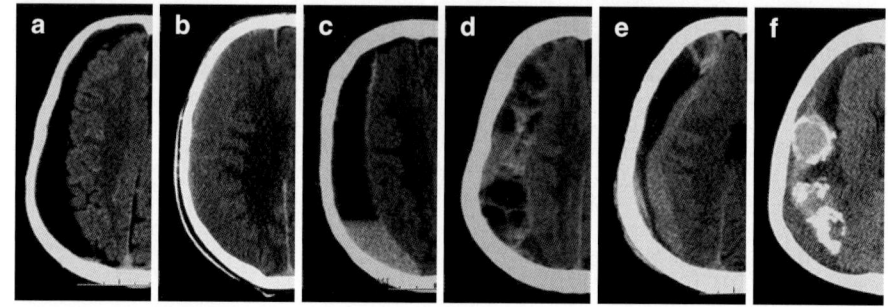

图 1.4　各种类型颅内慢性硬膜下血肿的 CT 扫描表现。（a）低密度。（b）等密度。（c）慢性 SDH 急性发作。（d）多层分布的混杂密度 SDH。（e）机化的 SDH。（f）钙化/骨化的 SDH

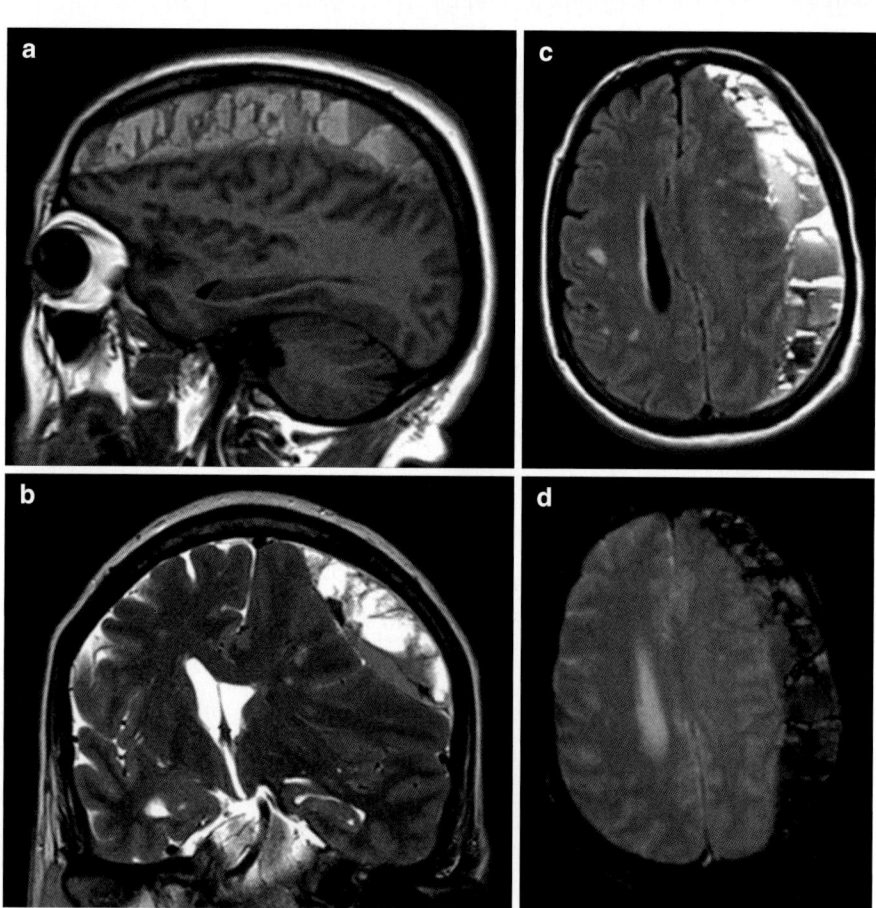

图 1.5　左侧多层异质混合性颅内慢性 SDH 的 MRI 表现（a～d）

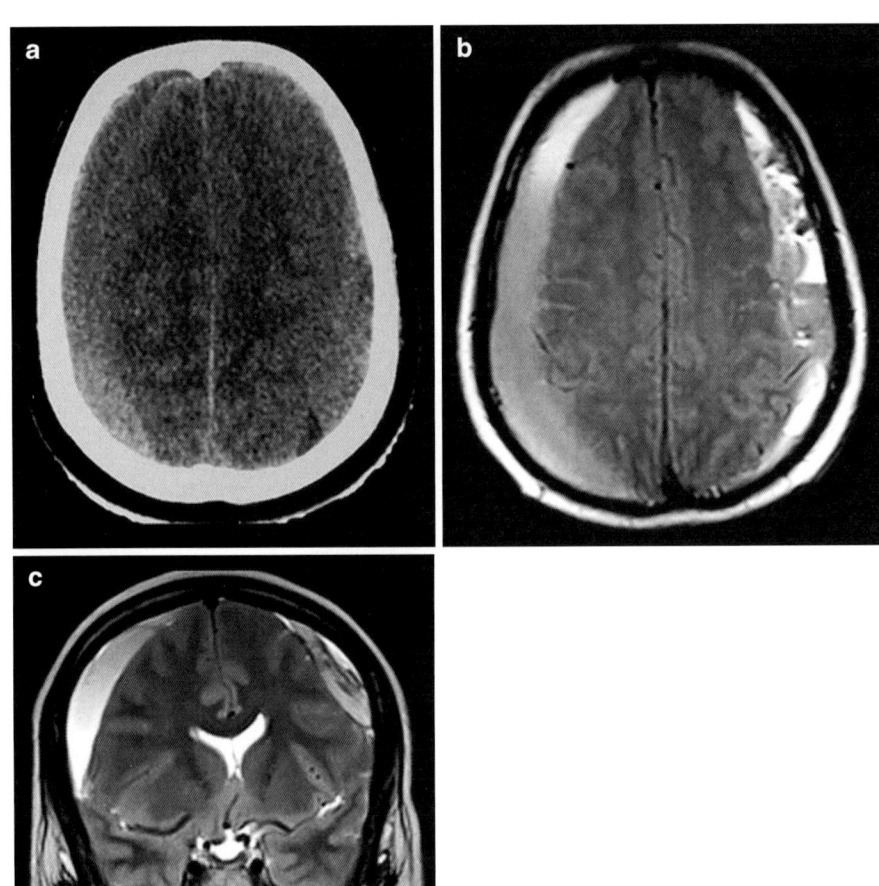

图 1.6 双侧等密度慢性硬膜下血肿的 CT 扫描（a）。MRI 上更好区别 SDH：轴向（b）和冠状（c）T2 加权像

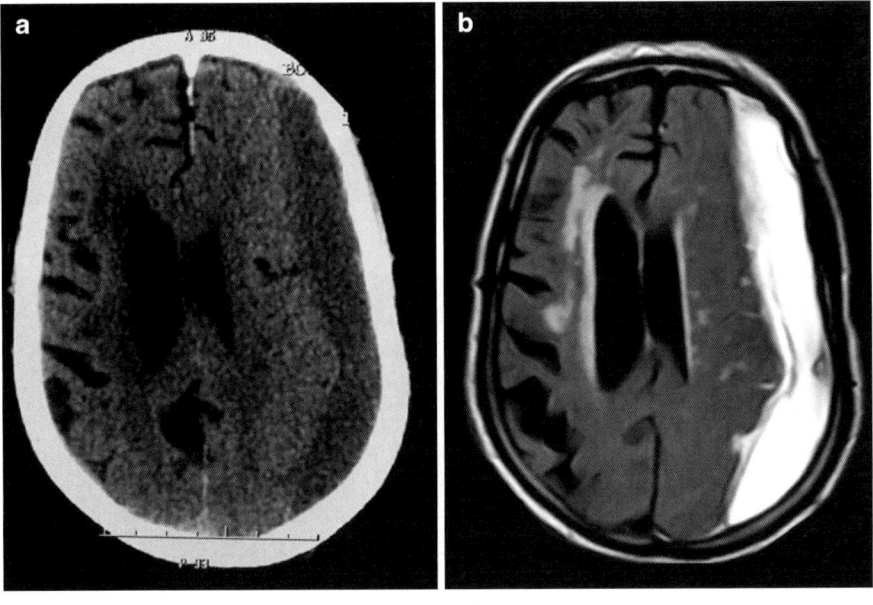

图 1.7 同一左侧颅内慢性 SDH 患者的轴向 CT 扫描（a）和 MRI IR 序列（b）

液的 Ommaya 囊、硬膜下钻孔引流系统（SEPS）、内镜血肿清除术以及脑膜中动脉栓塞术[14, 30, 78]。

慢性 SDH 手术清除术适用于有症状或者血肿最大厚度超过 10 mm 并有占位效应的患者。尽管慢性 SDH 的手术被认为是一项相对简单安全且并发症发生率低的操作，但根据目前报道仍有 38% 的手术患者可能会出现术后并发症（详情查阅本书第 33 章）。并发症包括与手术或手术方式直接相关的并发症（血肿复发、癫痫发作、新发颅内出血、张力性气颅以及感染），以及其他常见的非手术并发症。这些因素都

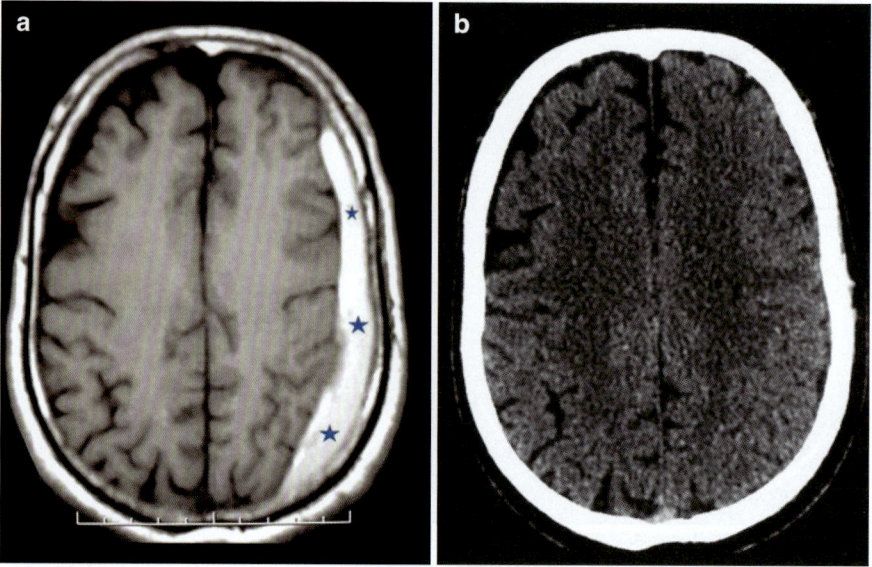

图 1.8　53 岁无症状颅内左侧慢性 SDH 的 T1 加权图像（a）。该患者使用皮质类固醇激素（氢化可的松）和口服补液治疗 8 周。对照 CT 扫描（第一次 MRI 检查后第 2 个月末）显示硬膜下血肿完全吸收

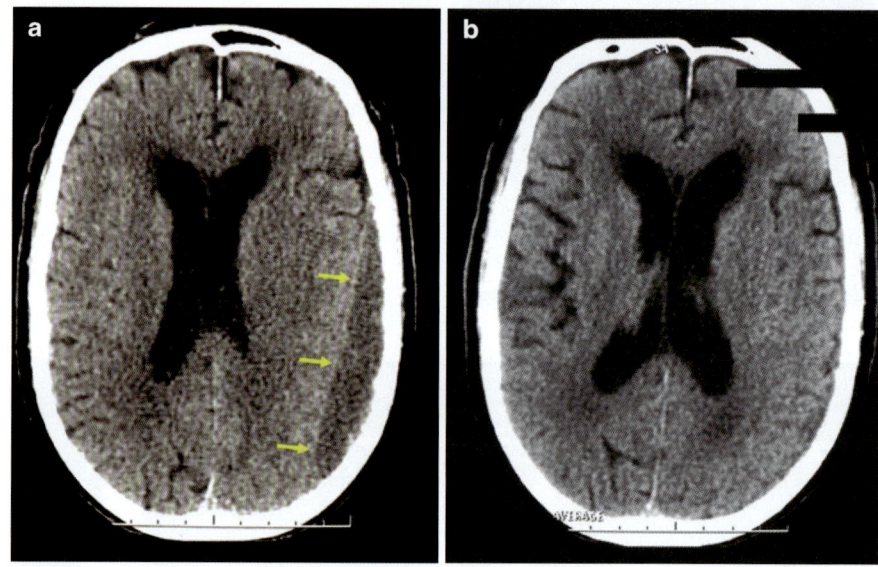

图 1.9　通过皮质类固醇激素和口服补液治疗 6 周的 72 岁无症状颅内慢性 SDH 男性患者。第一次 CT 扫描（a）和 2 个月后对照 CT 扫描结果显示血肿消失（b）

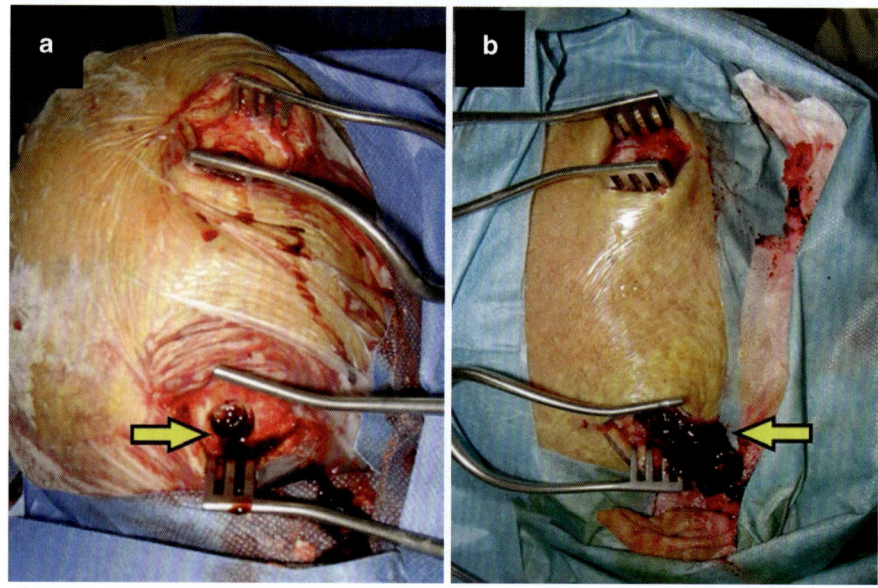

图 1.10　手术操作。需要通过两个钻孔来进行慢性硬膜下血肿的手术清除。第一个病例：清除棕褐色"机油样"硬膜下积液（箭头所指）（a）。第二个病例：慢性硬膜下血肿包含深色血凝块（箭头所指）（b）

第 1 章 急性、亚急性及慢性硬膜下血肿综述

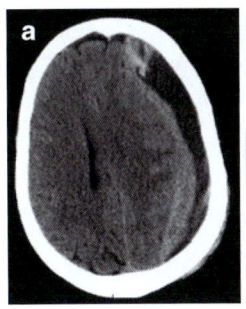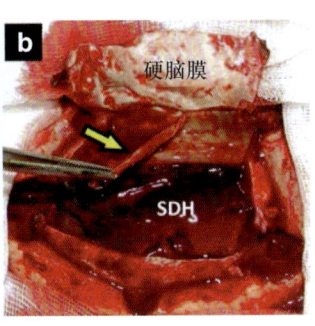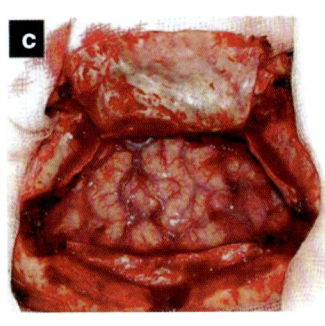

图 1.11 机化的慢性或亚急性硬膜下血肿轴向 CT 扫描（a）。该患者行大骨瓣开颅术和硬脑膜切开术进行治疗。我们可以看到有厚纤维囊的机化 SDH（箭头所指）（b）。血肿清除和扩大膜切除术的脑皮质实质手术视野（c）

会对发病率和死亡率产生不良影响，并且产生大量治疗费用和住院费用[65]。

目前对于抗癫痫药的疗效尚不明确。对于一些患者来说，应用抗癫痫药可系统性地预防癫痫发作。我们的研究结果与大多数神经外科医生得到的结论一致，如果没有癫痫发作不建议使用抗癫痫药。如果近期出现癫痫发作，那么长期抗癫痫治疗是必需的。糖皮质激素的疗效目前已得到认可[72]，可以作为单一疗法或手术的辅助。纠正凝血功能障碍应权衡治疗风险及获益。

一般情况下慢性 SDH 要比急性 SDH 预后更好。慢性 SDH 手术患者的发病率和死亡率在绝大多数情况下与手术技术、患者年龄和基础疾病情况以及初始神经功能状态有关。据报道，整体上年轻患者术后良好结局达到了 90%，与老年患者相比预后更佳[66]。而且，与硬膜外低压患者相比，高压患者的脑扩张更快、神经功能改善更好（图 1.12）。

1.4 脊髓硬膜下血肿

脊髓 SDH 的患病率远低于颅脑 SDH，原因在于椎管内硬膜下隙缺少导致硬膜下出血的重要血管或桥静脉[35,54,68]。然而，覆盖在硬膜下隙的神经根静脉损伤可能成为出血的原因[61]。硬膜下血肿是脊髓血肿中最不常见的类型，Kreppel 等在 2003 年对于 613 例脊髓血肿的系统性回顾研究中，只有 4.1% 病例为硬膜下血肿，75.2%（461 例患者）为硬膜外血肿，15.7%（96 例患者）为蛛网膜下腔血肿[46]。在最近更多的文献报道中，所有脊髓 SDH 报道病例为 259 例[35]。本书第 40 章深入回顾了相关脊髓 SDH 的诊疗知识。

存在多种情况及病因会导致脊髓 SDH，包括出血性疾病、血液系统疾病、抗凝治疗、创伤、医源性损伤（腰椎穿刺、硬膜外麻醉、脊柱或颅脑手术）、椎管内动静脉畸形以及椎管内肿瘤[1-2,8,20,35,39,48,51,53,55,61]。当出血病因不明确时，脊髓 SDH 被称为"特发性"[3,44]。

脊髓硬膜下血肿（SDH）的临床表现缺乏特异性，其症状取决于血肿体积、受累节段位置及病因。除了创伤性脊髓 SDH，大多数病例表现为急性或亚急性背痛和各种程度的神经症状如神经根病、下肢无力以及括约肌障碍。尽管罕见，极少数脊髓 SDH 患者可能表现为自发性颅内 SDH（见下文）。

脊髓 SDH 的病理变化长期以来未被完全认知，MR 扫描通常作为其诊断的首选方法[23]。MR 图像不仅能够显示硬膜下血肿及其发生部位，还能显示潜在的肿瘤或血管病因。血肿由于出血时间不同可能有多种 T1 和 T2 信号（图 1.13）。轴向 MRI

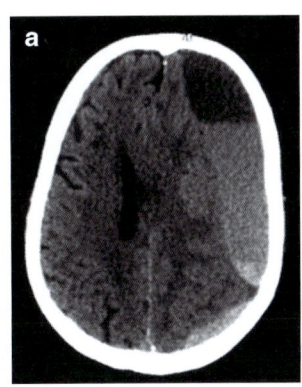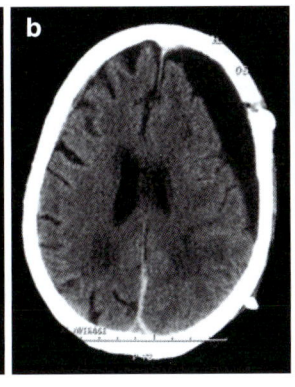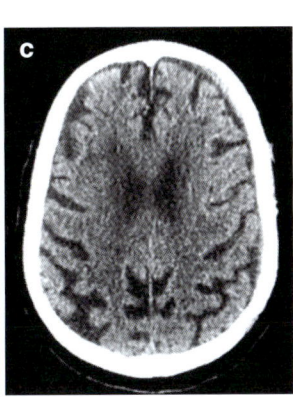

图 1.12 通过两个钻孔行慢性硬膜下血肿清除术并取得良好预后的 83 岁女性患者的术前（a）、术后第 3 天（b）以及术后 3 个月（c）轴向 CT 表现

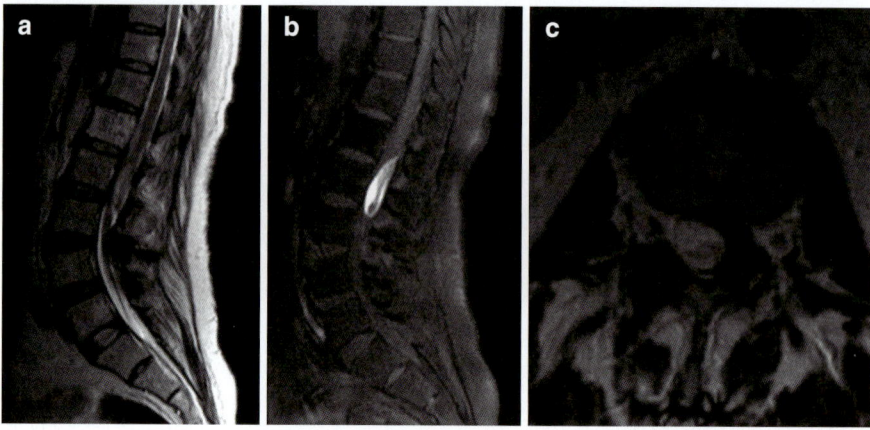

图 1.13 （a）术前矢状 T2 增强 MRI 图像，（b）矢状 T2 增强 FSE MRI，以及（c）轴向 T2 增强 MRI 表明在 L2 的脊髓硬膜下血肿（Reproduced from Kobayashi K et al. Eur Spine J（2017）26：2739-43；with permission）

图像对于硬膜下血肿和硬膜外血肿的鉴别尤为重要。脊髓硬膜外血肿通常位于脊髓后方呈凸透镜状，然而硬膜下血肿位于脊髓腹侧和周围呈半圆形"帽边征"或在腰部呈"倒置奔驰征"的三辐射状血肿[43, 47]。然而，术前很难准确鉴别硬膜下血肿和硬膜外血肿，许多患者仅能通过术中诊断。如果怀疑血管畸形，应立即行脊髓选择性血管造影，或者最好使用血管 MR 检查以减少医源性漏诊[1]。

在既往文献报道中，脊髓 SDH 有多种治疗方案[9, 49, 61]。当讨论手术治疗时，神经外科医生会考虑多种相关情况，如潜在出血病因、脊柱稳定性、患者一般状况，以及任何的凝血功能障碍。一般来说，当患者出现严重的神经功能状况，手术减压清除血肿能够取得良好效果（图 1.14），因此应当立即安排手术治疗，除非患者不能耐受麻醉或手术。对于无症状患者来说，保守治疗和手术治疗都能取得良好预后，因此对于这些病例可以保守治疗并密切随访。同时需要注意的是，腰椎穿刺（腰穿）可能导致腰椎或骶椎硬膜下血肿。

影响脊髓 SDH 预后的主要因素是初始神经功能障碍的严重程度。腰椎 SDH 患者较颈椎或胸椎 SDH 预后更佳。

1.5 颅脑合并脊髓硬膜下血肿

尽管罕见，神经外科医生应该意识到脊髓 SDH 与颅脑 SDH 同时发生的可能性。据我们所知，文献中报道的颅脑脊髓 SDH 不到 50 例（表 1.1）[17, 26, 29, 31, 35, 37, 42, 45, 57, 67, 68, 74, 77]。对于 Kokubo 等研究人员来说，颅脑脊髓 SDH 难以准确诊断。在他们的前瞻性研究中，接受颅脑慢性 SDH 手术治疗的患者中，1.19%（168 例中 2 例）伴有腰椎 SDH，但这些患者均为无症状患者[45]。

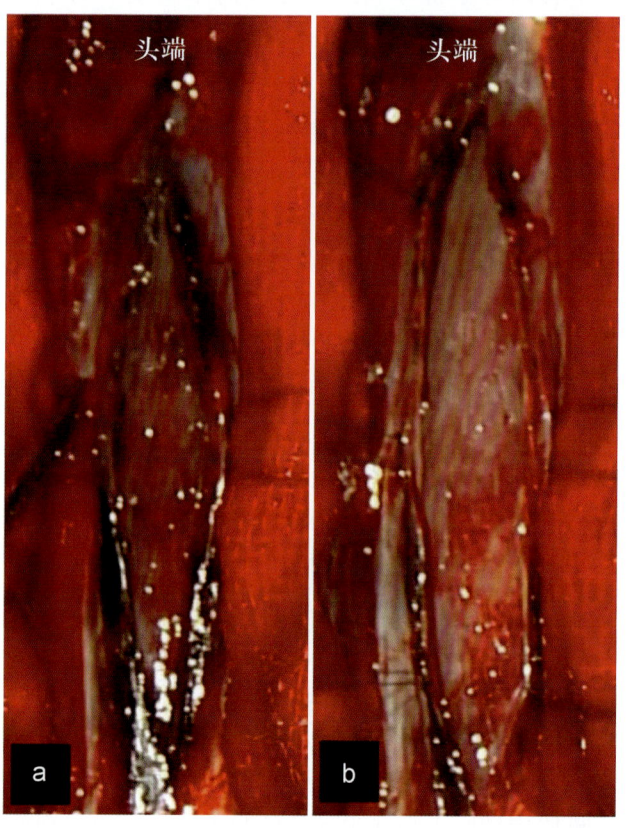

图 1.14 术中图像。（a）暴露硬脊膜和蛛网膜，脊髓中央回缩并且显示腹侧间隙有血肿。（b）血肿清除后，脊髓减压（Reproduced from Kobayashi K et al. Eur Spine J（2017）26：2739-43；with permission）

这些罕见的联系被分为三种类型，如下所示：

- 1 型：脊髓 SDH 合并颅脑 SDH
- 2 型：颅脑 SDH 后出现脊髓 SDH
- 3 型：脊髓 SDH 清除后出现颅脑 SDH

颅脑 SDH 合并脊髓 SDH 的发病机制仍不明确，

表 1.1　48 例颅脑脊髓硬膜下血肿的文献回顾

第一作者，发表时间[参考文献]	年龄、性别	诱发事件/因素	初始发现病变的部位	颅脑 SDH 位置	脊髓 SDH 位置	颅脑 SDH 治疗	脊髓 SDH 治疗	预后
Lee, 1996[49]	15 岁，男	创伤	颅脑	单侧，(ASDH)	腰部	保守	腰穿	良好
Shimada, 1996[35]	68 岁，不明	创伤	颅脑	单侧	T5-S2 (ASDH)	保守	手术	良好
Leber, 1997[37]	54 岁，男	创伤	颅脑	双侧	L1-S2	保守	手术	良好
Tillich, 1999[37]	54 岁，男	创伤	颅脑	双侧	T12-S2	保守	手术	良好
Kirsch, 2000[43]	42 岁，男	自杀未遂	脊髓	颅后窝	C1-L3 (ASDH)	保守	手术	不良
Hung, 2002[35]	12 岁，男	创伤	颅脑	单侧(ASDH)	L1-L5	保守	保守	良好
Lecouvet, 2003[68]	31 岁，男	转移性黑色素瘤治疗	脊髓	单侧，颅后窝	L1-S2	手术	保守	改善
Bortolotti, 2004[35]	23 岁，女	创伤	颅脑	单侧	L4-S2	保守	手术	良好
Ahn, 2005[3]	4 岁，男	创伤	同时	单侧，颅后窝	颈胸部	保守	保守	改善
Yamaguchi, 2005[37]	59 岁，男	抗血小板治疗	同时	双侧，颅后窝	T11-S1	保守	保守	良好
Jimbo, 2006[74]	72 岁，男	抗凝治疗	脊髓	多发	L4-S2	保守	手术	良好
Sari, 2006[67]	56 岁，男	创伤		大脑半球之间	L1-S2	保守	手术	良好
Lee, 2007[26]	68 岁，女	无	颅脑	单侧	L4-S1	手术	手术	良好
Morishige, 2007[56]	54 岁，男	无	同时	单侧，颅后窝	C1-S2	手术	腰穿	良好
Broc-Haro, 2008[68]	44 岁，男	无	颅脑	单侧(亚急性SDH)	L2-L5 (ASDH)	手术	保守	良好
Gruber, 2008[35]	4 个月，男	婴儿摇晃综合征	颅脑	单侧(ASDH)	T10-L4	脑室分流	手术	好转
Jain, 2008[37]	12 岁，男	再生障碍性贫血	同时	颅后窝	C1-S3	保守	保守	良好
Nakajima, 2009[37]	65 岁，女	创伤	同时	单侧	T12-S1	手术	保守	良好
Wong, 2009[29]	73 岁，女	创伤	颅脑	单侧	T4-T10	保守	保守	良好
Yang, 2009[37]	35 岁，女	无	同时	单侧	L3-S1	手术	手术	良好
Hagihara, 2010[31]	47 岁，男	创伤、抗血小板治疗	颅脑	双侧	L3-S1	手术	保守	良好
Kim K, 2010[37]	24 岁，女	创伤	同时	双侧	L4-S2	保守	保守	良好
Nagashima, 2010[37]	66 岁，男	无	脊髓	双侧	L1-S1	手术	手术	良好
Nagashima, 2010[37]	60 岁，男	无	颅脑	双侧	L3-S2	手术	保守	不明
Moscovici, 2011[57]	88 岁，男	创伤	颅脑	双侧(ASDH)	L5-S1	保守	手术	好转
Wajima, 2012[77]	78 岁，女	创伤、抗血小板治疗	颅脑	单侧，大脑半球之间、颅后窝(ASDH)	S1-S2	手术	保守	良好
Wang, 2012[37]	63 岁，女	抗血小板治疗	同时	单侧	L4-S1	手术	手术	良好
Ji, 2013[29]	47 岁，女	创伤	同时	小脑幕	L5-S2	保守	保守	良好
Jibu K, 2013[29]	73 岁，男	无		双侧	L3-S2	手术	保守	良好
Li, 2013[50]	26 岁，男	创伤	颅脑	单侧(ASDH)	T4-S1	保守	保守	良好
Moon, 2013[37]	39 岁，女	无	脊髓	单侧	L1-S2	手术	手术	良好
Kim, 2014[35]	62 岁，男	创伤	颅脑	单侧	L2-L5	保守	保守	良好

（续表）

第一作者，发表时间 [参考文献]	年龄、性别	诱发事件/因素	初始发现病变的部位	颅脑 SDH 位置	脊髓 SDH 位置	颅脑 SDH 治疗	脊髓 SDH 治疗	预后
Kokubo, 2014[45]	83 岁，男	骨髓异常综合征	颅脑	双侧	L5-S1	手术	保守	良好
Kokubo, 2014[45]	70 岁，男	无	颅脑	双侧	S1	手术	保守	良好
Lin, 2014[29]	70 岁，男	无	同时	双侧	L4-S1	手术	保守	良好
Treister, 2014[29]	15 岁，男	创伤	同时	单侧，大脑半球之间	T11-L4	保守	保守	良好
Cui, 2015[17]	45 岁，男	无	脊髓	双侧	L4-S3	保守	手术	良好
Kim MS, 2015[42]	82 岁，女	创伤	颅脑	双侧	L3-L4	手术	保守	良好
Köksal, 2015[35]	20 岁，男	创伤	颅脑	单侧（ASDH）	T10-L2	保守	保守	改善
Kwon, 2015[35]	57 岁，男	创伤	脊髓	单侧（ASDH）	L2-S1	手术	手术	良好
Kanamaru, 2016[37]	67 岁，男	创伤	颅脑	双侧	L4-S1	手术	手术	良好
Matsumoto, 2016[54]	58 岁，男	创伤	颅脑	单侧，颅后窝	T1-S1	手术	手术	良好
Ichinose, 2018[37]	40 岁，男	创伤	同时	双侧	L2-S1	手术	腰穿	良好
Satyarthee, 2018[68]	14 岁，男	再生障碍性贫血	同时	颅后窝	胸腰段	保守	保守	良好
Uto, 2018[74]	77 岁，男	抗血小板和抗凝治疗	脊髓	单侧	L4-S1	手术	保守	良好
Fugita, 2019[26]	63 岁，女	创伤	颅脑	单侧	L4-S1	保守	保守	良好
Golden, 2019[29]	56 岁，男	创伤	脊髓	双侧（亚急性）	T12-S1（亚急性）	手术	手术	良好
Hsieh, 2020[35]	35 岁，男	创伤	颅脑	双侧，大脑镰（ASDH）	胸腰段	保守	保守	改善

简写：ASDH，急性硬膜下血肿；CSDH，慢性硬膜下血肿；C，颈；L，腰；S，骶；T，胸

目前已经提出了基于上述三种形式的多种假说：

对于 1 型来说，血肿均是在创伤后发展形成的，而不是凝血疾病或非创伤因素而形成的常见孤立脊髓 SDH。对于 2 型来说，一直认为是颅脑 SDH 在重力作用下向下迁移至椎管（尤其是腰骶部）形成血肿[3, 45, 50]。同样推测新形成的脊髓 SDH 可能与颅后窝桥静脉撕裂尤其是在颅脑 SDH 外科手术清除血肿术后相关。对于 3 型来说，脊髓 SDH 清除后的低颅压可能会导致颅脑 SDH 的发展，老年患者常见的额叶萎缩也可能为颅脑 SDH 提供潜在空间[29, 35, 74]。

根据对文献的回顾（表 1.1），我们没有发现颅脑脊髓 SDH 确切的发病年龄。报道的颅脑脊髓 SDH 平均发病年龄为 49.37 岁（发病年龄范围从 4 个月到 88 岁），而且患者以男性居多，男女比例为 35:12（其中 1 例性别不明）。11 例患者（22.9%）没有诱发或危险因素；28 例（58.3%）硬膜下隙血肿患者的病因为创伤，并且 7 例（14.5%）患者使用抗凝或抗血小板治疗；3 例（6.2%）患者与血液疾病有关；14 例（29.1%）患者同时诊断为两种 SDH（1 型）。然而，25 例（52.2%）患者首先被诊断为颅脑 SDH，9 例（18.7%）患者在被诊断为颅脑 SDH 前先被诊断为脊髓 SDH（3 型）。颅内血肿绝大部分位于颅后窝及单侧，而脊髓 SDH 大多分布在腰骶部。

不管何种类型颅脑脊髓 SDH，针对 SDH 血肿部位的独立治疗都是错误的。既往报道中保守和外科治疗都有良好的预后。绝大部分病例尤其是脊髓 SDH 对于保守治疗反应较好，29 例（60.4%）脊髓 SDH 患者接受保守治疗；16 例（33.3%）患者行外科脊髓血肿清除术；仅有 3 例（6.3%）患者行腰穿治疗[37, 49, 56]。腰穿抽吸血肿液对于液化良好的脊髓 SDH 是简单有效的。

对于所有颅内 SDH 病例，当患者出现下肢神经症状时，神经外科医生应当格外警惕需行 MRI 检查鉴别诊断脊髓 SDH 的发生。如果有严重的神

经功能症状或患者病情恶化，应考虑行急诊手术清除血肿。

1.6 结论

硬膜下血肿是一种常见的具有多种临床表现的特殊疾病类型，其临床表现形式比以往人们对其的认知更为复杂。硬膜下血肿类型包括颅脑、脊髓、急性、亚急性、慢性以及各种类型的混合类型。由于人口老龄化、公共交通事故增加以及抗凝治疗的患者增多，硬膜下血肿尤其是颅脑硬膜下血肿的发病率在未来将会逐步升高。虽然可以采用保守治疗的方法，但硬膜下血肿的手术清除减压伴（或不伴）术后引流仍然是许多症状性病例最常用的治疗方法。然而，对于硬膜下血肿的最佳治疗方案仍有争论。因此，需要对硬膜下血肿的病因和病理生理学进行补充研究，以更好地了解该病。在讨论手术方案时，神经外科医生应考虑出血的潜在病因、临床体征和症状、血肿的外观和定位、患者的一般情况，以及任何可能相关的凝血功能障碍。

参考文献

1. Abut Y, Erkalp K, Bay B. Spinal subdural hematoma: a pre-eclamptic patient with a spinal arteriovenous malformation. Anesth Analg. 2006;103:1610. https://doi.org/10.1213/01.ane.0000246274.96202.c7.
2. Abuzayed B, Oğuzoğlu SA, Dashti R, Ozyurt E. Spinal chronic subdural hematoma mimicking intradural tumor in a patient with history of Hemophilia a: case report. Turk Neurosurg. 2009;19:189–91.
3. Ahn ES, Smith ER. Acute clival and spinal subdural hematoma with spontaneous resolution: clinical and radiographic correlation in support of a proposed pathophysiological mechanism. Case report. J Neurosurg. 2005;103(2 Suppl):175–9. https://doi.org/10.3171/ped.2005.103.2.0175.
4. Akhaddar A. The yin-yang shaped image following head injury. Pan Afr Med J. 2013;16:133. https://doi.org/10.11604/pamj.2013.16.133.3555.
5. Akhaddar A, Bensghir M, Abouqal R, Boucetta M. Influence of cranial morphology on the location of chronic subdural haematoma. Acta Neurochir (Wien). 2009;151:1235–40. https://doi.org/10.1007/s00701-009-0357-7.
6. Akhaddar A, Karouache A, Boucetta M. Bilateral chronic subdural hematoma misdiagnosed as neuroleptic malignant syndrome. Emerg Med J. 2010;27:233. https://doi.org/10.1136/emj.2008.071001.
7. Akhaddar A, Boucetta M. Reversible tetraparesis due to bilateral chronic subdural haematoma. Age Ageing. 2010;39(Suppl). https://doi.org/10.1093/ageing/el_105.
8. Akiyama Y, Koyanagi I, Mikuni N. Chronic spinal subdural hematoma associated with antiplatelet therapy. World Neurosurg. 2017;105:1032.e1–5. https://doi.org/10.1016/j.wneu.2016.11.128.
9. Al B, Yildirim C, Zengin S, Genc S, Erkutlu I, Mete A. Acute spontaneous spinal subdural haematoma presenting as paraplegia and complete recovery with non-operative treatment. BMJ Case Rep. 2009;2009:bcr02.2009.1599. https://doi.org/10.1136/bcr.02.2009.1599.
10. Amagasaki K, Takusagawa Y, Kanehashi K, Abe S, Watanabe S, Shono N, et al. Supratentorial acute subdural haematoma during microvascular decompression surgery: report of three cases. J Surg Case Rep. 2017;2017(2):rjx004. https://doi.org/10.1093/jscr/rjx004.
11. Balser D, Farooq S, Mehmood T, Reyes M, Samadani U. Actual and projected incidence rates for chronic subdural hematomas in United States Veterans Administration and civilian populations. J Neurosurg. 2015;123:1209–15. https://doi.org/10.3171/2014.9.JNS141550.
12. Berger A, Constantini S, Ram Z, Roth J. Acute subdural hematomas in shunted normal-pressure hydrocephalus patients—management options and literature review: a case-based series. Surg Neurol Int. 2018;9:238. https://doi.org/10.4103/sni.sni_338_18. PMID: 30595959; PMCID: PMC6287333.
13. Caton MT Jr, Wiggins WF, Nuñez D. Non-traumatic subdural hemorrhage: beware of ruptured intracranial aneurysm. Emerg Radiol. 2019;26:567–71. https://doi.org/10.1007/s10140-019-01691-2.
14. Chari A, Kolias AG, Santarius T, Bond S, Hutchinson PJ. Twist-drill craniostomy with hollow screws for evacuation of chronic subdural hematoma. J Neurosurg. 2014;121:176–83. https://

doi.org/10.3171/2014.4.JNS131212.
15. Cherif El Asri A, El Mostarchid B, Akhaddar A, Boucetta M. Chronic subdural hematoma revealing skull metastasis. Intern Med. 2011;50:791. https://doi.org/10.2169/internalmedicine.50.4654.
16. Chye CL, Lin KH, Ou CH, Sun CK, Chang IW, Liang CL. Acute spontaneous subdural hematoma caused by skull metastasis of hepatocellular carcinoma: case report. BMC Surg. 2015;15:60. https://doi.org/10.1186/s12893-015-0045-x.
17. Cui Z, Zhong Z, Wang B, Sun Q, Zhong C, Bian L. Coexistence of spontaneous spinal and undiagnosed cranial subdual hematomas. J Craniofac Surg. 2015;26:e118–9. https://doi.org/10.1097/SCS.0000000000001343.
18. de Aguiar GB, Veiga JC, Silva JM, Conti ML. Spontaneous acute subdural hematoma: a rare presentation of a dural intracranial fistula. J Clin Neurosci. 2016;25:159–60. https://doi.org/10.1016/j.jocn.2015.05.057.
19. de Amorim RL, Stiver SI, Paiva WS, Bor-Seng-Shu E, Sterman-Neto H, de Andrade AF, et al. Treatment of traumatic acute posterior fossa subdural hematoma: report of four cases with systematic review and management algorithm. Acta Neurochir (Wien). 2014;156:199–206. https://doi.org/10.1007/s00701-013-1850-6.
20. Edelson RN, Chernik NL, Posner JB. Spinal subdural hematomas complicating lumbar puncture. Arch Neurol. 1974;31:134–7. https://doi.org/10.1001/archneur.1974.00490380082011.
21. Edlmann E, Giorgi-Coll S, Whitfield PC, Carpenter KLH, Hutchinson PJ. Pathophysiology of chronic subdural haematoma: inflammation, angiogenesis and implications for pharmacotherapy. J Neuroinflammation. 2017;14:108. https://doi.org/10.1186/s12974-017-0881-y.
22. Evans LR, Jones J, Lee HQ, Gantner D, Jaison A, Matthew J, Fitzgerald MC, Rosenfeld JV, Hunn MK, Tee JW. Prognosis of acute subdural hematoma in the elderly: a systematic review. J Neurotrauma. 2019;36:517–22. https://doi.org/10.1089/neu.2018.5829.
23. Felber S, Langmaier J, Judmaier W, Dessl A, Ortler M, Birbamer G, et al. Magnetic resonance tomography in epidural and subdural spinal hematoma. Radiologe. 1994;34:656–61.
24. Fountain DM, Kolias AG, Lecky FE, Bouamra O, Lawrence T, Adams H, et al. Survival trends after surgery for acute subdural hematoma in adults over a 20-year period. Ann Surg. 2017;265:590–6. https://doi.org/10.1097/SLA.0000000000001682.
25. Fu S, Li F, Bie L. Drug therapy for chronic subdural hematoma: bench to bedside. J Clin Neurosci. 2018;56:16–20. https://doi.org/10.1016/j.jocn.2017.07.034.
26. Fujita T, Iwamoto Y, Takeuchi H, Tsujino H, Hashimoto N. Lumbar subdural hematoma detected after surgical treatment of chronic intracranial subdural hematoma. World Neurosurg. 2020;134:472–6. https://doi.org/10.1016/j.wneu.2019.11.053.
27. Gao X, Yue F, Zhang F, Sun Y, Zhang Y, Zhu X, et al. Acute non-traumatic subdural hematoma induced by intracranial aneurysm rupture: a case report and systematic review of the literature. Medicine (Baltimore). 2020;99:e21434. https://doi.org/10.1097/MD.0000000000021434.
28. Gaonkar VB, Garg K, Agrawal D, Chandra PS, Kale SS. Risk factors for progression of conservatively managed acute traumatic subdural hematoma: a systematic review and meta-analysis. World Neurosurg. 2021;146:332–41. https://doi.org/10.1016/j.wneu.2020.11.031. S1878-8750(20)32406-2.
29. Golden N, Asih MW. Traumatic subacute spinal subdural hematoma concomitant with symptomatic cranial subdural hematoma: possible mechanism. World Neurosurg. 2019;123:343–7. https://doi.org/10.1016/j.wneu.2018.12.053.
30. Golub D, Ashayeri K, Dogra S, Lewis A, Pacione D. Benefits of the subdural evacuating port system (SEPS) procedure over traditional craniotomy for subdural hematoma evacuation. Neurohospitalist. 2020;10:257–65. https://doi.org/10.1177/1941874420920520.
31. Hagihara N, Abe T, Kojima K, Watanabe M, Tabuchi K. Coexistence of cranial and spinal subdural hematomas: case report. Neurol Med Chir (Tokyo). 2010;50:333–5. https://doi.org/10.2176/nmc.50.333.
32. Hambra DV, de Danilo P, Alessandro R, Sara M, Juan GR. Meningioma associated with acute subdural hematoma: a review of the literature. Surg Neurol Int. 2014;5(Suppl 12):S469–71. https://doi.org/10.4103/2152-7806.143724.
33. Hiraizumi S, Shiomi N, Echigo T, Oka H, Hino A, Baba M, et al. Factors associated with poor outcomes in patients with mild or moderate acute subdural hematomas. Neurol Med Chir (Tokyo). 2020;60:402–10. https://doi.org/10.2176/nmc.oa.2020-0030.
34. Holl DC, Volovici V, Dirven CMF, Peul WC, van Kooten F, Jellema K, et al. Pathophysiology and nonsurgical treatment of chronic subdural hematoma: from past to present to future. World Neurosurg. 2018;116:402–11.e2. https://doi.org/10.1016/j.wneu.2018.05.037.

35. Hsieh JK, Colby S, Nichols D, Kondylis E, Liu JKC. Delayed development of spinal subdural hematoma following cranial trauma: a case report and review of the literature. World Neurosurg. 2020;141:44–51. https://doi.org/10.1016/j.wneu.2020.05.158.
36. Huang KT, Bi WL, Abd-El-Barr M, Yan SC, Tafel IJ, Dunn IF, et al. The neurocritical and neurosurgical care of subdural hematomas. Neurocrit Care. 2016;24:294–307. https://doi.org/10.1007/s12028-015-0194-x.
37. Ichinose D, Tochigi S, Tanaka T, Suzuki T, Takei J, Hatano K, et al. Concomitant intracranial and lumbar chronic subdural hematoma treated by fluoroscopic guided lumbar puncture: a case report and literature review. Neurol Med Chir (Tokyo). 2018;58:178–84. https://doi.org/10.2176/nmc.cr.2017-0177.
38. Jensen TSR, Andersen-Ranberg N, Poulsen FR, Bergholt B, Hundsholt T, Fugleholm K. The Danish Chronic Subdural Hematoma Study-comparison of hematoma age to the radiological appearance at time of diagnosis. Acta Neurochir (Wien). 2020;162:2007–13. https://doi.org/10.1007/s00701-020-04472-w.
39. Joubert C, Gazzola S, Sellier A, Dagain A. Acute idiopathic spinal subdural hematoma: what to do in an emergency? Neurochirurgie. 2019;65:93–7. https://doi.org/10.1016/j.neuchi.2018.10.009.
40. Karibe H, Kameyama M, Hayashi T, Narisawa A, Tominaga T. Acute subdural hematoma in infants with abusive head trauma: a literature review. Neurol Med Chir (Tokyo). 2016;56:264–73. https://doi.org/10.2176/nmc.ra.2015-0308.
41. Kaur G, Dakay K, Sursal T, Pisapia J, Bowers C, Hanft S, et al. Acute subdural hematomas secondary to aneurysmal subarachnoid hemorrhage confer poor prognosis: a national perspective. J Neurointerv Surg. 2021;13(5):426–9. https://doi.org/10.1136/neurintsurg-2020-016470.
42. Kim MS, Sim SY. Spinal subdural hematoma associated with intracranial subdural hematoma. J Korean Neurosurg Soc. 2015;58:397–400. https://doi.org/10.3340/jkns.2015.58.4.397.
43. Kirsch EC, Khangure MS, Holthouse D, McAuliffe W. Acute spontaneous spinal subdural haematoma: MRI features. Neuroradiology. 2000;42:586–90. https://doi.org/10.1007/s002340000331.
44. Kobayashi K, Imagama S, Ando K, Nishida Y, Ishiguro N. Acute non-traumatic idiopathic spinal subdural hematoma: radiographic findings and surgical results with a literature review. Eur Spine J. 2017;26:2739–43. https://doi.org/10.1007/s00586-017-5013-y.
45. Kokubo R, Kim K, Mishina M, Isu T, Kobayashi S, Yoshida D, et al. Prospective assessment of concomitant lumbar and chronic subdural hematoma: is migration from the intracranial space involved in their manifestation? J Neurosurg Spine. 2014;20:157–63. https://doi.org/10.3171/2013.10.SPINE13346.
46. Kreppel D, Antoniadis G, Seeling W. Spinal hematoma: a literature survey with meta-analysis of 613 patients. Neurosurg Rev. 2003;26:1–49. https://doi.org/10.1007/s10143-002-0224-y.
47. Krishnan P, Banerjee TK. Classical imaging findings in spinal subdural hematoma—"Mercedes-Benz" and "Cap" signs. Br J Neurosurg. 2016;30:99–100. https://doi.org/10.3109/02688697.2015.1071319.
48. Lee HS, Lee SH, Chung YS, Yang HJ, Son YJ, Park SB. Large spinal meningioma with hemorrhage after selective root block in the thoraco-lumbar spine. Korean J Spine. 2013;10:255–7. https://doi.org/10.14245/kjs.2013.10.4.255.
49. Lee JI, Hong SC, Shin HJ, Eoh W, Byun HS, Kim JH. Traumatic spinal subdural hematoma: rapid resolution after repeated lumbar spinal puncture and drainage. J Trauma. 1996;40:654–5. https://doi.org/10.1097/00005373-199604000-00026.
50. Li CH, Yew AY, Lu DC. Migration of traumatic intracranial subdural hematoma to lumbar spine causing radiculopathy. Surg Neurol Int. 2013;4:81. https://doi.org/10.4103/2152-7806.113647.
51. Liu J, Wu B, Feng H, You C. Spinal subdural hematoma following cranial surgery: a case report and review of the literature. Neurol India. 2011;59:281–4. https://doi.org/10.4103/0028-3886.79151.
52. Lv J, Qi X, Wang Y, Wu H, Wang K, Niu H, et al. Contralateral subdural hematoma following surgical evacuation of acute subdural hematoma: super-early intervention and clinical implications. World Neurosurg. 2019;122:24–7. https://doi.org/10.1016/j.wneu.2018.10.106.
53. Maddali P, Walker B, Fisahn C, Page J, Diaz V, Zwillman ME, et al. Subdural thoracolumbar spine hematoma after spinal anesthesia: a rare occurrence and literature review of spinal hematomas after spinal anesthesia. Cureus. 2017;9:e1032. https://doi.org/10.7759/cureus.1032.
54. Matsumoto H, Matsumoto S, Yoshida Y. Concomitant intracranial chronic subdural hematoma and spinal subdural hematoma: a case report and literature review. World Neurosurg.

2016;90:706.e1–9. https://doi.org/10.1016/j.wneu.2016.03.020.
55. Mattei TA, Rehman AA, Dinh DH. Acute spinal subdural hematoma after vertebroplasty: a case report emphasizing the possible etiologic role of venous congestion. Global Spine J. 2015;5:e52–8. https://doi.org/10.1055/s-0035-1544155.
56. Morishige M, Abe T, Ishii K, Fujiki M, Kobayashi H, Karashima A, et al. Spontaneous chronic head and spinal subdural haematoma. Acta Neurochir (Wien). 2007;149:1081–2. https://doi.org/10.1007/s00701-007-1256-4.
57. Moscovici S, Paldor I, Ramirez de-Noriega F, Itshayek E, Shoshan Y, Spektor S, et al. Do cranial subdural hematomas migrate to the lumbar spine? J Clin Neurosci. 2011;18:563–5. https://doi.org/10.1016/j.jocn.2010.07.116.
58. Mrfka M, Pistracher K, Augustin M, Kurschel-Lackner S, Mokry M. Acute subdural hematoma without subarachnoid hemorrhage or intraparenchymal hematoma caused by rupture of a posterior communicating artery aneurysm: case report and review of the literature. J Emerg Med. 2013;44:e369–73. https://doi.org/10.1016/j.jemermed.2012.11.073.
59. Neifert SN, Chaman EK, Hardigan T, Ladner TR, Feng R, Caridi JM, et al. Increases in subdural hematoma with an aging population-the future of American cerebrovascular disease. World Neurosurg. 2020;141:e166–74. https://doi.org/10.1016/j.wneu.2020.05.060.
60. Phan K, Moore JM, Griessenauer C, Dmytriw AA, Scherman DB, Sheik-Ali S, et al. Craniotomy versus decompressive craniectomy for acute subdural hematoma: systematic review and meta-analysis. World Neurosurg. 2017;101:677–85.e2. https://doi.org/10.1016/j.wneu.2017.03.024.
61. Porter ZR, Johnson MD, Horn PS, Ngwenya LB. Traumatic spinal subdural hematoma: an illustrative case and series review. Interdiscip Neurosurg. 2020;19:100570. https://doi.org/10.1016/j.inat.2019.100570.
62. Pradhan RR, Shrestha GS, Sedain G. Remote supratentorial subdural hematoma following craniectomy and evacuation of hypertensive cerebellar hematoma. Cureus. 2020;12:e6977. https://doi.org/10.7759/cureus.6977.
63. Putnam TJ, Cushing H. Chronic subdural hematoma: its pathology, its relation to pachymeningitis hemorrhagica interna and its surgical treatment. Arch Surg. 1925;11:329–39.
64. Raha A, Wadehra A, Sandhu K, Dasgupta A. Acute subdural hematoma causing neurogenic pulmonary edema following lumbar spine surgery. J Neurosurg Anesthesiol. 2017;29:63–4. https://doi.org/10.1097/ANA.0000000000000254.
65. Rauhala M, Luoto TM, Huhtala H, Iverson GL, Niskakangas T, Öhman J, et al. The incidence of chronic subdural hematomas from 1990 to 2015 in a defined Finnish population. J Neurosurg. 2019;22:1–11. https://doi.org/10.3171/2018.12.JNS183035.
66. Robinson D, Khoury JC, Kleindorfer D. Regional variation in the management of nontraumatic subdural hematomas across the United States. World Neurosurg. 2020;135:e418–23. https://doi.org/10.1016/j.wneu.2019.12.011.
67. Sari A, Sert B, Dinc H, Kuzeyli K. Subacute spinal subdural hematoma associated with intracranial subdural hematoma. J Neuroradiol. 2006;33:67–9. https://doi.org/10.1016/s0150-9861(06)77231-5.
68. Satyarthee GD, Ahmad F. Spontaneous concurrent intraspinal and intracranial subdural hematoma: management and review of literature. J Pediatr Neurosci. 2018;13:24–7. https://doi.org/10.4103/JPN.JPN_121_17.
69. Schachenmayr W, Friede RL. The origin of subdural neomembranes. Fine structure of dura-arachnoid interface in man. Am J Pathol. 1978;92:53–68.
70. Shin DS, Hwang SC. Neurocritical management of traumatic acute subdural hematomas. Korean J Neurotrauma. 2020;16:113–25. https://doi.org/10.13004/kjnt.2020.16.e43.
71. Trotter W. Chronic subdural hemorrhage of traumatic origin, and its relation to pachymeningitis hemorrhagica interna. Br J Neurosurg. 1914;2:271–91.
72. Turgut M, Akhaddar A. Dexamethasone for chronic subdural hematoma: a systematic review and meta-analysis. Acta Neurochir (Wien). 2017;159:2289–90. https://doi.org/10.1007/s00701-017-3341-7.
73. Turgut M, Akhaddar A, Turgut AT. Calcified or ossified chronic subdural hematoma: a systematic review of 114 cases reported during last century with a demonstrative case report. World Neurosurg. 2020;134:240–63. https://doi.org/10.1016/j.wneu.2019.10.153.
74. Uto T, Yonezawa N, Komine N, Tokuumi Y, Torigoe K, Koda Y, et al. A delayed-onset intracranial chronic subdural hematoma following a lumbar spinal subdural hematoma: a case report. Medicine (Baltimore). 2018;97:e12479. https://doi.org/10.1097/MD.0000000000012479.
75. Virchow R. Das haematom der dura mater. Verh Phys Med Ges Wuerzburg. 1857;7:134–42.

76. Vital RB, Hamamoto Filho PT, Oliveira VA, Romero FR, Zanini MA. Spontaneous resolution of traumatic acute subdural haematomas: a systematic review. Neurocirugia (Astur). 2016;27:129–35. https://doi.org/10.1016/j.neucir.2015.05.003.
77. Wajima D, Yokota H, Ida Y, Nakase H. Spinal subdural hematoma associated with traumatic intracranial interhemispheric subdural hematoma. Neurol Med Chir (Tokyo). 2012;52:636–9. https://doi.org/10.2176/nmc.52.636.
78. Waqas M, Vakhari K, Weimer PV, Hashmi E, Davies JM, Siddiqui AH. Safety and effectiveness of embolization for chronic subdural hematoma: systematic review and case series. World Neurosurg. 2019;126:228–36. https://doi.org/10.1016/j.wneu.2019.02.208.

第 2 章 颅内急性及亚急性硬膜下血肿

Ayhan Kanat

译者：刘伟明

2.1 引言

颅脑损伤是神经外科常见的疾病。在过去的几十年里，医疗水平已经发生重大进步[11]。在 20 世纪 90 年代，现代诊断方法和诊疗技术的提升[15, 35]极大改善了颅脑创伤患者的治疗方式[14]，并且深化了对脑血管疾病病理生理过程的认识[6, 28, 39]。对急性硬膜下血肿（ASDH）病理生理过程更好的理解能够帮助患者获得更好的预后。目前，创伤仍是导致高发病率[16]和高死亡率的主要公共卫生问题[7]。11%～20% 颅脑创伤患者患 ASDH[31]，在严重颅脑创伤患者中这一比例甚至可达 1/3[3]并且死亡率在 50%～90%[36]。在神经外科临床诊疗中，最危急的情况便是大范围的 ASDH[36]。本章旨在阐述目前对急性和亚急性 SDH 的认知。

2.2 急性硬膜下血肿

钝性颅脑外伤在任何群体和任何年龄组中都是常见的[27]。由于脑组织受到其外周颅骨的保护，因此颅骨也被认为是决定手术的关键因素[17]。颅脑外伤后，可出现生理、认知、心理和行为功能障碍及早期并发症[20]，如急性硬脑膜下出血，即硬脑膜和蛛网膜之间出现新鲜血液积聚，这通常是由于皮质桥静脉[2]撕裂所致。

2.3 亚急性硬膜下血肿

一些 ASDH 患者会在创伤后 24 h 内出现病情延迟恶化，期间可发生 ASDH 向亚急性硬膜下血肿（sASDH）的转化过程[33]，血肿通常会在形成的 2 周后液化[12]。在一些患者中，ASDH 血肿初期会被吸收并且体积减小，但是随着病情发展，蛛网膜下腔出血（SAH）的占位效应将会增加、血肿密度将会降低，在计算机断层成像（CT）上将会显示明显的中线偏移[33]。亚急性 SDH 可能会出现新的神经功能缺失。

2.4 病理生理学

老年患者脑萎缩以及较大硬膜下空间导致了硬膜下腔增大[19]。在这些患者中，增大的硬膜下腔能够在神经功能恶化发生前代偿血肿体积和脑水肿导致的脑组织体积增大[32]。在神经外科临床治疗中及时发现神经功能恶化非常重要[5]，因此对于颅脑外伤患者应密切进行神经功能监护[23]和影像学检查[21]。

位于颅腔内的大脑是人体最重要的器官之一，大脑控制着所有的中枢神经系统[8]。颅腔内的体积是固定的，颅腔内部脑实质、脑脊液以及脑血流量是相对恒定的[26]。Monro 和 Kellie 在 1783 年提出该原理，后被命名为 Monro-Kellie 学说（Monro-Kellie 假设）在没有发生 ASDH 的正常颅腔内部，颅内各部分会维持自身平衡。如果在 SDH 后使得颅内某一部分的体积改变，颅内压（ICP）将会升高并可能导致昏迷和脑疝的发生。正常颅内压是 5～15 mmHg。25%～50% 病例在严重颅脑损伤刚发生的时候会出现昏迷[2]。ASDH 的昏迷和高死亡率可能取决于多种因素，如格拉斯哥昏迷评分（GCS）、SDH 的占位效应程度、中线移位的程度、颅内压增加和脑水肿的存在。颅高压（大于 20 mmHg）可能导致神经功能损害及预后不良[32]。中线偏移程度和颅内压可用来评估 SDH 的严重程度。当血肿位于颅后窝时，血肿体积会是一个重要的影响因素[38]。血脑屏障对于维持正常的脑功能非常重要[4, 14]，急性和亚急性 SDH 可能会破坏血脑屏障的完整性。急性 SDH 患者的脑灌注压（CPP）也会发生改变。CPP 是向脑组织输送氧气的重要途径，它受到脑血流量的影响，发生 SDH 后脑血流量可能立即减少[22]。

GCS最初是为头部外伤患者设计的，用于评估患者意识受损或昏迷程度[18]。该评分量表已成为全球范围内评估颅脑创伤患者的标准。GCS存在一些缺点，如无法很好反映插管ASDH患者[23]的语言反应。交感和副交感神经系统紊乱会使患者瞳孔直径发生改变[5, 29]，SDH患者发生钩回疝产生的占位效应压迫视神经和脑干[24]也会导致瞳孔改变。因此，通过检查对光反射、对比瞳孔直径能够帮助诊断ASDH后视神经损伤，需要注意的是，直接眼眶或眼外伤也会导致瞳孔改变[24]。

2.5 影像学

CT平扫是诊断ASDH的重要影像学方法。脑磁共振成像（MRI）对于轻度ASDH以及小脑幕和大脑半球之间的ASDH判断更加准确。头颅MRI比头颅CT对于轻度ASDH的血肿判断更加敏感[2]。在ASDH中，跨过颅缝的新月形或半月形血肿区阴影可被观察到[12]，同时可能会检测到延迟性扩张血肿[32]。

2.6 治疗

SDH的治疗由于缺少循证指南和随机对照试验，目前仍具有争议[31]。是否手术取决于SDH定位、大小、占位效应、中线偏移程度、视力改变、患者年龄、基础疾病以及神经功能缺失情况[31]。一些因素如年龄、基础疾病以及是否清除SDH可以作为患者临床预后的预测因素[31]。

2.7 手术的作用

ASDH可能引起原发性或继发性脑损伤[27]。手术治疗的目的是避免患者出现脑疝并且最大程度避免出现继发性缺血性脑损伤[22]。在某些病例中，可能会观察到亚急性硬膜下血肿的明显吸收。而由于ASDH较大的血凝块会出现占位效应，去骨瓣减压术和血肿清除术会是有效的治疗手段。然而最近几十年间，去骨瓣减压术已发展成开颅减压术的一种替代手术方法[30]。一般来说，ASDH患者初诊时的神经功能状况、血肿大小以及相关中线偏移和CT上脑水肿的表现是影响选择如去骨瓣或开颅减压等手术方式[1]的重要因素。去骨瓣减压术的优势在于可以更有效控制颅高压以及提高脑灌注压和氧分压[1]。持续的氧供给与二氧化碳排出对于脑功能与组织完整性非常重要[14]。手术时间通常被认为是影响ASDH预后的重要因素[34]。ASDH的手术指征为ASDH的厚度>10 mm或中线偏移>5 mm、GCS<8分的病情恶化患者、单侧或双侧病变伴随瞳孔扩张或有证据表明颅内压升高>20 mmHg[9]。除了以上因素，无论患者GCS多少，存在占位效应就是手术干预的重要指征[25]。图2.1a展示了一名ASDH患者的CT图像，该患者的血肿厚度为12.88 mm，并且中线偏移9.46 mm。图2.1b展示了术后中线偏移恢复。

非手术治疗更适用于不伴明显中线偏移（中线偏移<5 mm），神经功能缺陷轻微甚至没有的轻度ASDH（血肿厚度<10 mm）[25]。

癫痫发作是SDH患者的严重并发症[37]。据报道在急性SDH中癫痫发作的发病率为24%，而在慢性SDH中的发病率为11%[37]。是否应该对ASDH患者使用抗癫痫药仍具有争议[32]。

2.8 结论

急性SDH患者的发病率和死亡率仍然很高。对于严重颅脑创伤患者出现意识障碍或单侧神经功能缺失（如瞳孔扩大、运动无力、体位异常等）应当怀疑出现了急性SDH[12]。密切的临床观察和影像学检查对于判断ASDH是否快速进展是必需的。由于ASDH的高发病率和死亡率，正确评估脑损伤是非常重要的。但是由于存在伦理问题，很难在ASDH患者中进行研究，因此需把研究重点放在实验研究上[28]。一些损伤模型被用于实验研究中，用于了解创伤性脑损伤的生物力学、分子和细胞效应[27]。与人体研究相比，这些实验研究能够更好地了解急性和亚急性SDH的病理生理机制。如果将神经系统看作是一个能够演奏出完整节奏、旋律以及最复杂和声组合的管弦乐队[10]，这会帮助我们更容易理解当创伤性急性硬膜下血肿发生后，血脑屏障被破坏以及脑灌注压发生改变，完整的神经系统发生了哪些节律改变。为了探究一项理论，提出可验证的假设是有必要的，并根据实验结果来判

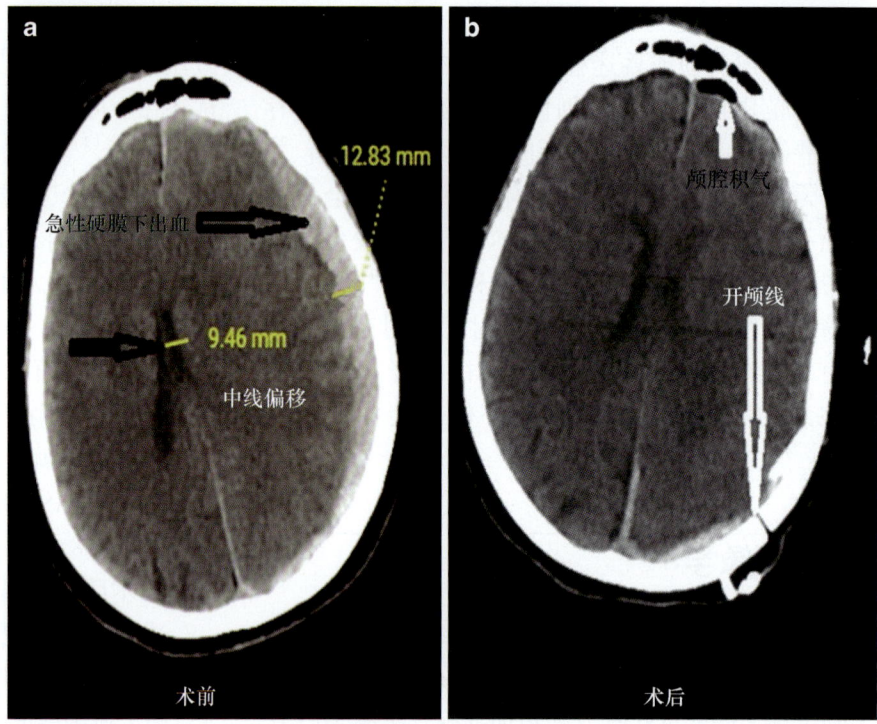

图 2.1 （a）急性硬膜下血肿患者的 CT 图像。该患者血肿厚度为 12.83 mm，中线偏移 9.46 mm。（b）展示了术后中线偏移得到纠正

断假设的正确性[13]。由于合并弥散性轴索损伤及 ICP 增高[32]，ASDH 患者的预后通常很差，因此需要认真规划、循证、多学科研究来实现 ASDH 患者的最佳预后。

参考文献

1. Ahmed N, Greenberg P, Shin S. Mortality outcome of emergency decompressive craniectomy and craniotomy in the management of acute subdural hematoma: a national data analysis. Am Surg. 2021;87(3):347–53. https://doi.org/10.1177/0003134820951463.
2. Al-Mufti F, Mayer SA. Neurocritical care of acute subdural hemorrhage. Neurosurg Clin N Am. 2017;28:267–78. https://doi.org/10.1016/j.nec.2016.11.009.
3. Altaf I, Shams S, Vohra AH. Role of surgical modality and timing of surgery as clinical outcome predictors following acute subdural hematoma evacuation. Pak J Med Sci. 2020;36:412–5. https://doi.org/10.12669/pjms.36.3.1771.
4. Aydin MD, Kanat A, Hacimuftuoglu A, Ozmen S, Ahiskalioglu A, Kocak MN. A new experimental evidence that olfactory bulb lesion may be a causative factor for substantia nigra degeneration; preliminary study. Int J Neurosci. 2021;131(3):220–7. https://doi.org/10.1080/00207454.2020.1737049.
5. Aydin MD, Kanat A, Yolas C, Soyalp C, Onen MR, Yilmaz I, Karaavci NC, Calik M, Baykal O, Ramazanoglu L. Spinal subarachnoid hemorrhage induced intractable miotic pupil. A reminder of ciliospinal sympathetic center ischemia based miosis: an experimental study. Turk Neurosurg. 2019;29:434–9. https://doi.org/10.5137/1019-5149.JTN.24446-18.1.
6. Celiker M, Kanat A, Aydin MDMD, Ozdemir D, Aydin N, Yolas C, Calik M, Peker HOHO. First emerging objective experimental evidence of hearing impairment following subarachnoid haemorrhage; Felix culpa, phonophobia, and elucidation of the role of trigeminal ganglion. Int J Neurosci. 2019;129:794–800. https://doi.org/10.1080/00207454.2019.1569651.
7. Celiker M, Kanat A, Ozdemir A, Celiker FB, Kazdal H, Ozdemir B, Batcik OE, Ozdemir D. Controversy about the protective role of volume in the frontal sinus after severe head trauma: larger sinus equates with higher risk of death. Br J Oral Maxillofac Surg. 2020;58:314–8. https://doi.org/10.1016/j.bjoms.2019.12.008.
8. Costa JMC, Fernandes FAO, Alves de Sousa RJ. Prediction of subdural haematoma based on a detailed numerical model of the cerebral bridging veins. J Mech Behav Biomed Mater.

2020;111:103976. https://doi.org/10.1016/j.jmbbm.2020.103976.
9. Fomchenko EI, Gilmore EJ, Matouk CC, Gerrard JL, Sheth KN. Management of subdural hematomas: part II. Surgical management of subdural hematomas. Curr Treat Options Neurol. 2018;20:34. https://doi.org/10.1007/s11940-018-0518-1.
10. Gasenzer ER, Kanat A, Neugebauer E. Neurosurgery and music; effect of Wolfgang Amadeus Mozart. World Neurosurg. 2017;102:313–9. https://doi.org/10.1016/j.wneu.2017.02.081.
11. Gasenzer ER, Kanat A, Ozdemir V, Rakici SY, Neugebauer E. Interesting different survival status of musicians with malignant cerebral tumors. Br J Neurosurg. 2020;34:264–70. https://doi.org/10.1080/02688697.2019.1701629.
12. Huang KT, Bi WL, Abd-El-Barr M, Yan SC, Tafel IJ, Dunn IF, Gormley WB. The Neurocritical and neurosurgical care of subdural hematomas. Neurocrit Care. 2016;24:294–307. https://doi.org/10.1007/s12028-015-0194-x.
13. Kanat A. Patient-evaluated outcome after surgery for basal meningiomas. Neurosurgery. 2002;51:1530–2.
14. Kanat A. Brain oxygenation and energy metabolism: part I—biological function and pathophysiology. Neurosurgery. 2003;52:1508–9.
15. Kanat A, Aydin MD, Akca N, Ozmen S: First histopathological bridging of the distance between Onuf's nucleus and substantia nigra after olfactory bulbectomy-new ideas about the urinary dysfunction in cerebral neurodegenerative disease: an experimental study Low Urin Tract Symptoms. 2021;13:383–9. https://doi.org/10.1111/luts.12371.
16. Kanat A, Aydin Y. Postcontrast magnetic resonance imaging to predict progression of traumatic epidural and subdural hematomas in the acute stage. Neurosurgery. 1999;44:685–6.
17. Kanat A, Aydin Y. Recurrent meningiomas. J Neurosurg. 1999;91:720–1.
18. Kanat A, Aydin Y. Prognostic value and determinants of ultraearly angiographic vasospasm after aneurysmal subarachnoid hemorrhage. Neurosurgery. 2000;46:505–7.
19. Kanat A, Kayaci S, Yazar U, Kazdal H, Terzi Y. Chronic subdural hematoma in adults: why does it occur more often in males than females? Influence of patient's sexual gender on occurrence. J Neurosurg Sci. 2010;54:99–103.
20. Kanat A, Romana Gasenzer E, Neugebauer E. A different aspect of the unexpected death of Mozart at the age of 35 years. CNS Spectr. 2019;24:628–31. https://doi.org/10.1017/S1092852918001736.
21. Kanat A, Yazar U, Kazdal H. Chronic subdural hygroma with thrombocythemia: first case report. J Neurosurg Sci. 2009;53:165–7.
22. Karibe H, Hayashi T, Hirano T, Kameyama M, Nakagawa A, Tominaga T. Surgical management of traumatic acute subdural hematoma in adults: a review. Neurol Med Chir (Tokyo). 2014;54:887–94. https://doi.org/10.2176/nmc.cr.2014-0204.
23. Kazdal H, Kanat A, Aydin MD, Yazar U, Guvercin AR, Calik M, Gundogdu B. Sudden death and cervical spine: a new contribution to pathogenesis for sudden death in critical care unit from subarachnoid hemorrhage; first report—an experimental study. J Craniovertebr Junction Spine. 2017;8:33.
24. Kerezoudis P, Goyal A, Puffer RC, Parney IF, Meyer FB, Bydon M. Morbidity and mortality in elderly patients undergoing evacuation of acute traumatic subdural hematoma. Neurosurg Focus. 2020;49:E22. https://doi.org/10.3171/2020.7.FOCUS20439.
25. Kvint S, Gutierrez A, Blue R, Petrov D. Surgical management of trauma-related intracranial hemorrhage—a review. Curr Neurol Neurosci Rep. 2020;20:63. https://doi.org/10.1007/s11910-020-01080-0.
26. Mokri B. The Monro-Kellie hypothesis: applications in CSF volume depletion. Neurology. 2001;56:1746–8. https://doi.org/10.1212/wnl.56.12.1746.
27. Ozdemir B, Kanat A, Kazdal H. Experimental cerebral injury models (in Turkish). Turk Norosirurji Derg. 2020;30:308–11.
28. Ozdemir B, Kanat A, Ozdemir V, Batcik OE, Yazar U, Guvercin AR. The effect of neuroscientists on the studies of autonomic nervous system dysfunction following experimental subarachnoid hemorrhage. J Craniofac Surg. 2019;30:2184–8. https://doi.org/10.1097/scs.0000000000005763.
29. Ozturk C, Ozdemir NG, Kanat A, Aydin MD, Findik H, Aydin N, Kabalar ME, Kazdal H, Yolas C, Baykal O, Calik M. How reliable is pupillary evaluation following subarachnoid hemorrhage? Effect of oculomotor nerve degeneration secondary to posterior communicating artery vasospasm: first experimental study. J Neurol Surg A Cent Eur Neurosurg. 2018;79:302–8. https://doi.org/10.1055/s-0037-1608841.

30. Rush B, Rousseau J, Sekhon MS, Griesdale DE. Craniotomy versus craniectomy for acute traumatic subdural hematoma in the United States: a national retrospective cohort analysis. World Neurosurg. 2016;88:25–31. https://doi.org/10.1016/j.wneu.2015.12.034.
31. Sharma R, Rocha E, Pasi M, Lee H, Patel A, Singhal AB. Subdural hematoma: predictors of outcome and a score to guide surgical decision-making. J Stroke Cerebrovasc Dis. 2020;29:105180. https://doi.org/10.1016/j.jstrokecerebrovasdis.2020.105180.
32. Shin D-S, Hwang S-C. Neurocritical management of traumatic acute subdural hematomas. Korean. J Neurotrauma. 2020;16:113–25. https://doi.org/10.13004/kjnt.2020.16.e43.
33. Tao Z-Q, Ding S-H, Huang J-Y, Zhu Z-G. The pathogenesis of subacute subdural hematoma: a report of 3 cases and literature review. World Neurosurg. 2018;114:e22–8. https://doi.org/10.1016/j.wneu.2018.01.147.
34. Trevisi G, Sturiale CL, Scerrati A, Rustemi O, Ricciardi L, Raneri F, Tomatis A, Piazza A, Auricchio AM, Stifano V, Romano C, De Bonis P, Mangiola A. Acute subdural hematoma in the elderly: outcome analysis in a retrospective multicentric series of 213 patients. Neurosurg Focus. 2020;49:E21. https://doi.org/10.3171/2020.7.FOCUS20437.
35. Turk O, Ozdemir NG, Demirel N, Atci IB, Kanat A, Yolas C. Nontraumatic intradiploic epidermoid cyst and older age: association or causality? J Craniofac Surg. 2018;29:e143–6. https://doi.org/10.1097/SCS.0000000000003897.
36. Vega RA, Valadka AB. Natural history of acute subdural hematoma. Neurosurg Clin N Am. 2017;28:247–55. https://doi.org/10.1016/j.nec.2016.11.007.
37. Won S-Y, Konczalla J, Dubinski D, Cattani A, Cuca C, Seifert V, Rosenow F, Strzelczyk A, Freiman TM. A systematic review of epileptic seizures in adults with subdural haematomas. Seizure. 2017;45:28–35. https://doi.org/10.1016/j.seizure.2016.11.017.
38. Yilmaz A, Musluman AM, Kanat A, Cavusoglu H, Terzi Y, Aydin Y. The correlation between hematoma volume and outcome in ruptured posterior fossa arteriovenous malformations indicates the importance of surgical evacuation of hematomas. Turk Neurosurg. 2011;21:152–9. https://doi.org/10.5137/1019-5149.JTN.3401-10.0.
39. Yolas C, Kanat A, Aydin MD, Altas E, Kanat IF, Kazdal H, Duman A, Gundogdu B, Gursan N. Unraveling of the effect of nodose ganglion degeneration on the coronary artery vasospasm after subarachnoid hemorrhage: an experimental study. World Neurosurg. 2016;86:79–87. https://doi.org/10.1016/j.wneu.2015.09.004.

第 3 章 颅内硬膜下血肿研究发展史

Nikolaos Ch. Syrmos, Vaitsa Giannouli, Sotirios Kottas 和 Mehmet Turgut

译者：刘伟明

3.1 引言

硬膜下血肿（SDH）是指积聚在硬脑膜和蛛网膜之间，包围和保护位于颅骨内脑组织的血液。SDH 分为三种类型：急性、亚急性和慢性。在这些类型中，慢性 SDH 多为轻度或中度颅脑创伤后 2～3 周发展形成并伴随慢性炎症和多种症状（行为改变、头痛、局灶神经功能缺失、偏瘫、癫痫发作等）。本章目的旨在探究从古至今慢性 SDH 重要的历史研究发现。

3.2 古代史

人类治疗 SDH 最古老的外科手术方式是颅脑钻孔术或环锯术。在许多地区如非洲、南美以及美拉尼西亚，我们发现了旧石器时代和新石器时代关于钻孔术的记载。钻孔术的应用从石器时代、青铜器时代和铁器时代一直延续到希腊时期[1, 3, 12, 22]。

希波克拉底（Hellenic Hippocrates，Ιπποκράτης）（公元前 460—370 年），来自希腊科斯岛（Κώς），是人类历史上第一位有记载的医生和第一位神经外科医生。在他的著作中详细记载了在他的时代中，他和他的学生一起进行精确的神经外科手术如各种类型颅骨钻孔术（图 3.1）[3, 7, 20-22]。

在世界其他地方，如中美、拉美、北非、地中海地区、中东以及其他重要人类文明（玛雅人、印加人、阿兹特克人、扎波特人、米诺斯人、埃及人、巴比伦人、苏美尔人、亚述人、赫梯人、波斯人、以色列人等）SDH 的治疗同样得到了发展[3, 7, 20-22]。根据各种研究以及通过绘画和其他考古发现，数百年来这些地区通过神经外科颅脑手术和如献祭等宗教行为发展了关于颅骨钻孔术的知识[1, 3, 7, 12, 20, 22]。

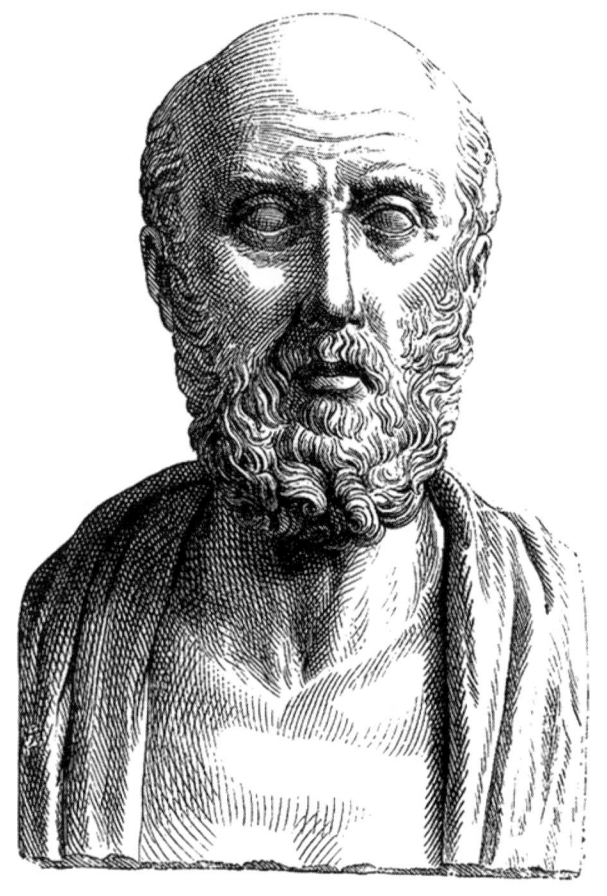

图 3.1 希波克拉底（公元前 460—370 年）

3.3 现代史

3.3.1 15 世纪

安布列斯·帕雷（Ambroise Paré，1510—1590）是一位来自法国的外科理发师，为国王亨利二世、弗朗西斯二世、查理九世和亨利三世服务（图 3.2）。他还是一名法医病理学家和那个时代的解剖学家。据帕雷记载，亨利二世因在 1559 年左右的一次比武中受伤，而患有 SDH[3, 12, 17]。

3.3.2 16 世纪

约翰·雅各布·维普夫（Johann Jakob Wepfer，1620 年 12 月 23 日—1695 年 1 月 26 日）是一名来

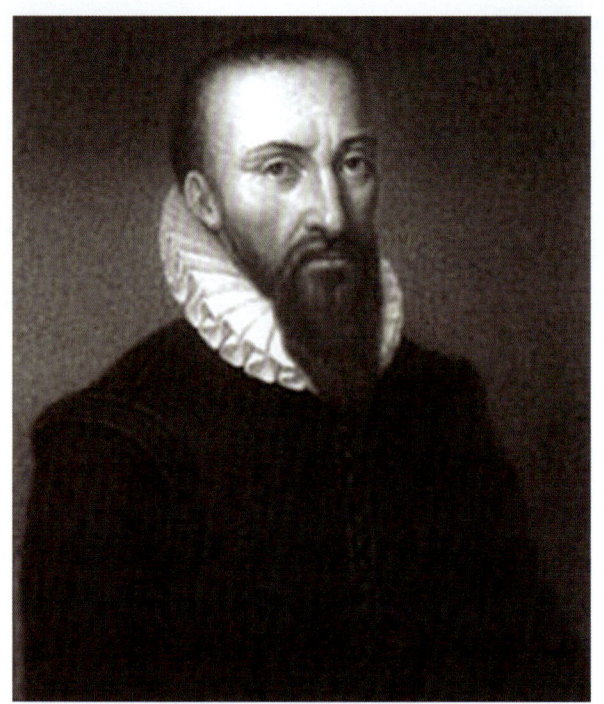

图 3.2　安布列斯·帕雷（1510—1590）

自瑞士沙夫豪森的内科医生。在他自己的国家（巴塞尔）和国外（斯特拉斯堡、帕多瓦）进行了几次医学研究后，他于 1647 年返回祖国[3-4, 12]。为了更好地了解脑血管疾病，他学习了脑血管解剖学和生理学知识。他对尸体进行了解剖从而探究大脑血供以及卒中的发病机制。他也是其生活年代的一位著名科学家（药理学家和毒理学家）[2-4, 12, 17]。根据德埃里克和杰尔曼（Errico 和 German）的记载，维普夫是第一位将慢性 SDH 描述为患者经历过所谓的"卒中"发作后积聚在硬脑膜下一个充满血的大囊肿[5, 12]。

乔瓦尼·巴蒂斯塔·莫尔加尼（Giovanni Battista Morgagni，1682 年 2 月 25 日—1771 年 12 月 6 日）是一名意大利解剖学家（图 3.3），他被认为是现代解剖病理学之父。他曾在意大利北部威尼托地区的帕多瓦大学担任解剖学教授多年。1761 年，在约翰·雅各布·维普夫去世 60 年后，他记载了一名被诊断为"卒中发作"的慢性 SDH 患者[3-4, 6, 12, 17]。

在 1772 年，伊尔（Hill）将钻孔术看作是慢性 SDH 的一种治疗方法[3, 8, 12, 17]。

3.3.3　18—19 世纪

在 18 世纪，一些重大研究结果的发现，帮助我们更好地了解 SDH：

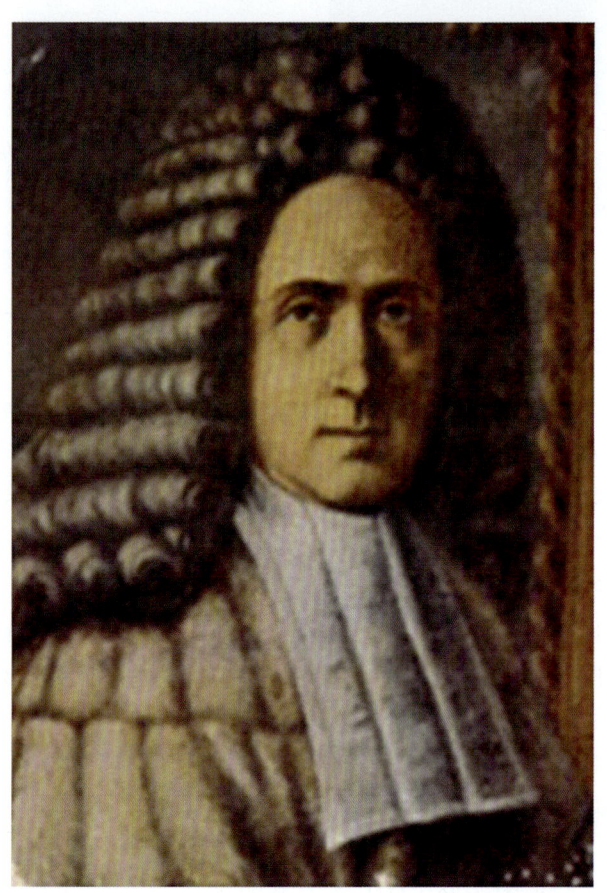

图 3.3　乔瓦尼·巴蒂斯塔·莫尔加尼（1682—1771）

- 1800 年，比沙（Bichat M）在他的解剖著作《论膜》（*Traité des membranes engénéral et de diverses membranes en particulier*）中描述了大量与脑膜有关的内容[3, 9, 12, 17]。
- 1817 年，在乌萨尔（Houssard）的描述中阐述了血块和脑膜的性质[3, 11-12, 17]。
- 1822 年，蒂贝尔（Thubert）描述了在最初创伤 9 年后出现症状的病变。这种创伤可能是导致血液在硬膜下积聚的主要因素[3, 10, 12-13, 17]。
- 1826 年，根据贝勒（Bayle）病理、生理和形态学研究，他提出慢性再出血是该病的主要致病因素[2-3, 12, 14-15, 17]。
- 1840 年，奥诺雷·德·巴尔扎克（Honore de Balzac）描述了一例 SDH 的疑似病例，包括他的外伤病因以及手术治疗[2-3, 12, 14-15, 17]。
- 1845 年，休伊特（Hewit）发表了一篇题为《关于蛛网膜外腔渗血》（*On extravasations of blood into the cavity of the arachnoid*）的文章，他相信覆盖在血凝块上的膜是血液

直接流入腔隙的结果，而不是蛛网膜或硬脑膜的特定成分[3, 12, 17]。

- 1855 年，赫舍尔（Heschl）反对出血是形成病变首要原因的观点，相反他认为膜发生炎症先于出血[3, 12, 16-17]。
- 1857 年，魏尔肖进行了病因学和组织学研究[3, 12, 17-18]。

道夫·路德维希·卡尔·魏尔肖（Rudolf Ludwig Carl Virchow，1821 年 10 月 13 日—1902 年 9 月 5 日）是一名来自德国的学者（图 3.4）。他同时是一名内科医生、人类学家、病理学家以及多个其他科学领域的专家（历史学和生物学）。他是一名作家、编辑和政治家[3, 12, 17, 19]。他以"现代病理学之父"而闻名世界。魏尔肖通过对组织学的研究阐释了脑膜的形成，他认为 SDH 通常是由硬脑膜慢性炎症引起的，称为"慢性出血性脑膜炎"，有血液外溢到硬膜下间隙，并在硬脑膜内表面形成一层纤维蛋白膜[3, 12, 17, 23]。

1868 年，克莱明斯基（Kremiansky）认为脑膜中动脉病变是出血的主要病因，可能是由全身疾病所导致。他也意识到局部刺激和全身疾病都会对 SDH 的发生发展发挥作用[3, 12, 17, 24]。

1872 年，斯珀林（Sperling）重新采纳了早期的观点，即认为出血是首要病因，而硬脑膜炎性假膜是由溢出物质形成的。他在犬中进行了多次实验研究[3, 12, 15, 17]。

霍格尼（Huegenin）在他的研究中认为大脑退化萎缩在该过程中起到重要作用。1862 年，威格尔斯沃斯（Wigelsworth）在他的实验报告中提出了相同的观点[3, 12, 15, 17]。

1883 年，哈尔克（Hulke）报道了一例经过神经外科手术成功治疗的慢性 SDH。然而，1911 年，奥本海姆（Oppenheim）仍将该病变看作是炎症过程[3, 12, 15, 17]。

严格意义上来说，创伤仅是从 19 世纪后期到 20 世纪初期被看作慢性 SDH 的可能病因[3, 12, 15, 17, 25-26, 28]。

3.3.4 20 世纪

1902 年，巴雷特（Barret）进行了对 SDH 的病因的实验研究。他在猫中进行了多种研究[3, 12, 15, 17, 27, 29-30]。

威廉·福特·罗伯逊（William Ford Robertson，1867—1923）详细描述了血肿膜形成的组织学过程[12, 16-17, 23]。

威尔弗里德·特罗特（Wilfrid Trotter，1872—1939）出生在英国。尽管童年时因严重的肌肉骨骼问题而长期卧床，但他首先在伦敦大学学习医学，并成为大学学院医院的教授和外科主任。他进行了许多外科学和肿瘤学研究。1914 年，特罗特的研究聚焦于创伤领域和慢性 SDH 的病因[12, 16-17, 23]。

特雷西·杰克逊·普特南（1894 年 4 月 14 日—1975 年 3 月 9 日）是一名美国医生。普特南在波士顿市立医院和哥伦比亚大学纽约神经学研究所工作（图 3.5）[12, 16-17, 23]。

哈维·威廉姆斯·库欣（1869 年 4 月 8 日—1939 年 10 月 7 日）既是美国神经外科先驱，又是内分泌学等其他科学领域的专家（图 3.6）。在他的影响下，神经外科成为一门独立的医学学科，他被认为是神经外科之父。在他的领导下，培养了许多伟大的神经外科医生：

- 沃尔特·丹迪（Walter Dandy），第一位小儿神经外科医生和气脑造影术的研发者[12, 16-17]。
- 利奥·大卫杜夫（Leo M.Davidoff），爱因斯

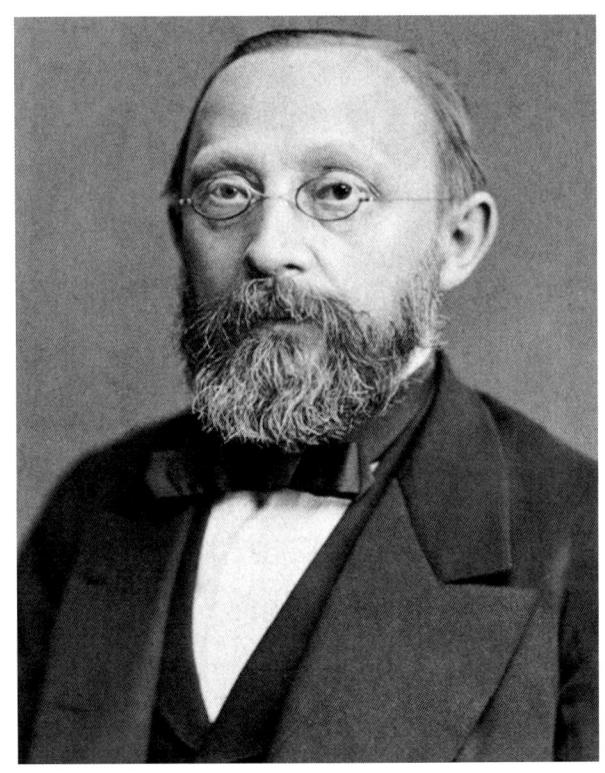

图 3.4　路德维希·魏尔肖（1821—1902）

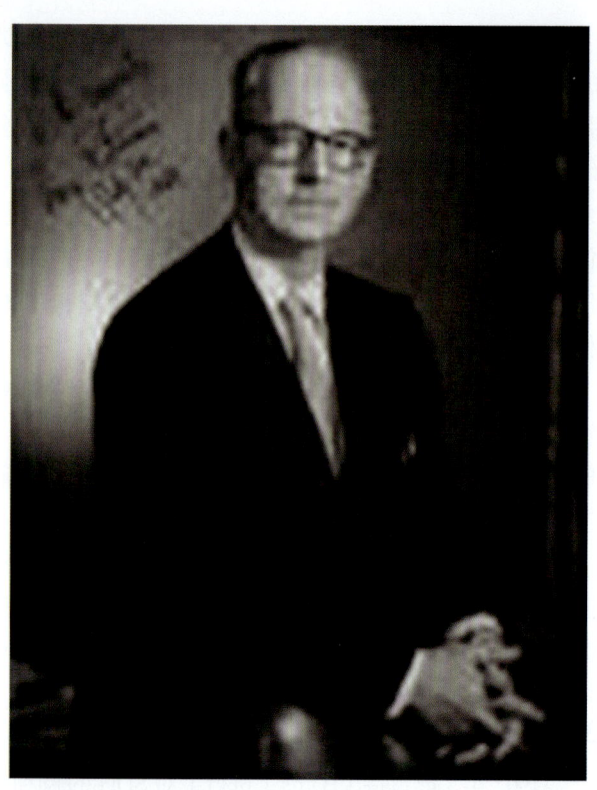

图 3.5　特雷西·杰克逊·普特南（1894—1975）

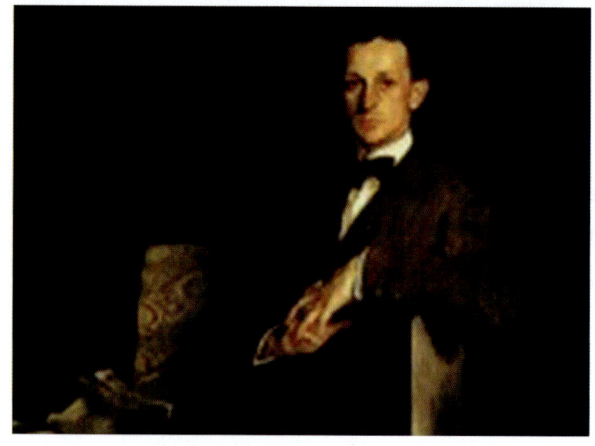

图 3.6　哈维·威廉姆斯·库欣（1869—1939）

坦医学院神经外科系创始人[12, 16-17]。
- 诺曼·多特（Norman Dott）[12, 16-17]。
- 怀尔德·彭菲尔德（Wilder Penfeld），蒙特利尔神经学研究所创始人[12, 16-17]。

哈维·威廉姆斯·库欣同样将急性 SDH 定义为一种损伤性疾病，并描述这种损伤情况下需要的相应治疗[12, 16-17]。1925 年 9 月，特雷西·杰克逊·普特南和哈维·库欣共同发表了一篇题为《慢性硬膜下血肿的病因，与出血性硬脑膜炎的关系及其手术治疗》（*Chronic Subdural Hematoma. Its Pathology, Its Relation to Pachymeningitis Hemorrhagica and Its Surgical Treatment*）的论文。在这篇科学报告中，他们阐述了复发性出血会导致血肿进行性增大。根据普特南和库欣的研究，该病变被称为慢性 SDH，而不是内出血性硬脑膜炎[12, 16-17]。

1920 年，萨克斯（Sachs）发表了在婴儿中该类型疾病的综述。他提出脑外伤后存活下来的婴儿可能会发展成一种慢性疾病[12, 17]。

1924 年，斯蒂芬森（Stephenson）报道了一例合并梅毒的硬脑膜炎。他认为这两种疾病具有相关性[12, 17]。

1928 年，克雷格（Craig）指出在硬脑膜间隙中发现的间皮细胞可被归类为网状间皮系统的一部分，因为其具有能够与血红蛋白反应的能力，这种相互作用会分解血液中的色素从而使血液呈现最后的深色[12, 17]。

在接下来的几十年，各种各样的 SDH 发病理论被提出，其中渗透压理论是近 40 年来最被广泛接受的观点：

- 1932 年，加德纳（Gardner）提出半透性血肿内膜的血液对脑脊液的渗透吸引导致硬膜下血凝块扩大的观点[12, 17]。
- 1934 年，佐林格（Zollinger）同样提出胶体渗透压理论[30]。
- 1936 年，门罗和梅里特（Munro 和 Merritt）研究了关于这种病变进展的 105 例患者[12, 17]。
- 同一时间，汉娜和坎普（Hannah 和 Kaump）也进行了关于硬脑膜内膜二次形成的研究[12, 17]。
- 1955 年，吉尔汀（Giltin）提出了渗透学说[12]。

20 世纪 70 年代：

- 威尔（Weir）反对胶体渗透压理论并且发现在血液、脑脊液和慢性 SDH 的液体之间没有胶体渗透压差异（1971）[25-30]。
- 渡边（Watanabe）通过将混合血液和脑血管内液的血凝块注射到实验犬和实验猴的硬膜下腔隙构建慢性 SDH 临床模型（1972）[25-30]。
- 阿普费鲍姆（Apfelbaum）未能证实脑血管内液是导致慢性 SDH 的必要因素（1974）[25-30]。
- 佐藤和铃木（Sato 和 Suzuki）报道了来自血

肿膜外毛细血管重复微出血与慢性SDH扩大有关（1975）[25-30]。

- 拉巴迪和格洛弗（Labadie和Glover）证实了注射进入脑脊液的地塞米松会阻碍膜的形成（1976）[25-30]。
- 山田（Yamada）报道了从积液到血肿的转化（1979）[25-30]。

20世纪80年代：

- 1980年，威尔（Weir）否认胶体渗透压理论。然而，在他的研究中并没有解释血肿扩大的机制[25-30]。
- 1981年，马克瓦尔德（Markwalder）支持血肿膜再出血是形成慢性SDH的理论。马克瓦尔德对膜再出血理论的综述被广泛接受[25-30]。
- 无症状急性SDH被怀疑是慢性SDH的起源（1985）[25-30]。

20世纪90年代和21世纪：

- 李（Lee）的研究（1996、1998和2004）揭示了硬膜下病变及其起源与慢性SDH自然进展之间的关系[10-12]。

20世纪末：

- 所有使用的实验模型都无法证明慢性SDH会逐渐扩大，除非创造相同的病理环境，即在液化的血肿外包裹了一层新膜[12]。
- 关于该病变的起源以及自然进展仍有争议[12]。

3.4 结论

慢性SDH仍然是一种重要的神经外科疾病。从古代人类最初的描述到现代，人类关于该疾病的认识也在不断提高。神经外科作为一门独立的医学学科不断在发展，慢性SDH最初在17世纪和18世纪被描述为脑卒中，随后在19世纪被看作是炎症，最后在20世纪被认为是一种创伤性损伤。尽管慢性SDH的病因被证明为创伤，但是该疾病仍有许多值得研究的内容：①无症状的急性SDH如何成为慢性SDH的主要来源；②最初的颅脑损伤和症状发作之间为什么会存在潜伏期未得到明确解释。

参考文献

1. Andrushko VA, Verano JW. Prehistoric trepanation in the Cuzco region of Peru: a view into an ancient Andean practice. Am J Phys Anthropol. 2008;137:4–13.
2. Apfelbaum RI, Guthkelch AN, Shulman K. Experimental production of subdural hematomas. J Neurosurg. 1974;40:336–46.
3. Castiglioni A. Storia della Medicina. Milan: A. Mondadori; 1936.
4. D'Abbondanza JA, Loch Macdonald R. Experimental models of chronic subdural hematoma. Neurol Res. 2014;36:176–88.
5. D'Errico AP, German WJ. Chronic subdural hematoma. Yale J Biol Med. 1930;3:11–20.
6. Ellis H. The Cambridge illustrated history of surgery. Cambridge: Cambridge University Press; 2009.
7. Giannouli V, Syrmos N. Information about Macedonian medicine in ancient Greece. Hell J Nucl Med. 2011;14:324–5.
8. Kaufman MH, Whitaker D, McTavish J. Differential diagnosis of holes in the calvarium: application of modern clinical data to palaeopathology. J Archaeol Sci. 1997;24:193–218.
9. Kim DJ. The appeal of holes in the head. In: Whitelaw WA, editor. The Proceedings of the 13th annual history of medicine days. Calgary: Faculty of Medicine; University of Calgary; 2004. p. 17–24.
10. Lee KS. The pathogenesis and clinical significance of traumatic subdural hygroma. Brain Inj. 1998;12:595–603.
11. Lee KS. Natural history of chronic subdural haematoma. Brain Inj. 2004;18:351–8.
12. Lee K-S. History of chronic subdural hematoma. Korean J Neurotrauma. 2015;11:27–34.
13. Marino R Jr, Gonzales-Portillo M. Preconquest Peruvian neurosurgeons: a study of Inca and pre-Columbian trephination and the art of medicine in ancient Peru. Neurosurgery. 2000;47:940–50.

14. Oka H, Motomochi M, Suzuki Y, Ando K. Subdural hygroma after head injury. A review of 26 cases. Acta Neurochir (Wien). 1972;26:265–73.
15. Oppenheim H. Textbook of nervous diseases for physicians and students. 5th ed. New York: Otto Schulze and Company; 1911.
16. Putnam TJ, Cushing H. Chronic subdural hematoma: its pathology, its relation to pachymeningitis hemorrhagica, and its surgical treatment. Arch Surg. 1925;11:329–93.
17. Richards CE. Chronic subdural hematoma with special reference to etiology, diagnosis, and treatment. MD Thesis. 1940.
18. Sato S, Suzuki J. Ultrastructural observations of the capsule of chronic subdural hematoma in various clinical stages. J Neurosurg. 1975;43:569–78.
19. Schachenmayr W, Friede RL. The origin of subdural neomembranes. I. Fine structure of the dura-arachnoid interface in man. Am J Pathol. 1978;92:53–68.
20. Syrmos N. Microcephaly in ancient Greece-the Minoan microcephalus of Zakros. Childs Nerv Syst. 2011;27:685–6.
21. Syrmos N. Historical back training in most important points of neurosurgery. Master Thesis. Aristotle University of Thessaloniki, Thessaloniki, Macedonia, Greece. 2009.
22. Syrmos N, Ampatzidis G, Fachantidou A, Mouratidis A, Syrmos C. Historical back training in most important points of neurosurgery. Ann General Psychiatry. 2010;9(Suppl 1):S89.
23. Trotter W. Chronic subdural hæmorrhage of traumatic origin, and its relation to pachymeningitis hæmorrhagica interna. Br J Surg. 1914;2:271–91.
24. Tullo E. Trepanation and Roman medicine: a comparison of osteoarchaeological remains, material culture and written texts. J R Coll Physicians Edinb. 2010;40:165–71.
25. Velasco-Suarez M, Bautista Martinez J, Garcia Oliveros R, Weinstein PR. Archaeological origins of cranial surgery: trephination in Mexico. Neurosurgery. 1992;31:313–8.
26. Watanabe S, Shimada H, Ishii S. Production of clinical form of chronic subdural hematoma in experimental animals. J Neurosurg. 1972;37:552–61.
27. Weir B. The osmolality of subdural hematoma fluid. J Neurosurg. 1971;34:528–33.
28. Weir B. Oncotic pressure of subdural fluids. J Neurosurg. 1980;53:512–5.
29. Wilberger JE. Pathophysiology of evolution and recurrence of chronic subdural hematoma. Neurosurg Clin N Am. 2000;11:435–8.
30. Zollinger R, Gross RE. Traumatic subdural hematoma: an explanation of the late onset of pressure symptoms. J Am Med Assoc. 1934;103:245–9.

第 4 章　慢性硬膜下血肿：病理生理学

George W. Koutsouras，Sydney Colvin 和 Satish Krishnamurthy

译者：王李傲

4.1　引言

慢性硬膜下血肿（chronic subdural hematoma，CSDH）是一种常见的神经系统疾病，发病率为 10～18 人/10 万人，在老年人中发病率有逐年增加的趋势[2]。CSDH 的病理生理机制复杂多样，亟待探索。CSDH 患病率相当高，但尚未确定一种有效的治疗方法能够显著降低其复发率[4]。

硬脑膜边界细胞参与维持了硬脑膜下间隙的稳态，同时将硬脑膜与蛛网膜连接在一起。CSDH 的发生正是始于这个间隙的破坏，这种损伤可以是自发性的，也可以是外伤引起的[10, 23, 28]。损伤发生后，一系列病理生理反应将发生，包括炎症过程导致新膜生成，以及血肿不完全吸收进而形成 CSDH。我们描述了一系列参与 CSDH 发生的病理生理过程（图 4.1）。

4.2　临床特征

CSDH 通常在发生发展后的 4～7 周引起症状。患者出现头痛、恶心、精神状态改变、肢体无力、癫痫甚至昏迷等症状，这是由皮质刺激、脑组织受

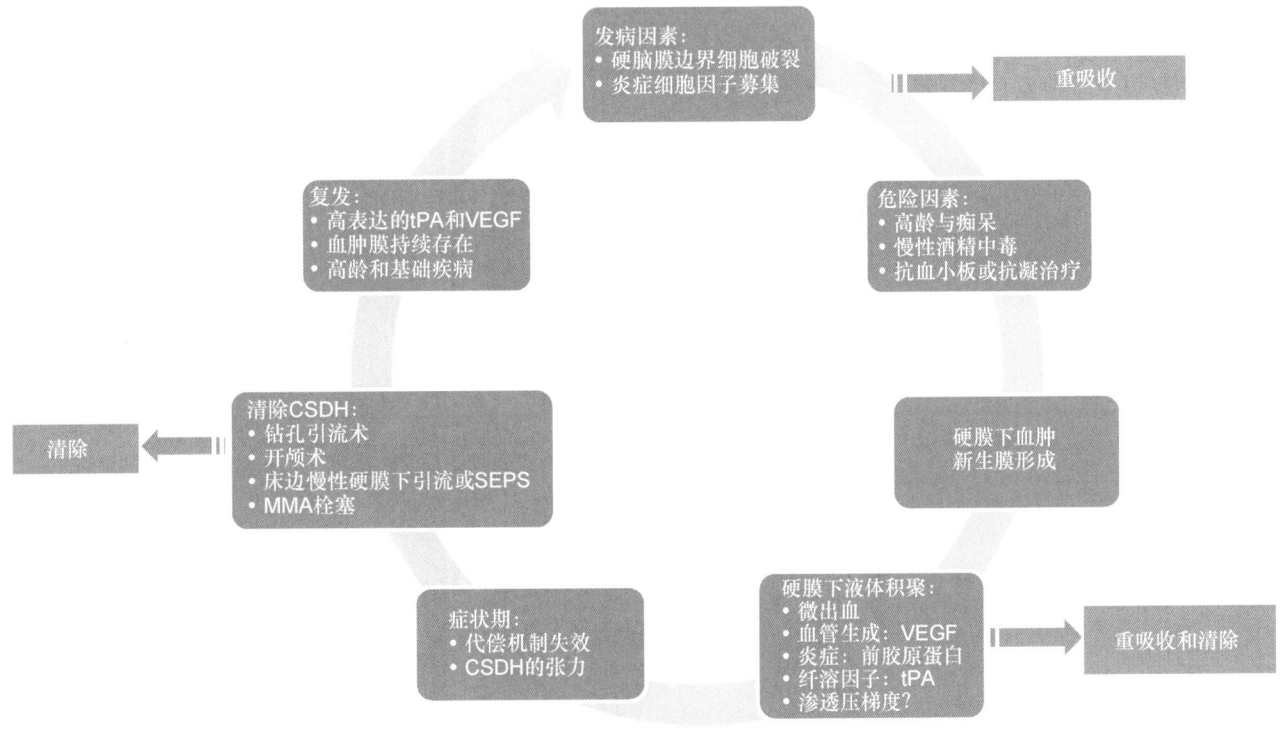

图 4.1　慢性硬膜下血肿（CSDH）的病程。患者发病为外伤，当同时存在罹患 CSDH 的风险因素，如老年、使用抗凝药物以及慢性酒精中毒，将会导致新生膜的形成，继而红细胞和脑脊液渗入硬膜下间隙，但硬膜下组织无法吸收渗入的液体，导致代偿机制失衡和症状的发生发展。症状的出现提示患者出现手术指征。防止复发的因素包括清除血肿并去除新生膜，或通过栓塞脑膜中动脉（MMA）以减少 CSDH 的血流。SEPS，硬膜下引流系统；VEGF，血管内皮生长因子；tPA，组织型纤溶酶原激活剂

压或颅内压增高所致。

通常认为，CSDH 的形成是由急性硬膜下血肿演变而来的，然而仅有 3%～26% 的急性硬膜下血肿患者发展为 CSDH[20]。这表明 CSDH 具有一定潜伏性并存在无症状期，可见有其他因素通过特定病理生理机制促进了 CSDH 的形成。CSDH 中凝固的血液会液化，留下血清样液体在硬膜下间隙中被逐步吸收。这个过程是由脑实质压力导致的，它会减小硬膜下间隙的大小。在颅内压较低的患者或患有脑萎缩的患者中，例如晚期痴呆症或慢性酗酒者，硬膜下间隙更有可能积聚这种液体[19]。高龄是硬膜下血肿发生的一个风险因素，超过 60% 的 CSDH 患者年龄在 65 岁以上[2]。硬膜下血肿也可能出现在婴儿和儿童身上，通常与人为性头部外伤有关，但也可能出现在外部性脑积水、蛛网膜下腔良性扩大、特发性巨颅畸形甚至脱水的患儿中[40]。男性比女性更容易出现 CSDH[1]。服用抗凝药物或抗血小板药物的患者在外伤后发展成急性硬膜下血肿和 CSDH 的风险较高，而不服用抗血栓药物的患者则风险较低[1]（图 4.2）。

4.3 影像学特征

计算机断层成像（CT）是诊断 CSDH 的理想检查方法，CSDH 在 CT 上呈现为不同于脑实质密度的轴外液体积聚（图 4.3）。等密度病变最为常见。此外，由于炎症过程的发生，混合密度也常见，它们被认为是持续微出血和新生膜形成的结果。混合密度也可见于急性和慢性创伤事件[10]。磁共振成像（MRI）在区分不同病程的 CSDH 以及鉴别 CSDH 与硬膜下积液或儿童蛛网膜下腔良性扩张等方面具有一定意义[31, 48]。

4.4 病理生理机制

自 19 世纪初 CSDH 被首次报道以来，研究者们应用组织病理学明确了硬膜下血肿的内部结构，此外，外科手术技术的进步也揭示了影响该疾病发展和复发的诸多因素[20]。CSDH 最早在 1857 年被 Virchow 描述为"内出血性硬脑膜炎"，Virchow 认为它是细菌感染介导慢性炎症后促进了新生血管

图 4.2 头部 CT 上显示了不同血肿密度。（a）低密度，（b）等密度，（c）高密度（左侧凸面），（d）双侧混合密度，右侧凸面局限性血肿

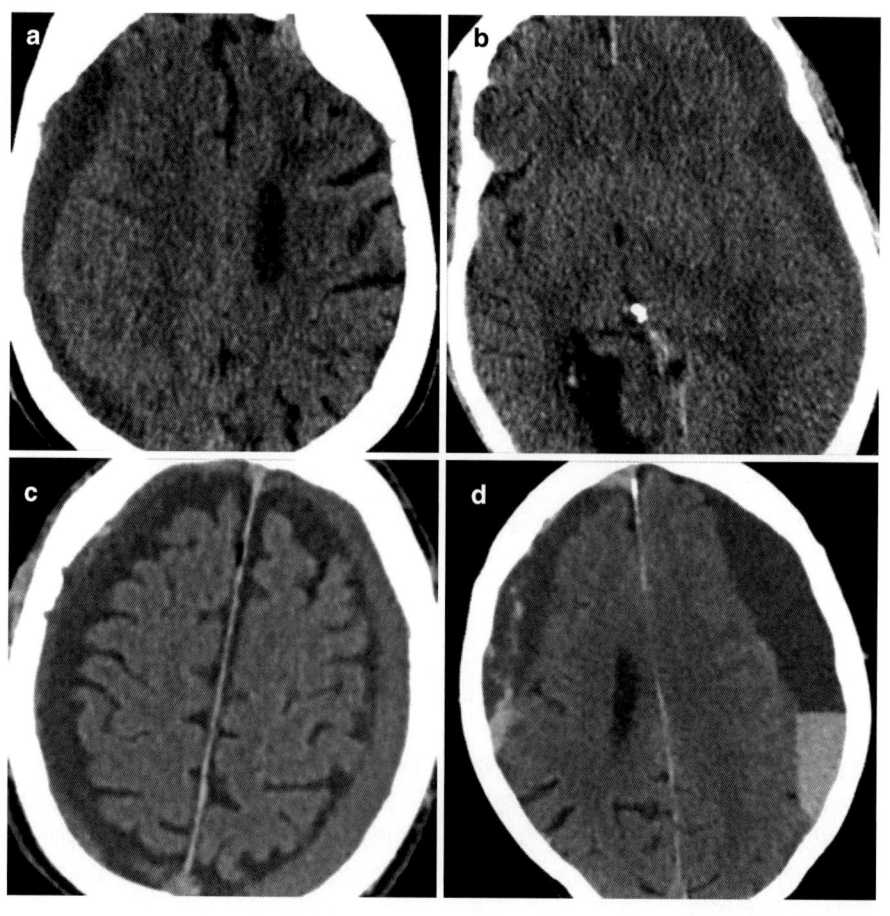

的形成和纤维素渗出[6]。在 20 世纪初，Schwartz、Trotter、Putnam 和 Cushing 都描述了一种创伤后引发的慢性炎症过程[32-33]。1936 年，来自华盛顿大学的神经外科医生 Furlow 进一步扩展了 Putnam 和 Cushing 的病例报道，描述了两种类型的硬膜下血肿，他根据组织病理学表现将它们分为反应/创伤型和血管型[42]。

1946 年，Inglis 定义了衬覆于硬脑膜的硬脑膜边界细胞[14]。当这些细胞受损时，会吸引炎症细胞聚集，并能在硬膜下间隙形成新生膜。一旦膜形成，血液和脑脊液（CSF）的混合物便会填充硬膜下腔[5]。当硬脑膜边界细胞被破坏时触发炎症级联反应，而新生膜在硬膜下血液、脑脊液积聚中起到了关键作用。

CSDH 的新生膜由外层和内层组成。早在 1936 年，研究者发现硬脑膜细胞在致病事件后大约 1 周形成外层膜，在 3 周内形成内层膜[24]。随着 CSDH 的发展，脑脊液和血液填充硬膜下间隙，引发了一系列纤维蛋白沉积和纤溶反应循环，这一循环最初通过组织型纤溶酶原激活剂（tPA）的激活来启动。通过激活血管内皮生长因子（VEGF），导致血管生成，以及硬膜下血肿的重组或液化[5]。CSDH 液体中已经发现了大量的 1 型和 3 型前胶原蛋白、纤维蛋白、血管生成素-2、其他细胞因子和趋化因子（图 4.3）。

外层膜中的血管和毛细血管均流向 CSDH 的血肿腔。外层膜中包含成纤维细胞、胶原纤维和迁移细胞（图 4.4）[7]。血管也参与炎症反应，毛细血管和蛛网膜下间隙的存在允许血液和脑脊液进入硬膜下腔。有文献表明，外层新生膜可以分为几种组织学亚型，与影像学特征相关。例如，Ⅱ型或出血性新生膜更常与血肿的快速扩张和最大血肿厚度相关[29]。这些微血管虽然很小，但会持续出血和促进血肿进展。VEGF 是 CSDH 进展中的重要血管生成因子。作为炎症过程的一部分，VEGF 的表达上调参与了新生膜形成的蛋白质修饰过程[35, 37, 41]。VEGF 导致高渗透性，从而形成不成熟的毛细血管，引起微出血和血肿形成。手术引流被认为可以减少血肿腔内的 VEGF 含量，从而缓解其刺激作用[35]。血管生成素是调节血管生成和血管通透性的生长因子。血管生成素-2（Ang-2）是一种促血管生成因子，可能对血管生成过程产生负面影响[12]。

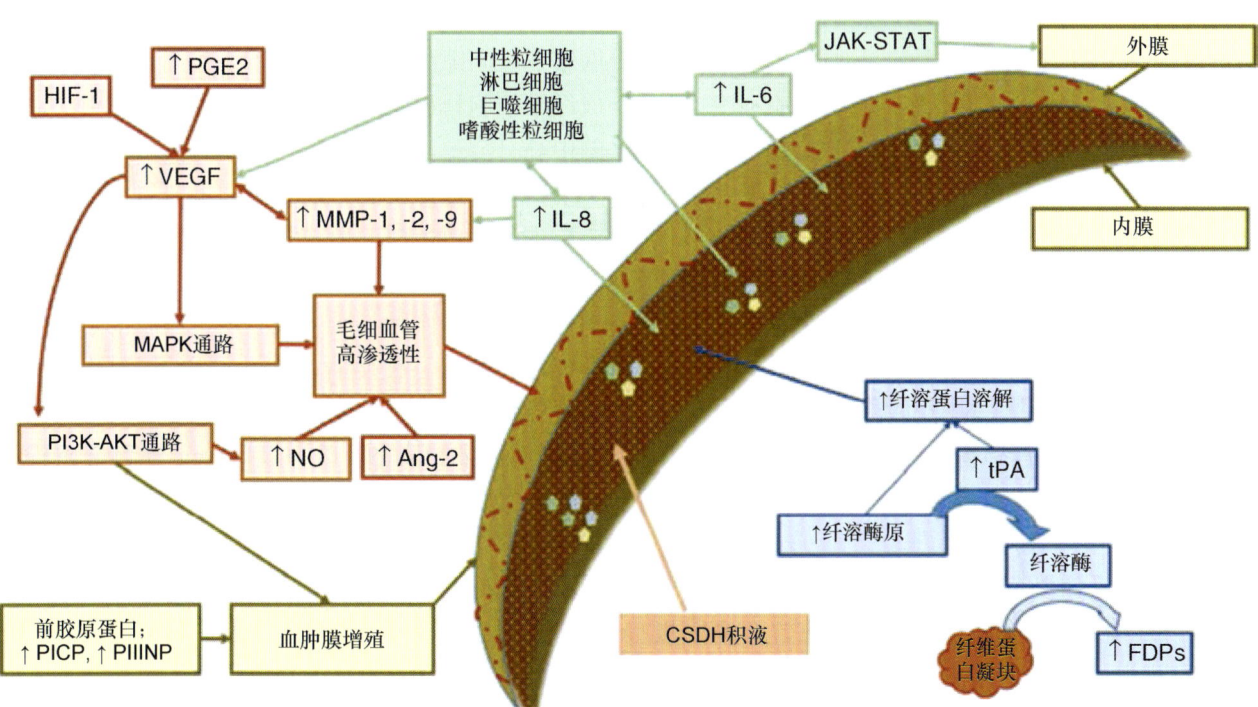

图 4.3 慢性硬膜下血肿的发病机制和炎症级联反应。Ang，血管生成素；FDPs，纤维蛋白/纤维蛋白原降解产物；HIF，缺氧诱导因子；IL，白细胞介素；JAK-STAT，Janus 激酶-信号传导与转录激活因子；MAPK，丝裂原活化蛋白激酶；MMP，基质金属蛋白酶；NO，一氧化氮；PGE，前列腺素 E；PI3K-AKT，磷脂酰肌醇 3-激酶-丝氨酸/苏氨酸激酶；PICP，前胶原蛋白Ⅰ型；PIIINP，前胶原蛋白Ⅲ型；tPA，组织型纤溶酶原激活剂；VEGF，血管内皮生长因子。版权引自 Edlmann et al. 2017[5] http://creativecommons.org/licenses/by/4.0/

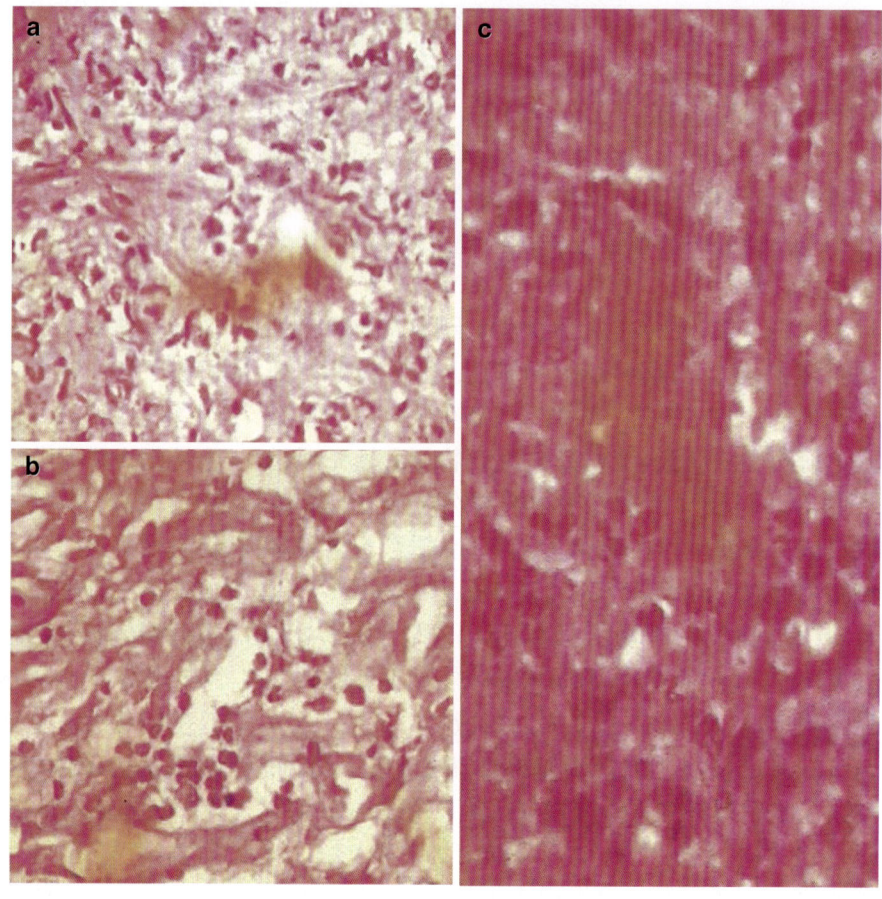

图 4.4 慢性硬膜下血肿外层膜的组织学分类。(a) Ⅱ型炎症膜由一层未成熟结缔组织组成，伴有明显的血管生成和细胞浸润。(b) Ⅲ型出血性炎症膜由多层组成，伴有大直径毛细血管和明显的细胞浸润，伴随着向膜内的血液渗出和新生血管。(c) Ⅳ型瘢痕性炎症膜中存在瘢痕组织和炎症细胞浸润。Copyright from Gandhoke et al. 2013[7] (Copyright reprint granted)

Ang-2 的过度表达导致 CSDH 膜中脆弱血管的形成，当与 VEGF 结合时，血管呈现高渗透性，在 CSDH 的发展过程中起重要作用。目前有研究关注 VEGF，旨在确定正常和异常 VEGF 功能之间的差异，以期减轻 CSDH 的进展。研究者发现脑膜中动脉供应了新生膜的微血管[16, 26, 36]。CSDH 同侧扩张的脑膜中动脉（MMA）是 CSDH 治疗的重要靶点。MMA 栓塞是一种旨在减少血液成分渗漏的技术。两项病例研究发现，MMA 栓塞后 CSDH 的复发率为 3.6%[16, 36]。对于可能存在其他潜在健康问题或正在服用抗栓药物的老年人来说，这种技术非常有意义。关于选择栓塞剂、麻醉类型和栓塞程序的明确指征，尚待确定。

当硬膜下血肿的发展成为慢性过程时，纤维蛋白形成和溶解循环出现，逐渐形成含有高密度隔膜的新生内膜[3, 7, 27]。新生内膜的内层包含四层：血肿层、中间层、蛛网膜表面和最终层。随着 CSDH 的发展，血管结构减少，而纤维组织数量增加。新生内膜中含有多种介质，包括细胞因子、IL-6 和高水平表达的趋化因子。炎症反应释放的细胞因子可以用作血肿发展的标志物。IL-6 在扩大蛛网膜下腔间隙的过程中发挥重要作用。内膜内的肌成纤维细胞释放趋化因子，会将炎症细胞引向血肿的中心[5, 11]。

CSDH 富含血液、脑脊液和蛋白质。富含的蛋白质主要以白蛋白的形式存在，相对于蛛网膜下腔的脑脊液更具高渗性。正如 Zollinger 等在 1934 年描述的那样，血肿基质中较高的蛋白质水平会导致形成渗透梯度，使脑脊液渗入硬膜下腔[49]。由于新生外膜内存在毛细血管，我们有必要研究硬膜下血肿和血清之间的渗透梯度。Weir 等测量比较了硬膜下血肿液和血液之间的渗透压，然而他们没有发现两者之间存在渗透梯度[43-44]。学者们坚持认为，渗透梯度在不同区域之间会迅速均衡，因此很难检测到这一梯度。硬膜下血肿液较高的大分子物质含量增加了渗透负荷，将周围血管（尤其是渗漏的小毛细血管）内的液体抽吸到 CSDH 血肿腔内。Thomas 等指出，渗透梯度很可能既存在于 CSDH 的生成又存在于 CSDH 的吸收过程中。尽管人们没有发现 CSDH 和血管内存在渗透压差异，但如果新生膜的表面积大于硬膜下血肿的表面积，新生膜上的毛细血管很可能会在 CSDH 吸收中起到关键作用。与血肿体积相比，新生膜表面积越大，血肿吸收的机会越大[38]。

硬膜下积液是一种在成人和儿童中都能见到的疾病。对于颅骨、脑实质比例过大的群体，他们可能存在过大的硬膜下间隙，尤其是在脑积水时，硬膜下间隙可以积聚脑脊液[30-31]。此外，对于一些巨颅症患儿和脑萎缩的老年人这些颅骨、脑实质比例失调的人群来说，静水压在蛛网膜下腔、硬膜下腔和新生血肿膜之间的液体流向中起着关键作用[31]。因此，在 CSDH 的病理生理学中必须考虑渗透压和静水压。此外，Nakaguchi 指出，在蛛网膜破裂的情况下，脑脊液可以积聚在硬膜下腔隙中[8]。当存在硬膜下积液时，CSDH 发生的可能性增加，因为硬膜下积液的病理生理过程可能存在新生膜的形成和微出血[18-20]。

4.5 复发

CSDH 的复发可能性很高，治疗医生应对此予以考虑。导致复发的一些与患者相关的因素包括年龄较大、慢性酒精中毒、脑萎缩、脑积水和糖尿病。其他因素包括血肿密度、血肿存在时间、双侧 CSDH 的存在、手术后残留血肿的程度，甚至是手术腔内存在硬膜下积气[15, 17, 25, 34, 39, 45, 47]。相悖于常规观点，CSDH 手术引流后重新使用抗凝药物与高复发率无关[9, 21, 46]。Jeong 及其团队证明了高密度或混合密度 CSDH 与高复发率之间的相关性[15]。

人们对硬膜下新生膜及其与 CSDH 复发的关系非常关注。正如前面提到的，新生膜的营养主要由新生的毛细血管供应。中国的 Xin Liu 及其团队证明了在开颅时切除较厚的内层新生膜可以降低 CSDH 的复发率。他们发现开颅时存在较厚的内层新生膜与 CSDH 复发率之间存在显著关联[22]，他们还论证了存在的较厚内层新生膜与 CT 上血肿呈现混合密度之间显著关联。其他研究表明，随着血肿膜厚度的增加以及对脑皮质施加的张力增加，无症状患者或潜伏期患者出现症状的可能性增加[39]。

许多研究表明，在手术引流过程中给予地塞米松可以降低 CSDH 的复发率。地塞米松是一种合成的类固醇激素，其功能是减少 CSDH 导致的炎症反应。地塞米松可以减少血凝块的形成，并阻止炎症反应，从而停止新生膜的发展[17]。类固醇激素抑制与 CSDH 发展有关的细胞因子和趋化因子等炎症蛋白的表达。研究人员仍在分析类固醇在老年人群中的副作用。最近由 Hutchinson 和 Dex-CSDH 试验研究人员发表的研究发现，在治疗慢性硬膜下血肿方面，地塞米松利大于弊[13]。

4.6 结论

CSDH 是一种相当常见且需要及时治疗的神经外科疾病，对该疾病复杂的病理生理机制的理解为改善治疗策略、降低复发率铺平了道路。本章概述了血肿形成的起始，即硬脑膜边界细胞的破坏、血凝块的积聚，导致了一系列级联事件的发生，其中炎症反应促成了新生膜的形成。此外，本章还介绍了外层膜和内层膜形成的机制和时间线，以及 VEGF 和血管生成素在新生膜的血管生成和血肿渗透性中的重要作用。本章还讨论了 CSDH 的复发机制和预测复发的因素，以及一些新型治疗方法（如 MMA 栓塞）背后的理论基础。随着我们对该疾病形成机制的理解加深，潜在的药物和外科干预措施也将逐步进入临床。

参考文献

1. Baechli H, Nordmann A, Bucher HC, Gratzl O. Demographics and prevalent risk factors of chronic subdural haematoma: results of a large single-center cohort study. Neurosurg Rev. 2004;27(4):263–6.
2. Balser D, Farooq S, Mehmood T, Reyes M, Samadani U. Actual and projected incidence rates for chronic subdural hematomas in United States Veterans Administration and civilian populations. J Neurosurg. 2015;123(5):1209–15.
3. Bokka S, Trivedi A. Histopathological study of the outer membrane of the dura mater in

chronic sub dural hematoma: its clinical and radiological correlation. Asian J Neurosurg. 2016;11(1):34–8.
4. Ducruet AF, Grobelny BT, Zacharia BE, Hickman ZL, DeRosa PL, Andersen KN, et al. The surgical management of chronic subdural hematoma. Neurosurg Rev. 2012;35(2):155–69.
5. Edlmann E, Giorgi-Coll S, Whitfield PC, Carpenter KLH, Hutchinson PJ. Pathophysiology of chronic subdural haematoma: inflammation, angiogenesis and implications for pharmacotherapy. J Neuroinflammation. 2017;14(1):108.
6. Feghali J, Yang W, Huang J. Updates in chronic subdural hematoma: epidemiology, etiology, pathogenesis, treatment, and outcome. World Neurosurg. 2020;141:339–45.
7. Gandhoke GS, Kaif M, Choi L, Williamson RW, Nakaji P. Histopathological features of the outer membrane of chronic subdural hematoma and correlation with clinical and radiological features. J Clin Neurosci. 2013;20(10):1398–401.
8. Gitlin D. Pathogenesis of subdural collections of fluid. Pediatrics. 1955;16(3):345–52.
9. Glover D, Labadie EL. Physiopathogenesis of subdural hematomas. Part 2: inhibition of growth of experimental hematomas with dexamethasone. J Neurosurg. 1976;45(4):393–7.
10. Haines DE, Harkey HL, al-Mefty O. The "subdural" space: a new look at an outdated concept. Neurosurgery. 1993;32(1):111–20.
11. Heula AL, Ohlmeier S, Sajanti J, Majamaa K. Characterization of chronic subdural hematoma fluid proteome. Neurosurgery. 2013;73(2):317–31.
12. Holl DC, Volovici V, Dirven CMF, Peul WC, van Kooten F, Jellema K, et al. Pathophysiology and nonsurgical treatment of chronic subdural hematoma: from past to present to future. World Neurosurg. 2018;116:402–11.e2.
13. Hutchinson PJ, Edlmann E, Bulters D, Zolnourian A, Holton P, Suttner N, et al. Trial of dexamethasone for chronic subdural hematoma. N Engl J Med. 2020;383(27):2616–27.
14. Inglis K. Subdural haemorrhage, cysts and false membranes; illustrating the influence of intrinsic factors in disease when development of the body is normal. Brain. 1946;69(3):157–94.
15. Jeong SI, Kim SO, Won YS, Kwon YJ, Choi CS. Clinical analysis of risk factors for recurrence in patients with chronic subdural hematoma undergoing Burr hole trephination. Korean J Neurotrauma. 2014;10(1):15–21.
16. Jumah F, Osama M, Islim AI, Jumah A, Patra DP, Kosty J, et al. Efficacy and safety of middle meningeal artery embolization in the management of refractory or chronic subdural hematomas: a systematic review and meta-analysis. Acta Neurochir. 2020;162(3):499–507.
17. Kamenova M, Lutz K, Schaedelin S, Fandino J, Mariani L, Soleman J. Does early resumption of low-dose aspirin after evacuation of chronic subdural hematoma with Burr-hole drainage lead to higher recurrence rates? Neurosurgery. 2016;79(5):715–21.
18. Knox B, Rorke-Adams L, Luyet F. Subdural hematoma rebleeding in relation to abusive head trauma. J Fam Violence. 2016;31(7):815–21.
19. Lee K-S. History of chronic subdural hematoma. Korean J Neurotrauma. 2015;11(2):27–34.
20. Lee KS, Bae WK, Park YT, Yun IG. The pathogenesis and fate of traumatic subdural hygroma. Br J Neurosurg. 1994;8(5):551–8.
21. Liu LX, Cao XD, Ren YM, Zhou LX, Yang CH. Risk factors for recurrence of chronic subdural hematoma: a single center experience. World Neurosurg. 2019;132:e506–e13.
22. Lutz K, Kamenova M, Schaedelin S, Guzman R, Mariani L, Fandino J, et al. Time to and possible risk factors for recurrence after Burr-hole drainage of chronic subdural hematoma: a subanalysis of the cSDH-drain randomized controlled trial. World Neurosurg. 2019;132:e283–e9.
23. Mori K, Maeda M. Surgical treatment of chronic subdural hematoma in 500 consecutive cases: clinical characteristics, surgical outcome, complications, and recurrence rate. Neurol Med Chir. 2001;41(8):371–81.
24. Munro D, Merritt HH. Surgical pathology of subdural hematoma: based on a study of one hundred and five cases. Arch Neurol Psychiatr. 1936;35(1):64–78.
25. Nagatani K, Wada K, Takeuchi S, Nawashiro H. Corticosteroid suppression of vascular endothelial growth factor and recurrence of chronic subdural hematoma. Neurosurgery. 2012;70(5):E1334; author reply E1334–6.
26. Nakagawa I, Park HS, Kotsugi M, Wada T, Takeshima Y, Matsuda R, et al. Enhanced hematoma membrane on DynaCT images during middle meningeal artery embolization for persistently recurrent chronic subdural hematoma. World Neurosurg. 2019;126:e473–e9.
27. Nakaguchi H, Tanishima T, Yoshimasu N. Factors in the natural history of chronic subdural hematomas that influence their postoperative recurrence. J Neurosurg. 2001;95(2):256–62.

28. Park H-R, Lee K-S, Shim J-J, Yoon S-M, Bae H-G, Doh J-W. Multiple densities of the chronic subdural hematoma in CT scans. J Korean Neurosurg Soc. 2013;54(1):38–41.
29. Park MH, Kim CH, Cho TG, Park JK, Moon JG, Lee HK. Clinical features according to the histological types of the outer membrane of chronic subdural hematoma. Korean J Neurotrauma. 2015;11(2):70–4.
30. Piatt JH Jr. A pitfall in the diagnosis of child abuse: external hydrocephalus, subdural hematoma, and retinal hemorrhages. Neurosurg Focus. 1999;7(4):e4.
31. Pittman T. Significance of a subdural hematoma in a child with external hydrocephalus. Pediatr Neurosurg. 2003;39(2):57–9.
32. Putnam TJ, Cushing H. Chronic subdural hematoma: its pathology, its relation to pachymeningitis hemorrhagica and its surgical treatment. Arch Surg. 1925;11(3):329–93.
33. Schwartz AB. The etiology of pachymeningitis hemorrhagica interna in infants. Am J Dis Child. 1916;XI(1):23–32.
34. Schwarz F, Loos F, Dunisch P, Sakr Y, Safatli DA, Kalff R, et al. Risk factors for reoperation after initial burr hole trephination in chronic subdural hematomas. Clin Neurol Neurosurg. 2015;138:66–71.
35. Shono T, Inamura T, Morioka T, Matsumoto K, Suzuki SO, Ikezaki K, et al. Vascular endothelial growth factor in chronic subdural haematomas. J Clin Neurosci. 2001;8(5):411–5.
36. Srivatsan A, Mohanty A, Nascimento FA, Hafeez MU, Srinivasan VM, Thomas A, et al. Middle meningeal artery embolization for chronic subdural hematoma: meta-analysis and systematic review. World Neurosurg. 2019;122:613–9.
37. Suzuki K, Takano S, Nose T, Doi M, Ohashi N. Increased concentration of vascular endothelial growth factor (VEGF) in chronic subdural hematoma. J Trauma. 1999;46(3):532–3.
38. Thomas PAW, Marshman LAG, Rudd D, Moffat C, Mitchell PS. Growth and resorption of chronic subdural hematomas: Gardner, Weir, and the osmotic hypothesis revisited. World Neurosurg. 2019;132:e202–e7.
39. Tomita Y, Yamada SM, Yamada S, Matsuno A. Subdural tension on the brain in patients with chronic subdural hematoma is related to hemiparesis but not to headache or recurrence. World Neurosurg. 2018;119:e518–e26.
40. Vinchon M, Delestret I, DeFoort-Dhellemmes S, Desurmont M, Noulé N. Subdural hematoma in infants: can it occur spontaneously? Data from a prospective series and critical review of the literature. Childs Nerv Syst. 2010;26(9):1195–205.
41. Weigel R, Hohenstein A, Schilling L. Vascular endothelial growth factor concentration in chronic subdural hematoma fluid is related to computed tomography appearance and exudation rate. J Neurotrauma. 2014;31(7):670–3.
42. Weigel R, Krauss JK, Schmiedek P. Concepts of neurosurgical management of chronic subdural haematoma: historical perspectives. Br J Neurosurg. 2004;18(1):8–18.
43. Weir B. Oncotic pressure of subdural fluids. J Neurosurg. 1980;53(4):512–5.
44. Weir B. The osmolality of subdural hematoma fluid. J Neurosurg. 1971;34(4):528–33.
45. Xu FF, Chen JH, Leung GK, Hao SY, Xu L, Hou ZG, et al. Quantitative computer tomography analysis of post-operative subdural fluid volume predicts recurrence of chronic subdural haematoma. Brain Inj. 2014;28(8):1121–6.
46. Yamamoto H, Hirashima Y, Hamada H, Hayashi N, Origasa H, Endo S. Independent predictors of recurrence of chronic subdural hematoma: results of multivariate analysis performed using a logistic regression model. J Neurosurg. 2003;98(6):1217–21.
47. You W, Zhu Y, Wang Y, Liu W, Wang H, Wen L, et al. Prevalence of and risk factors for recurrence of chronic subdural hematoma. Acta Neurochir (Wien). 2018;160(5):893–9.
48. Zahl SM, Wester K, Gabaeff S. Examining perinatal subdural haematoma as an aetiology of extra-axial hygroma and chronic subdural haematoma. Acta Paediatr (Oslo, Norway: 1992). 2020;109(4):659–66.
49. Zollinger R, Gross RE. Traumatic subdural hematoma: an explanation of the late onset of pressure symptoms. J Am Med Assoc. 1934;103(4):245–9.

第 5 章　慢性硬膜下血肿的实验模型

Sinan Sağıroğlu，Mehmet Turgut 和 R. Shane Tubbs

译者：王李傲

5.1　引言

慢性硬膜下血肿（CSDH）是临床实践中最常见的神经外科疾病之一。由于患者较为高龄，且多存在合并症，手术治疗常常会导致各种并发症[14, 18]。CSDH 的理想治疗方法仍存在争议[14, 18]。尽管已经有许多关于动物模型建立的研究，但这些模型研究对发病机制的解释仍然不够完善[5]。在本章中，我们将回顾 CSDH 实验模型的发展和演变。

5.2　慢性硬膜下血肿的实验模型

对硬膜下血肿（SDH）的实验研究始于 1819 年，Serres 撕裂了上矢状窦的硬膜下间隙，并检查了紧邻硬脑膜的纤维囊[16]。1864 年，Laborde 在犬和猫的硬膜下间隙注入了血液，但他没有对形成的 CSDH 进行组织学检查[10]。之后，Sperling 和 Van Vleuten 分别在 1872 年和 1898 年的兔子实验中将血液注射到兔子的硬膜下间隙[17, 19]。尽管这两项研究在产生 SDH 的特征性膜方面取得了一定的成功，但组织学结果尚未得到很好的证明[12]。此外，有关慢性酒精中毒与 CSDH 关系的动物研究也多次被报道，并由 Saltykow 进行了总结[15]。但是，这些研究未能让模型产生典型的 CSDH 膜结构。

接下来的章节中，实验性 CSDH 模型被分为以下几类：（a）硬膜下注射血液模型，（b）硬膜下植入血凝块模型，（c）降低颅内压且硬膜下植入血液或血凝块模型，（d）皮下植入模型，（e）血管损伤模型，（f）脑萎缩模型。然后，我们将详细总结每个模型的构建过程。

5.2.1　硬膜下注射血液模型

下文详细介绍了六项硬膜下注射血液模型的实验研究摘要作为示例（表 5.1）[4, 6-7, 11-13]：

- **Putnam 和 Putnam 的研究**

  Putnam 和 Putnam 在犬和猫的硬膜下间隙注入自体血液，并在 5～50 天后处死动物。一些动物产生了一个薄的间皮膜，位于蛛网膜上方，但它们既没有形成液化的血肿腔，也没有显示出血肿体积增加[12]。此外，学者们注意到动物模型的组织学发现与创伤性 SDH 的病理发现相似[12]。

- **Gardner 的研究**

  Gardner 提出渗透作用是 SDH 扩大的机制。他将 5 只实验犬的自体血液注入其硬膜下间隙[6]。在另外 5 只实验犬中，他用弯曲的针将血液注入对侧[6]。他还植入了含有自体血液的半透性纤维素袋，测量了操作前和操作后 3～18 天袋子的重量[6]。他发现袋子的重量增加了 39%～103%，由此推断液化血液中的高蛋白含量产生了渗透压梯度，增加了血肿体积[6]。他还注意到间皮细胞覆盖的硬膜下区域缺乏淋巴引流[6]。在这项研究之后，渗透压假说得到了广泛的认可。

- **Christensen 的研究**

  Christensen 进行了 4 种类型的动物实验[4]。第一个实验中，他在 4 只实验犬的硬膜下间隙注入了含枸橼酸盐的血液，并在第 8～11 天将其处死[4]。他的结果与 Putnam 的研究结果相似[4]。在第二个实验中，他每周给 2 只实验犬的硬膜下间隙注射血液，连续进行 3 周，并在最后一次注射后 1 周将动物处死[4]。他发现硬膜下的血肿膜上有直径高达 50 μm 的毛细血管以及新形成的膜，其中包含巨噬细胞、残破的红细胞和成纤维细胞，与慢性硬膜下血肿中的血肿膜情况类似，但没有出现血凝块的液化[4]。在第三个实验中，他对 4 只实验犬使用了与第二个实验相同的流程，并在枕骨区域制造创伤[4]。结果与前述实验结果相同，但在枕骨区域

表 5.1 硬膜下注射血液动物实验模型

作者/引用	年份	研究物种/研究时间	研究方法	部位	结论
Putnam and Putnam[12]	1927	犬（$n=3$）和猫（$n=15$）/1 天至 3 个月	1～2 ml 自体全血，去纤维血，去纤维蛋白血注入硬膜下腔	距窦角纵、横相交处 1～2 cm 环钻开口	在外观上类似于 CSDH 的病变，但不能复制其病变过程
Gardner[6]	1932	犬（$n=5$），犬（$n=7$）和犬（$n=8$）	硬膜下注射，对侧硬膜下注射，硬膜下腔含有自体全血	在顶骨凸面处环钻开口或钻孔	如果不能复制 SDH 在犬的病程，对 CSDH 的研究将是困难的
Christensen[4]	1944	犬（$n=2$）、犬（$n=4$）、犬（$n=4$）、犬（$n=4$）/8 天至 2 个月	单次和多次硬膜下血液注射，有或无外伤，有或无矢状窦结扎	未说明，大多为双侧	CSDH 的发病原因是创伤；上矢状窦结扎有助于囊肿的形成
Goodell and Mealy[7]	1963	犬（$n=8$）/8～72 天 犬（$n=4$）/36 天	硬膜下注射血液，静脉尿素给药	顶叶凸面	硬膜下出血、脑容积减少、桥静脉撕裂等均不足以诱发 CSDH；渗透的作用尚不清楚
Ohshima[11]	1982	犬（$n=22$）/30 天	硬膜下自体全血，混合 CSF 的血液	颅顶凸起处硬膜下间隙开口和使用球囊扩张	SDH 的扩大需要 CSF 混合血液和低颅内压（甘露醇和脑脊液排液）
Quan 等[13]	2015	大鼠（$n=144$）	硬膜下自体全血注射	通过钻孔处重复硬膜下注射	血液循环中血浆炎症标志物水平与 CSDH 的生成和清除过程平行

CSDH，慢性硬膜下血肿；CSF，脑脊液；SDH，硬膜下血肿。

还出现了创伤性蛛网膜下腔出血[4]。在第四个实验中，他对 4 只实验犬部分结扎了上矢状窦，但在 5 天至 2 个月后未能产生任何慢性硬膜下血肿[4]。他结扎了上矢状窦，并同时在双侧硬膜下间隙注射血液[4]。在 11 天至 3 周后，出现了类似慢性硬膜下血肿的病变，其具有大的囊性腔和血管丰富的新生膜[4]。他在结论中认同了 Gardner 的渗透压假说[4]。

• **Goodell 和 Mealy 的研究**

Goodell 和 Mealy 在 2 个试验组中各进行了 4 个实验，包括硬膜下注射血液或血块、撕裂桥静脉、使用减小颅内容积的试剂、分流和注射抗炎药物[7]。本章稍后会提到该研究中的一些实验。在第一个实验中（A 组），8 只实验犬被注射新鲜血液，并静脉注射尿素以减少脑容积。注射的血液体积平均为 6.7 ml，动物在注射后的 8～72 天被处死，硬膜下积液未形成[7]。在第 4 个实验中（A 组），7 只实验犬被注射了混合血块、脑脊液、氢化可的松和链激酶，实验动物没有出现延迟症状，处理方案与之前的实验类似[7]。在 B 组中，冷冻和解冻的血液被注射到 4 只实验犬中，存活的 2 只实验犬分别在第 24 天和第 36 天被处死，显示血肿吸收和硬脑膜增厚[7]。Goodell 和 Mealy 尝试了多种方法来建立慢性硬膜下血肿模型，但始终未能复制病变的进展或血肿的液化[7]。他们得出的结论是，渗透机制导致血肿扩大是不成立的[7]。

• **Ohshima 的研究**

Ohshima 将 45 只实验犬分到 4 个试验组进行了实验，使用了类似 Watanabe 等的开窗和球囊技术，植入 3～4 ml 的血液或血块[11]。他还在一些实验犬身上使用了甘露醇和脑脊液引流以增加硬膜下间隙的体积，与 Goodell 和 Mealy 的实验类似，注射了 8～10 ml 的血液[11]。第一组包括 9 只实验犬，在硬膜下间隙接种自体新鲜血液[11]。第二组注射了血块（10 只实验犬），第三组给予了混合脑脊液的血液（13 只实验犬）[11]。在第四组中，接种了血、脑脊液混合物，并在接种第 7 天开始每天给予甘露醇 3 g/kg 和肝素 200 U/kg[11]。第一和第二组在第 3～4 天显示高密度血块，随访时在计算机断层成像（CT）图像中血肿体积和密度减小，组织学检查提示血肿吸收[11]。在第三组中，低密度和等密度病变显现，随访时 CT 图像中血肿减小，第 18 天 CT 扫描时，病变已经大部分消退。

在 2～3 周时处死动物进行组织学检查，显示血肿膜类似 CSDH 的新生血管膜和纤维层[11]。第四个实验组将在下一节中描述。

- **Quan 等的研究**

    Quan 等在 4 个组的 144 只大鼠中使用了钻孔反复注射血液造模，注射部位位于额顶区域[13]。每只大鼠最初注射 400 μl 的自体新鲜血液，然后在 72 h 后在同一区域注射额外的 300 μl[13]。通过体内磁共振成像（MRI）评估确认颅下间隙存在血液[13]。作者分别在第 3 天、第 10 天、第 17 天和第 24 天处死了 4 个组的动物。每组包括 12 只对照鼠，它们在没有血液输注的情况下进行了相同的程序处理[13]。所有病变都遵循典型的 SDH 分解模式，形成血管新生膜和炎症过程[13]。在第 24 天，所有血肿几乎完全消退[13]。外周血酶联免疫吸附试验（ELISA）检测显示，炎症因子如白细胞介素 -6（IL-6）、IL-8 和肿瘤坏死因子 -α 的水平在第 10 天达到峰值[13]。IL-10、IL-13 和其他抗炎因子在第 17 天和第 24 天增加，与 CSDH 的消退过程相平行[13]。

5.2.2 硬膜下植入血凝块模型

下面将介绍 4 个硬膜下植入血凝块模型的实验研究摘要（表 5.2）[3, 7, 11, 20]：

- **Goodell 和 Mealy 的研究**

    Goodell 和 Mealy 在第二组实验中使用了 21 只实验犬（组 A），他们向硬膜下间隙注射大量的血凝块。他们还使用了尿素、脑脊液引流和低温来减少脑容积，并向动物注射了至多 12.2 ml 的血凝块[7]。尽管最初实验犬表现出倦怠和不稳定，但临床症状有所改善，它们在第 15 小时到第 20 天之间被处死[7]。这一组记录了血肿的再机化和吸收的情况[7]。B 组中，8 只实验犬每周重复接种血液或植入血块，过程持续 12～35 天。实验者们再次使用了尿素、脑脊液引流和低温来减少脑容积[7]。在随访期间，有 3 只实验犬因不同原因死亡，尸检结果显示血肿大小"并不大"[7]。后来又有 5 只实验犬被处死，血肿的消退情况与第一次实验类似[7]。

- **Watanabe 等的研究**

    Watanabe 等研究了存在 CSF 时对血凝块形成

表 5.2 硬膜下植入血凝块动物实验模型

作者/引用	年份	研究物种/研究时间	研究方法	部位	结论
Goodell and Mealy[7]	1963	犬（n = 21）/20 天，犬（n = 8）/35 天（译者注：原文有误）	硬膜下植入血凝块和静脉尿素给药；硬膜下植入血凝块，多次尿素给药 6 天；多次硬膜下植入血凝块/注射尿素	顶叶凸面	硬膜下出血、脑容积减少、桥静脉撕裂等均不足以诱发 CSDH；渗透的作用尚不清楚
Watanabe 等[20]	1972	犬（n = 14）和猴（n = 5）/7～21 天	单次硬膜下植入体外形成的血凝块，有或无脑脊液（n = 2）	右额颞区环钻开孔和球囊扩张	CSF 存在时形成的血凝块具有不同的弹性纤维囊，这些囊的存在是血肿扩大所必需的。渗透作用对血肿扩大没有明显的效果
Apfelbaum 等[3]	1974	犬（n = 2）和猫（n = 40）/8～30 天	硬膜下植入不同类型的血凝块	额颞隆起处环钻开孔和球囊扩张	CSF 对扩大血肿体积没有作用，纤维蛋白和随后硬膜表面的形成以及再出血是血肿体积进展的关键因素
Ohshima[11]	1982	犬（n = 10）/30 天	硬膜下植入血凝块	颅顶凸起处硬膜下间隙开孔和球囊扩张	SDH 体积扩大需要 CSF 混合血液和低颅内压（甘露醇和 CSF 排液）

CSDH，慢性硬膜下血肿；CSF，脑脊液；SDH，硬膜下血肿。

的影响，并通过离体实验证明了血凝块的纤维膜渗透性良好，因此极不可能参与病变进展，否定了渗透性假说[20]。作者使用了 12 只实验犬和 5 只猴进行硬膜下血凝块接种，并将另外 50 只实验犬分为 6 组进行皮下血凝块接种[20]。血液与 CSF 混合在 37℃下孵育 24 h，形成了 1～5 ml 的血凝块，作者随后将血凝块接种到 12 只实验犬和 5 只猴的硬膜下间隙中[20]。3 只实验犬出现了进行性症状，9 只实验犬和 5 只猴未出现临床症状[20]。所有动物在 7～21 天内被处死。作者展示了 CSDH 的组织学水平发现，指出血肿囊膜内含有红褐色液体，血肿容积增加。囊膜附着于硬膜，显微镜下可见迂曲充血的血管[20]。另外 2 只接受没有混合 CSF 的全血凝块的实验犬，未表现出血肿发展的证据，但出现轻度的硬膜增厚，与先前的研究结果一致[20]。

- Apfelbaum 等的研究

Apfelbaum 按照 Watanabe 等的研究步骤进行重复实验[3]。他们使用了 2 只实验犬和 40 只猫[3]。他们为 4 组猫制备了 4 ml 血液样本，分别与 1 ml CSF、人工 CSF、生理盐水或未稀释的血液混合，并在 37℃下孵育 24 h[3]。与 Watanabe 等的研究一样，作者在颅骨隆起处进行了开孔和球囊扩张，并将离体血肿块植入硬膜下间隙[3]。他们还在 2 只猫的硬膜上做了一个大圆形切口，以研究硬膜的血管[3]。每组动物在第 8、10、13 和 21 天随机选取一只被处死。2 只接受 CSF/血液处理的猫在第 29 和 30 天被处死，1 只接受生理盐水/血液混合物的猫在第 27 天被处死[3]。2 只实验犬接受与猫相同的处理，并在第 13 天被处死[3]。所有病变都表现出典型的硬膜下血肿演变和消退模式。到了第 21 天，只能看到轻度的硬膜增厚，血肿基本上已经消退[3]。10 只猫被植入人类或牛纤维蛋白原与人类或人工 CSF、人血清、生理盐水或 5% 葡萄糖混合物的血凝块。每个样本在 37℃下经过凝血酶处理和离体凝固[3]。人类和人工 CSF 样本经过草酸盐处理以去除钙离子，生理盐水和葡萄糖溶液中添加了氯化钙[3]。2 只猫被植入明胶海绵，其中一只被注入去纤维蛋白血液[3]。这些动物也出现典型新生膜形成和消退模式[3]。4 只猫的血凝块和硬膜间使用聚乙烯隔开，其中有 3 只动物既没有形成新生膜，也没有出现血肿吸收[3]。由于技术操作问题，聚乙烯屏障在 1 只猫身上未能阻止血肿边缘与硬脑膜接触，因而产生了新生膜[3]。

Apfelbaum 批判了 Watanabe 等的研究，因为在他们的实验方案中只有脑脊液含有钙离子。只有存在钙离子的情况下，纤维蛋白原才能转化为双键连接的纤维蛋白[3]。他们未能获得相同的结果，并推断血肿硬膜侧新生膜的产生是由纤维蛋白介导的；此外，随着血肿老化，新生血管会渗出血液进入腔内，这支持了 Putnam 和 Putnam 的研究结果[3]。Apfelbaum 等还指出，由于病变的表面积/体积比增加不成比例，当血肿体积过大时，吸收机制不能有效促成血肿的吸收[3]。作者假设在动物中复制人类慢性硬膜下血肿是困难的，因为动物在 Monro 孔上下具有较大的颅内压差异[3]，且人类的直立姿势对于区域压力差异也是有影响的[3]。

- Ohshima 的研究

Ohshima 在第二组也进行了血凝块植入实验，内容如前文所述[11]。

5.2.3 降低颅内压且硬膜下植入血液或血凝块模型

下面介绍硬膜下植入血液或血凝块并同时降低颅内压的模型案例（表 5.3）[7, 11]：

- Goodell 和 Mealy 的研究

在针对 15 只实验犬的第三部分实验中，Goodell 和 Mealy 进行了脑室胸膜聚乙烯分流术，并同时进行了硬膜下血液凝块植入（组 A）[7]。其中有 9 只实验犬产生了 SDH。这 9 只实验犬中的 4 只还参与了第二部分实验的组 B，接受了重复注射。在其中的 5 只实验犬身上还使用了尿素和低温作为附加变量[7]。在这项研究中，所有植入的导管在实验动物被处死时都部分阻塞或移位，因此颅内压降低效果不确切[7]。组 B 包括 2 只实验犬，它们接受了硬膜下血凝块注射和重复静脉尿素给药，2 个血肿均以预期的方式消退[7]。

- Ohshisima 的研究

在该研究的第四组中，作者给予了 13 只实验犬 d-甘露醇和肝素。其中 13 只实验犬中有 10 只

表 5.3　硬膜下植入血液或血凝块并降低颅内压动物实验模型

作者/引用	年份	研究物种/研究时间	研究方法	部位	结论
Goodell and Mealy[7]	1963	犬（$n=15$）	硬膜下重复注射血液或植入血凝块，行脑池胸膜分流术，并静脉注射尿素，或降低体温	顶叶凸面	硬膜下出血、脑容积减少、桥静脉撕裂等均不足以诱发 CSDH；渗透的作用尚不清楚
Ohshima[11]	1982	犬（$n=13$）/30 天	自体硬膜下注射全血混合 CSF，静脉甘露醇、肝素给药	颅顶凸起处硬膜下间隙开孔和球囊扩张	SDH 体积扩大需要 CSF 混合血液和低颅内压（甘露醇和 CSF 排液）

缩写：CSDH 慢性硬膜下血肿、CSF 脑脊液、SDH 硬膜下血肿。

没有出现症状，血肿自行消退[11]。2 只实验犬的病变扩大，并在 CT 扫描中显示血肿进展。尸检时发现了出血性外层新生膜[11]。在 1 只实验犬中，硬膜下肿块扩大，CT 上呈现低密度血肿，类似于人类的 CSDH[11]。作者得出结论，脑脊液与血液的混合是一个重要过程，与低颅内压和机械因素起到协同作用[11]。

5.2.4　皮下植入模型

下面介绍三项皮下植入模型的案例（表 5.4）[3, 9, 20]：

- **Watanabe 等的研究**

  Watanabe 等将血凝块皮下注射到 50 只实验犬中，分为以下 5 组：存在脑脊液时形成的血凝块；正常血凝块；存在脑脊液时形成的并经过纤溶酶处理的血凝块；无脑脊液时形成的纤维蛋白凝块；存在脑脊液时形成的纤维蛋白凝块[20]。作者得出结论，存在脑脊液时形成的血肿纤维膜比那些没有脑脊液参与形成的纤维膜更加细腻，并具有不同的特性。他们认为渗入包膜形成的新生毛细血管窦道可能是血肿扩张的原因[20]。

- **Apfelbaum 等的研究**

  Apfelbaum 等也重复了对前述不同类型的血凝块的皮下植入的实验。少数动物的血肿略微增大，最多达到原始大小的 2 倍；这种效应与任何类型的血凝块无关[3]。

- **Labadie 和 Glover 的研究**

  Labadie 和 Glover 在 154 只大鼠中进行了 5 个实验。他们将不同组合的血液制品和化学物质注射或外科植入到背部皮下组织中[9]。使用了无血小板的人类血浆、低温溶血的自体抗凝鼠全血或 4℃的全血、人类脑脊液和卡拉胶（Chonduru crispus 的提取物）的不同组合[9]。此外，他们还进行了体外对照，使用 12 ml 无血小板、富血小板、溶血和全血对照制备并在 37℃孵育 100 h。所有血液和血浆凝块均由人类凝血酶诱导[9]。所有动物在植入血凝块后的第 9 天被处死。在第一个实验中，作者研究了脑脊液对外科植入血凝块的影响[9]。他们在体外通过人凝血酶诱导形成血块，之后迅速植入 52 只大鼠的背部皮下。其中，32 只大鼠接种了 2 ml 无血小板血浆和 1.5 ml 事先通过 0.22 μm 滤器过滤的人类脑脊液，20 只大鼠只接种凝固的血浆。植入后比较显示，有无脑脊液的存在没有产生差异[9]。在第二个实验中，他们比较了外科切口和针头注射的效果。30 只大鼠在 12 ml 无血小板血浆和 2 ml 人类凝血酶溶液混合后立即注射，之后形成原位凝块。21 只大鼠进行了体内植入凝块的手术[9]。在尸检时，手术植入的凝块几乎总会被发现，其中 43% 的凝块扩大并液化。组织学呈现出新生膜、纤维蛋白凝块和新生毛细血管。相比之下，原位注射的血凝块几乎总是被重吸收[9]。在第三个实验中，测试了一种无菌的促炎剂卡拉胶的效果。作者假设炎症刺激有助于新生膜形成和病变生长[9]。作者给 13 只大鼠注射了卡拉胶溶液，其中 9 只立即在同一部位注射了 8 ml 人类血浆凝血酶混合物，4 只注射了 12 ml，均形成原位凝块。在尸检时，这些病变具有与手术植入相似的膜，其中成纤维细胞的反应最为显著。一些组织显示出中心性出血[9]。在第四个实验中，作者注射了不同量的冷冻、解冻和原位凝固的自体血液，以比较病变初始体积产生的影响。他们还分别向 8 只、

表 5.4　皮下植入血凝块动物实验模型

作者 / 引用	年份	研究物种 / 研究时间	研究方法	部位	结论
Watanabe 等[20]	1972	犬（$n=50$）/ 7～21 天	将不同条件下形成的血凝块植入皮下	腹部皮下接种	CSF 存在时形成的血凝块具有不同的弹性纤维囊，这些囊的存在是血肿扩大所必需的。渗透作用对血肿扩大没有明显的效果
Apfelbaum 等[3]	1974	犬（$n=2$）和猫（$n=40$）/ 8～30 天	硬膜下植入不同类型的血凝块	皮下腹部包含 4 个开口切口	CSF 对扩大血肿体积没有作用，纤维蛋白和随后血肿膜的形成以及再出血是血肿体积进展的关键因素
Labadie 和 Glover[9]	1976	大鼠（$n=154$）/ 9 天	注射或手术植入血块、血液、血浆、不同组合的卡拉胶	背部皮下注射或手术植入	植入血凝块的初始体积是影响病变吸收或扩大的主要因素。CSF 无明显作用

CSF，脑脊液。

15 只和 11 只大鼠注射了 8 ml、12 ml 和 15 ml 的溶血血液和凝血酶混合物，并注入 1 ml 空气。注射 12 ml 和 15 ml 的大鼠出现扩大的血肿，并带有液化物[9]。在第五个实验中，向大鼠注射了相对较大量的自体血液。有 4 只大鼠注射了 16 ml 的血液和凝血酶溶液，大鼠形成原位凝块。这些结果与第四个实验相似[9]。

通过这些实验，Labadie 和 Glover 提出血肿大小在第三天有所减小，但之后逐渐增大的结论[9]。"初始大小越大，后续扩大的可能性就越大"[9]。他们没有发现脑脊液与病变大小之间的关系。然而，他们指出实验性凝块的解剖位置可能是病变大小不同的原因[9]。在所有样本中，血肿液中的白蛋白 / 球蛋白比值增加，但所有标本的渗透压保持在 289～295 mOsm/kg[9]。

5.2.5　血管损伤模型

以下讨论血管损伤模型的实验案例，详细内容见表 5.5[7]：

- **Goodell 和 Mealy 的研究**

在第一个实验 B 组中，Goodell 和 Mealy 缝合了 7 只实验犬的桥静脉，并在手术后第三天撕裂了该静脉[7]。在静脉撕裂之前，对 2 只实验犬进行了静脉内尿素和肝素的注射[7]。2 只接受肝素治疗的实验犬在静脉撕裂后急性死亡[7]。幸存的实验犬在第 11 至 72 天被处死。尽管有机化和血肿吸收的证据，但没有出现慢性硬膜下积血[7]。

5.2.6　脑萎缩模型

以下是两项有关慢性硬膜下血肿脑萎缩模型的研究案例，详细内容见表 5.6[1, 8]：

- **Aikawa 和 Suzuki 的研究**

Aikawa 和 Suzuki 使用了 48 只哺乳的小鼠，其中 38 只注射了 6-氨基烟酰胺（6-AN），10 只作为对照组[1]。在出生后第 5 天，将 6-AN 以每千克体重 25 mg 的剂量腹腔注射。对照组接受相同的处理，

表 5.5　血管损伤动物实验模型

作者 / 引用	年份	研究物种 / 研究时间	研究方法	部位	结论
Goodell and Mealy[7]	1963	犬（$n=7$）/ 11～72 天	提前对撕裂桥静脉的实验组静脉注射尿素（2 例在给予肝素治疗后的 72 h 后死亡）	顶叶凸面	硬膜下出血、脑容积减少、桥静脉撕裂等均不足以诱发 CSDH；渗透的作用尚不清楚

CSDH，慢性硬膜下血肿。

表 5.6 脑萎缩动物实验模型

作者/引用	年份	研究物种/研究时间	研究方法	部位	结论
Aikawa and Suzuki[1]	1987	小鼠（$n=48$）/30 天	无注射	腹腔注射 6-AN 引起脑积水，后演变成为 SDH	因为侧脑室突然减压，颅内压剧烈变化导致桥静脉撕裂
Kaneko 等[8]	1993	犬（$n=10$）/7 周	硬膜下注射自体全血	脑池注射 6-OHDA 后出现脑萎缩，后钻孔注射血液	血肿的产生、新血肿膜的形成和脑萎缩是 CSDH 发生的关键因素

6-AN，6-氨基烟酰胺；6-OHDA，6-羟基多巴胺；CSDH，慢性硬膜下血肿；SDH，硬膜下血肿。

但使用生理盐水代替[1]。作者之前的研究表明，6-AN 对小鼠具有神经毒性，并导致脑积水[2]。第 9 天，38 只小鼠中有 37 只发生了脑积水[1]。其中 11 只小鼠在注射后的第 20～23 天被处死，8 只在第 25～26 天被处死，4 只在第 29～30 天被处死。作者分别将这些治疗组归类为早期、中期和晚期[1]。在组织学和显微镜检查中，早期组的大脑皮质上有一层薄膜覆盖于硬膜下血肿外，此阶段未见炎症变化[1]。在中期组中，有一块附着在硬脑膜上的棕色血块，伴有宽阔的硬膜下腔和新生膜形成[1]。在晚期组中，发现一个充分机化的球形血肿，内含非机化的棕色血块。较厚的外膜中有新鲜的出血，并伴有许多血管[1]。作者认为，在这个模型中，CSDH 的发生机制是由神经毒素引起的枕叶皮质穿孔，随后导致侧脑室的急剧减压引起桥静脉撕裂[1]。血肿的增长归因于外膜的反复机化和出血[1]。

- **Kaneko 等的研究**

Kaneko 等也探索了利用脑萎缩模型构建 CSDH 模型。他们从 10 只实验犬的枕大池中排出 10～15 ml 的脑脊液，并将 1 mg/kg 的 6-羟基多巴胺（6-OHDA）溶于含有 0.01% 抗坏血酸的人工脑脊液中注射入枕大池[8]。经过 3～4 周后，确认脑室明显扩大[8]。他们还在麻醉状态下对 5 只实验犬进行实验，采用了微球法测量局部脑血流量（rCBF），灰质和白质的 rCBF 分别比对照组低 49% 和 47%。

此外，白质和灰质的水含量也降低。因此，脑室扩大是由脑萎缩引起的[8]。在 6-OHDA 给药后第 3 周，通过顶骨隆起钻孔注射 2～3 ml 的自体血液，随后对实验犬进行随访，观察症状和进行 CT 检查。在注射血液后的 2～4 周，4 只实验犬逐渐出现血肿并不断增大[8]。2 只实验犬临床情况恶化，CT 结果显示血肿扩大分别出现在第 7～30 天和第 14～28 天。将这两只动物处死，作者观察到有囊血肿和血肿外部纤维、窦道丛生的新生膜[8]。作者把血肿产生称为 α 因子，新生膜形成称为 β 因子，CSDH 形成的重要条件之一脑容积减少是 γ 因子[8]。

5.3 结论

尽管 CSDH 是临床实践中最常见的神经外科疾病之一，但其理想的治疗方式仍存在争议。构建 CSDH 的动物模型非常困难且具有挑战性。

许多学者尝试创建可验证 CSDH 的模型，但目前的文献中尚没有记载任何可重复、建模效果良好的 CSDH 动物模型[5]。自 19 世纪初到现在的研究表明，在特定条件下，SDH 会演变为慢性血肿形式。尽管每项实验都因技术的进步而使科学家更接近真相，但该疾病的病理生理学还有许多未解之谜，需要研究者们进一步研究该疾病的形态学和炎症进展过程。

参考文献

1. Aikawa H, Suzuki K. Experimental chronic subdural hematoma in mice. Gross morphology and light microscopic observations. J Neurosurg. 1987;67:710–6.
2. Aikawa H, Suzuki K, Ito N, Iwasaki Y, Nonaka I. 6-Aminonicotinamide-induced hydrocephalus in suckling mice. J Neuropathol Exp Neurol. 1984;43:511–21.

3. Apfelbaum RI, Guthkelch AN, Shulman K. Experimental production of subdural hematomas. J Neurosurg. 1874;40:336–46.
4. Christensen E. Studies on chronic subdural hematoma. Acta Psychiatr Neurol. 1944;19:69–148.
5. D'Abbondanza JA, Loch Macdonald R. Experimental models of chronic subdural hematoma. Neurol Res. 2014;36:176–88.
6. Gardner WJ. Traumatic subdural hematoma with particular reference to the latent interval. Arch Neurol Psychiatr. 1932;27:847–58.
7. Goodell CL, Mealey J Jr. Pathogenesis of chronic subdural hematoma. Experimental studies. Arch Neurol. 1963;8:429–37.
8. Kaneko F, Ohbayashi M, Ohshima T, Matsumoto K. An experimental chronic subdural hematoma in dogs-with a brain atrophy model. In: Nakamura N, Hashimoto T, Yasue M, editors. Recent advances in neurotraumatology. Tokyo: Springer; 1993. p. 45–8.
9. Labadie EL, Glover D. Physiopathogenesis of subdural hematomas. Part 1: histological and biochemical comparisons of subcutaneous hematoma in rats with subdural hematoma in man. J Neurosurg. 1976;45:382–92.
10. Laborde J. Contribution a l'etude des conditions pathogeniques des kystes sanguines de l'arachnoide; recherches experimentales sur les animaux. Cr Soc Biol Paris. 1864;1:70.
11. Ohshima T. Experimental study on the evolution of chronic subdural hematoma. Neurol Med Chir (Tokyo). 1982;22:696–706.
12. Putnam TJ, Putnam IK. The experimental study of pachymeningitis hemorrhagica. J Nerv Ment Dis. 1927;65:260–2.
13. Quan W, Zhang Z, Tian Q, Wen X, Yu P, Wang D, Cui W, Zhou L, Park E, Baker AJ, Zhang J, Jiang R. A rat model of chronic subdural hematoma: insight into mechanisms of revascularization and inflammation. Brain Res. 2015;1625:84–96.
14. Rovlias A, Theodoropoulos S, Papoutsakis D. Chronic subdural hematoma: surgical management and outcome in 986 cases: a classification and regression tree approach. Surg Neurol Int. 2015;6:127.
15. Saltykow. Referat, alcoholismus chronicus. Centralbl. f. allg. Path. u. path. Anat. 1911;22:849.
16. Serres A. Nouvelle division des apoplexies. Annuaire Med Chir Hop. 1819;1:246.
17. Sperling H. Ueber pachymeningitis haemorrhagica interna. Inaug.-Diss., Univ. Konigsberg. 1872.
18. Turgut M, Akhaddar A, Turgut AT. Calcified or ossified chronic subdural hematoma: a systematic review of 114 cases reported during last century with a demonstrative case report. World Neurosurg. 2020;134:240–63.
19. Van Vleuten CF. Ueber pachymeningitis haemorrhagica interna traumatica. Inaug.-Diss., Univ. Bonn. 1898.
20. Watanabe S, Shimada H, Ishii S. Production of clinical form of chronic subdural hematoma in experimental animals. J Neurosurg. 1972;37:552–61.

第 6 章 颅腔形态对慢性硬膜下血肿好发部位的影响

Ali Akhaddar

译者：王李傲

6.1 引言

颅内慢性硬膜下血肿（CSDH）是神经外科临床中常见的疾病，其存在多种潜在病因。然而，CSDH的病理生理机制尚未被完全解释清楚[6, 25-26]。三个世纪以前，CSDH被认为是卒中的一种。一个世纪后，它被视为一种炎症。然后，在20世纪初，人们接受了其外伤起源的观点[9]。此后，出现了许多其他的假说，例如渗透压或渗液假说[11, 18]。一些研究者还发现，CSDH中凝血和纤溶系统都存在过度活化[15, 26]。此外，研究者们已经确定了与这种颅内血肿发生相关的多个危险因素。自2001年Lee KS等首次提及[17]，许多作者已经开始探讨"颅形"（对称或非对称）对CSDH好发位置的意义[2, 10, 16-17, 22]。

在本章中，我们将全面介绍颅腔形态对CSDH发病位置的可能作用。

6.2 评估颅腔对称性/非对称性的方法

Lee等对颅骨对称性的评估采用了一种简单的方法。他们将计算机断层成像（CT）和（或）磁共振成像（MRI）获取的轴位图像调整成为黑白对比色呈现，从顶枕区的一个单一点开始，画出三条线：一条通过中线，另外两条接触外部颅骨（外层骨板）的两侧，比较中线和每侧接触外部颅骨的线形成的两个角度，较小角度所在的一侧是颅骨扁平的一侧[10, 17, 19]。

在我们的个人经验中[2]，我们改进了Lee的测量方法。选择内层骨板（而不是外层骨板）以避免后部（枕骨突起）和前部（额骨突起）区域颅骨厚度的影响（图6.1）。如果颅腔凸度两侧角度的差异小于2°，则认为颅腔是对称的（图6.2），较小角

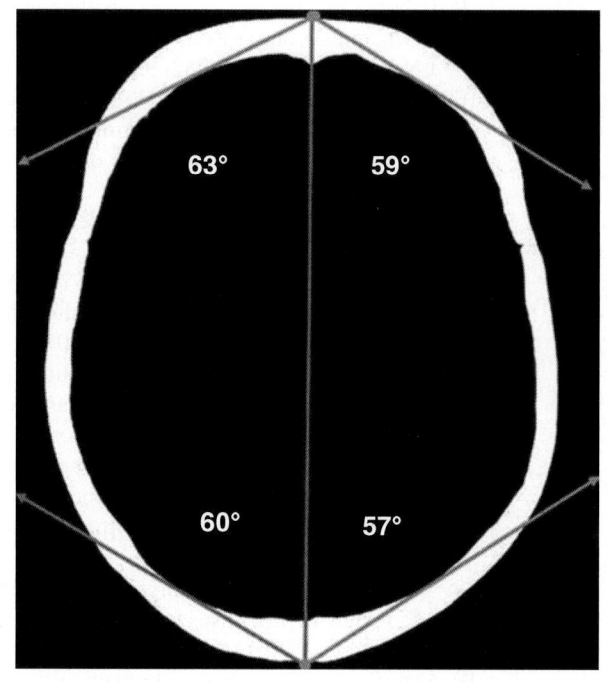

图6.1 从颅骨顶部的一个单一点开始，画出三条线：一条通过中线，另外两条接触颅骨两侧的内层骨板。较小角度所在的一侧是非对称颅骨中较平坦的额叶凸起。在枕骨突起的区域进行相同的测量（Reproduced from Akhaddar A et al. Acta Neurochir（Wien）（2009）151: 1235-40；with permission）

度所在的一侧是较平坦的额骨或枕骨（图6.3）。所有角度的测量都在CT轴位的相同水平上进行（成年人大约在眶-鼻外线上方平行的一个平面上）[2]。Khursheed的研究中，这个CT扫描平面是在眶-鼻外线上方7 cm处[16]。在Oh等的另一项研究中，颅骨对称性/非对称性的测量方法如下：在能清晰显示第三脑室的最佳轴向CT扫描图像上，将大脑镰从前到后设为中线，并计算每侧的最大半径[22]。

最近，Hsieh和同事们[10]使用了一种新的半自动化测量方法，该方法符合Zonenshayn在2004年提出的斜颅测量的概念[27]。CT图像被加载到LabVIEW软件系统（National Instruments，美国得

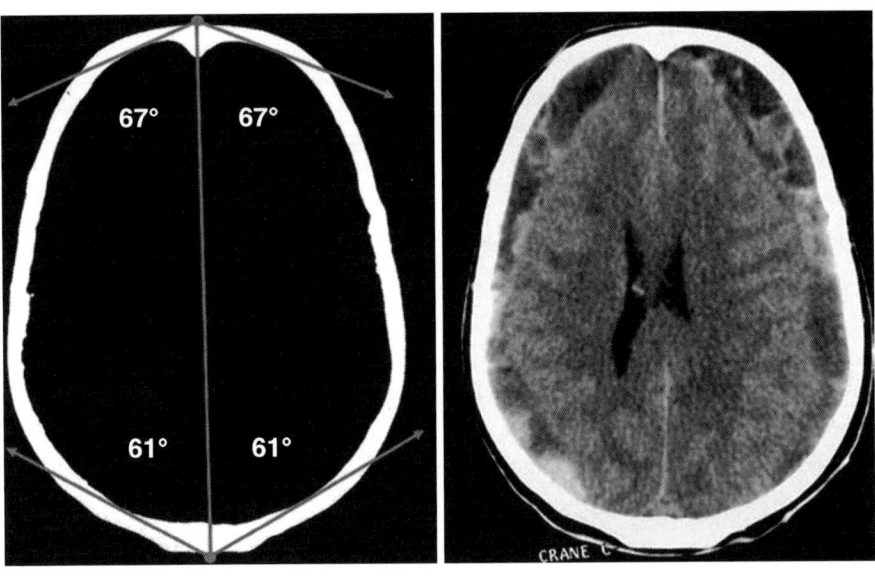

图 6.2 具有对称的前额和枕骨颅形的患者；慢性硬膜下血肿（CSDH）为双侧性（Reproduced from Akhaddar A et al. Acta Neurochir（Wien）(2009) 151：1235-40；with permission）

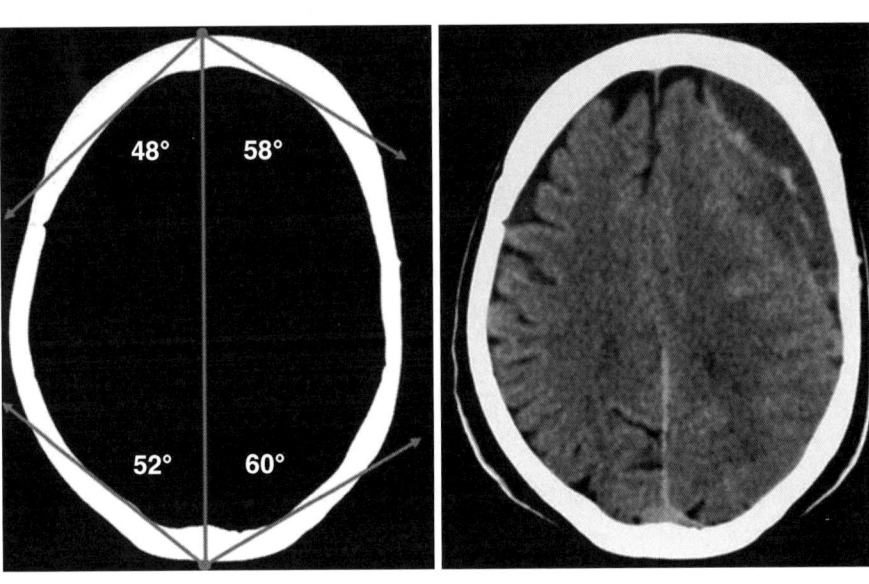

图 6.3 具有不对称前额和枕骨颅形的患者，慢性硬膜下血肿（CSDH）位于角度较大的一侧（左侧）（Reproduced from Akhaddar A et al. Acta Neurochir（Wien）(2009) 151：1235-40；with permission）

克萨斯州）中，他们人工标记鼻尖和枕尖连线并定义其为中线。随后他们进行自动化处理，包括去除颅骨、编码像素数以及确定每个颅骨区域。中线被视为轴，颅骨的一侧可以水平翻转到另一侧以建立重叠和非重叠区域。较大的非重叠区域的一侧被定义为优势的非重叠侧。颅骨对称指数比由 2 倍的重叠面积除以颅脑总面积来确定[10]。

6.3 单侧慢性硬膜下血肿

在一般人群中，颅骨凸起的形状并不总是左右两侧对称[13-14, 19, 23]。当颅骨不对称时，脑组织倾向于位于扁平的一侧。如果颅骨右侧扁平，脑组织将位于右侧，然后慢性硬膜下血肿有发展在左侧的倾向，因为左侧颅骨凸起更加突出（图 6.3）。这个假设至少在四项先前的研究中得到验证：其中三项在韩国进行，一项在摩洛哥进行[2, 16-17, 19]。

如果我们考虑慢性硬膜下血肿发展的经典病理生理学（请参阅第 4 章和第 5 章关于慢性硬膜下血肿的病理生理学和实验模型），上述四项研究的作者假设当内脑凸面更为显著/曲度更大时，脑膜-蛛网膜界面更容易分离[2, 16-17, 19]。此外，当有明显的硬膜下腔存在时，桥静脉也更容易破裂。脑实质的移动使得这些桥静脉在更为凸曲一侧更容易出血。

6.4 双侧慢性硬膜下血肿

正如前文所述，完全对称的颅骨凸起是不常见的。对"颅形"与 CSDH 之间关系感兴趣的学者假设，在对称的弯曲的颅骨凸起处，当发生直接或间接损伤时，分离力在两侧是相等的（图6.2）。事实上，和其他研究者一样，我们相信间接头部创伤似乎比直接损伤在颅骨慢性硬膜下血肿的形成中更为重要[1]。这种分离可能是引发硬脑膜边缘细胞层增生、随后形成新生膜的初始因素。此外，桥静脉更有可能双侧破裂，从而在左右两侧形成慢性硬膜下血肿的机会相等。根据Lee的观点，因为重力的作用，颅后窝必须考虑对称性，特别是当患者处于俯卧位时[18-19]。我们认为，Lee的观点同时涉及前（额）和后（枕）凸度，这个假设在后来得到了证实[2]。这些结果也在2015年由Khursheed等重复得到：对称的前额和枕骨凸起与双侧慢性硬膜下血肿相关[16]。

6.5 慢性硬膜下血肿发生的侧别倾向

在提及慢性硬膜下血肿（CSDH）的发生侧别倾向的几个系列文献回顾中，似乎左侧慢性硬膜下血肿比右侧更常见（表6.1）。MacFarlane及其团队试图解释左侧CSDH确诊率更高的原因[20]。

许多研究表明，右侧的卒中较为隐匿，因为非主导半球的右侧病变较少与沟通困难相关（在大多数右利手的群体中，语言和言语中心以及优势手功能主要位于左半球）[4-5, 7, 12, 24]。类似于缺血性卒中，非主导半球（最常见于右侧）上的其他脑病变可能会表现出更为微妙的神经症状和体征，因此可能会被漏诊或至少延迟诊断[3]。根据这一假

表6.1 文献中提及慢性硬膜下血肿好发侧别倾向的四个系列研究

作者［参考文献］	病例总数	左侧发病病例数（%）	右侧发病病例数（%）
Mori 等[21]	500	260（52.0%）	152（30.4%）
Gelabert-Gonzalez 等[8]	1000	471（47.1%）	432（43.2%）
Akhaddar 等[2]	110	47（42.7%）	32（29.1%）
MacFarlane 等[20]	258	123（47.6%）	92（35.6%）

设，MacFarlane等认为相比右侧，左侧CSDH更容易被识别和发现[20]。根据他们的理论，发生在右侧但未经诊断的CSDH可能会自行消散或吸收，或者患者在未经诊断的情况下可能会死亡。然而，同样的假设并不能解释其他一些系列研究中右侧CSDH的发生率[10, 17]。

6.6 结论

颅盖对称性/不对称性的概念试图解释CSDH的好发侧别或双侧性CSDH，这个相对较新的解剖参数可能有助于更好地了解CSDH的病因和发病机制。然而，需要神经放射科医生和神经外科医生进行进一步的前瞻性研究，纳入更多的患者人群，以确定颅骨形态对CSDH发生发展的作用。

除了需要考虑颅骨形状的种族差异外，还必须考虑颅骨的冠状重建和三维重建差异。

参考文献

1. Adhiyaman V, Asghar M, Ganeshram KN, Bhowmick BK. Chronic subdural haematoma in the elderly. Postgrad Med J. 2002;78:71–5. https://doi.org/10.1136/pmj.78.916.71.
2. Akhaddar A, Bensghir M, Abouqal R, Boucetta M. Influence of cranial morphology on the location of chronic subdural haematoma. Acta Neurochir (Wien). 2009;151:1235–40. https://doi.org/10.1007/s00701-009-0357-7.
3. Baumann C, Tichy J, Schaefer JH, Steinbach JP, Mittelbronn M, Wagner M, et al. Delay in diagnosing patients with right-sided glioblastoma induced by hemispheric-specific clinical presentation. J Neurooncol. 2020;146:63–9. https://doi.org/10.1007/s11060-019-03335-4.
4. Brott T, Tomsick T, Feinberg W, Johnson C, Biller J, Broderick J, et al. Baseline silent cerebral infarction in the Asymptomatic Carotid Atherosclerosis Study. Stroke. 1994;25:1122–9. https://doi.org/10.1161/01.str.25.6.1122.
5. Dimopoulos VG, Kapsalakis IZ, Fountas KN. Skull morphology and its neurosurgical implications in the Hippocratic era. Neurosurg Focus. 2007;23:E10. https://doi.org/10.3171/foc.2007.23.1.10.
6. Drapkin AJ. Chronic subdural hematoma: pathophysiological basis for treatment. Br J Neurosurg. 1991;5:467–73. https://doi.org/10.3109/02688699108998475.
7. Foerch C, Misselwitz B, Sitzer M, Berger K, Steinmetz H, Neumann-Haefelin T, Arbeitsgruppe

Schlaganfall Hessen. Difference in recognition of right and left hemispheric stroke. Lancet. 2005;366:392–3. https://doi.org/10.1016/S0140-6736(05)67024-9.
8. Gelabert-González M, Iglesias-Pais M, García-Allut A, Martínez-Rumbo R. Chronic subdural haematoma: surgical treatment and outcome in 1000 cases. Clin Neurol Neurosurg. 2005;107:223–9. https://doi.org/10.1016/j.clineuro.2004.09.015.
9. Haines DE, Harkey HL, al-Mefty O. The "subdural" space: a new look at an outdated concept. Neurosurgery. 1993;32:111–20. https://doi.org/10.1227/00006123-199301000-00017.
10. Hsieh CT, Huang CT, Chen YH, Sun JM. Association between cranial asymmetry severity and chronic subdural hematoma laterality. Neurosciences (Riyadh). 2020;25:205–9. https://doi.org/10.17712/nsj.2020.3.20190125.
11. Ito H, Yamamoto S, Saito K, Ikeda K, Hisada K. Quantitative estimation of hemorrhage in chronic subdural hematoma using the 51Cr erythrocyte labeling method. J Neurosurg. 1987;66:862–4. https://doi.org/10.3171/jns.1987.66.6.0862.
12. Ito H, Kano O, Ikeda K. Different variables between patients with left and right hemispheric ischemic stroke. J Stroke Cerebrovasc Dis. 2008;17:35–8. https://doi.org/10.1016/j.jstrokecerebrovasdis.2007.11.002.
13. Kanat A, Kayaci S, Yazar U, Kazdal H, Terzi Y. Chronic subdural hematoma in adults: why does it occur more often in males than females? Influence of patient's sexual gender on occurrence. J Neurosurg Sci. 2010;54:99–103.
14. Kanat A, Yazar U, Ozdemir B, Coskun ZO, Erdivanli O. Frontal sinus asymmetry: is it an effect of cranial asymmetry? X-ray analysis of 469 normal adult human frontal sinus. J Neurosci Rural Pract. 2015;6:511–4. https://doi.org/10.4103/0976-3147.168436.
15. Kawakami Y, Chikama M, Tamiya T, Shimamura Y. Coagulation and fibrinolysis in chronic subdural hematoma. Neurosurgery. 1989;25:25–9. https://doi.org/10.1097/00006123-198907000-00005.
16. Khursheed N, Jain A, Haneef M, Tanki H, Ramzan A, Shaheen F, et al. Skull vault morphology in subdural hematomas: a geometrical analysis. Indian J Neurotrauma. 2015;12:107–10. https://doi.org/10.1055/s-0035-1570092.
17. Kim BG, Lee KS, Shim JJ, Yoon SM, Doh JW, Bae HG. What determines the laterality of the chronic subdural hematoma? J Korean Neurosurg Soc. 2010;47:424–7. https://doi.org/10.3340/jkns.2010.47.6.424.
18. Lee KS. Chronic subdural hematoma in the aged, trauma or degeneration? J Korean Neurosurg Soc. 2016;59:1–5. https://doi.org/10.3340/jkns.2016.59.1.1.
19. Lee KS, Bae WK, Yoon SM, Doh JW, Bae HG, Yun IG. Location of the chronic subdural haematoma: role of the gravity and cranial morphology. Brain Inj. 2001;15:47–52. https://doi.org/10.1080/02699050150209129.
20. MacFarlane MR, Weerakkody Y, Kathiravel Y. Chronic subdural haematomas are more common on the left than on the right. J Clin Neurosci. 2009;16:642–4. https://doi.org/10.1016/j.jocn.2008.07.074.
21. Mori K, Maeda M. Surgical treatment of chronic subdural hematoma in 500 consecutive cases: clinical characteristics, surgical outcome, complications, and recurrence rate. Neurol Med Chir (Tokyo). 2001;41:371–81. https://doi.org/10.2176/nmc.41.371.
22. Oh JS, Shim JJ, Yoon SM, Lee KS. Influence of gender on occurrence of chronic subdural hematoma; Is it an effect of cranial asymmetry? Korean J Neurotrauma. 2014;10:82–5. https://doi.org/10.13004/kjnt.2014.10.2.82.
23. Pesce Delfino V, Potente F, Chiarelli B. Evaluation of skull vault asymmetry using methods of analytical morphometry. Boll Soc Ital Biol Sper. 1990;66:405–11.
24. Portegies ML, Selwaness M, Hofman A, Koudstaal PJ, Vernooij MW, Ikram MA. Left-sided strokes are more often recognized than right-sided strokes: the Rotterdam study. Stroke. 2015;46:252–4. https://doi.org/10.1161/STROKEAHA.114.007385.
25. Sambasivan M. An overview of chronic subdural hematoma: experience with 2300 cases. Surg Neurol. 1997;47:418–22. https://doi.org/10.1016/s0090-3019(97)00188-2.
26. Suzuki M, Kudo A, Kitakami A, Doi M, Kubo N, Kuroda K, Ogawa A. Local hypercoagulative activity precedes hyperfibrinolytic activity in the subdural space during development of chronic subdural haematoma from subdural effusion. Acta Neurochir (Wien). 1998;140:261–5. https://doi.org/10.1007/s007010050093.
27. Zonenshayn M, Kronberg E, Souweidane MM. Cranial index of symmetry: an objective semiautomated measure of plagiocephaly. Technical note. J Neurosurg. 2004;100(5 Suppl Pediatrics):537–40. https://doi.org/10.3171/ped.2004.100.5.0537.

第 7 章 慢性硬膜下血肿的解剖病理学和组织病理学变化

Lorenzo Gitto 和 Timothy E. Richardson

译者：王李傲

7.1 引言

在正常的生理条件下，大脑悬浮在颅腔中，由脑脊液（CSF）提供缓冲和保护，硬脑膜窦和其他颅内血管位置是固定的。硬膜下血肿（SDH）通常是头部外伤的结果，伴或不伴直接冲击。因此需要注意的是，即使缺乏外部直接冲击损伤证据也不一定能排除创伤性病因。例如，严重的机动车事故没有直接的头部创伤也可能会导致头部的旋转运动，从而导致血管撕裂和 SDH。这种情况在幼儿和老年人中特别常见，SDH 可能在头部外伤极度轻微的情况下发生。

通常情况下，SDH 会在远离冲击点的部位发生发展。创伤的惯性可以解释这一发现：由于头部是自由移动的，头部外伤会产生显著的加速/减速力量，导致颅骨和大脑移动不同步。这会导致血管的拉伸和撕裂，形成 SDH。然而，也有一些 SDH 是由脑挫伤引起的。在这种情况下，脑压的增加会导致小脑皮质静脉的扭曲和撕裂，随后形成 SDH。

此外，与线性或凹陷骨折相关的皮质撕裂也可以导致 SDH，因为尖锐的骨片可以撕裂颅内血管。在这些情况下，SDH 通常会发生在冲击点。文献中很少描述自发性 SDH，其病因可能涉及动脉出血（如严重高血压）[23, 34]、凝血功能障碍[6]或其他慢性疾病。大多数 SDH 是由矢状中线旁的桥静脉间接撕裂和拉伸所致。因此，了解这些特殊静脉的解剖和组织学特征有助于理解相关的损伤机制[20]。

7.2 桥静脉和硬膜下间隙的解剖学和组织学，以及损伤的基本机制

颅内桥静脉负责脑部的静脉引流，它们是神经外科重要的手术标志，与许多病理情况特别是 SDH 相关联。

软脑膜静脉负责引流大脑半球的静脉血液。这些血管具有环形平滑肌层，位于皮质表面。它们从皮质静脉收集静脉血液，并从脑的中线区域离开软脑膜。然后，这些血管穿过蛛网膜下间隙，穿破蛛网膜进入潜在的硬膜下间隙。最后，它们到达并穿破硬脑膜，在那里汇合并引流到最近的脑静脉，继而汇入硬脑膜窦。位于软脑膜和矢状窦之间的静脉被称为"桥静脉"（图 7.1）[33]。

桥静脉的分布比矢状旁凸面静脉更广泛。桥静脉根据其在颅腔内的位置进行分类。

颅后窝桥静脉位于小脑幕表面，包括蚓部组和半球组。蚓部组位于小脑下蚓部之上，负责引流下蚓静脉和山坡静脉的末端血液。半球组位于小脑幕半球面的侧面，收集来自上半球静脉和下半球静脉

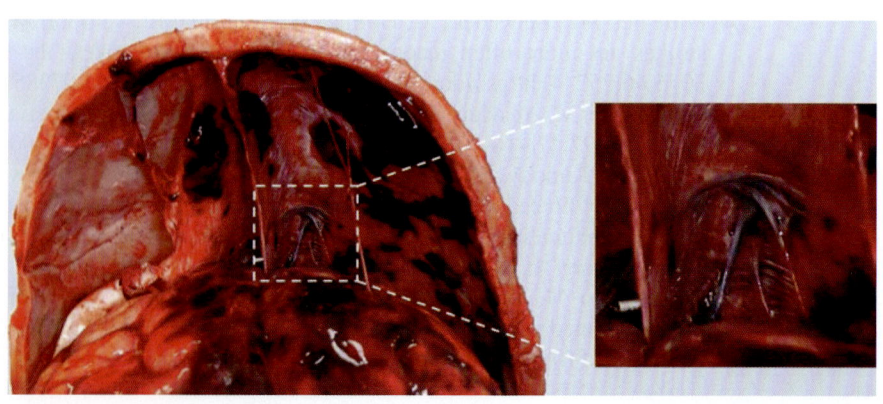

图 7.1 尸体解剖头部检查显示位于硬脑膜和蛛网膜之间的桥静脉

的末端血液[18-19]。

有三种类型的半球桥静脉[35]：

- 类型1：由上、下半球静脉汇合形成。
- 类型2：由上半球静脉汇合形成。
- 类型3：由下半球静脉汇合形成。

上、下半球静脉有许多侧支血管通路，将枕下表面的下部与下蚓部静脉连接起来。解剖观察到颅后窝中其他桥静脉是围绕颈静脉孔的小静脉，它们收集来自颅后窝的微小静脉血液，并排入硬脑膜窦。

颞叶桥静脉位于颞叶的侧面，它们通过其静脉入口处的静脉复合体来识别，这些结构组成特定的颞叶桥静脉模式。其中一种是"烛台"型，包括多个静脉复合体汇合成一个单一静脉；还有一种"分离"型，每一根静脉独立进入同一区域[29]。颞叶桥静脉可分为流入矢状窦的中背静脉组，以及流入外侧窦的后中脑静脉组。颞叶桥静脉有三个主要组别。

- 横窦组，位于横窦的内侧1 cm，并包括后颞底静脉、中颞静脉和后颞静脉。这些静脉在通过窦硬膜点（乙状窦与岩上窦的交界点）向后行进1 cm后汇入脑静脉窦。
- 小脑幕组，位于窦硬膜点的后方，并汇入小脑幕的硬膜窦[22]。
- 岩部组，位于窦硬膜点的前方，靠近岩脊（将颅中窝和颅后窝分开）。这些静脉收集来自小脑和脑干前部的血液，并汇入岩上、下静脉窦[13]。

额叶桥静脉位于颅前窝，引流大脑凸面、中部和底部。它们分为两种类型[30]。

- 类型1：通过单一静脉干汇入上矢状窦。
- 类型2：通过≥2个静脉干汇入上矢状窦。

桥静脉向上矢状窦引流的方向极其多变。它可以是顺行的、垂直的、逆行的、发夹状的（在进入窦腔前不久改变方向）或蜂窝状的（大的静脉腔）[2, 26]。此外，在通向上矢状窦的桥静脉入口也存在很大的变异性。它可以分为四个段，每段接收不同数量的桥静脉。其中1、2段为5 cm左右，3和4段为7 cm左右。1段和4段各接收到一簇桥静脉，而2段和3段只接收到几条静脉[12]。

桥静脉壁的结构类似于一般静脉壁的结构，不过在组织学上很难鉴定[8]。静脉从外到内有三层：

- 外膜，由致密的纤维组织、胶原蛋白、弹力纤维组成，保护血管免受过度伸展。
- 中膜，可能由平滑肌细胞组成[37]，尽管关于中膜是否存在仍面临争议[14]。
- 内膜，由光滑的内皮细胞组成，覆盖着弹力组织。内皮细胞通过紧密连接而连在一起，可以是扁平或收缩的细胞。

桥静脉的直径根据其位置而异，范围从0.5 mm到约5.0 mm。在静脉的蛛网膜下部分，其直径是恒定的，但在外流的袖套段之前会扩大。外流袖套段是位于大脑桥静脉和上矢状窦交界处的狭窄区域，表现为球状膨胀。在这个区域，外流袖套段的桥静脉直径和长度较小，厚度高于脑桥静脉的厚度[27]。

在桥静脉发育过程中，其血管壁结构发生变化。不同部分的静脉壁厚度有所差异。在通过蛛网膜下间隙时，桥静脉的壁厚度相对一致，范围在$50 \sim 200$ μm之间，但随着进入硬脑膜，其厚度增加，已发现其厚度在$10 \sim 600$ μm之间[39]。不同部分之间的胶原纤维含量也有所不同。与蛛网膜下间隙中较紧密的纤维相比，硬脑膜桥静脉显示出较松散的纤维网。此外，硬脑膜桥静脉表现出环状胶原纤维增加，而非纵向胶原纤维。无论位于血管何段，桥静脉都被致密的纤维组织和松散的结缔组织所包围。

桥静脉的特殊结构使其对加速/减速的力特别敏感。角加速度是旋转物体在单位时间内发生角速度变化程度的量化参数。高角加速度的损伤（例如，严重头部冲击导致的跌倒）可能导致急性硬膜下血肿和弥漫性轴索损伤。加速度或减速度越大，速度变化的时间越短，患者罹患硬膜下血肿而非弥漫性轴索损伤的可能性就越大。旋转和剪切力（如剧烈摇晃或面部受击造成的头部旋转）也可以导致硬膜下血肿。旋转主要导致桥静脉沿横向或斜向前轴撕裂，但围绕垂直轴的旋转与平移加速度也可能导致硬膜下血肿发生。研究者经过大量尸检后估计，在外力持续时间小于10 ms时，旋转加速度耐受度约为10 000 rad/s^2 [3]。

硬膜下间隙的概念随着时间的推移而发展，并且由于硬膜下间隙这一定义并未统一，其是否存在经常受到质疑。Haines 等[10-11]证明了真正的硬膜下间隙并不存在,而是在与蛛网膜交界处存在由松散细胞层组成的硬脑膜边界。在生理条件下,由于硬脑膜与蛛网膜之间有一层薄的硬脑膜边界细胞,所以并不存在硬膜下间隙[7]。这层细胞细长扁平,未与大量细胞外基质紧密连接,同时其胶原纤维含量有限。电镜研究表明,蛛网膜屏障层跟一层硬脑膜边界细胞松散地交织在一起,界面上没有真正的间隙。因此,只存在着一个"潜在的"或"虚拟的"硬膜下间隙。在外伤、颅内各种病理情况或缺乏脑脊液的情况下,它可以扩展成为一个真正的空间(在许多尸检中可以观察到)。出血时,这层松散的细胞很容易分离,使血液积聚在这个位置,形成血肿(图 7.2)。硬膜下血肿是由于血液渗入这些"层"之间而形成的,实际上是在硬脑膜内形成的(也称 Intradural)[32]。因此,硬膜下间隙(或硬膜下腔)只被定义为一个"潜在的"腔体,它是两个直接相邻结构之间的空间。

7.3 解剖病理学和组织病理学

尸检中,硬脑膜通常与颅骨松散连接,可以通过向后拉拔而将其从额头处轻松分离。另一方面,在老年和婴儿时期,硬脑膜可能与颅骨紧密粘连,因此难以移除。务必小心地移除硬脑膜,保留硬膜下血肿的潜在区域,并避免由于强行分离而产生的伪迹。

尸检中,SDH 表现为不明确的部分凝固的血块,通常覆盖在大脑半球的凸面上(图 7.3)。既往研究将硬膜下血肿分为三个临床阶段(急性、亚急性和慢性),它们在形态上可以区分开来[16, 25]。尸检中,可以观察到:

- 急性。急性硬膜下血肿在受伤后的 72 h 内出现临床症状(图 7.4)。凝胶状血液或液态血液中的红色薄膜在蛛网膜和硬脑膜之间形成。当尸检打开颅腔时,硬脑膜是紧张的,很容易看到血液存于硬膜下。凝固的血液厚度各异,从几毫米到大量硬膜下出血导致严重颅内高压。新鲜凝固的血液容易从硬脑膜表面分离,几乎不留残余物。根据血肿的大小,大脑可以发生变形,同侧的脑回受压加深,对侧的脑回扁平。蛛网膜下腔通常清晰,血肿没有扩展到脑沟深处。如果急性硬膜下血肿迅速发展,可能会危及生命,并需要紧急减压手术。如果出血缓慢,会发展成亚急性血肿。
- 亚急性。硬膜下血肿的亚急性阶段在急性受伤后的 3～7 天开始出现临床症状,不超过 3 周(图 7.5)。如果硬膜下血肿发展缓慢,颅内则可以容纳更大体积的血液,形成亚急性血肿。血肿由混合液体和凝固血液组成,局部附着于硬脑膜表面。随着进行性血液自溶和含铁血黄素沉积,逐渐发生组织变化,血肿呈现出铁锈色至金棕色的外观,并产生凝胶状物质粘连在硬脑膜上(图 7.6)。

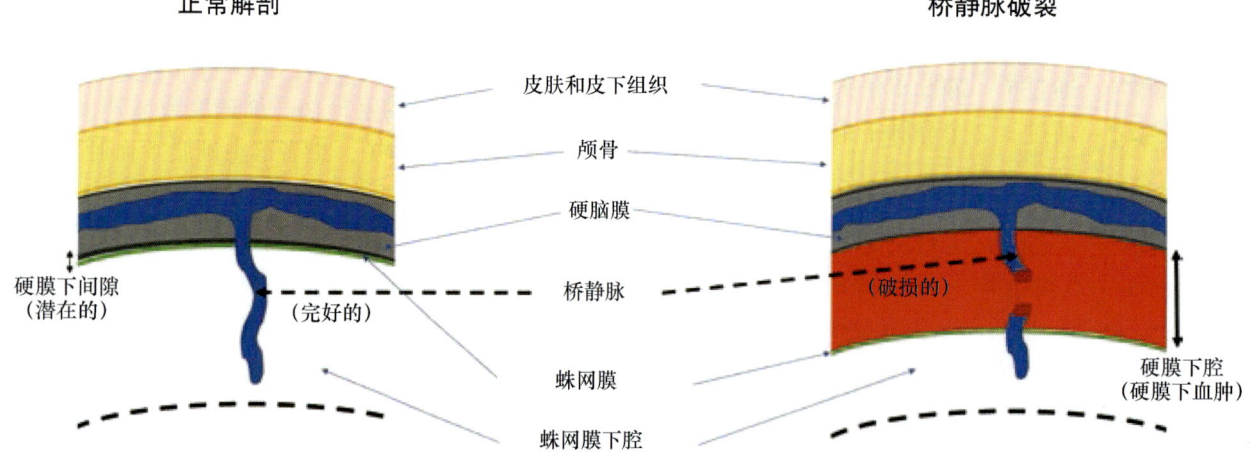

图 7.2 在生理条件下,由于硬脑膜通过一层松散的细胞基质与蛛网膜直接相连,所以没有真正的硬膜下间隙。因此,硬膜下间隙被视为一个潜在的空间(左图)。如果发生损伤,血液可以轻易地分离这层松散的细胞,使血液在硬脑膜的层内积聚,形成硬膜下血肿(SDH)(右图)

第 7 章 慢性硬膜下血肿的解剖病理学和组织病理学变化 49

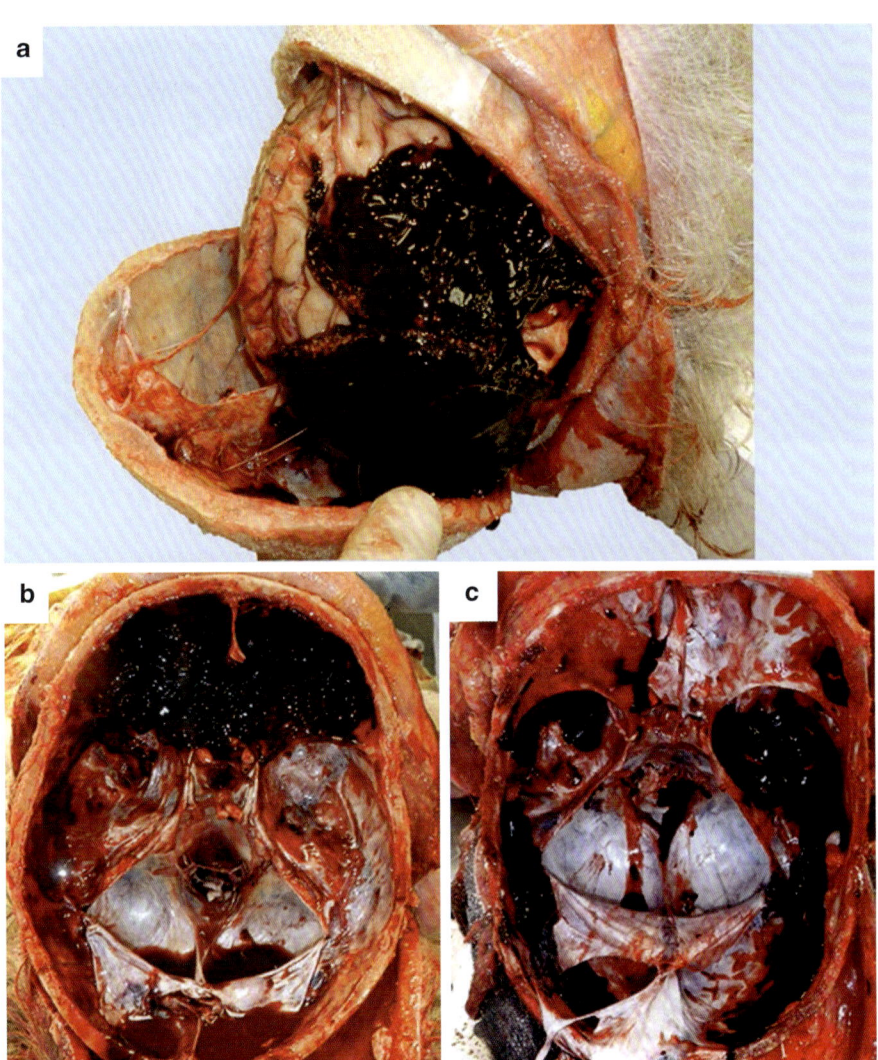

图 7.3 经典的硬膜下血肿在脑半球凸面上形成（a）。然而，在严重头部受伤的情况下，前颅底（b）、中颅底和后颅底（c）也可能受到影响

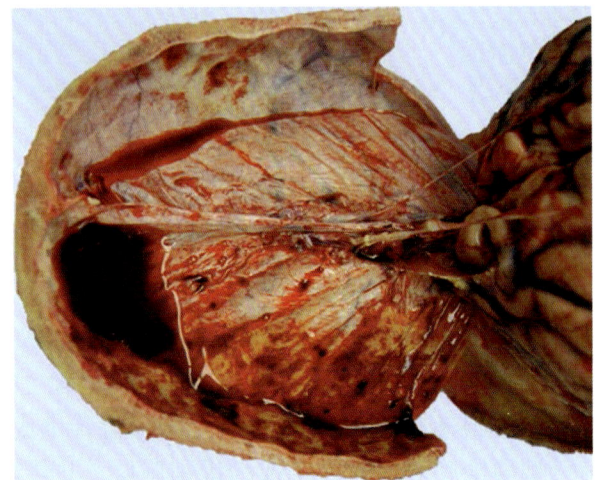

图 7.4 急性硬膜下血肿，出现硬膜下积液

- 慢性。受伤后超过 3 周才出现明显临床表现，被临床定义为慢性硬膜下血肿（CSDH）。慢性硬膜下血肿的典型形态特征是凝血块被纤维膜包裹。如果血肿从亚急性阶段继续发展，组织机化过程会在软膜侧和硬膜侧同时进行，形成坚韧的纤维组织。新生膜似乎是血肿上缘硬膜边界细胞增殖的产物。CSDH 的另一个特征是新生膜内液化的出血残留物。CSDH 的肉眼外观随血肿存在时间而异。新鲜血肿通常难以与亚急性血肿区分开来，呈棕黄色或红棕色，硬脑膜表面存在凝胶状物质粘连，可见近期出血区域。较早期的血肿（数月至数年）呈厚实坚硬的外膜，内含液体，类似于装有果冻或油的橡胶热水袋。内部液体通常呈稻草色（如"机油"），但可能被不同时期出血产生的坚硬的杂色组织所替代（图 7.7 和图 7.8）。我们也经常可以观察到多腔外观，每个小室中的液体量和颜色不同。

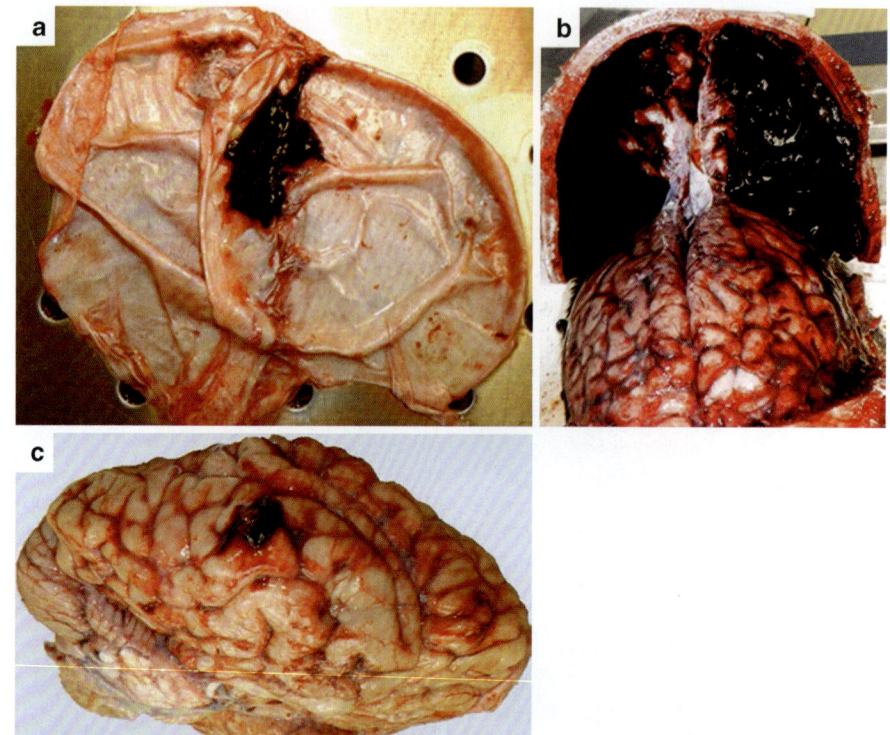

图 7.5 亚急性硬膜下血肿。血肿由混合的液体和凝血块组成，具有早期组织变化。通常观察到典型的深红色胶状外观，伴有硬脑膜粘连（a）。随着组织变化的发展，血肿开始紧密附着于硬脑膜表面（b），并开始附着于蛛网膜层。根据血肿的"年龄"，可以在脑表面观察到局部残留物（c）

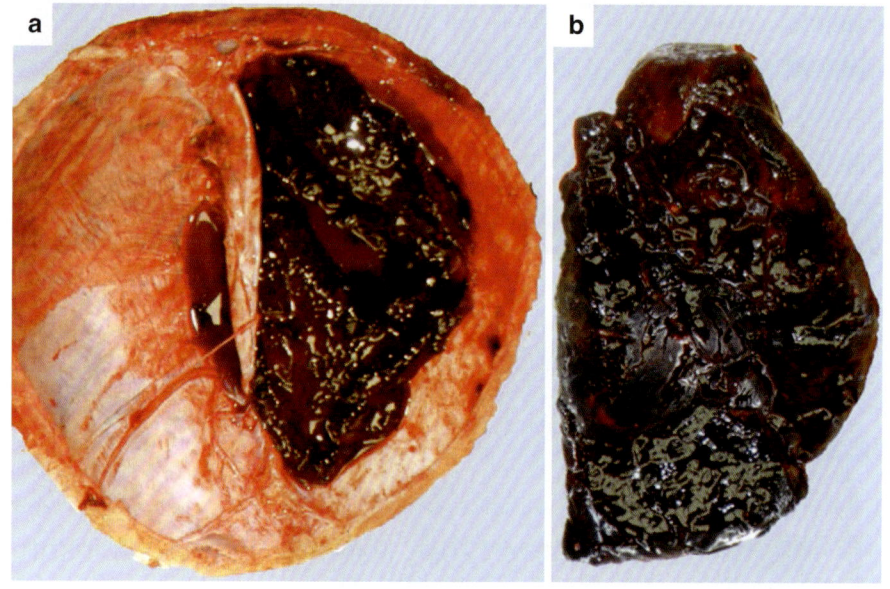

图 7.6 机化的硬膜下血肿，该图显示了血肿的下部（a）。上部分牢固地附着在硬脑膜上。血肿从硬脑膜剥离后的上部表现（b）。外膜呈深褐色，不规则，并显示出因不同时期的出血而呈现的多种颜色

常规组织病理学检查是一种相对可靠的评估硬膜下血肿时间的方法，在法医学案件中具有重要意义[36]。有关血肿存在时间的问题在文献中已多有报道。Munro 和 Merritt 在 1936 年首次尝试估算硬膜下血肿的存在时间[21]，此后发表了多篇论文。

Nagahori 等研究了 CSDH 外层膜的组织学特征[24]。他们根据炎症反应和血肿的成熟度和强度提出了 4 种不同类型的组织学特征。第一型不显示炎症迹象，但含有不成熟的成纤维细胞、胶原纤维、新生毛细血管和稀疏的细胞浸润。第二型炎症变化显著，有明显的细胞浸润和血管生成。第三型硬脑膜表面有多个成纤维细胞层，并伴有大血管以及血肿内小的新生血管和明显的细胞浸润。第四型存在瘢痕组织，有细胞浸润、新生血管和出血[1]。

通过显微镜检查硬膜下血肿的特定形态学特征，可以进行血肿存在时间的评估（表 7.1）[4-5, 15, 17, 31, 38]。

第 7 章 慢性硬膜下血肿的解剖病理学和组织病理学变化

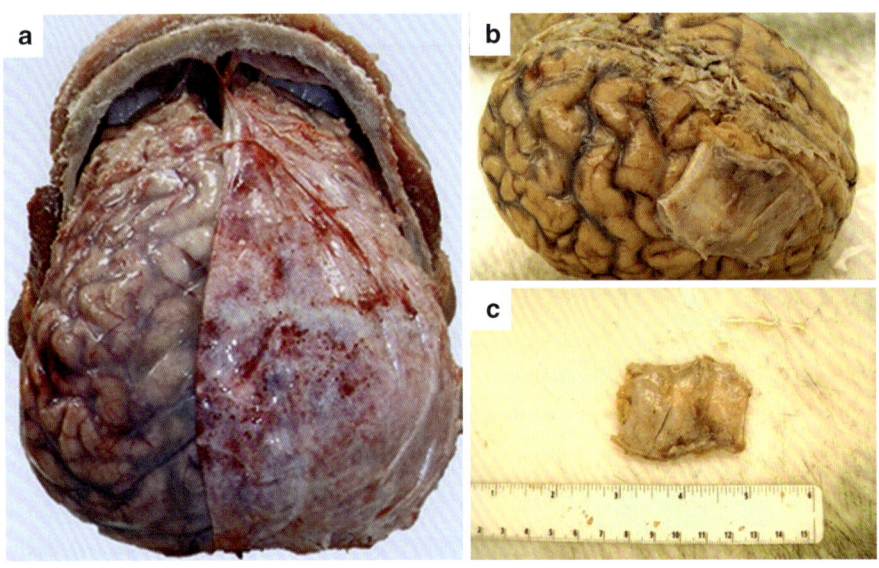

图 7.7 慢性硬膜下血肿。血肿会逐渐被重吸收（a），或者可能再次出血，导致纤维组织形成、硬脑膜变厚和永久变色，并伴有粘连的纤维新生膜（b、c）

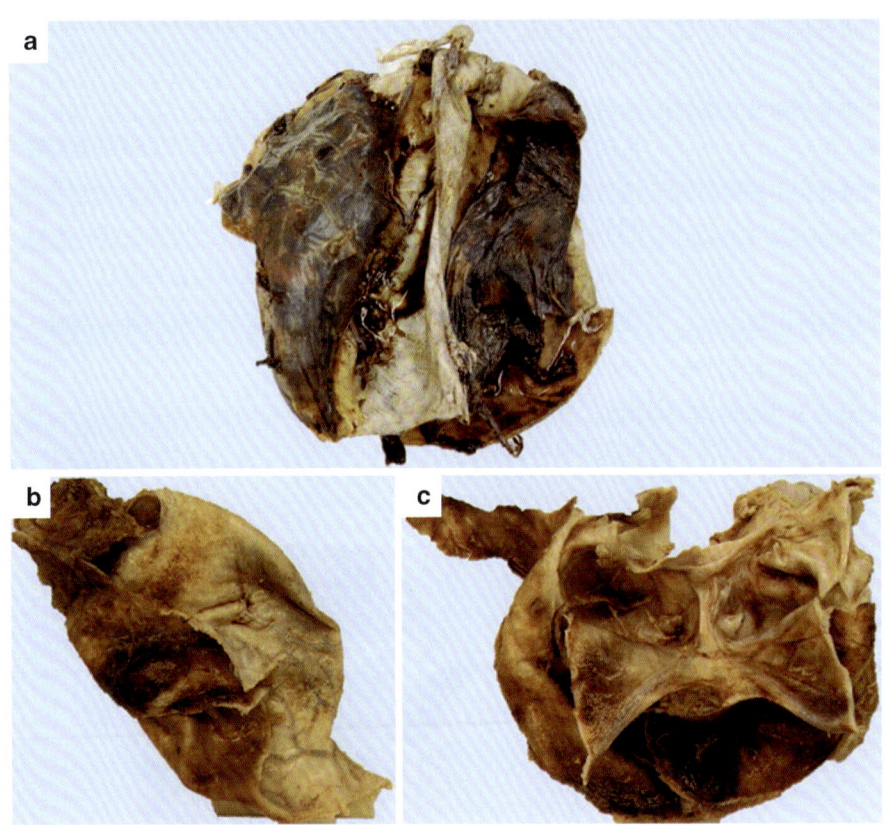

图 7.8 固定在福尔马林中的硬脑膜伴硬膜下血肿。（a）双侧粘连的机化血液。（b、c）硬脑膜标本的绝大部分呈棕红色，中间大脑镰位置颜色较深

受伤后几个小时内，硬膜下便会出现出血反应。在血凝块中可观察到完整的红细胞（图 7.9）。在损伤发生后不久，可以检测到不同数量的中性粒细胞，这被认为是损伤的结果而不是对损伤本身的反应。理论上讲，在损伤发生时，一些血液循环中的中性粒细胞可能会从断裂的桥静脉中流出[28]。相反，反应性中性粒细胞通常在几天后出现，与血管的其他炎症变化一起形成肉芽组织，表示 SDH 进入了组织学上的"机化"阶段（图 7.10）。组织学上，可以见到含铁血黄素点缀的巨噬细胞吞噬并降解红细胞。肉芽组织由许多毛细血管、成纤维细胞、胶原纤维和巨噬细胞组成，并形成血肿的初始薄外膜。在接下来的几天到几周内，密集的纤维蛋白网络将血肿限制在一块，成纤维细胞从外层穿过血肿形成没有血管的内膜。最初的外膜通常在大约 1 周后能通过肉眼

表 7.1　硬膜下血肿显微分期

时间间隔	显微镜下结果		
	血肿	硬脑膜表面	蛛网膜表面
0 h	完整的红细胞	/	/
24 h	完整的红细胞	薄的纤维蛋白层（硬脑膜和血块之间）	薄的纤维蛋白层（蛛网膜和血块之间）
36 h	完整的红细胞	早期成纤维细胞活跃	薄的纤维蛋白层
48～72 h	完整的红细胞	连接处成纤维细胞少见（梭形细胞）	薄的纤维蛋白层
4 天	红细胞分解（失去锐利轮廓和染色变性）	2～4 层成纤维细胞	薄的纤维蛋白层，偶见梭形细胞
5 天	红细胞分解（失去锐利轮廓和染色变性）	3～6 层成纤维细胞，血凝块边缘出现噬铁细胞	薄的纤维蛋白层，偶见梭形细胞
7～8 天	红细胞裂解，早期毛细血管/肉芽组织、成纤维细胞进入血凝块，血凝块液化	12～15 层成纤维细胞，血凝块外膜大致可以辨认	主要由纤维蛋白层和一些成纤维细胞组成
10～12 天	血凝块被毛细血管、成纤维细胞和纤维蛋白分解	成纤维细胞在凝块的边缘移动	出现噬铁细胞
14～17 天	仍可辨认出进行性红细胞裂解及其降解产物，巨大毛细血管	成纤维层大约是硬脑膜厚度的 1/2	出现成纤维层，形成早期的血肿薄膜，凝块可以被完全包裹
18～28 天	血块在新出血区域被液化，出现更大的血管	成纤维层的厚度与硬脑膜相似，膜中出现噬铁细胞	与硬脑膜厚度相似的成形良好的血肿膜，膜中含有噬铁细胞
29～36 天	大量毛细血管	可观察到新生血肿膜	可观察到新生血肿膜
1～3 个月	毛细血管扩张伴继发性新鲜出血	透明膜，胶原蛋白含量增加	透明膜，胶原蛋白含量增加
3～6 个月	可能出现局部再出血，原始红细胞消失	透明膜	透明膜
>6 个月（慢性）	在这个时间点上，估计血凝块的时间变得困难。没有红细胞或明显残留的炎症细胞，新膜变厚，可能发生钙化。膜可类似硬脑膜，并可保留局灶含铁血黄素巨噬细胞		

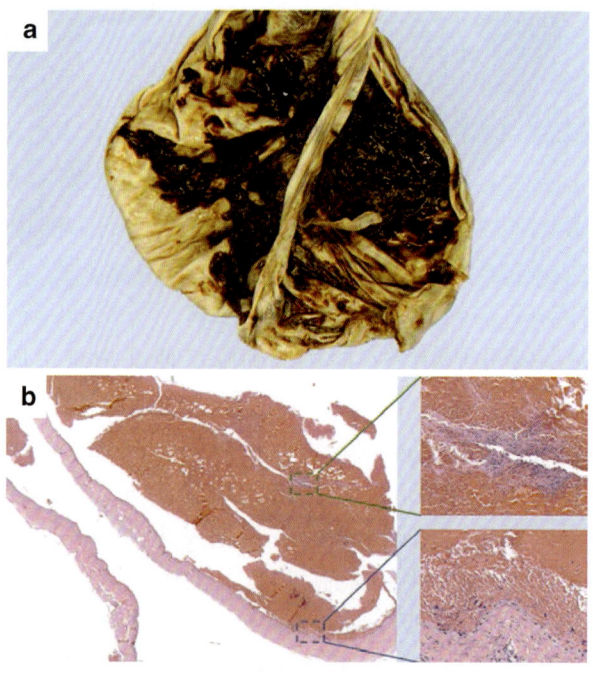

图 7.9　急性硬膜下血肿。硬脑膜（a）外观完整，在双侧硬膜下表面附有红褐色血液，没有新生膜的证据。（b）显微镜检查硬脑膜切片显示在硬膜下表面有附着的血液，没有明显的成纤维细胞增殖（蓝色方框）。血肿区域内存在局部的细胞浸润和纤维蛋白（绿色方框）

看到，而内层膜通常在 2 周后可见。当血肿不再扩张时，膜纤维化程度增加，呈现出上述典型的肉眼外观。大约 6 个月后，SDH 在组织学上变为"慢性"。这种慢性 CSDH 的组织学表现为硬膜下的纤维新生膜，通常有散在的富含含铁血黄素的巨噬细胞（图 7.11），但没有活动性炎症或红细胞，除非 CSDH 上有继发性出血的情况。此时通常无法进一步估计血肿的存在时间。

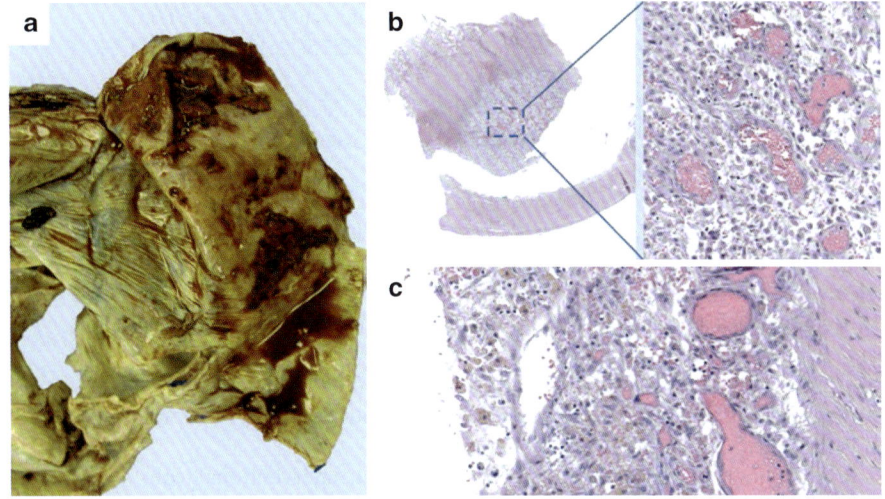

图 7.10 机化的硬膜下血肿。硬脑膜（a）基本完整，双侧有不规则的粘连血液。对硬脑膜切片进行显微镜检查（b）发现黏附的红细胞，有明显的成纤维细胞生长和新血管生成，提示血肿机化（蓝色方框）。其他区域显示偏急性出血区域和纤维层上有含铁血黄素沉积的局部区域（c）

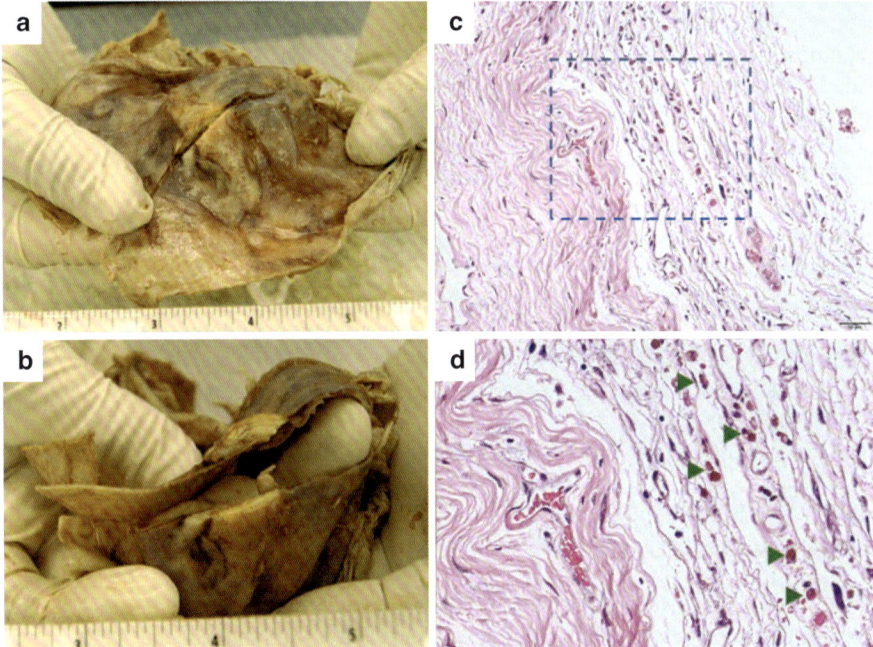

图 7.11 慢性硬膜下血肿。肉眼观察，硬脑膜上有附着的硬膜下新生膜（a、b），显微镜下显示硬脑膜（左）和新生膜（右）的外观（c），可见散在的含铁血黄素（绿色三角箭头）（d）

参考文献

1. Bokka S, Trivedi A. Histopathological study of the outer membrane of the dura mater in chronic sub dural hematoma: its clinical and radiological correlation. Asian J Neurosurg. 2016;11(1):34–8.
2. Brockmann C, Kunze S, Scharf J. Computed tomographic angiography of the superior sagittal sinus and bridging veins. Surg Radiol Anat. 2011;33(2):129–34.
3. Depreitere B, Van Lierde C, Sloten JV, Van Audekercke R, Van der Perre G, Plets C, et al. Mechanics of acute subdural hematomas resulting from bridging vein rupture. J Neurosurg. 2006;104(6):950–6.

4. Dettmeyer RB. Forensic histopathology: fundamentals and perspectives. 2nd ed. Cham: Springer International Publishing; 2018. p. 519–29.
5. DiMaio VJM, Dana MD. Handbook of forensic pathology. 2nd ed. Boca Raton: CRC Press; 2006. p. 165–9.
6. Dobran M, Iacoangeli M, Scortichini AR, Mancini F, Benigni R, Nasi D, et al. Spontaneous chronic subdural hematoma in young adult: the role of missing coagulation facto. G Chir. 2017;38(2):66–70.
7. Ducruet AF, Grobelny BT, Zacharia BE, Hickman ZL, DeRosa PL, Andersen KN, et al. The surgical management of chronic subdural hematoma. Neurosurg Rev. 2012;35(2):155–69; discussion 169.
8. Famaey N, Ying Cui Z, Umuhire Musigazi G, Ivens J, Depreitere B, Verbeken E, et al. Structural and mechanical characterisation of bridging veins: a review. J Mech Behav Biomed Mater. 2015;41:222–40.
9. Gu S-X, Yang D-L, Cui D-M, Xu Q-W, Che X-M, Wu J-S, et al. Anatomical studies on the temporal bridging veins with Dextroscope and its application in tumor surgery across the middle and posterior fossa. Clin Neurol Neurosurg. 2011;113(10):889–94.
10. Haines DE. On the question of a subdural space. Anat Rec. 1991;230(1):3–21.
11. Haines DE, Harkey HL, al-Mefty O. The "subdural" space: a new look at an outdated concept. Neurosurgery. 1993;32(1):111–20.
12. Han H, Tao W, Zhang M. The dural entrance of cerebral bridging veins into the superior sagittal sinus: an anatomical comparison between cadavers and digital subtraction angiography. Neuroradiology. 2007;49(2):169–75.
13. Harrigan MR, Deveikis JP. Handbook of cerebrovascular disease and neurointerventional technique. 3rd ed. Cham: Springer International Publishing; 2018. p. 73.
14. Kiliç T, Akakin A. Anatomy of cerebral veins and sinuses. Front Neurol Neurosci. 2008;23:4–15.
15. Leestma JE. Forensic neuropathology. 3rd ed. Boca Raton: CRC Press; 2014. p. 484–502.
16. Love S, Perry A, Ironside JW, Budka H. Greenfield's neuropathology, ninth edition—two volume set. 9th ed. London: CRC Press; 2016. p. 646–52.
17. Madea B. Handbook of forensic medicine. 1st ed. Hoboken: Wiley-Blackwell; 2014. p. 293–6.
18. Matsushima T, Rhoton AL Jr, de Oliveira E, Peace D. Microsurgical anatomy of the veins of the posterior fossa. J Neurosurg. 1983;59(1):63–105.
19. Matsushima T, Suzuki SO, Fukui M, Rhoton AL Jr, de Oliveira E, Ono M. Microsurgical anatomy of the tentorial sinuses. J Neurosurg. 1989;71(6):923–8.
20. Mortazavi MM, Denning M, Yalcin B, Shoja MM, Loukas M, Tubbs RS. The intracranial bridging veins: a comprehensive review of their history, anatomy, histology, pathology, and neurosurgical implications. Childs Nerv Syst. 2013;29(7):1073–8.
21. Munro D. Surgical pathology of subdural hematoma: based on a study of one hundred and five cases. Arch Neurol Psychiatr. 1936;35(1):64.
22. Muthukumar N, Palaniappan P. Tentorial venous sinuses: an anatomic study. Neurosurgery. 1998;42(2):363–71.
23. Naama O, Belhachmi A, Ziadi T, Boulahroud O, Abad Elasri C, Elmostarchid B, et al. Acute spontaneous subdural hematoma: an unusual form of cerebrovacular accident. J Neurosurg Sci. 2009;53(4):157–9.
24. Nagahori T, Nishijima M, Takaku A. Histological study of the outer membrane of chronic subdural hematoma: possible mechanism for expansion of hematoma cavity. No Shinkei Geka. 1993;21(8):697–701.
25. Oehmichen M, Auer RN, König HG. Forensic neuropathology and associated neurology. Berlin: Springer; 2006. p. 126–38.
26. Oka K, Rhoton AL Jr, Barry M, Rodriguez R. Microsurgical anatomy of the superficial veins of the cerebrum. Neurosurgery. 1985;17(5):711–48.
27. Pang Q, Wang C, Hu Y, Xu G, Zhang L, Hao X, et al. Experimental study of the morphology of cerebral bridging vein. Chin Med Sci J. 2001;16(1):19–22.
28. Rao MG, Singh D, Vashista RK, Sharma SK. Dating of acute and subacute subdural haemorrhage: a histo-pathological study. J Clin Diagn Res. 2016;10(7):HC01–7.
29. Sakata K, Al-Mefty O, Yamamoto I. Venous consideration in petrosal approach: microsurgical anatomy of the temporal bridging vein. Neurosurgery. 2000;47(1):153–61.
30. Sampei T, Yasui N, Okudera T, Fukasawa H. Anatomic study of anterior frontal cortical bridging veins with special reference to the frontopolar vein. Neurosurgery. 1996;38(5):971–5.
31. Saukko PJ, Knight B. Knight's forensic pathology. 4th ed. London: Hodder Arnold; 2015.

p. 185–8.
32. Schachenmayr W, Friede RL. The origin of subdural neomembranes. I. Fine structure of the dura-arachnoid interface in man. Am J Pathol. 1978;92(1):53–68.
33. Schaller B. Physiology of cerebral venous blood flow: from experimental data in animals to normal function in humans. Brain Res Brain Res Rev. 2004;46(3):243–60.
34. Sung SK, Kim SH, Son DW, Lee SW. Acute spontaneous subdural hematoma of arterial origin. J Korean Neurosurg Soc. 2012;51(2):91–3.
35. Ueyama T, Al-Mefty O, Tamaki N. Bridging veins on the tentorial surface of the cerebellum: a microsurgical anatomic study and operative considerations. Neurosurgery. 1998;43(5):1137–45.
36. van den Bos D, Zomer S, Kubat B. Dare to date: age estimation of subdural hematomas, literature, and case analysis. Int J Legal Med. 2014;128(4):631–40.
37. Vignes J-R, Dagain A, Guérin J, Liguoro D. A hypothesis of cerebral venous system regulation based on a study of the junction between the cortical bridging veins and the superior sagittal sinus: laboratory investigation. J Neurosurg. 2007;107(6):1205–10.
38. Whitwell HL, editor. Forensic neuropathology. London: Hodder Arnold; 2005.
39. Yamashima T, Friede RL. Why do bridging veins rupture into the virtual subdural space? J Neurol Neurosurg Psychiatry. 1984;47(2):121–7.

第8章 慢性硬膜下血肿的流行病学和诱发因素

Abad Cherif El Asri，Ali Akhaddar 和 Miloudi Gazzaz

译者：李锦平

8.1 引言

慢性硬膜下血肿（CSDH）是神经外科临床实践中最常见的疾病之一，其病理特征是硬脑膜下出现积血，发病过程隐匿。鉴于CSDH在老年人群中的发病率增加，随着人口老龄化其发病率一直在上升，预计到2030年发病率将是现在的2倍[40,47]。这种增长趋势以前归因于欧美人口老龄化[25,40,42,47]，然而不能排除其他因素，例如医生的临床经验积累和CT检查的普及而提高了诊断能力[27,44]。在20%~25%的病例中，CSDH是双侧的[27]。文献报道了很多慢性硬膜下血肿发生发展的危险因素，并且CSDH在发病过程中可能不止一个危险因素，可能是多个危险因素累加导致的，这些危险因素包括高龄、直接或间接头部创伤、凝血功能障碍以及抗血小板药物和抗凝治疗。其中，头部外伤史通常被认为是最重要的危险因素[22,24,32]。其他重要的危险因素包括出血倾向、肾脏疾病、血液透析、肝功能障碍、癫痫、分流手术史、使用化疗药物和蛛网膜囊肿[22,32]。近年来，由于预期寿命的提高导致人口老龄化，接受抗凝和抗血小板药物治疗的人数在逐步增加，CSDH的发生率也随之逐年上升。

8.1.1 发病率

慢性硬膜下血肿的发病率在全球范围内呈上升趋势。Foelholm 和 Waltimo 在1967年的研究中发现，在7年的时间内赫尔辛基市64名居民被诊断患有CSDH，其年发病率约为1.72/10万人[13]。Rauhala 等在2015年提出，在芬兰的普通人群中，CSDH的年发病率从8.2/10万人增长了1倍，增至17.6/10万人[37]。另外，近期由 Balser 及其同事在研究美国退伍军人中CSDH的发病率时发现，CSDH总发病率为每年79.4/10万人[47]。

在亚洲，特别是日本，也有相同的研究结果发现。日本的老龄化人口数目超过世界上任何一个国家。因此，日本的CSDH发病率呈上升趋势。Kudo 等在1992年报道在日本 Awagishima 地区 CSDH 的年发生率是13.1/10万人[27]。此外，有日本学者以2005年至2007年国家登记处数据资料为基础研究了CSDH的发病率，作者报道了日本CSDH的发病率正在以每年20.6/10万人的趋势增加，在70~79岁年龄组年发病率为76.5/10万人，80岁年龄组年发病率为127.1/10万人[23]。因此，根据日本目前约1.2亿的人口[44]，日本的CSDH年发病率（新诊断病例数）约为24 000例。

由于在非洲没有特定的研究，CSDH的发病率没有确切的数据，所有的研究均引用西方CSDH的发病率作为参考。

8.1.2 年龄

流行病学研究结果表明老年人CSDH的发病率显著高于其他年龄组。此外，大多数CSDH病例组报道了其纳入人群为中老年患者，平均年龄55~60岁，部分患者年龄大于70岁[3,10-11,14]。据报道，CSDH患者的平均年龄在印度为60岁[34]，巴西为64.3岁[43]，瑞士为68.9岁[31]，韩国为69.0岁[38]，加拿大为69.3岁[19]，德国为71.4岁[41]，西班牙为72.7岁[15]，摩洛哥为62岁[8]。随着相关数据不断完善，CSDH的发病率预期到2030年将达到目前的2倍[11,27,50]。一项大规模人口统计学研究发现CSDH在65岁以上患者中的发病率显著升高（69% vs. 31%）[4]。另一项基于北威尔士的研究报告了在1996—1999年间，65岁以上人群的CSDH发病率相对较低，为每年8.2/10万人[1]。相比之下，2005年至2007年使用日本国家登记处数据进行的一项最新研究分析显示，日本CSDH

的年发病率为 20.6/10 万人（70～79 岁人口年发病率为 76.5/10 万人），相对较高[23]。

CSDH 在老年人群中的高发病率的潜在病因尚未完全清楚，但可能和老年人群更易摔伤有关。

8.1.3 性别

男性比女性更容易患上 CSDH。芬兰关于 CSDH 发病率的流行病学研究表明，男性的总体发病率高于女性，这一趋势在进行年龄分层数据研究后没有改变[13]。同样，在其他 CSDH 的研究中发现男性的发病率和流行率要高于女性[10, 33]。男性/女性的发病比率在巴西为 4.8∶1[43]，加拿大为 4.2∶1[19]，印度为 3.4∶1[34]，韩国为 2.6∶1[38]，德国为 2.4∶1[41]，瑞士为 1.9∶1[31]，西班牙为 1.7∶1[15]，摩洛哥为 5.3∶1[8]。近期，日本报道了女性 CSDH 的患病比率有上升趋势，同时男性 CSDH 的患病比率相应下降。随着老龄化社会的到来，女性 CSDH 的发病率也有上升趋势，而男性已被认为是 CSDH 的潜在危险因素[35]。

8.1.4 慢性硬膜下血肿的危险因素

文献研究表明，CSDH 不是一种孤立的疾病，CSDH 的发生、发展和复发可能受到多种危险因素的共同影响[11, 40, 50]。

8.1.4.1 头部外伤

文献报道指出，头部外伤史是导致 CSDH 发生的主要诱发因素，在 50%～70% 的患者中均可发现头部外伤史[5, 20, 22, 24]。尽管曾经轻微的头部外伤有时被忽略，但在 CSDH 发生之前通常均存在外伤史[5, 22, 30, 35]。芬兰一项全国性、以人口为基础的研究纳入了 1991—2005 年全部脑外伤患者，发现 CSDH 总发生率是每年 101/10 万人，显著低于其他国家（包括荷兰、爱沙尼亚和新西兰）的报道[12, 26, 46]。在纳入人群为创伤性脑损伤高发的退伍军人的研究中发现，CSDH 的发病率显著高于普通人群，预计 CSDH 的发病率达到每年 121.4/10 万人；相反，在同一研究中，基于民用模型的 CSDH 预测发病率为每年 17.4/10 万人[4]。然而，有报道指出创伤后出血的确切血管来源于从大脑皮质延伸到硬脑膜静脉窦的桥静脉，这些静脉在老年脑萎缩患者中因为受到牵拉而格外脆弱[36, 44]。

这种观点存在争议，因为在外伤和实际症状出现之间有着很长的时间间隔（平均 4～7 周），即使是缓慢的静脉出血也会在几天内出现相应症状。静脉出血后随着新毛细血管的生长、纤维蛋白酶的溶解以及凝血块的液化，使纤维蛋白降解产物进入新的血凝块中，进一步抑制止血[7, 44]。

8.1.4.2 高龄

既往研究证实，CSDH 是老年患者中的常见病。由于脑萎缩，老年人更易患 CSDH[20, 22, 28-29]。脑萎缩程度是老年人发生 CSDH 的独立预测因素，因为脑萎缩增加了蛛网膜下腔的空间并牵拉桥静脉，这导致了在轻度颅脑外伤后桥静脉撕裂并出血进入硬脑膜下腔脑脊液中[4, 11, 25, 47]。根据脑萎缩分级量表的视觉评分，将脑萎缩分为四个阶段[11, 33, 47]，严重的脑萎缩可能会导致误诊。

此外，老年人比年轻人更容易跌倒并导致头部轻度创伤。最后，随着年龄增长，使用抗凝疗法的概率增加，导致出血的风险增加。文献报告 CSDH 的发病高峰年龄在 70～80 岁[11, 20, 22, 24, 32]。随着老龄化社会的到来，高龄作为 CSDH 的危险因素的重要性也将会增加。

一项对 1990—2015 年芬兰人口进行的时序分析也证实了这一趋势，报道证实了研究时段内 CSDH 的发病率增长了 1 倍，从每年 8.2/10 万人增长至 17.6/10 万人，其中大部分发生在 80 岁及 80 岁以上人口中[37]。此外，除了人口老龄化因素外，抗凝和抗血小板药物使用率的增加也解释了这一趋势[2, 39]。正如 Toi 等学者的报道所述，CSDH 患者的患病年龄峰值也随着时间的推移而上升。在日本，1972 年的一项研究报道的 CSDH 发生年龄峰值在 50～59 岁，而在 Toi 等学者 2010—2013 年的研究中 63 358 例患者年龄峰值为 80～89 岁[44]。

8.1.4.3 慢性酒精中毒

众所周知，酗酒和 CSDH 的发生有关。慢性酒精中毒患者易导致慢性硬膜下血肿形成的机制尚不清楚。一些学者提出，持续的酒精摄入会导致脑萎缩和凝血功能障碍（继发于肝脏功能障碍）[11, 20, 24, 42]，同时慢性酒精中毒还会导致隐匿性脑外伤的发生率增加。报道指出慢性酒精中毒患者发生 CSDH 的概率为 6%～35%，上述原因在

CSDH 的发生中可能发挥着重要作用[24, 30, 42]。

8.1.4.4 男性

所有年龄段的男性患 CSDH 的比例都高于女性[11, 42, 45, 50]。虽然具体原因无法证实，可能的理论包括外伤、形态原因和激素因素。CSDH 的性别分布差异可能与跌倒因素无关，一项研究发现两性之间跌倒风险无显著差异。但是也有学者提出男性更有可能遭受外伤或是其他 CSDH 的相关危险因素[3]。Giuffrè 等学者在血肿外膜的研究中发现，发病男性的雌激素受体和孕激素受体含量高于女性[16]。饮酒和癫痫可能也是解释男性较女性易患 CSDH 的相关因素[40]。

8.1.4.5 凝血功能障碍

除人口统计学相关的患病危险因素以外，凝血功能障碍，包括抗凝治疗（AC）和抗血小板治疗（AP），也是目前已知的 CSDH 致病因素。其他诱发疾病包括败血症、肝功能衰竭、各种类型的血友病、弥散性血管内凝血和肾衰竭[11, 42, 50]。由于 CSDH 的患者多为老年人，增加了使用抗凝药物和合并其他全身性疾病的患者比例。有文献报道，超过 1/3 的 CSDH 患者在确诊时同时在使用抗凝药物或抗血小板药物[11, 40, 42, 50]。Lindvall 和 Koskinen 报道了类似发现，71% 的非创伤组接受抗凝或抗血小板治疗，而创伤组仅为 18%[30]。基于抗凝和抗血小板治疗在预防心血管事件方面的成本效益和易获得性，抗凝和抗血小板治疗的应用深切改变了脑出血和硬膜下血肿的发病率[39]。Rust 等学者报道，与未服用药物的病例对比，服用华法林发生 CSDH 的可能性提高 42.5 倍[2, 18-19, 30, 39]。研究结果提示抗凝或抗血小板治疗在 CSDH 的发生中具有一定的致病作用，与颅脑外伤无关，也与 CSDH 的 8 个流行病学和易感因素无关。除 CSDH 的发生外，抗凝和抗血小板药物可能也与血肿的扩大有关[45]。这两种药物与 CSDH 复发的关系尚不清楚，同时许多研究报道 CSDH 的复发与这两种药物无关[17, 40, 45]。

尽管这些抗凝或抗血小板治疗药物的益处众所周知，但近期对其副作用、出血性并发症和出血性卒中的关注也有所增加。随着抗凝或抗血小板治疗的广泛使用，其关注度也会逐渐增加[2, 5, 11, 45, 49-50]。

8.1.4.6 低颅内压

低颅内压主要是由于外伤性或术后脑脊液漏、腰椎穿刺或引流、脑室腹腔分流术后的过度引流，医源性或是相关疾病导致的脱水或自发性事件[21, 42, 48]。正常颅内压型脑积水分流术后的患者中有 8% 的患者可能会发生硬膜下血肿，其原因可能是对桥静脉的牵拉导致张力增加，桥静脉破裂出血，导致血肿形成的可能性增加[6, 21, 48]。尽管可调压分流管的应用减少了出血并发症的发生，过度引流导致的低颅内压仍是一个重要的问题[21]。

8.1.4.7 其他的原因

其他罕见的自发性硬膜下血肿的原因有：血管畸形（如脑动脉瘤和动静脉畸形）[11, 42, 50]，良性肿瘤（如大脑凸面脑膜瘤）和恶性肿瘤，转移癌/肉瘤，脑膜炎和感染性疾病（如细菌性和结核性脑膜炎）[9]。

8.2 结论

CSDH 的发病率在世界范围内逐年上升。许多学者认为这是由合并基础疾病和老年衰弱造成的，而不是老年患者的特定情况[33]。他们将这一神经外科疾病和髋关节骨折进行了比较，后者具有很高的短期和长期死亡率。高发病率的原因包括人口老龄化、影像学检查的普及以及抗血栓药物的广泛应用。对于确定为易患 CSDH 的高风险人群，即使症状轻微也应怀疑出现慢性硬膜下血肿。患者的预后取决于早期诊断以及合理的治疗。

参考文献

1. Asghar M, Adhiyaman V, Greenway MW, Bhowmick BK, Bates A. Chronic subdural haematoma in the elderly—a North Wales experience. J R Soc Med. 2002;95(6):290–2.
2. Aspegren O, Åstrand R, Lundgren MI, Romner B. Anticoagulation therapy a risk factor 323 for the development of chronic subdural hematoma. Clin Neurol Neurosurg. 2013;115(7):981–4.

3. Baechli H, Nordmann A, Bucher HC, Gratzl O. Demographics and prevalent risk factors of chronic subdural haematoma: results of a large single-center cohort study. Neurosurg Rev. 2004;27:263–6.
4. Balser D, Farooq S, Mehmood T, et al. Actual and projected incidence rates for chronic subdural hematomas in United States veterans administration and civilian populations. J Neurosurg. 2015;123(5):1209–15.
5. Choi WW, Kim KH. Prognostic factors of chronic subdural hematoma. J Korean Neurosurg Soc. 2002;32:18–22.
6. Dietrich U, Lumenta C, Sprick C. Subdural hematoma in a case of hydrocephalus and macrocrania. Experience with a pressure-adjustable valve. Childs Nerv Syst. 1987;3(4):242–4.
7. Edlmann E, Giorgi-Coll S, Whitfield PC, Carpenter KLH, Hutchinson PJ. Pathophysiology of chronic subdural haematoma: inflammation, angiogenesis and implications for pharmacotherapy. J Neuroinflammation. 2017;14(1):108.
8. El Asri AC, Benzagmout M, Chakour K, Chaoui MF, Laaguili J, Gazzaz M, Baallal H, El Mostarchid B. Variation of ventricular size after surgical treatment of chronic subdural hematoma. Asian J Neurosurg. 2019;14(1):122–5.
9. El Asri AC, El Mostarchid B, Akhaddar A, Boucetta M. Chronic subdural hematoma revealing skull metastasis. Intern Med. 2011;50(7):791.
10. Farhat Neto J, Araujo JLV, Ferraz VR, et al. Chronic subdural hematoma: epidemiological and prognostic analysis of 176 cases. Rev Col Bras Cir. 2015;42(5):283–7.
11. Feghali J, Yang W, Huang J. Updates in chronic subdural hematoma: epidemiology, etiology, pathogenesis, treatment and outcome. World Neurosurg. 2020;141:339–45.
12. Feigin VL, Theadom A, Barker-Collo S, et al. Incidence of traumatic brain injury in New Zealand: a population-based study. Lancet Neurol. 2013;12(1):53–64.
13. Foelholm R, Waltimo O. Epidemiology of chronic subdural haematoma. Acta Neurochir (Wien). 1975;32(3–4):247–50.
14. Fujioka S, Matsukado Y, Kaku M, Sakurama N, Nonaka N, Miura G. CT analysis of 100 cases with chronic subdural hematoma with respect to clinical manifestation and the enlarging process of the hematoma (author's transl). Neurol Med Chir (Tokyo). 1981;21:1153–60.
15. Gelabert-González M, Iglesias-Pais M, García-Allut A, Martínez-Rumbo R. Chronic subdural haematoma: surgical treatment and outcome in 1000 cases. Clin Neurol Neurosurg. 2005;107:223–9.
16. Giuffrè R, Palma E, Liccardo G, Sciarra F, Pastore FS, Concolino G. Sex steroid hormones in the pathogenesis of chronic subdural haematoma. Neurochirurgia (Stuttg). 1992;35:103–7.
17. Gonugunta V, Buxton N. Warfarin and chronic subdural haematomas. Br J Neurosurg. 2001;15(6):514–7.
18. Hirakawa K, Hashizume K, Fuchinoue T, Takahashi H, Nomura K. Statistical analysis of chronic subdural hematoma in 309 adult cases. Neurol Med Chir (Tokyo). 1972;12:71–83.
19. Jack A, O'Kelly C, McDougall C, Findlay JM. Predicting recurrence after chronic subdural haematoma drainage. Can J Neurol Sci. 2015;42:34–9.
20. Jeong JE, Kim GK, Park JT, Lim YJ, Kim TS, Rhee BA, et al. A clinical analysis of chronic subdural hematoma according to age factor. J Korean Neurosurg Soc. 2000;29:748–53.
21. Kamano S, Nakano Y, Imanishi T. Management with a programmable pressure valve of subdural hematomas caused by ventriculoperitoneal shunt: case report. Surg Neurol. 1991;35:381–3.
22. Kang HL, Shin HS, Kim TH, Hwang YS, Park SK. Clinical analysis of recurrent chronic subdural hematoma. J Korean Neurosurg Soc. 2006;40:262–6.
23. Karibe H, Kameyama M, Kawase M, et al. Epidemiology of chronic subdural hematomas. No Shinkei Geka. 2011;39(12):1149–53.
24. Ko BS, Lee JK, Seo BR, Moon SJ, Kim JH, Kim SH. Clinical analysis of risk factors related to recurrent chronic subdural hematoma. J Korean Neurosurg Soc. 2008;43:11–5.
25. Kolias AG, Chari A, Santarius T, Hutchinson PJ. Chronic subdural haematoma: modern management and emerging therapies. Nat Rev Neurol. 2014;10(10):570–8.
26. Koskinen S, Alaranta H. Traumatic brain injury in Finland 1991-2005: a nationwide register study of hospitalized and fatal TBI. Brain Inj. 2008;22(3):205–14.
27. Kudo H, Kuwamura K, Izawa I, Sawa H, Tamaki N. Chronic subdural hematoma in elderly people: present status on Awaji Island and epidemiological prospect. Neurol Med Chir. 1992;32(4):207–9.
28. Kwon HJ, Youm JY, Kim SH, Koh HS, Song SH, Kim Y. Postoperative radiological changes in chronic subdural hematoma and its relation to recurrence. J Korean Neurosurg Soc. 2004;35:410–4.

29. Lee JK, Choi JH, Kim CH, Lee HK, Moon JG. Chronic subdural hematomas: a comparative study of three types of operative procedures. J Korean Neurosurg Soc. 2009;46:210–4.
30. Lindvall P, Koskinen LO. Anticoagulants and antiplatelet agents and the risk of development and recurrence of chronic subdural haematomas. J Clin Neurosci. 2009;16:1287–90.
31. MacFarlane MR, Weerakkody Y, Kathiravel Y. Chronic subdural haematomas are more common on the left than on the right. J Clin Neurosci. 2009;16:642–4.
32. Markwalder TM. Chronic subdural hematomas: a review. J Neurosurg. 1981;54:637–45.
33. Miranda LB, Braxton E, Hobbs J, Quigley MR. Chronic subdural hematoma in the elderly: not a benign disease. J Neurosurg. 2011;114(1):72–6.
34. Nayil K, Ramzan A, Sajad A, Zahoor S, Wani A, Nizami F, et al. Subdural hematomas: an analysis of 1181 Kashmiri patients. World Neurosurg. 2012;77:103–10.
35. Nioka H, Matsuda M, Handa J. [A review of cases of a chronic subdural hematoma: an analysis of findings in two age groups]. Jpn J Neurosurg (Tokyo). 1995;4:359–63.
36. Ommaya AK, Yarnell P. Subdural haematoma after whiplash injury. Lancet (London, England). 1969;2(7614):237–9.
37. Rauhala M, Luoto TM, Huhtala H, et al. The incidence of chronic subdural hematomas from 1990 to 2015 in a defined Finnish population. J Neurosurg. 2019;132(4):1147–57.
38. Ro HW, Park SK, Jang DK, Yoon WS, Jang KS, Han YM. Preoperative predictive factors for surgical and functional outcomes in chronic subdural hematoma. Acta Neurochir (Wien). 2016;158:135–9.
39. Rust T, Kiemer N, Erasmus A. Chronic subdural haematomas and anticoagulation or antithrombotic therapy. J Clin Neurosci. 2006;13(8):823–7.
40. Santarius T, Kirkpatrick PJ, Kolias AG, Hutchinson PJ. Working toward rational and evidence based treatment of chronic subdural hematoma. Clin Neurosurg. 2010;57:112–22.
41. Schwarz F, Loos F, Dünisch P, Sakr Y, Safatli DA, Kalff R, et al. Risk factors for reoperation after initial burr hole trephination in chronic subdural hematomas. Clin Neurol Neurosurg. 2015;138:66–71.
42. Sim YW, Min KS, Lee MS, Kim YG, Kim DH. Recent changes in risk factors of chronic subdural hematoma. J Korean Neurosurg Soc. 2012;52:234–9.
43. Sousa EB, Brandão LFS, Tavares CB, Borges IBC, Freire Neto NG, Kessler IM. Epidemiological characteristics of patients who underwent surgical drainage of chronic subdural hematomas in Brasília, Brazil. BMC Surg. 2013;13:5.
44. Toi H, Kinoshita K, Hirai S, et al. Present epidemiology of chronic subdural hematoma in Japan: analysis of 63,358 cases recorded in a national administrative database. J Neurosurg. 2018;128(1):222–8.
45. Torihashi K, Sadamasa N, Yoshida K, et al. Independent predictors for recurrence of chronic subdural hematoma: a review of 343 consecutive surgical cases. Neurosurgery. 2008;63(6):1125–9; discussion: 1129.
46. Ventsel G, Kolk A, Talvik I, et al. The incidence of childhood traumatic brain injury in Tartu and Tartu County in Estonia. Neuroepidemiology. 2008;30(1):20–4.
47. Welling LC, Welling MS, Teixeira MJ, Figueiredo EG. Chronic subdural hematoma: so common and so neglected. World Neurosurg. 2018;111:393–4.
48. Weiner HLCS, Cohen H. Current treatment of normal-pressure hydrocephalus: comparison of flow-regulated and differential-pressure shunt valves. Neurosurgery. 1995;37:877–84.
49. Wintzen AR, Tijssen JG. Subdural hematoma and oral anticoagulant therapy. Arch Neurol. 1982;39:69–72.
50. Yang W, Huang J. Chronic subdural hematoma epidemiology and natural history. Neurosurg Clin N Am. 2017;28:205–10.

第 9 章 慢性硬膜下血肿的主要临床表现

Michelle E. De Witt 和 Walter A. Hall

译者：郭鹏

9.1 引言

慢性硬膜下血肿（CSDH）是一种常见的神经外科疾病，在世界范围内其发病率逐渐增加[3, 69]，具有较高的发病率和死亡率[44, 50]。解剖学上，血肿位于蛛网膜和硬脑膜之间的硬脑膜边缘细胞层内[40, 56]。影像学表现为凹形或新月形病灶，可跨越颅缝，相较于脑实质呈低密度或等/高密度表现[44, 57]。患者到医院就诊的最常见症状是头痛、行走不稳、意识障碍以及行为异常。临床体检经常可以发现肢体活动障碍、定向力障碍和意识障碍等典型表现[21, 46, 58]。CSDH 患者的临床表现相当多变，不典型临床症状伴随其他合并症时可能会给诊断带来难度和挑战[40, 58]。对 CSDH 患者临床症状的鉴别具有多重重要性，有临床症状的 CSDH 患者可以通过及时的手术干预来减少发病率和死亡率。除此之外，CSDH 的诊断可以作为患者"脆弱"的标志，具有一定的预后评估价值[44]。在多项研究中表明，相比于普通人群，CSDH 患者具有更高的死亡率[44, 50]。

9.2 症状和体征

很多临床症状和体征与慢性硬膜下血肿（CSDH）相关。而大多数症状和体征来源于血肿的占位效应或颅内压升高[58]。文献报告的症状包括虚弱无力、步态不稳、头晕、书写困难、语言障碍、疲劳加重、易怒、性格改变、头痛、谵妄、记忆力减退、意识障碍、食欲减退、活动减弱、感觉异常、恶心/呕吐、尿失禁、行为改变、耳鸣或听力障碍、晕厥、眩晕和视物模糊。体征包括肌力下降、感觉减退、癫痫、双侧瞳孔不等大、视乳头水肿、复视、其他局限性神经功能障碍、帕金森综合征、嗜睡及昏迷[3, 7, 13, 16, 21, 28, 31, 42, 44, 56, 58-59, 66]。不同年龄患者可表现为不同的临床体征和症状（表 9.1）。不

表 9.1 慢性硬膜下血肿不同年龄患者的临床表现

年轻患者	老年患者
常见症状： 头痛、恶心、呕吐	常见症状： 意识障碍、认知功能障碍、肢体活动障碍
双侧 CSDH 的发生率较低	双侧 CSDH 的发生率较高
血肿厚度较小	血肿厚度较大
男：女比例增加	男：女比例减小

CSDH，慢性硬膜下血肿。

同研究报道的症状和体征存在显著差异，这种情况阻碍了对 CSDH 临床表现的交叉研究评估[8]。尽管如此，仔细回顾文献仍然可以发现这些患者临床表现的共性，如下文所述。

9.2.1 头痛

头痛是 CSDH 患者最常见的症状之一。在大多数研究中，头痛的发生率为 25%～90%[7, 28, 31, 42, 46, 58]。然而，根据 2017 年来自威尔士北部的一篇报道，Adhiyaman 等研究报道 66 例 CSDH 患者未发现头痛症状[3]。

CSDH 患者头痛的病因不尽相同，常见的病因是颅内压升高[36, 39, 58]。另外，也有人认为头痛是硬脑膜动静脉受牵拉所致[66]。还有一种不太常见的原因是当颅内压低时导致的直立性头痛，这种病因已在很多报道中得到明确描述[48, 59, 66]，可通过详细询问病史和检查进行明确。

Yamada 等对 1080 例接受外科手术治疗的 CSDH 患者进行回顾性分析，其中 22.6% 的患者有头痛症状。值得注意的是，研究发现头痛症状在年轻患者中更为显著[66]，此现象在先前其他研究中也有体现[16, 21, 36, 42, 46]。此外，他们还发现中线移位长度与血肿厚度的比值是头痛症状的重要影响因素。通过测量部分患者血肿内压力，发现血肿内压力大小与头痛并不相关[66]。这些发现可能支持头痛症状

的发生是由于颅内对于疼痛敏感的动静脉牵拉所致这一理论；然而，血肿内压力不能反映颅内压的真实水平。

9.2.2 步态异常

步态异常是 CSDH 患者就诊时的常见主诉，这可能与患者多次跌倒的病史有关。几项研究报告表明，跌倒病史在多达 2/3 的慢性硬膜下血肿患者中出现[3, 46]。其他研究也报道了在确定 CSDH 为病因的患者中，有跌倒史患者占了相似比例。然而，文献中报告的出现跌倒情况也可能是因为已经存在了颅内血肿，导致一系列的相关临床症状[3]。步态异常也可能与检查中发现的运动障碍有关。

9.2.3 恶心/呕吐

恶心/呕吐是 CSDH 患者的另一种症状。在这些患者中，恶心和呕吐往往提示颅内压升高。在几个大型研究中，有 3.0%~12.5% 的患者存在颅内压升高的情况[42, 46, 64, 66]。其中年轻患者更容易出现恶心、呕吐。以上发现说明年轻患者更容易出现颅内压升高的症状[36, 39]。

9.2.4 行为障碍

行为改变在 24.8%~35% 的 CSDH 患者中出现[7, 42, 58]，其包括易怒、容易疲劳、性格改变或思维紊乱。Gelabert 等在对 1000 例 CSDH 患者进行回顾性分析时发现，行为改变是老年人群中最常见的主诉，该研究中将老年人定义为 > 70 岁[21]。

9.2.5 意识改变

意识障碍、定向力障碍和智能障碍在 CSDH 患者中经常出现。这些症状在文献报道中的发生比例为 17%~70%，其中老年患者更为常见[3, 28, 31, 46, 66]。

在 CSDH 患者中，与精神状态轻微改变相比，意识水平出现下降（包括昏迷）较为少见。CSDH 患者中出现意识水平下降的比率从 10.9% 到 28.8% 不等[7, 28, 42, 46, 66]。由于部分文献中术语的使用不够精确，某种程度上对于意识水平下降并没有一个准确的定义。在多个病例报道中，昏迷的发生率从 2.5% 到 12.6% 不等[19, 21, 31, 42, 46]。

与许多研究一致，入院时的意识状态是患者预后的重要预测因素，意识状态下降与不良预后相关[21, 44, 52]，同时与该人群较高的死亡率相关[50]。

9.2.6 肢体活动障碍

CSDH 患者最突出的临床表现之一是体格检查中发现肢体无力。患者自述症状为肢体无力、活动笨拙和（或）运动失衡，这些描述与体格检查发现一致。对侧肢体活动障碍在 CSDH 患者中常见，根据报道有 40.3%~60.6% 的患者存在肢体活动障碍[5, 28, 42, 46, 66]。在大多数患者中会出现对侧肢体偏瘫症状，即对侧的上肢和下肢都受到影响。也有一些患者下肢偏瘫症状较上肢更明显，或者仅仅出现对侧下肢偏瘫，而上肢未受累，这种情况常在颅内血肿位于两大脑半球之间、靠近旁中央小叶的患者中出现[17, 55]。单纯对侧上肢偏瘫也可能出现。此外，有病例报告显示，CSDH 患者的肢体无力可仅局限于对侧手或脚，首次诊断时可能与周围神经病变相混淆[30, 63]。极其罕见的情况下，患者可能出现截瘫或四肢瘫痪的症状[24, 28, 33, 35]。

9.2.7 癫痫

癫痫发作在 CSDH 患者中并不常见。在一系列关于 CSDH 的临床表现的报道中，癫痫发生率从 0.4% 到 42% 不等[12, 21, 31-32, 42, 46, 53, 58, 64, 66]，发生率的巨大差异可能与诊断不规范相关。在许多研究中，CSDH 患者未常规进行脑电图（EEG）检查，而是根据临床医生的判断进行相关检查。在多达 2% 的病例中，患者可能出现癫痫持续状态。最近 Won 等对 375 例 CSDH 患者的病例分析中发现 Glasgow 昏迷评分（GCS）≤ 13 和既往卒中病史是癫痫发作的独立预测因子[64]。

9.3 患者人口统计学特征

9.3.1 性别

CSDH 在男性人群中更为常见。这种性别倾向性在全球范围内的许多研究中都有所报道，根据报道 CSDH 患者的男女比例范围从 1.7∶1 到 4.4∶1 不等[6, 9, 14-16, 19, 21, 28, 31, 38, 42, 46-47, 51, 58, 66]。在低收入和中低收入国家中也发现 CSDH 患者的男性比例占优势[31,43]。一些研究进一步分析了性别与年龄的关系。这些研究表明，男性患者所占比例随着年龄的增加而降低[16,28,38,62,66]。一项包含 1080 例 CSDH 患者的研究显示，年龄＞90 岁的患者中，女性患者的数量超过了男性[66]，男女比例的变化可能与 CSDH 的病因相关。年轻患者（＜65 岁）因外伤原因导致 CSDH 更多，而且其中大多数男性患者有外伤史[31,58]。然而在老年人群中，外伤一般都比较轻微，比较典型的情况就是跌倒[31,42,44]，而大约 1/3 的患者并没有外伤或其他病因[44]。因此，目前还无法解释在老年人群中随着年龄增长女性患者数量增加的现象。同时，也有人认为这与女性有更长的寿命相关[20-21]。

9.3.2 年龄

虽然 CSDH 可以发生在任何年龄段，从新生儿[18,37,49]到老年人[22,66]，但绝大多数 CSDH 患者为老年人。其首次发病的年龄在全球不同地区各不相同，中高收入或高收入国家的数据显示首次发病的平均年龄较高。事实上，来自这些地区的一些研究显示，老年人占所有 CSDH 患者的 90% 以上，平均发病年龄从 62.9 岁到 83.8 岁不等[19,21,26,42,62]。来自中低收入国家（世界银行集团数据中人均国民总收入≤4045 美元的国家[23]）的数据显示，这些国家的平均发病年龄更小[1,13,31]。然而，随着这些国家人口平均年龄逐渐增长，CSDH 的发病年龄也在增加[43]，呈现出与发达国家类似的发病情况[62]。

年龄与 CSDH 的联系是多方面的。首先，随着年龄的增长，脑实质萎缩，硬脑膜细胞边界层和穿过它的桥静脉受到牵拉。在这种情况下，被牵拉的桥静脉极易受到损伤，造成静脉破裂出血[2,9,34,54,56,67]，从而导致硬脑膜下腔的急性出血，随着时间的推移形成慢性硬膜下血肿。有文献根据头部 CT 数据对 CSDH 患者的硬膜下腔体积进行测算，通过与对照组比较分析证实了脑萎缩与 CSDH 的发病率呈正相关[27,68]，而 Ju 等认为硬膜下容积是预测慢性硬脑膜血肿形成的间接标志物[27]。其次，跌倒和轻微头部创伤的发生率随着年龄的增长而增加[52,57-58]。最后，随着年龄增长，使用抗血小板药物或抗凝药物的患者也越来越普遍，因此增加了此人群的出血风险[52,57]。

9.4 影像学表现

CSDH 位于蛛网膜和硬脑膜之间的硬膜下间隙，可被包裹在一个血肿囊中[40]。通常可用头部 CT 平扫来诊断。在 CT 扫描上，CSDH 通常表现为凹陷或新月形的硬膜下病变，可跨越颅缝[57,65]；少数情况下表现为梭形，形态与硬膜外血肿类似[4,65]。CSDH 在平扫 CT 上表现为低密度或等密度影[44,57,65]，少数情况下可见钙化影[61]。发生于硬脑膜的原发或转移性肿瘤也可导致慢性硬膜下血肿的发生，虽然不常见[10,65]，但增强头部 CT 可协助诊断。

脑磁共振成像很少应用于此类患者。在 T1 加权像或液体衰减反转序列像（FLAIR）上，CSDH 表现为等信号或高信号的硬膜下病灶。MRI 有助于分辨硬膜下血肿病灶内血肿的分隔情况，对双侧少量等信号血肿或急性出血更加敏感[56,65]。增强 MRI 可以通过强化硬脑膜来评估疑似脑脊液低容量综合征的患者[11,59]或用于评估硬脑膜原发性或转移性肿瘤。增强 MRI 和弥散加权像（DWI）有助于诊断感染性硬膜下血肿[65]。

9.4.1 血肿位置

绝大多数 CSDH 位于幕上大脑半球表面，其他的部位如镰旁[17,55]、硬脊膜下腔[25,41]和后颅窝[45,60]也有报道。大脑半球表面 CSDH 可以为单侧（左侧或右侧）或双侧。有文献报道左侧 CSDH 的发病率更高[14,39,42,46,66]。学者们提出了多种假设来解释这一现象，其中一个假设认为右侧 CSDH 的诊断率低于左侧，但真实的发生率可能是相等的[39]；其他人则认为这种现象是由颅骨形态不对称引起的[29,34]。

双侧 CSDH 比单侧 CSDH 少见，双侧 CSDH 发生率为 9.7%～34.8%[7,14,42,46,62,66]。几项研究发现，双侧硬膜下血肿更容易出现在老年患者中[6,46,62]，由于老年患者脑萎缩，使得桥静脉在双侧半球上受到更多牵拉，从而导致双侧硬膜下血肿形成。

9.4.2 血肿大小

影像学研究显示，CSDH 的厚度与发病时长[16,36,66]和是否是双侧硬膜下血肿[46]相关，这种关联可能是由脑实质萎缩导致的。如前所述，脑萎缩与年龄直接相关，并且脑萎缩与双侧 CSDH 形成密切相关。当脑萎缩患者合并慢性硬膜下血肿时，则需要更大的血肿量才能产生明显的占位效应，从而导致患者出现临床症状，促使患者就诊。

9.5 结论

CSDH 的发病率在全球范围内逐渐上升，因此对 CSDH 的临床表现的认识越来越重要。年轻患者更有可能出现颅内压升高的症状和体征，而老年患者通常表现为认知功能改变和局灶性神经功能障碍，主要症状是肢体活动障碍。大多数 CSDH 患者为老年人，这类人群中 CSDH 的发生与脑萎缩、血肿大小及是否为双侧血肿相关。临床医生熟悉 CSDH 的临床表现可及时诊断和治疗该疾病，以减少患者的发病率和死亡率。

参考文献

1. Adeolu AA, Rabiu TB, Adeleye AO. Post-operative day two versus day seven mobilization after burr-hole drainage of subacute and chronic subdural haematoma in Nigerians. Br J Neurosurg. 2012;26:743–6.
2. Adhiyaman V, Chatterjee I. Increasing incidence of chronic subdural haematoma in the elderly. QJM. 2017;110:775.
3. Adhiyaman V, Chattopadhyay I, Irshad F, Curran D, Abraham S. Increasing incidence of chronic subdural haematoma in the elderly. QJM. 2017;110:375–8.
4. Agrawal A. Bilateral biconvex frontal chronic subdural hematoma mimicking extradural hematoma. J Surg Tech Case Rep. 2010;2:90–1.
5. Akakin A, Yilmaz B, Ekşi M, Özcan-Ekşi EE, Demir MK, Toktaş ZO, Konya D. Recurrent cranial chronic subdural hematoma due to cervical cerebrospinal fluid fistula: repair of both entities in the same session. J Craniofac Surg. 2016;27:e578–80.
6. Baechli H, Nordmann A, Bucher HC, Gratzl O. Demographics and prevalent risk factors of chronic subdural haematoma: results of a large single-center cohort study. Neurosurg Rev. 2004;27:263–6.
7. Cameron MM. Chronic subdural haematoma: a review of 114 cases. J Neurol Neurosurg Psychiatry. 1978;41:834–9.
8. Chari A, Hocking KC, Edlmann E, Turner C, Santarius T, Hutchinson PJ, Kolias AG. Core outcomes and common data elements in chronic subdural hematoma: a systematic review of the literature focusing on baseline and peri-operative care data elements. J Neurotrauma. 2016;33:1569–75.
9. Chen JC, Levy ML. Causes, epidemiology, and risk factors of chronic subdural hematoma. Neurosurg Clin N Am. 2000;11:399–406.
10. Cheng YK, Wang TC, Yang JT, Lee MH, Su CH. Dural metastasis from prostatic adenocarcinoma mimicking chronic subdural hematoma. J Clin Neurosci. 2009;16:1084–6.
11. Chung SJ, Kim JS, Lee MC. Syndrome of cerebral spinal fluid hypovolemia: clinical and imaging features and outcome. Neurology. 2000;55:1321–7.
12. Cole M, Spatz E. Seizures in chronic subdural hematoma. N Engl J Med. 1961;265:628–31.
13. Dakurah TK, Iddrissu M, Wepeba G, Nuamah I. Chronic subdural haematoma: review of 96 cases attending the Korle Bu Teaching Hospital, Accra. West Afr J Med. 2005;24:283–6.
14. de Araújo Silva DO, Matis GK, Costa LF, Kitamura MA, de Carvalho Junior EV, de Moura Silva M, Barbosa BJ, Pereira CU, da Silva JC, Birbilis TA, de Azevedo Filho HR. Chronic subdural hematomas and the elderly: surgical results from a series of 125 cases: old "horses" are not to be shot! Surg Neurol Int. 2012;3:150.
15. Ernestus RI, Beldzinski P, Lanfermann H, Klug N. Chronic subdural hematoma: surgical treatment and outcome in 104 patients. Surg Neurol. 1997;48:220–5.
16. Fogelholm R, Heiskanen O, Waltimo O. Chronic subdural hematoma in adults. Influence of patient's age on symptoms, signs, and thickness of hematoma. J Neurosurg. 1975;42:43–6.
17. Fruin AH, Juhl GL, Taylon C. Interhemispheric subdural hematoma. Case report. J Neurosurg. 1984;60:1300–2.
18. Gabaeff SC. Investigating the possibility and probability of perinatal subdural hematoma progressing to chronic subdural hematoma, with and without complications, in neonates, and its potential relationship to the misdiagnosis of abusive head trauma. Leg Med (Tokyo). 2013;15:177–92.

19. Gastone P, Fabrizia C, Homere M, Cacciola F, Alberto M, Nicola DL. Chronic subdural hematoma: results of a homogeneous series of 159 patients operated on by residents. Neurol India. 2004;52:475–7.
20. Gelabert-González M, Fernández-Villa JM, López-García E, García-Allut A. [Chronic subdural hematoma in patients over 80 years of age]. Neurocirugia (Astur). 2001;12:325–30.
21. Gelabert-González M, Iglesias-Pais M, García-Allut A, Martínez-Rumbo R. Chronic subdural haematoma: surgical treatment and outcome in 1000 cases. Clin Neurol Neurosurg. 2005;107:223–9.
22. Gelabert-González M, Román-Pena P, Arán-Echabe E. Chronic subdural hematoma in the oldest-old population. Neurosurg Rev. 2018;41:983–4.
23. Group TWB. World Bank Country and Lending Groups. 2020. Accessed 28 Dec 2020.
24. Herath H, Matthias AT, Kulatunga A. Acute on chronic bilateral subdural hematoma presenting with acute complete flaccid paraplegia and urinary retention mimicking an acute spinal cord injury: a case report. BMC Res Notes. 2017;10:627.
25. Ichinose D, Tochigi S, Tanaka T, Suzuki T, Takei J, Hatano K, Kajiwara I, Maruyama F, Sakamoto H, Hasegawa Y, Tani S, Murayama Y. Concomitant intracranial and lumbar chronic subdural hematoma treated by fluoroscopic guided lumbar puncture: a case report and literature review. Neurol Med Chir (Tokyo). 2018;58:178–84.
26. Jones S, Kafetz K. A prospective study of chronic subdural haematomas in elderly patients. Age Ageing. 1999;28:519–21.
27. Ju MW, Kim SH, Kwon HJ, Choi SW, Koh HS, Youm JY, Song SH. Comparison between brain atrophy and subdural volume to predict chronic subdural hematoma: volumetric CT imaging analysis. Korean J Neurotrauma. 2015;11:87–92.
28. Kak VK, Gleadhill CA. Chronic subdural haematoma (a review of 66 cases). Ulster Med J. 1971;40:163–8.
29. Kim BG, Lee KS, Shim JJ, Yoon SM, Doh JW, Bae HG. What determines the laterality of the chronic subdural hematoma? J Korean Neurosurg Soc. 2010;47:424–7.
30. Kim HI, Oh YJ, Cho YN, Choi YC. Subdural hemorrhage mimicking peripheral neuropathy. J Korean Neurosurg Soc. 2014;56:166–7.
31. Kitya D, Punchak M, Abdelgadir J, Obiga O, Harborne D, Haglund MM. Causes, clinical presentation, management, and outcomes of chronic subdural hematoma at Mbarara Regional Referral Hospital. Neurosurg Focus. 2018;45:E7.
32. Kotwica Z, Brzeiński J. Epilepsy in chronic subdural haematoma. Acta Neurochir (Wien). 1991;113:118–20.
33. Kumar AS, Alugolu R. Chronic subdural hematoma presenting as diplegia—a rare presentation. J Neurosci Rural Pract. 2014;5:445–6.
34. Lee KS. Chronic subdural hematoma in the aged, trauma or degeneration? J Korean Neurosurg Soc. 2016;59:1–5.
35. Lesoin F, Destee A, Jomin M, Warot P, Wilson SG. Quadriparesis as an unusual manifestation of chronic subdural haematoma. J Neurol Neurosurg Psychiatry. 1983;46:783–5.
36. Liliang PC, Tsai YD, Liang CL, Lee TC, Chen HJ. Chronic subdural haematoma in young and extremely aged adults: a comparative study of two age groups. Injury. 2002;33:345–8.
37. Lin CL, Hwang SL, Su YF, Tsai LC, Kwan AL, Howng SL, Loh JK. External subdural drainage in the treatment of infantile chronic subdural hematoma. J Trauma. 2004;57:104–7.
38. Luxon LM, Harrison MJ. Chronic subdural haematoma. Q J Med. 1979;48:43–53.
39. MacFarlane MR, Weerakkody Y, Kathiravel Y. Chronic subdural haematomas are more common on the left than on the right. J Clin Neurosci. 2009;16:642–4.
40. Markwalder TM. Chronic subdural hematomas: a review. J Neurosurg. 1981;54:637–45.
41. Matsumoto H, Matsumoto S, Yoshida Y. Concomitant intracranial chronic subdural hematoma and spinal subdural hematoma: a case report and literature review. World Neurosurg. 2016;90:706.e1–9.
42. Mekaj AY, Morina AA, Mekaj YH, Manxhuka-Kerliu S, Miftari EI, Duci SB, Hamza AR, Gashi MM, Xhelaj MR, Kelmendi FM, Morina Q. Surgical treatment of 137 cases with chronic subdural hematoma at the university clinical center of Kosovo during the period 2008-2012. J Neurosci Rural Pract. 2015;6:186–90.
43. Mezue WC, Ohaebgulam SC, Chikani MC, Erechukwu AU. Changing trends in chronic subdural haematoma in Nigeria. Afr J Med Med Sci. 2011;40:373–6.
44. Miranda LB, Braxton E, Hobbs J, Quigley MR. Chronic subdural hematoma in the elderly: not a benign disease. J Neurosurg. 2011;114:72–6.
45. Mochizuki Y, Kobayashi T, Kawashima A, Funatsu T, Kawamata T. Chronic subdural hema-

toma of the posterior fossa treated by suboccipital craniotomy. Surg Neurol Int. 2018;9:20.
46. Mori K, Maeda M. Surgical treatment of chronic subdural hematoma in 500 consecutive cases: clinical characteristics, surgical outcome, complications, and recurrence rate. Neurol Med Chir (Tokyo). 2001;41:371–81.
47. Nakaguchi H, Tanishima T, Yoshimasu N. Factors in the natural history of chronic subdural hematomas that influence their postoperative recurrence. J Neurosurg. 2001;95:256–62.
48. Osada Y, Shibahara I, Nakagawa A, Sakata H, Niizuma K, Saito R, Kanamori M, Fujimura M, Suzuki S, Tominaga T. Unilateral chronic subdural hematoma due to spontaneous intracranial hypotension: a report of four cases. Br J Neurosurg. 2020;34:632–7.
49. Powers CJ, Fuchs HE, George TM. Chronic subdural hematoma of the neonate: report of two cases and literature review. Pediatr Neurosurg. 2007;43:25–8.
50. Rauhala M, Helén P, Seppä K, Huhtala H, Iverson GL, Niskakangas T, Öhman J, Luoto TM. Long-term excess mortality after chronic subdural hematoma. Acta Neurochir (Wien). 2020;162:1467–78.
51. Robinson RG. Chronic subdural hematoma: surgical management in 133 patients. J Neurosurg. 1984;61:263–8.
52. Rozzelle CJ, Wofford JL, Branch CL. Predictors of hospital mortality in older patients with subdural hematoma. J Am Geriatr Soc. 1995;43:240–4.
53. Rubin G, Rappaport ZH. Epilepsy in chronic subdural haematoma. Acta Neurochir (Wien). 1993;123:39–42.
54. Santarius T, Kirkpatrick PJ, Kolias AG, Hutchinson PJ. Working toward rational and evidence-based treatment of chronic subdural hematoma. Clin Neurosurg. 2010;57:112–22.
55. Schilder JC, Weisfelt M. Ataxia associated with an interhemispheric subdural hematoma: a case report. Cases J. 2009;2:8876.
56. Soleman J, Nocera F, Mariani L. The conservative and pharmacological management of chronic subdural haematoma. Swiss Med Wkly. 2017;147:w14398.
57. Soleman J, Taussky P, Fandino J, Muroi C. Evidence based treatment of chronic subdural hematoma. In: Sadaka DF, editor. Traumatic brain injury. InTechOpen; 2014.
58. Sousa EB, Brandão LF, Tavares CB, Borges IB, Neto NG, Kessler IM. Epidemiological characteristics of 778 patients who underwent surgical drainage of chronic subdural hematomas in Brasília, Brazil. BMC Surg. 2013;13:5.
59. Takahashi K, Mima T, Akiba Y. Chronic subdural hematoma associated with spontaneous intracranial hypotension: therapeutic strategies and outcomes of 55 cases. Neurol Med Chir (Tokyo). 2016;56:69–76.
60. Takemoto Y, Matsumoto J, Ohta K, Hasegawa S, Miura M, Kuratsu J. Bilateral posterior fossa chronic subdural hematoma treated with craniectomy: case report and review of the literature. Surg Neurol Int. 2016;7:S255–8.
61. Turgut M, Akhaddar A, Turgut AT. Calcified or ossified chronic subdural hematoma: a systematic review of 114 cases reported during last century with a demonstrative case report. World Neurosurg. 2020;134:240–63.
62. Uno M, Toi H, Hirai S. Chronic subdural hematoma in elderly patients: is this disease benign? Neurol Med Chir (Tokyo). 2017;57:402–9.
63. Weisberg SD, Houten JK. An unusual presentation of chronic subdural hematoma with isolated footdrop. World Neurosurg. 2019;121:166–8.
64. Won SY, Dubinski D, Sautter L, Hattingen E, Seifert V, Rosenow F, Freiman T, Strzelczyk A, Konczalla J. Seizure and status epilepticus in chronic subdural hematoma. Acta Neurol Scand. 2019;140:194–203.
65. Yadav YR, Parihar V, Namdev H, Bajaj J. Chronic subdural hematoma. Asian J Neurosurg. 2016;11:330–42.
66. Yamada SM, Tomita Y, Murakami H, Nakane M, Yamada S, Murakami M, Hoya K, Nakagomi T, Tamura A, Matsuno A. Headache in patients with chronic subdural hematoma: analysis in 1080 patients. Neurosurg Rev. 2018;41:549–56.
67. Yamashima T, Friede RL. Why do bridging veins rupture into the virtual subdural space? J Neurol Neurosurg Psychiatry. 1984;47:121–7.
68. Yang AI, Balser DS, Mikheev A, Offen S, Huang JH, Babb J, Rusinek H, Samadani U. Cerebral atrophy is associated with development of chronic subdural haematoma. Brain Inj. 2012;26:1731–6.
69. Yang W, Huang J. Chronic subdural hematoma: epidemiology and natural history. Neurosurg Clin N Am. 2017;28:205–10.

第 10 章 慢性硬膜下血肿与癫痫

Amal Satté 和 Jamal Mounach

译者：郭旭飞

10.1 引言

癫痫发作是慢性硬膜下血肿（CSDH）的常见并发症之一，然而目前关于癫痫发作的许多方面仍然存在争议，包括其定义、分类、病理生理学，以及诊断标准和治疗等。首个癫痫及癫痫发作类型的分类是由 Gatsaut 于 1969 年提出的，多年来，癫痫和癫痫发作的定义及其分类也逐步变化。国际抗癫痫联盟（ILAE）在综合临床、脑电图（EEG）、影像学以及遗传学发现后，对该标准进行了多次修订。癫痫发作的定义为由于大脑内异常、过度或同步的神经元活动而导致的一过性体征和（或）症状[13]。

在过去，癫痫被定义为一种以至少两次无诱因发作为特征的疾病，其发病间隔需超过 24 h[13]。ILAE 和国际癫痫署（IBE）最近一致认为，最好将癫痫视为一种疾病，而非功能紊乱。修订后的定义表明癫痫可以在以下情况被诊断：①至少两次非诱发性或反射性发作，间隔 > 24 h；②一次非诱发性发作或反射性发作，且在未来 10 年内再次发作的概率大于 60%；③诊断为癫痫综合征。

诱发性癫痫发作是由作用于正常大脑的暂时性降低癫痫发作阈值的因素，如低血糖、高血糖、酗酒或滥用药物等所引起的发作。"非诱发性"则是指在该时间点不存在导致癫痫发作的短暂性诱发因素[11-12]。

急性症状性癫痫是由外伤、脑炎和卒中等急性病程所引起的。一些作者将急性症状性癫痫发作与诱发性癫痫发作归为一类，因为两者后续癫痫发作的风险都很低。然而，与诱发性癫痫发作不同的是，急性症状性癫痫发作可能引起脑部改变，从而导致远期症状性癫痫发作[7, 16]。

在 CSDH 中，癫痫发作应分为急性期以及远期症状性癫痫发作。急性症状性癫痫发作定义为在系统性损伤时发生的或与病案记录的脑损伤有密切时间关系的临床癫痫发作。如果癫痫发作发生在受伤后的前 7 天内，则被认为是急性症状[5-6, 25]。在 CSDH 中，癫痫发作发生为 CSDH 首次临床诊断或血肿复发后 1 周内，则被认为是癫痫发作急性期[48]。远期症状性癫痫发作发生在没有急性诱发因素的情况下（即非诱发性癫痫发作），但有既往静止性损伤的证据[25]。在 CSDH 中，远期症状性癫痫被定义为发生在确定 CSDH 临床诊断的 1 周后，且与血肿复发及任何其他急性脑损伤无关[48]。

值得注意的是，大多数关于 CSDH 的研究没有区分早期或远期症状性癫痫发作[49]。需要更大规模的研究来区分两种类型的癫痫发作，以更好地了解其危险因素、临床特征以及患者预后。

10.2 CSDH 患者癫痫发作的流行病学

CSDH 患者急性症状性癫痫发作的发生率为 2%～42%。总体而言，其发生率低于急性硬膜下血肿（SDH）[26, 49]。创伤后癫痫发作的临床危险因素包括酗酒、既往卒中史、精神状态异常、入院时格拉斯哥昏迷评分（GCS 评分）低、出院时平均格拉斯哥预后评分（GOS 评分）。影像危险因素包括脑萎缩和混合密度 SDH。接受开颅手术的患者癫痫发作的风险也更高，尤其是晚期症状性癫痫发作。年龄、中线移位程度和血肿大小不是癫痫发作的预测因素[17, 39, 49]。

10.3 病理生理学

CSDH 癫痫发作有几种可能机制。其中可能的机制之一是由于血肿的占位效应直接刺激大脑皮质，从而减少了局部脑血流量[21, 39]。此外，纤维蛋白原降解产物可以促使血肿膜的形成并刺激大脑皮质[49]。接受血肿膜切开术的患者比接受钻孔引流的患者更容易出现癫痫发作，这表明 SDH 或手术操作引起的神经胶质增生可能在癫痫的发生发展中发挥作用。混合密度血肿的占位效应更明显，同时产生更多的纤维蛋白原降解产物，从而导致更显著的皮质刺激和更剧烈的神经元兴奋刺激[39, 49]。最后，相关的脑损伤也可能起重要作用，包括并发的脑损伤，如脑挫伤，也包括由卒中、酗酒或脑萎缩引起的既往脑部病变[39, 49]。

10.4 癫痫发作类型

2017年ILAE将癫痫的发作分为局灶性、全面性和原因不明性发作[12]。然而，目前大多数关于CSDH的研究都没有描述癫痫发作的类型。由于CSDH刺激局部皮质，因此预计引起局灶性而非全身性癫痫发作。部分描述了患者临床特征的研究表示，只有20%~40%的癫痫发作是局灶性的，60%~80%是全身性的[8, 17]。然而，这些研究并未明确将癫痫发作定为全身性发作或是局灶性意识障碍发作（以前被称为继发性全身性发作）[39]。报告的局灶性癫痫为Jackson发作或感觉性发作。在CSDH中，发作性言语障碍如失语症、言语错乱或命名障碍等很少见[2]。Levin报道了一例双侧慢性硬膜下血肿患者，其表现为精神运动性癫痫，曾被误诊为功能性神经系统疾病[40]。癫痫持续状态（SE）非常少见，但其与患者不良预后相关[38, 48]。在一项为期23年的研究中，诊断为SDH的患者超过1 583 255人，其中SE的患病率为0.5%。Seif在此研究中表明，老年患者、黑人以及呼吸、代谢、血液和肾脏功能障碍患者的死亡率更高[38]。也有研究报道了非惊厥性癫痫持续状态表现为意识水平下降或局灶性功能缺陷[10]。癫痫发作症状通常与影像学表现不匹配，因此这也凸显了脑电图的重要作用。

10.5 CSDH的脑电图表现

很少有研究描述过CSDH的脑电图表现。随着影像技术的出现和发展，脑电图对诊断CSDH的重要性不断下降。然而，脑电图作为一项重要的工具，仍能为CSDH患者的治疗提供有价值的信息。CSDH会导致皮质和记录电极之间的距离增加，导致血肿侧与对侧半球相比振幅降低。另一方面，CSDH通过过滤脑部快速活动，导致优势波减慢、中断或消失。双侧弥漫性减慢是CSDH中最常见的脑电异常，在血肿侧的半球更为突出[19]。脑电减慢和衰减虽是CSDH的典型表现，但非CSDH特有，也可由头皮肿胀、脑膜瘤、脑梗死、积液等引起[23]（图10.1和图10.2）。

周期性偏侧癫痫样放电（PLED）或偏侧周期性放电（LPD）也在CSDH中有报道，可以在血肿清除之前或之后观察到[35, 44]。这种癫痫放电模式由周期或类周期尖峰波组成，间隔为1~3秒。PLED的发生机制尚不完全清楚，大多数研究表明它们可能是由于大脑皮质部分功能、解剖位置隔离，或是大脑皮质传入神经阻滞导致的[44]。因为并不总是与癫痫发作有关，因此该理论较难用于解

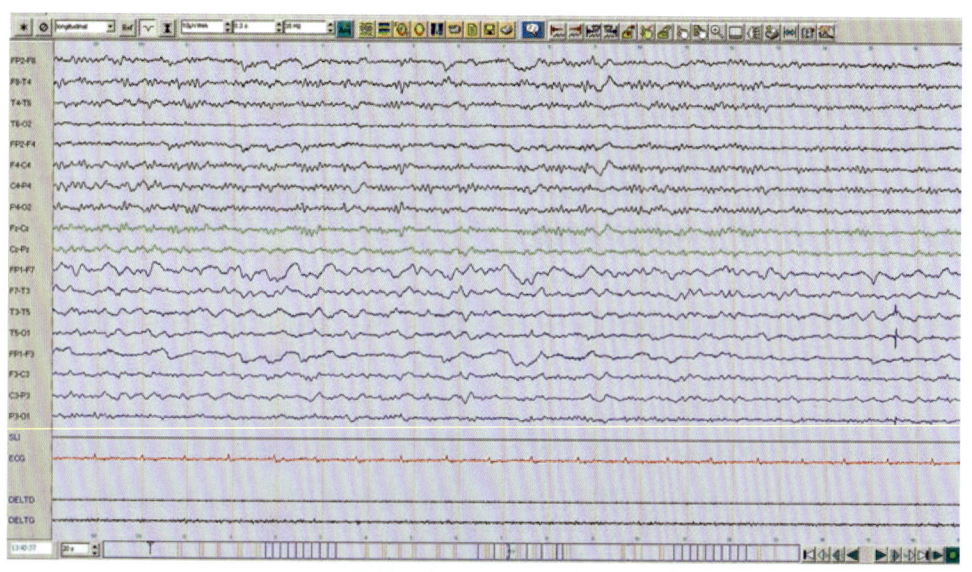

图10.1 64岁女性左侧大脑半球脑电减慢与左侧CSDH相关

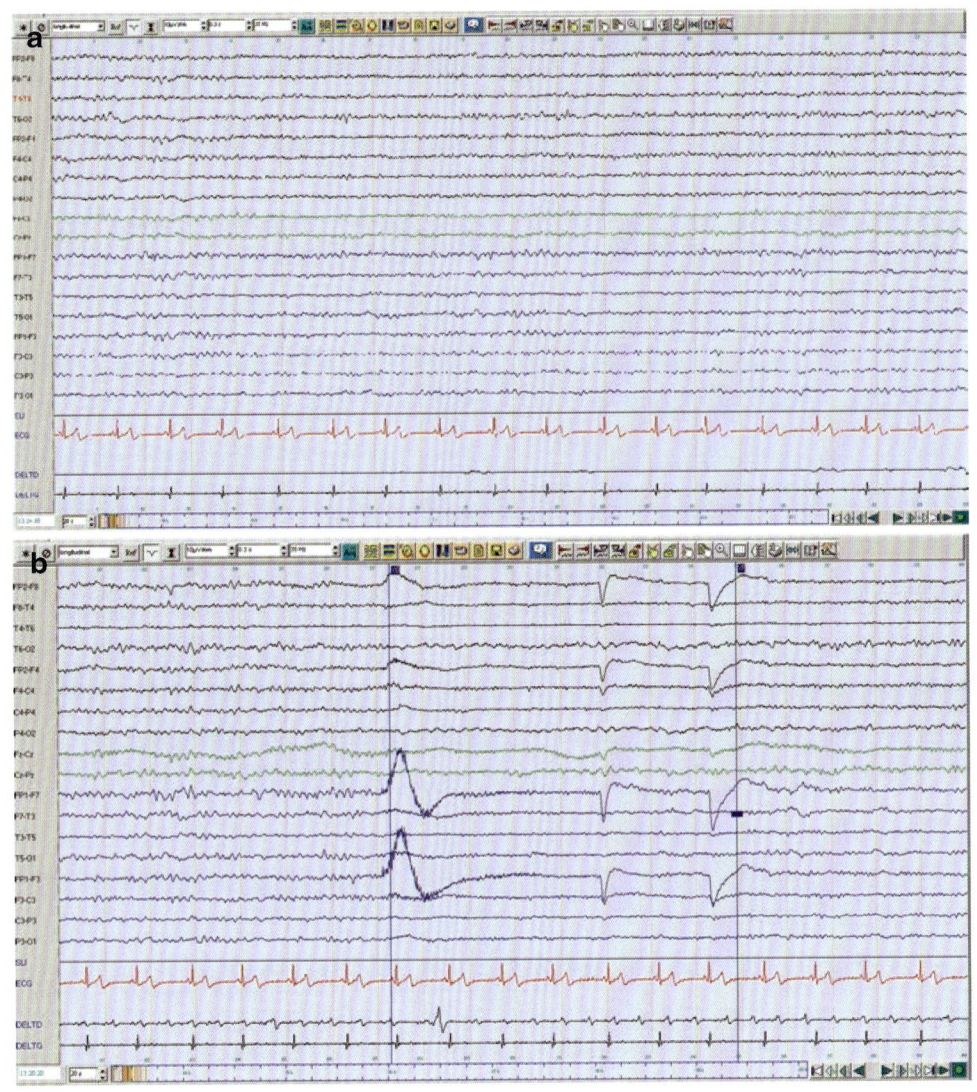

图 10.2（a，b）：男性，58 岁，双侧硬膜下血肿，表现为意识不清。脑电图显示双侧弥漫性脑电减慢

释癫痫发作。临床诊治重点是要区分致痫与非致痫性放电，以更好地指导治疗。周期性偏侧放电可细分为 PLED plus 和 PLED proper。PLED plus 的特点是放电节律快，并有单个或数个尖峰，与癫痫发作（发作前兆/发作）有关，特别是当放电周期很短（1 hz 或更短）时，振幅较高，频率和形态有所波动，并且出现宽大期。PLED proper 较少与癫痫发作相关（6%，而 PLED plus 则为 74%），特别是当 PLED 的脑电形态单一，周期长（0.5 Hz 或更长）以及振幅较低时[14,31]。详见图 10.3a、b。

在 PLED 患者中，长时间的脑电监测可以提供重要信息，并可能检测到亚临床癫痫发作（图 10.4）。

癫痫样放电很常见，既可以在血肿侧，也可以双侧出现。中线癫痫样放电可作为中线移位的标志。对侧放电也有报道，可能与肿块效应、相关损伤或先前的脑部疾病有关（图 10.4）[34,39]。

局灶性间歇性节律性 δ 波（FIRDA）可被视为局灶致痫性电位[39]（图 10.4）。

癫痫持续状态的典型特征是持续的节律性活动。然而，在一些非惊厥性癫痫持续状态和亚临床癫痫发作中，标准脑电图可能不提示癫痫发作。对于 CSDH 患者，特别是在意识障碍患者中，强烈建议进行长期脑电图监测，这样可以更好地研究 PLED 并识别癫痫发作[3,10,19,38]。

10.6 CSDH 癫痫发作的鉴别诊断

CSDH 癫痫发作的鉴别诊断应包括所有可能引起短暂性或波动性功能神经症状的情况。因为许多患者尽管检查结果呈阴性，但仍被诊断为癫痫，因

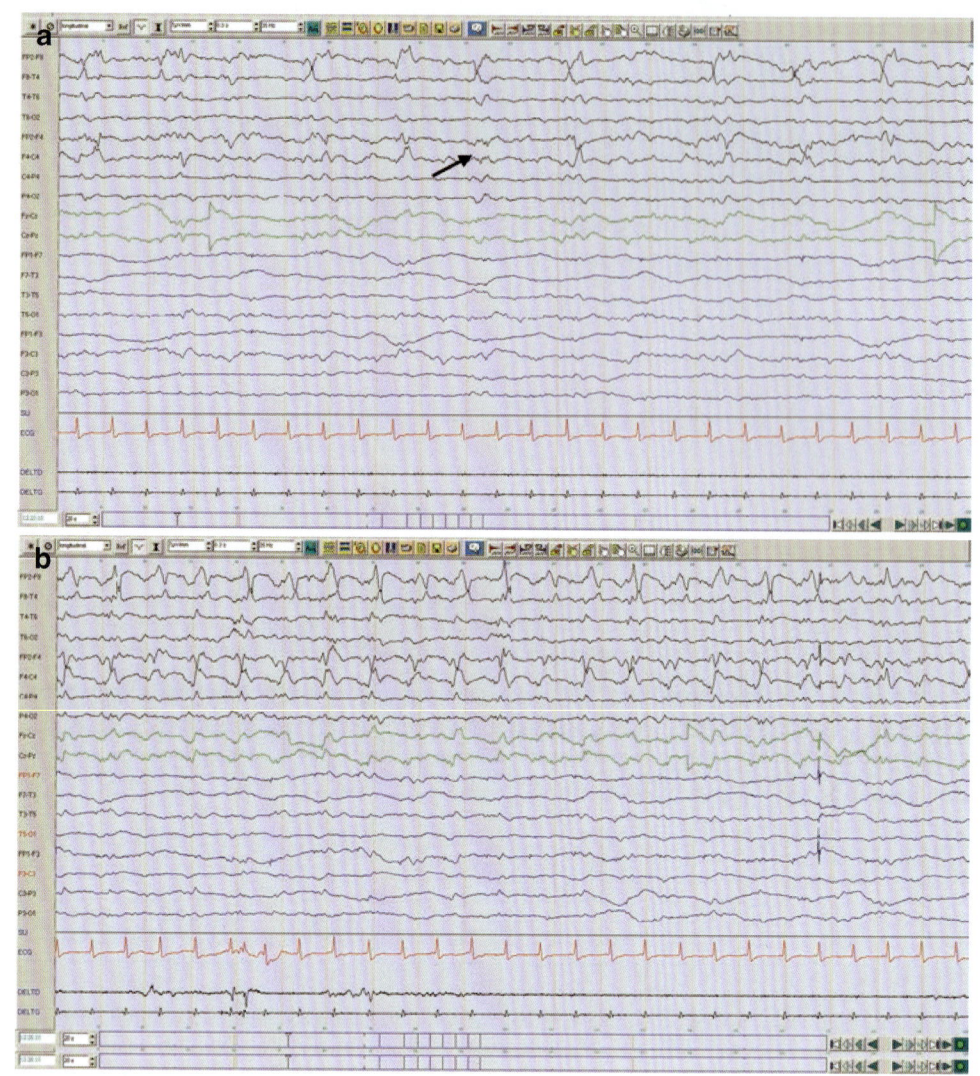

图 10.3 （a，b）65 岁右侧 CSDH 患者术后的延长脑电图，其表现为单次短暂的左侧阵挛性运动，随后意识受损。脑电图显示右侧周期性偏侧癫痫样放电，因为它们有时与复合波形内的尖峰波相关（箭头）可归类为 PLED plus。图 10.3b 的周期为 1 hz，幅值较高，图 10.3a 与 b 之间的频率和形态有明显的函数关系。所有这些脑电图特征都预示癫痫发作，需要紧急处理以避免发展为癫痫持续状态

此确定癫痫发作的潜在机制虽然困难但很重要。

CSDH 后脑损伤可能由血肿量、颅内压（ICP）升高或血液代谢物等多种因素引起。

皮质扩散性去极化是大脑灰质中神经元和胶质细胞的一种扩散性去极化波，其后是电活动的一过性抑制[43]。最近，在一项对 40 名接受 CSDH 清除术的患者进行的前瞻性观察研究中，Mohammad 等发现有 6 名（15%）患者检测到皮质扩散性去极化（SD），并与手术后神经恶化相关[24]。在另一项研究中，Levesque 对 59 例 SDH 患者的临床表现和脑电图特征进行了比较分析，研究发现阵挛性运动、意识障碍、阳性症状、对抗癫痫药物的反应以及死亡率与脑电图异常具有相关性，而语言障碍和长时间发作则与阴性脑电图结果相关。研究者提出使用"NESIS"（非癫痫性、刻板性、间歇性症状，non epileptic, stereotypical and intermittent symptoms）这一术语来界定后一类脑电图阴性患者群体，强调其与癫痫发作现象的鉴别诊断具有重要临床意义，因为这类症状具有特定的临床预后与治疗意义[22]。

CSDH 可出现短暂性缺血，也可导致症状反复。脑电图监测和经颅多普勒超声可以为 CSDH 的血流动力学机制提供相关的证据[1]。

最后，患者的自身相关情况也可能引起短暂的神经系统症状，如住院期间低血糖、高血糖、住院期间酒精或药物戒断等。

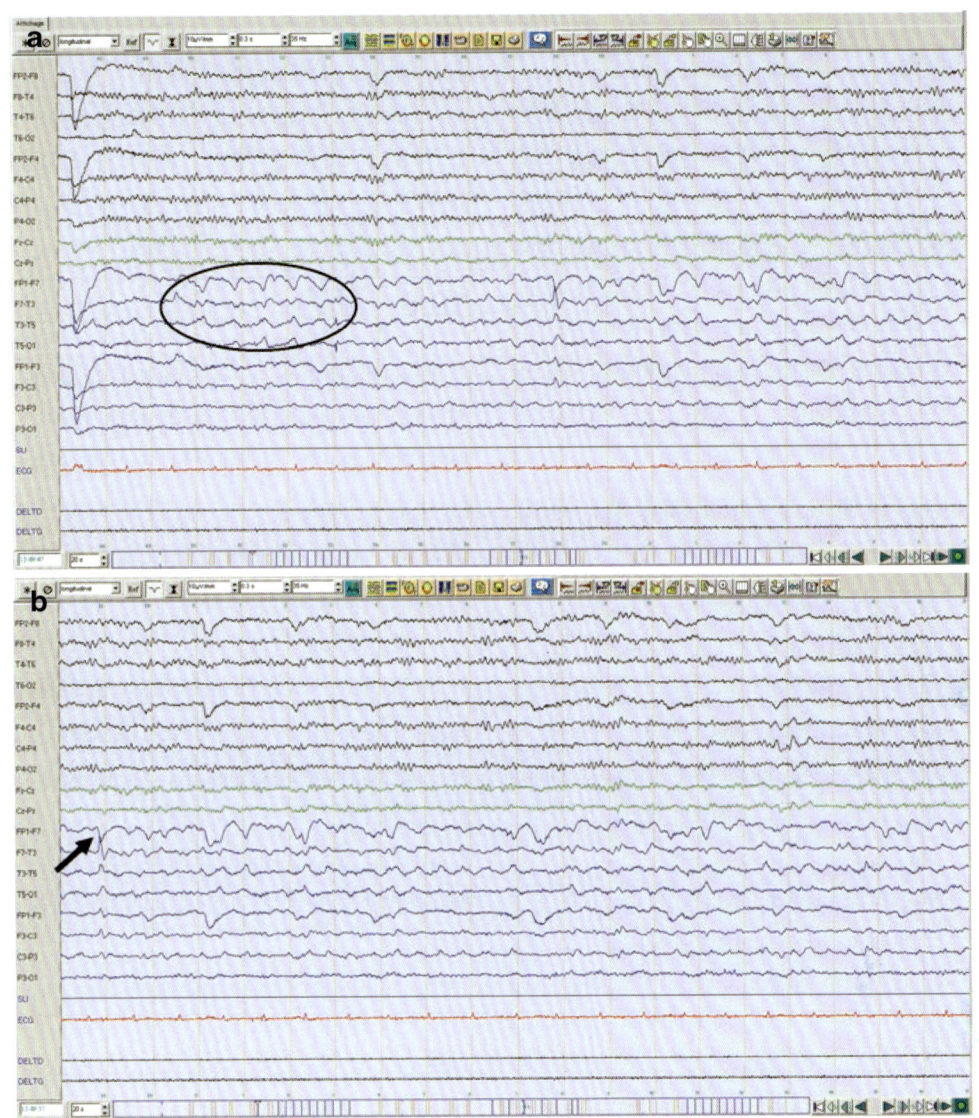

图 10.4 （a，b）48 岁男性，表现为全身性强直-阵挛性发作，左侧 CSDH。脑电图显示左额叶间歇性节律性 δ 波（FIRDA）（椭圆形标识）和 F7 上的尖峰（箭头指示）

10.7 治疗

目前对于 CSDH 的预防性抗癫痫药物治疗没有共识性建议，也缺乏随机对照试验。由于在部分研究中，CSDH 术前和术后癫痫发作的发生率很高，并且与不良的临床结局和较高死亡率相关，因此建议预防性使用抗癫痫药物[15, 46]。而不建议使用抗癫痫药物的原因是抗癫痫药物不能改善患者出院时的预后[42, 47-48]，在许多患者中清除血肿可以控制癫痫发作症状，无需给予抗癫痫药物[33, 50]。另一方面，使用抗癫痫药物也有不良影响，因为多数药物都存在副作用以及药物间的相互作用。Cochrane 的一篇综述研究了 CSDH 中预防性抗癫痫药物的使用。结果显示，从目前的研究中无法得出任何结论，未来需要进行随机对照试验[30]。在共识达成之前，临床医生应该权衡药物与这些疗法相关的风险，还要考虑到癫痫发作的危险因素以及患者的临床病史、体格检查等。此外，脑电图（包括术前脑电图、术后脑电图和必要情况下的长期脑电图监测）应作为决定是否开始抗癫痫治疗评估标准中的重要组成部分。

关于 CSDH，目前尚缺乏关于优先选择何种抗癫痫药物以及治疗剂量与使用时间的循证证据，因此多由临床医生基于经验决定，而非指南指导。目前苯妥英被广泛用于预防癫痫发作，然而更推荐使用副作用较小的新型抗癫痫药物。多项研究表明，左乙拉西坦在脑外伤（TBI）和 CSDH 患者中与苯妥英效果相近[20, 29, 32]。相较于左乙拉西坦，由于苯妥英副作用更多、药物相互作用更显著，使用时需要更密切的监测。

在癫痫持续状态中，一线治疗包括苯二氮䓬类药物，而二线抗癫痫药物包括苯妥英静注、磷苯妥英、丙戊酸钠、苯巴比妥、左乙拉西坦和拉科酰胺等。美国和许多其他国家更习惯于使用苯妥英或磷苯妥英[27]。然而，最近的一项meta分析和效益研究表明，现有证据并不支持使用苯妥英，无论是在有效性方面还是在成本方面。根据这项研究，丙戊酸盐和苯巴比妥治疗癫痫持续状态更有效，且苯巴比妥优于苯妥英[37]。

在老年人中，药物的选择应更加谨慎，不仅要考虑患者诊断，还要考虑患者的既往史以及药物的不良反应和药物间相互作用。对于肝病患者，应首选非肝脏代谢类药物，如左乙拉西坦。相反，对于肾功能不全的患者，应给予卡马西平或丙戊酸钠。部分新型药物（加巴喷丁、普瑞巴林、左乙拉西坦）因不与其他药物、肝酶、血浆蛋白产生相互作用，因此更适合该年龄段的患者使用[18]。

预防性抗癫痫治疗的持续时间仍然存在争议，除非癫痫发作，否则疗程范围从3个月到2年不等[17, 26, 39, 41, 48]。未来有必要在相关领域进行对照临床研究，以指导临床使用。

最后，目前缺乏CSDH急性症状性癫痫发作患者的长期预后数据。对于在CSDH数月后才出现癫痫发作的患者，治疗方法与其他癫痫相似[39]。

10.8 预后

一些研究认为，CSDH癫痫发作的患者出院后其预后比无癫痫发作的患者更差[4, 17, 28, 48, 50]。癫痫发作是躯体、认知和社会心理等方面的不良预后的独立预测因素[48]。虽然癫痫发作会影响早期功能结局，但存在晚期良好恢复的可能[17, 28]。CSDH癫痫发作患者的死亡率更高[4, 36]。

现仍缺乏关于CSDH患者长期癫痫控制和预后的数据[39]。急性症状性癫痫发作患者有迟发性发作可能，并有后期发展为慢性癫痫的趋势[17]。

根据Won等的研究，癫痫发作是CSDH复发的危险因素之一，其比值比（OR）为2.5[9, 45]。

脑电图结果有助于预测功能预后，脑电图显示癫痫样放电的患者在出院时和随访6个月时功能预后较差[28, 35, 39]。

参考文献

1. Alkhachroum AM, Fernandez-Baca Vaca G, Sundararajan S, Degeorgia M. Post-subdural hematoma transient ischemic attacks: hypoperfusion mechanism supported by quantitative electroencephalography and transcranial Doppler sonography. Stroke. 2017;48(3):e87–90.
2. Alliez J-R, Balan C, Kaya J-M, Leone M, Reynier Y, Alliez B. Hématome sous-dural chronique de l'adulte. EMC—Neurol. 2007;4(4):1–9.
3. Banoczi W. ICU-cEEG monitoring. Neurodiagn J. 2020;60(4):231–71.
4. Battaglia F, Lubrano V, Ribeiro-Filho T, Pradel V, Roche PH. Incidence et impact clinique des crises comitiales périopératoires pour les hématomes sous-duraux chroniques. Neurochirurgie. 2012;58(4):230–4.
5. Beghi E, Carpio A, Forsgren L, Hesdorffer DC, Malmgren K, et al. Recommendation for a definition of acute symptomatic seizure. Epilepsia. 2010;51(4):671–5.
6. Beleza P. Acute symptomatic seizures: a clinically oriented review. Neurologist. 2012;18(3):109–19.
7. Bergey GK. Management of a first seizure. Contin Lifelong Learn Neurol. 2016;22:38–50.
8. Chen CW, Kuo JR, Lin HJ, Yeh CH, Wong BS, et al. Early post-operative seizures after burr-hole drainage for chronic subdural hematoma: correlation with brain CT findings. J Clin Neurosci. 2004;11(7):706–9.
9. Chon KH, Lee JM, Koh EJ, Choi HY. Independent predictors for recurrence of chronic subdural hematoma. Acta Neurochir (Wien). 2012;154(9):1541–8.
10. Driver J, DiRisio AC, Mitchell H, Threlkeld ZD, Gormley WB. Non-electrographic seizures due to subdural hematoma: a case series and review of the literature. Neurocrit Care. 2019;30(1):16–21.
11. Fisher RS, Acevedo C, Arzimanoglou A, Bogacz A, Cross JH, et al. ILAE Official Report: a practical clinical definition of epilepsy. Epilepsia. 2014;55(4):475–82.

12. Fisher RS, Cross JH, French JA, Higurashi N, Hirsch E, et al. Operational classification of seizure types by the International League Against Epilepsy: position paper of the ILAE Commission for Classification and Terminology. Epilepsia. 2017;58(4):522–30.
13. Fisher RS, Van Emde Boas W, Blume W, Elger C, Genton P, et al. Response: definitions proposed by the International League Against Epilepsy (ILAE) and the International Bureau for Epilepsy (IBE) [4]. Epilepsia. 2005;46(10):1701–2.
14. Gelisse P, Crespel A, Genton P. Atlas of electroencephalography. In: Neurology and critical care. Montrouge: John Libbey Eurotext; 2019. p. 3346.
15. Grobelny BT, Ducruet AF, Zacharia BE, Hickman ZL, Andersen KN, et al. Preoperative antiepileptic drug administration and the incidence of postoperative seizures following bur hole-treated chronic subdural hematoma: clinical article. J Neurosurg. 2009;111(6):1257–62.
16. Hesdorffer DC, Benn EKT, Cascino GD, Hauser WA. Is a first acute symptomatic seizure epilepsy? Mortality and risk for recurrent seizure. Epilepsia. 2009;50(5):1102–8.
17. Huang YH, Yang TM, Lin YJ, Tsai NW, Lin WC, et al. Risk factors and outcome of seizures after chronic subdural hematoma. Neurocrit Care. 2011;14(2):253–9.
18. Jankovic SM, Dostic M. Choice of antiepileptic drugs for the elderly: possible drug interactions and adverse effects. Expert Opin Metab Toxicol. 2012;8(1):81–91.
19. Kaminski HJ, Hlavin ML, Likavec MJ, Schmidley JW. Transient neurologic deficit caused by chronic subdural hematoma. Am J Med. 1992;92(6):698–700.
20. Khan NR, Vanlandingham MA, Fierst TM, Hymel C, Hoes K, et al. Should levetiracetam or phenytoin be used for posttraumatic seizure prophylaxis? A systematic review of the literature and meta-analysis. Neurosurgery. 2016;79(6):775–81.
21. Kwon TH, Park YK, Lim DJ, Cho TH, Chung YG, et al. Chronic subdural hematoma: evaluation of the clinical significance of postoperative drainage volume. J Neurosurg. 2000;93(5):796–9.
22. Levesque M, Iorio-Morin C, Bocti C, Vézina C, Deacon C. Nonepileptic, stereotypical, and intermittent symptoms (NESIS) in patients with subdural hematoma: proposal for a new clinical entity with therapeutic and prognostic implications. Neurosurgery. 2020;87(1):96–103.
23. Marcuse LV, Fields MC, Yoo J, Rowan AJ. Rowan's primer of EEG. 2nd ed. Elsevier; 2016. p. 87–9.
24. Mohammad LM, Abbas M, Shuttleworth CW, Ahmadian R, Bhat A, et al. Spreading depolarization may represent a novel mechanism for delayed fluctuating neurological deficit after chronic subdural hematoma evacuation. J Neurosurg. 2020;134(3):1294–302.
25. Nowacki TA, Jirsch JD. Evaluation of the first seizure patient: key points in the history and physical examination. Seizure. 2017;49:54–63.
26. Ohno K, Maehara T, Ichimura K, Suzuki R, Hirakawa K, Monma S. Low incidence of seizures in patients with chronic subdural haematoma. J Neurol Neurosurg Psychiatry. 1993;56(11):1231–3.
27. Pichler M, Hocker S. Management of status epilepticus, vol. 140. 1st ed. Elsevier B.V.; 2017. p. 131–51.
28. Rabinstein AA, Chung SY, Rudzinski LA, Lanzino G. Seizures after evacuation of subdural hematomas: incidence, risk factors, and functional impact: clinical article. J Neurosurg. 2010;112(2):455–60.
29. Radic JAE, Chou SHY, Du R, Lee JW. Levetiracetam versus phenytoin: a comparison of efficacy of seizure prophylaxis and adverse event risk following acute or subacute subdural hematoma diagnosis. Neurocrit Care. 2014;21(2):228–37.
30. Ratilal BO, Pappamikail L, Costa J, Sampaio C. Anticonvulsants for preventing seizures in patients with chronic subdural haematoma. Cochrane Database Syst Rev. 2013;2013(6):CD004893.
31. Reiher J, Rivest J, Maison FG, Leduc CP. Periodic lateralized epileptiform discharges with transitional rhythmic discharges: association with seizures. Electroencephalogr Clin Neurophysiol. 1991;78(1):12–7.
32. Rowe AS, Goodwin H, Brophy GM, Bushwitz J, Castle A, et al. Seizure prophylaxis in neurocritical care: a review of evidence-based support. Pharmacotherapy. 2014;34(4):396–409.
33. Rubin G, Rappaport ZH. Epilepsy in chronic subdural haematoma. Acta Neurochir (Wien). 1993;123:39–42.
34. Rudzinski LA, Rabinstein AA. Response to "epileptiform discharges in acute subdural hematoma: to treat or not to treat". J Clin Neurophysiol. 2012;29(3):287.
35. Rudzinski LA, Rabinstein AA, Chung SY, Wong-Kisiel LC, Burrus TM, et al. Electroencephalographic findings in acute subdural hematoma. J Clin Neurophysiol.

2011;28(6):633–41.
36. Sabo RA, Hanigan WC, Aldag JC. Chronic subdural hematomas and seizures: the role of prophylactic anticonvulsive medication. Surg Neurol. 1995;43(6):579–82.
37. Sánchez Fernández I, Gaínza-Lein M, Lamb N, Loddenkemper T. Meta-analysis and cost-effectiveness of second-line antiepileptic drugs for status epilepticus. Neurology. 2019;92(20):E2339–48.
38. Seifi A, Asadi-Pooya AA, Carr K, Maltenfort M, Emami M, et al. The epidemiology, risk factors, and impact on hospital mortality of status epilepticus after subdural hematoma in the United States. Springerplus. 2014;3(1):1–10.
39. Shihabuddin B, Hinduja A, Yaghi S. Seizures in cerebrovascular disorders. In: Koubeissi MZ et al., editors. Seizures in subdural hematoma. Springer science+business media; 2015. p. 55–69.
40. Levin S. Psychomotor epilepsy as a manifestation of subdural hematoma. Am J Psychiatry. 1951;107(7):501–2.
41. Song Y, Cao C, Xu Q, Gu S, Wang F, et al. Piperine attenuates TBI-induced seizures via inhibiting cytokine-activated reactive astrogliosis. Front Neurol. 2020;11:431.
42. Spoelhof B, Sanchez-Bautista J, Zorrilla-Vaca A, Kaplan PW, Farrokh S, et al. Impact of antiepileptic drugs for seizure prophylaxis on short and long-term functional outcomes in patients with acute intracerebral hemorrhage: a meta-analysis and systematic review. Seizure. 2019;69:140–6.
43. Taş YÇ, Solaroğlu İ, Gürsoy-Özdemir Y. Spreading depolarization waves in neurological diseases: a short review about its pathophysiology and clinical relevance. Curr Neuropharmacol. 2018;17(2):151–64.
44. Westmoreland BF. Periodic lateralized epileptiform discharges after evacuation of subdural hematomas. J Clin Neurophysiol. 2001;18(1):20–4.
45. Won SY, Dubinski D, Eibach M, Gessler F, Herrmann E, et al. External validation and modification of the Oslo grading system for prediction of postoperative recurrence of chronic subdural hematoma. Neurosurg Rev. 2021;44(2):961–70.
46. Won SY, Dubinski D, Freiman T, Seifert V, Gessler F, et al. Acute-on-chronic subdural hematoma: a new entity for prophylactic anti-epileptic treatment? Eur J Trauma Emerg Surg. 2020. https://doi.org/10.1007/s00068-020-01508-9.
47. Won SY, Dubinski D, Herrmann E, Cuca C, Strzelczyk A, et al. Epileptic seizures in patients following surgical treatment of acute subdural hematoma—incidence, risk factors, patient outcome, and development of new scoring system for prophylactic antiepileptic treatment (GATE-24 score). World Neurosurg. 2017;101:416–24.
48. Won SY, Dubinski D, Sautter L, Hattingen E, Seifert V, et al. Seizure and status epilepticus in chronic subdural hematoma. Acta Neurol Scand. 2019;140(3):194–203.
49. Won SY, Konczalla J, Dubinski D, Cattani A, Cuca C, et al. A systematic review of epileptic seizures in adults with subdural haematomas. Seizure. 2017;45:28–35.
50. Yamada T. Evaluation of seizures in patients with chronic subdural hematoma treated by Burr-hole surgery and risk factors for seizures. Int J Brain Disord Treat. 2017;3(1):1–8.

第 11 章 伴精神障碍的慢性硬膜下血肿

Umut Kirli，Öykü Özçelik 和 Osman Vırıt

译者：郭旭飞

11.1 CSDH 伴精神障碍病因学

饮酒与慢性硬膜下血肿（CSDH）之间的关系已被许多研究证实，过量饮酒是 CSDH 发生发展中最常见的危险因素之一。一项关于无头部创伤的亚急性或慢性硬膜下血肿患者的病因研究表明，饮酒与癫痫一样是最常见的 CSDH 诱发因素[8]。此外，一个较大样本量的 CSDH 病例系列（$n=1000$）研究表明，除高血压和糖尿病外，患者最常见的既往史是过量饮酒（$n=132$，13.2%）[19]。过量饮酒也与 CSDH 患者预后较差相关[39]。文献目前提出了几种过量饮酒导致 CSDH 的机制。首先，饮酒会增加跌倒和头部受伤的风险，尤其是老年群体[30]。过量饮酒还会导致其他相关危险因素，如脑萎缩[38]、高血压[23]、糖尿病[49]、血小板及凝血功能改变[2]等。

文献报道药物滥用，特别是兴奋剂类（如安非他明、甲基苯丙胺、摇头丸、阿拉伯茶和可卡因等）与颅内出血风险相关，血压骤升被认为是一种可能的机制。此外，药物滥用与颅内出血之间的关联可能部分由过量饮酒所介导[3, 7, 34, 36, 40, 43, 52]。目前药物滥用与 CSDH 之间的关联还没有得到很好的解释，尚缺乏相关的研究。文献报道了两个病案报告，一例患者可卡因滥用并合并广泛脑梗死以及硬膜下血肿，另一例患者由于服用安非他明引起血管炎及硬膜下和蛛网膜下腔出血[10, 37]。此外，跌落、意外和斗殴等造成的创伤也与药物滥用有间接关联[22]。要对这个问题得出确切的结论，还需要进一步的研究。临床医生应该意识到 CSDH 与药物滥用的潜在联系。

选择性 5-羟色胺再摄取抑制剂（SSRI）的使用可能导致出血时间延长，这是由于 5-羟色胺再摄取进入血小板，导致血小板的聚集性和活性受抑制[4, 21]。因此这些药物的使用也存在问题，即是否可能与颅内出血的风险有关，特别是在老年人中[14]。Meta 分析显示，与 SSRI 相关的颅内出血风险升高，然而该类出血的绝对风险非常低[20, 32]。新发抑郁症本身也可能与颅内出血风险相关，这提示可能存在适应证偏倚[12]。然而，与使用三环类抗抑郁药相比，使用 SSRI 的颅内出血风险更高。这一结果表明，个体风险与使用 SSRI 类药物有关，这可能是由血小板功能改变介导的。目前使用的与 5-羟色胺转运体亲和力较强的抗抑郁药（帕罗西汀、舍曲林、福西汀、度洛西汀和氯丙咪嗪）比对 5-羟色胺再摄取抑制较弱的抗抑郁药（阿戈美拉汀、阿莫沙平、地塞帕明、多舒平、多塞平、异氨基脲、伊普林多、洛非普拉明、马普替林、米安色林、米氮平、莫氯贝胺、奈法唑酮、去甲替林、瑞波西汀、苯乙肼、扑尔敏、曲奈普明、曲美拉明、奥沙津）具有更高的风险[41]。此外，在使用 SSRI 或与抗凝药联合使用的前 30 天内，颅内出血的风险相对较高。尽管存在争议，一些证据表明 SSRI 与抗血小板药物联合使用会增加出血风险[9, 20, 28, 32, 41]。

虽然 SSRI 会轻微增加颅内出血的风险，特别是在使用的第一个月，但这些研究并没有提供硬膜下出血风险的具体数据。CSDH 的病因在某些方面可能与其他类型的颅内出血不同[29]。最近的一项大样本研究表明，使用抗抑郁药物会增加硬膜下出血的风险。风险的增加程度在使用的第一个月最高，第三年后接近于零。与非 SSRI 相比，使用 SSRI 的风险略高。此外，与抗凝血药或非甾体抗炎药（NSAID）等联合使用会增加出血风险，然而出血绝对风险非常低[18]。选择不使用抗抑郁药也会带来其他一些风险。因此，在老年人使用抗抑郁药时应考虑平衡可能的风险与收益。

一些抗抑郁药，尤其是三环类抗抑郁药和 SSRI 类抗抑郁药，与跌倒风险相关[46]，这表明抗抑郁药与硬膜下血肿之间的关联可能不仅仅归因于对血小板功能的影响。此外，抗精神病药、抗焦虑药、催眠药和镇静剂，特别是具有较长半衰期的苯二氮䓖类药物，也与跌倒的风险有关，尤其是在老年人中[30-31, 50]。因此，这些药物也可能通过增加跌倒的风险从而增加 CSDH 的风险。因此这些药物应谨慎使用，特别是在老年人中，并尽可能以最低剂量使用这些药物。

电休克疗法（ECT）是一种常用且相对安全的精神障碍治疗方法。然而，ECT 已被证明会提高大脑代谢，增加颅内压[44]。因此，ECT 可能与硬膜下血肿有关，特别是在存在其他危险因素的情况下，如硬膜下血肿史、脑萎缩、过量饮酒以及使用抗血小板或抗凝药物史[13]。文献报道了与 ECT 相关的罕见硬膜下血肿病例（5 例），其中 1 例死亡[13, 42]。另外，也有文献提出，ECT 可以应用于没有占位效应的硬膜下血肿患者中[51]，然而需要 RCT 研究进行进一步验证。但在开始 ECT 治疗之前，需要进行脑部影像学检查，根据每个病例的特点衡量患者的风险与收益。ECT 后患者若出现谵妄、局灶性神经缺损或意识改变等，临床医生应注意可能出现的硬膜下血肿。

智力障碍和痴呆患者也被报道是 CSDH 的高危人群[1, 15]。此外，痴呆患者出现硬膜下血肿其预后可能更差[1]。相反，CSDH 患者的进行性精神症状可能类似于痴呆，具体见下文。因此，在某些被诊断为"非典型"痴呆的病例中，临床医生应考虑 CSDH 的可能性，这些病例的症状在适当治疗后可能是可逆的。

11.2 慢性硬膜下血肿的精神症状

对于慢性硬膜下血肿（CSDH），从最初的损伤到明确的病理表现之间存在一段时间间隔。一项回顾性研究评估了 1000 例 CSDH 病例的病历，发现平均间隔时间为 49.1 天[19]。此外，据报道，约有一半的 CSDH 患者以精神症状为首发临床表现[24]。因此，由于早期的精神症状，CSDH 患者常被误转入精神科治疗，故而明确与 CSDH 相关的精神症状是很重要的。然而，关于 CSDH 的精神症状的文献目前并不充分。

一项回顾性研究调查了 79 例亚急性或慢性硬膜下血肿患者的临床表现，结果表明 58% 的患者入院时有精神障碍，符合 DSM-Ⅲ 标准。值得注意的是，在 1/5 的患者中，精神障碍是最初的表现。谵妄是最常见的诊断，其次是痴呆和器质性情感综合征[5]。同样，一项纳入 70 例 CSDH 患者的研究表明，人格或智力改变是最常见的临床表现，同时伴有偏瘫[8]。

CSDH 引起的患者认知变化包括注意力、语言、记忆、判断等的细微改变到思维混乱、痴呆和谵妄等。性格和行为的变化通常会被家庭成员注意到，这些变化表现为睡眠障碍、昼夜节律改变、自理能力下降、易冲动疲劳、语言增多、情绪易激动及精神病症状[35]。

精神症状进行性加重在老年人中比年轻患者更常见[47-48]。年轻患者更容易出现急性症状，这种与年龄相关的差异可以解释为因为年轻患者的脑内体积较大，血肿发展的空间更受限[35]。伴有阳性精神病症状（妄想和幻觉）的 CSDH 病例主要发生于 70 岁以上的人群中[6, 17, 26]，然而在较年轻的年龄组中也有例外情况，其表现可为阴性的精神错乱症状[27]。精神症状常随着血肿的吸收而消失。有文献提出，在 CSDH 发病前从未出现过精神症状的年轻患者有更大的治愈机会[24]。

对于 CSDH 精神症状的治疗，在必要时可以适当使用精神类药物。然而需要注意的是，这些药物的副作用（即低钠血症、锥体外系副作用）风险可能较大[27, 33, 45]。一项病例报告报道了 CSDH 患者使用氯氮平（一种低 D2 受体亲和力的抗精神病药）后出现的抗精神病药恶性综合征[16]。

精神类专科医院可能会遗漏 CSDH 的诊断。一项基于 200 例精神病院死亡患者尸检的经典研究显示，14 例（7%）患者有硬膜下血肿，其中 8 例为慢性或亚急性硬膜下血肿。然而，这些患者中只有 1 例死前通过计算机断层成像（CT）得到了诊断[11]，最常见的误诊包括痴呆（阿尔茨海默病或血管性痴呆）以及情感性和精神病综合征。在大多数情况下，痴呆被认为是不可逆转的。然而如果得到有效治疗，CSDH 引起的认知和情感障碍可能会得到治愈[25]，因此尽早诊断 CSDH 至关重要。一些特征表现可能有助于阿尔茨海默病痴呆和 CSDH 的鉴别诊断。阿尔茨海默病患者在对新信息进行优先编码方面存在问题，然而慢性硬膜下血肿患者在提取早期编码信息方面存在缺陷。此外，阿尔茨海默病患者的记忆缺陷史通常以月至年为单位，而 CSDH 患者的记忆缺陷史通常以周为单位[35]。

11.3 结论

因为 CSDH 的临床表现可能为一系列无神经系统症状的精神障碍，因此临床医生更应注意对该病的鉴别诊断[5]。针对精神障碍患者，特别是在老年人和过度饮酒、癫痫和痴呆的患者中，应仔细评估 CSDH 的可能性。在下列情况时，应考虑进行神经影像学检查：

1. 患者出现神经系统症状的同时伴有精神障碍或有头部创伤病史。
2. 认知改变，如意识、合作、注意力、定向力改变；进行性智力障碍或人格变化。
3. 非典型的精神症状并且经治疗后改善有限。
4. 非典型的药物副作用（如低效力 D2 阻滞剂或低剂量下出现的锥体外系副作用）。

参考文献

1. Arca R, Ricchi V, Murgia D, Melis M, Floris F, Mereu A, Contu P, Marrosu F, Cossu G. Parkinsonism and dementia are negative prognostic factors for the outcome of subdural hematoma. Neurol Sci. 2016;37(8):1299–303.
2. Ballard HS. The hematological complications of alcoholism. Alcohol Health Res World. 1997;21(1):42–52.
3. Bede P, El-Kininy N, O'Hara F, Menon P, Finegan E, Healy D. 'Khatatonia'—cathinone-induced hypertensive encephalopathy. Neth J Med. 2017;75(10):448–50.
4. Bismuth-Evenzal Y, Gonopolsky Y, Gurwitz D, Iancu I, Weizman A, Rehavi M. Decreased serotonin content and reduced agonist-induced aggregation in platelets of patients chronically medicated with SSRI drugs. J Affect Disord. 2012;136(1–2):99–103.
5. Black DW. Mental changes resulting from subdural haematoma. Br J Psychiatry. 1984;145:200–3.
6. Brunekreeft JA, Peerdeman SM, Rhebergen D. Subdural hematoma and depression (in German). Tijdschr Psychiatr. 2008;50(5):295–9.
7. Bruno A. Cerebrovascular complications of alcohol and sympathomimetic drug abuse. Curr Neurol Neurosci Rep. 2003;3(1):40–5.
8. Cameron MM. Chronic subdural haematoma: a review of 114 cases. J Neurol Neurosurg Psychiatry. 1978;41(9):834–9.
9. Castro VM, Gallagher PJ, Clements CC, Murphy SN, Gainer VS, Fava M, Weilburg JB, Churchill SE, Kohane IS, Iosifescu DV, Smoller JW, Perlis RH. Incident user cohort study of risk for gastrointestinal bleed and stroke in individuals with major depressive disorder treated with antidepressants. BMJ Open. 2012;2(2):e000544.
10. Chaudhary SC, Sawlani KK, Malhotra HS, Apurva, Nanda S, Rao PK. Cocaine abuse: an unusual association. J Assoc Physicians India. 2016;64(11):77–9.
11. Cole G. Intracranial space-occupying masses in mental hospital patients: necropsy study. J Neurol Neurosurg Psychiatry. 1978;41(8):730–6.
12. Daskalopoulou M, George J, Walters K, Osborn DP, Batty GD, Stogiannis D, Rapsomaniki E, Pujades-Rodriguez M, Denaxas S, Udumyan R, Kivimaki M, Hemingway H. Depression as a risk factor for the initial presentation of twelve cardiac, cerebrovascular, and peripheral arterial diseases: data linkage study of 1.9 million women and men. PLoS One. 2016;11(4):e0153838.
13. Dauleac C, Vinckier F, Bourdillon P. Subdural hematoma and electroconvulsive therapy: a case report and review of the literature. Neurochirurgie. 2019;65(1):40–2.
14. de Abajo FJ. Effects of selective serotonin reuptake inhibitors on platelet function: mechanisms, clinical outcomes and implications for use in elderly patients. Drugs Aging. 2011;28(5):345–67.
15. de Las Heras J, Aldamiz-Echevarria L, Cabrera A. Frontoparietal subdural hematoma in a child with mental regression. JAMA Neurol. 2018;75(6):759–60.
16. Duggal HS. Clozapine-induced neuroleptic malignant syndrome and subdural hematoma. J Neuropsychiatry Clin Neurosci. 2004;16(1):118–9.
17. Feki I, Abida I, Baati I, Masmoudi J, Jaoua A. Chronic subdural hematoma and neuropsychiatric disorders: report of a case. Eur Psychiatry. 2015;30:1271.
18. Gaist D, Garcia Rodriguez LA, Hald SM, Hellfritzsch M, Poulsen FR, Halle B, Hallas J, Pottegard A. Antidepressant drug use and subdural hematoma risk. J Thromb Haemost. 2020;18(2):318–27.

19. Gelabert-Gonzalez M, Iglesias-Pais M, Garcia-Allut A, Martinez-Rumbo R. Chronic subdural haematoma: surgical treatment and outcome in 1000 cases. Clin Neurol Neurosurg. 2005;107(3):223–9.
20. Hackam DG, Mrkobrada M. Selective serotonin reuptake inhibitors and brain hemorrhage: a meta-analysis. Neurology. 2012;79(18):1862–5.
21. Halperin D, Reber G. Influence of antidepressants on hemostasis. Dialogues Clin Neurosci. 2007;9(1):47–59.
22. Heninger M. Subdural hematoma occurrence. Am J Forensic Med Pathol. 2013;34(3):237–41.
23. Husain K, Ansari RA, Ferder L. Alcohol-induced hypertension: mechanism and prevention. World J Cardiol. 2014;6(5):245–52.
24. Iliescu IA, Constantinescu AI. Clinical evolutional aspects of chronic subdural haematomas—literature review. J Med Life. 2015;8(Spec Issue):26–33.
25. Ishikawa E, Yanaka K, Sugimoto K, Ayuzawa S, Nose T. Reversible dementia in patients with chronic subdural hematomas. J Neurosurg. 2002;96(4):680–3.
26. Jomli R, Zgueb Y, Nacef F, Douki S. Chronic subdural hematoma and psychotic decompensation (in France). Encéphale. 2012;38(4):356–9.
27. Kar SK, Kumar D, Singh P, Upadhyay PK. Psychiatric manifestation of chronic subdural hematoma: the unfolding of mystery in a homeless patient. Indian J Psychol Med. 2015;37(2):239–42.
28. Kharofa J, Sekar P, Haverbusch M, Moomaw C, Flaherty M, Kissela B, Broderick J, Woo D. Selective serotonin reuptake inhibitors and risk of hemorrhagic stroke. Stroke. 2007;38(11):3049–51.
29. Kolias AG, Chari A, Santarius T, Hutchinson PJ. Chronic subdural haematoma: modern management and emerging therapies. Nat Rev Neurol. 2014;10(10):570–8.
30. Laberge S, Crizzle AM. A literature review of psychotropic medications and alcohol as risk factors for falls in community dwelling older adults. Clin Drug Investig. 2019;39(2):117–39.
31. Landi F, Onder G, Cesari M, Barillaro C, Russo A, Bernabei R. Psychotropic medications and risk for falls among community-dwelling frail older people: an observational study. J Gerontol A Biol Sci Med Sci. 2005;60(5):622–6.
32. Laporte S, Chapelle C, Caillet P, Beyens MN, Bellet F, Delavenne X, Mismetti P, Bertoletti L. Bleeding risk under selective serotonin reuptake inhibitor (SSRI) antidepressants: a meta-analysis of observational studies. Pharmacol Res. 2017;118:19–32.
33. Lazarus A. Neuroleptic malignant syndrome and preexisting brain damage. J Neuropsychiatry Clin Neurosci. 1992;4(2):185–7.
34. Levine SR, Brust JC, Futrell N, Ho KL, Blake D, Millikan CH, Brass LM, Fayad P, Schultz LR, Selwa JF, et al. Cerebrovascular complications of the use of the "crack" form of alkaloidal cocaine. N Engl J Med. 1990;323(11):699–704.
35. Machulda MM, Haut MW. Clinical features of chronic subdural hematoma: neuropsychiatric and neuropsychologic changes in patients with chronic subdural hematoma. Neurosurg Clin N Am. 2000;11(3):473–7.
36. McEvoy AW, Kitchen ND, Thomas DG. Intracerebral haemorrhage and drug abuse in young adults. Br J Neurosurg. 2000;14(5):449–54.
37. Nagele EP, Ross A, Then RK, Kavi T. Interhemispheric subdural and subarachnoid haemorrhage in a patient with amphetamine-induced vasculitis. BMJ Case Rep. 2017;2017:bcr2017222918.
38. Nutt D. Alcohol and the brain. Pharmacological insights for psychiatrists. Br J Psychiatry. 1999;175:114–9.
39. Pencalet P. [Clinical forms and prognostic factors of chronic subdural hematoma in the adult]. Neurochirurgie. 2001;47(5):469–72.
40. Pozzi M, Roccatagliata D, Sterzi R. Drug abuse and intracranial hemorrhage. Neurol Sci. 2008;29(Suppl 2):S269–70.
41. Renoux C, Vahey S, Dell'Aniello S, Boivin JF. Association of selective serotonin reuptake inhibitors with the risk for spontaneous intracranial hemorrhage. JAMA Neurol. 2017;74(2):173–80.
42. Saha D, Bisui B, Thakurta RG, Ghoshmaulik S, Singh OP. Chronic subdural hematoma following electro convulsive therapy. Indian J Psychol Med. 2012;34(2):181–3.
43. Schlaeppi M, Prica A, de Torrente A. Cerebral hemorrhage and "ecstasy" (in German). Praxis (Bern 1994). 1999;88(13):568–72.
44. Taylor S. Electroconvulsive therapy: a review of history, patient selection, technique, and medication management. South Med J. 2007;100(5):494–8.
45. Taylor D, Barnes TRE, Young AH. The Maudsley prescribing guidelines in psychiatry. 13th

ed. New York: Wiley; 2018.
46. Thapa PB, Gideon P, Cost TW, Milam AB, Ray WA. Antidepressants and the risk of falls among nursing home residents. N Engl J Med. 1998;339(13):875–82.
47. Toi H, Kinoshita K, Hirai S, Takai H, Hara K, Matsushita N, Matsubara S, Otani M, Muramatsu K, Matsuda S, Fushimi K, Uno M. Present epidemiology of chronic subdural hematoma in Japan: analysis of 63,358 cases recorded in a national administrative database. J Neurosurg. 2018;128(1):222–8.
48. Uno M, Toi H, Hirai S. Chronic subdural hematoma in elderly patients: is this disease benign? Neurol Med Chir (Tokyo). 2017;57(8):402–9.
49. van de Wiel A. Diabetes mellitus and alcohol. Diabetes Metab Res Rev. 2004;20(4):263–7.
50. Vitry AI, Hoile AP, Gilbert AL, Esterman A, Luszcz MA. The risk of falls and fractures associated with persistent use of psychotropic medications in elderly people. Arch Gerontol Geriatr. 2010;50(3):e1–4.
51. Wijeratne C, Shome S. Electroconvulsive therapy and subdural hemorrhage. J ECT. 1999;15(4):275–9.
52. Wong S, Afshani M. Intracranial vascular complications of "molly" usage: case report and review of the literature. Conn Med. 2016;80(8):467–9.

第 12 章　小儿慢性硬膜下血肿

Murat Ö. Yay，Daniel Wittschieber 和 Mehmet Turgut
译者：欧云尉

12.1　引言

慢性硬膜下血肿（CSDH）被认为是神经外科临床中最常见的疾病之一[20]。慢性硬膜下积液的首次报道可追溯到 1916 年，Payr 描述了一例硬膜下病理性液体积聚（SDHy），他称之为"创伤性浆液性脑膜炎"[65]。Cohen 在 1927 年报告了相同的临床疾病，并将其称为"硬膜下积液"[15]。1932年，丹迪开始使用 SDHy 这个术语，现如今它被认为是一个独立的临床疾病[16, 65, 90]。

CSDH 通常发病于老年人，在极少数情况下也可能发生在婴儿中，发生在婴儿中通常是外伤造成的[28, 78]。虽然 CSDH 的确切发病率尚不清楚，但它在男性中更常见[28, 54, 63]。尽管在影像学研究中观察到显著的占位效应，但需要注意的是在儿科人群中，某些病例的临床症状和体征可能是隐匿的[1, 63]。这种病例在不同诊所的儿童和青少年中均有出现。从儿科医生的角度来看，慢性硬膜下积液这一专业术语是应用于一组以脑外或轴外区域内液体过量积聚为特征的病症[20]。目前的神经影像学技术已经极大地推进了我们对这一疾病的理解，但其确切的发病机制和适当的治疗方案仍然存在争议[36, 78]。在这一章中，我们的目的是探讨慢性硬膜下血肿的解剖、病理生理、病因、诊断和治疗。

12.2　解剖学与病理生理学

硬膜下腔是指硬膜下存在的潜在空间，在病理条件下，蛛网膜与硬脑膜之间可以被分离，CSDH 将会在该空间中发展[68]。正常情况下硬膜下和硬膜外区域不像蛛网膜下腔那样存在自然腔隙，这两个腔隙中的积液均为病理性的[30, 78]。解剖学上，硬膜下血肿（SDH）可穿过颅缝边缘出现在任何颅内位置，大脑镰和小脑幕等硬脑膜内结构可限制 SDH 的范围。因此，它在非增强计算机断层成像（NECT）上通常表现为一个新月形或凹陷型轴外病变[68]。

从病理生理学角度来看，应考虑以下六种常见硬膜下积液的类型：（a）急性 SDH；（b）SDHy；（c）混合型硬膜下血肿（SDHHy）；（d）CSDH（作为独立类型）；（e）硬膜下积液；（f）硬膜下积脓[90-91]。然而，即使在今天，尽管慢性硬膜下积液是一个众所周知的慢性疾病，但是上文提到的不同慢性硬膜下积液的发病机制和发展机制仍未被完全了解。

尽管硬膜下假膜再出血是神经病理学家熟知的病理因素，但硬膜下和蛛网膜下腔之间关系在许多方面仍然未知[23, 75]。在 CSDH 中，硬脑膜下腔出血大约 2 周后，硬脑膜中胶原蛋白的合成受到刺激，许多成纤维细胞向硬脑膜内表面移动，生成增厚的硬脑膜外膜[51, 72]。随后，更薄的血肿内膜形成，包裹住血凝块[51]。当怀疑儿童因受到虐待而头部受伤时，这种估计 CSDH 形成时间的方法经常被用作法医证据，这些作用于儿童头部的伤害主要是以"摇晃婴儿综合征"（SBS）的形式出现，也就是所谓的"虐待性头部创伤"（AHT）的一种常见变体[68]。随着时间的推移，SDH 可能会液化、分解或形成 SDHy 或 SDHHy，这些被认为是 CSDH 的前体，在某些情况下假膜可能会钙化[51, 90-91]。有人认为，所有 SDH 中的绝大多数会液化[84]，然后 SDH 会逐渐增大，而不是保持固体和稳定[84]。

目前，有学者认为，硬膜下腔内液体的持续积聚可能取决于以下详细描述的病理机制（表 12.1）[30, 38, 41, 48, 71, 85, 90-91]。

12.2.1　急性 SDH 后

许多学者认为再出血是引起急性 SDH 持续存在的主要原因[55]。研究表明，急性 SDH 周围可见血管化膜，膜内血管易碎，出现持续性创伤和血管压力改变时膜内血管可出血至血肿腔内[78]。事实

表 12.1 CSDH 发生发展的病理生理学

	原因	可能的病理机制
1	急性 SDH 后	急性 SDH 颗粒膜脆性新生血管向硬膜下反复出血[38,48,90-91]。然而,急性 SDH 向 CSDH 的直接转化很少能被观察到,在急性 SDH 和 CSDH 之间可能存在一个称为"SDHy"或"SDHHy"的中间过程[90-91]
2	脑脊液渗漏	脑脊液通过蛛网膜的开口渗漏,使脑脊液进入硬膜下腔。脑脊液与血液混合,形成薄薄的黄色硬脑膜下积液,分别称为"SDHy"或"SDHHy"[85,90-91]
3	脑萎缩	脑萎缩的婴儿可能更容易发展为 CSDH,这是由于蛛网膜随着脑萎缩而塌陷时硬脑膜外层的张力增加[30]
4	感染或炎症过程	在感染或炎症过程之后,鼻窦炎或中耳炎可导致硬膜下脓肿[41]

CSDH,慢性硬膜下血肿;CSF,脑脊液;SDH,硬膜下血肿;SDHy,硬膜下积液;SDHHy,混合型硬膜下血肿。

上,这种病理机制被认为是罕见的,在研究中未能重现[90-91]。更有可能的情况是,在 SDH 和 CSDH 之间有一个称为 SDHy 或 SDHHy 的中间过渡发展阶段[90-91]。

许多学者认为,反复出血会导致硬膜下腔内分隔的形成,从而使血凝块机化(或血凝块随着时间的推移因血清分离而改变)[55,91]。一般情况下,所有液化的血液都可以被吸收;然而在一些少见的病例中,血凝块可能会产生比最初期急性 SDH 更严重的症状。在这种情况下,由于压力平衡被打破,导致血肿(或积液)体积扩大,临床症状加重[78]。

12.2.2 脑脊液渗漏

一位作者在书中已详细解释了脑脊液渗漏的相关机制[91]。该作者认为蛛网膜撕裂可能会形成一个活瓣,阻碍脑脊液回流[9,44]。这种在硬膜下腔内的积液类型称为 SDHy,可能发生在蛛网膜撕裂后,CSF 进入硬膜下腔,SDHy 也是 CSDH 的主要初期形式[90-91]。SDHy 也可发生于脑室系统分流后扩张的硬膜下间隙[78](图 12.1)。一般来说,在 SDHy 中看不到分隔[78]。在这些病例中,考虑到硬膜下积液黄染的特性,可以将硬膜下积液与蛛网膜下液体和脑室内液区分开来[34]。据推测,在皮质表面可观察到小出血灶,是持续的轻度创伤或自发性桥静脉破裂造成的[78]。

12.2.3 脑萎缩

一些患有线粒体或溶酶体相关疾病的儿童在磁共振成像(MRI)检查中仅显示为脑萎缩[45,73]。1 型戊二酸尿症的特征是小头畸形,同时急性 SDH 也可能发生在这些患儿身上,这可能是由于脑萎缩导致桥静脉牵拉破裂所致,正如本章的一位作者在以前关于 SBS 成像的综述中所指出的(图 12.2)[54,89]。

12.2.4 感染或炎症过程

化脓性积液继发于感染或炎症或两者兼而有之[71]。硬膜下积脓也是硬膜下积液的一种,可能是由于感染从中耳或鼻窦首先扩展到硬膜外空间,然后通过邻近途径进入硬膜下腔[78]。硬膜下积脓

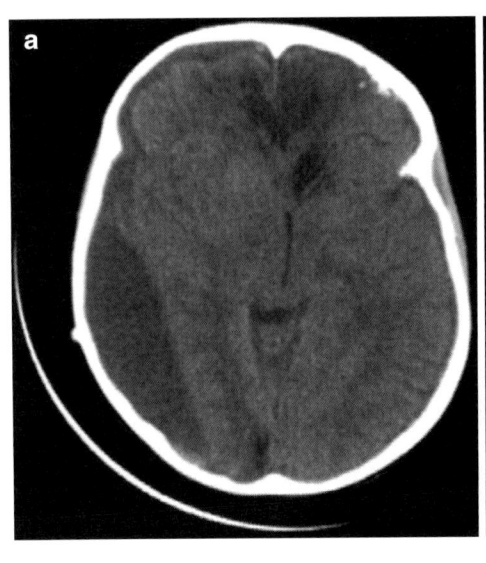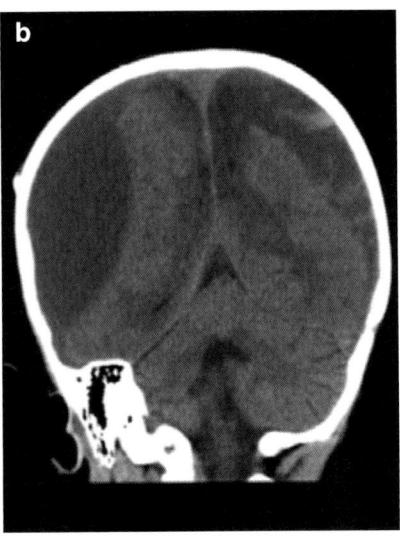

图 12.1 轴向(a)、冠状面(b)非增强计算机断层成像(NECT)切片,显示 10 岁男性患儿分流术后的双侧慢性硬膜下血肿(CSDH)

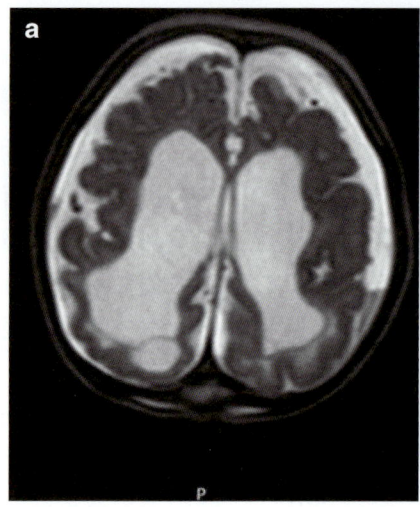
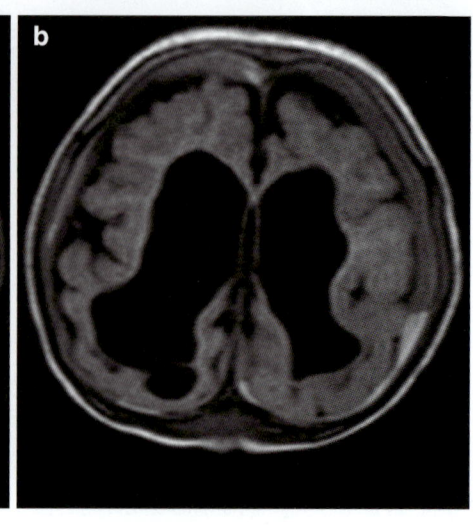

图 12.2 患有代谢性疾病的 2 岁患儿。T2 加权磁共振成像（MRI）扫描（a）显示覆盖双侧大脑半球的 CSDH，与脑脊液（CSF）相比呈高信号和等信号；然而，在 FLAIR 图像（b）上，信号强度高于 CSF，表明蛋白质含量不同

也可在链球菌属和肺炎双球菌导致的细菌性脑膜炎中观察到（图 12.3）[22, 33, 46, 60]。如果在取样培养前没有给予抗生素治疗，化脓性硬膜下积液的培养结果可能会提示相应的致病微生物[78]。

12.3 病因学

从专业角度，CSDH 被归类为硬脑膜和蛛网膜之间的持续性颅内出血。CSDH 常见于老年人，在儿童中罕见[1]。老年人的 CSDH 不在本章的讨论范围。已报道了婴儿期 CSDH 的几种病因，包括产伤、维生素 K 缺乏、虐待伤和凝血病[2-3, 42, 50, 93]。从病因学上讲，导致 CSDH 发生的原因有很多，但在儿童中最常见的原因是头部外伤，且在男性儿童中更为常见[63, 66]。AHT 作为一种常见的头部创伤，在婴儿年龄组的发病率为（14～30）/10 万[21, 31, 40]。AHT 这一定义主要用于儿科人群中由非意外（人为施加的）创伤引起的头部损伤[14, 31, 40, 49]。根据一些学者的看法，"SBS" 可视为 AHT 的一种常见变体[14, 49]。

儿科人群（婴儿年龄组和 2 岁以下人群）中急性 SDH 的发病率分别为（20～25）/10 万和每 12/10 万[7, 10, 32, 39, 52]。创伤性原因可能是意外或非意外，2 岁以下儿童 SDH 的最常见原因是非意外性损伤[63, 81]。一般来说，创伤发生阶段往往被忽视，研究更多关注 CSDH 而忽视了它的急性发生期[78]。如上所述，SDH 似乎不是 CSDH 的直接前身[90-91]。本章进一步的病因学讨论将着眼于 SDH 的发病机制，而不是 CSDH。下文将详细描述蛛网膜囊肿（AC）和蛛网膜下腔良性扩大（BESS）是 SDH 的原因，其然后可以经由 SDHy 发展为 CSDH[90-91]。

临床上，SDH 的其他原因包括血液学凝血疾病和各种颅内形态异常，如 AC[78, 92]。应首先评估患者的凝血功能状态[78]。在大多数此类病例中，颅中窝的 AC 可能是 SDH 发展的危险因素之一[78]。据报道，合并 AC 的 CSDH 病例的流行病学、人口统计学和临床特征与没有合并 AC 的病例不同[92]。AC 患者出血真实发生率尚不清楚，但 AC 外壁破裂可能使 CSF 进入硬膜下腔[64, 78]。目前研究表明，AC 是先天性或获得性的蛛网膜内 CSF 聚集，虽然

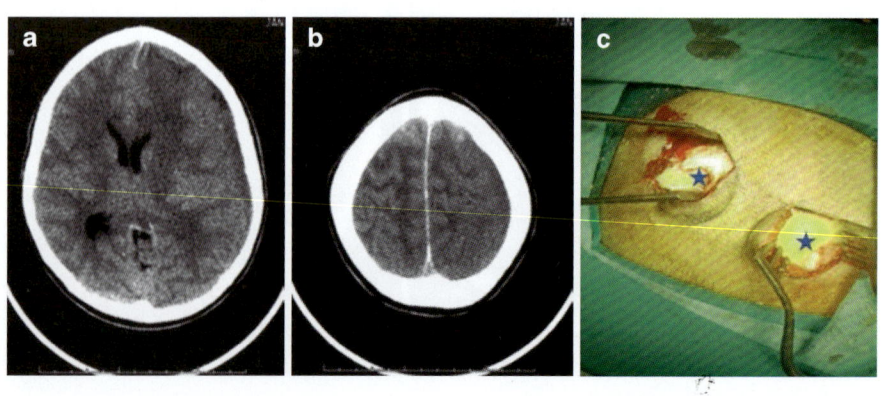

图 12.3 NECT（a，b）显示左侧硬膜下积液，钻孔后可见脓性积液（c）

很少发生，但先前存在的任何 AC 都可能由于 AHT 或 SBS 或突然的短期颅内压升高（IICP）而发生破裂[24, 69, 90-91]。尽管迄今为止尚未在婴儿中观察到 AC 的破裂，但推测 AC 破裂可能会导致 SDHy 而不是 SDH 的发展[69, 90-91]。Gelabert-González 等的综述报告了 SDHy 的发病年龄范围为 5~25 岁[24]。根据这些信息推测，婴儿的 AC 破裂是 AHT、SBS 或自发性的结果是合乎逻辑的[90-91]。

即使在今天，是否所谓的 BESS 可能会导致 SDH 仍存在争论。在宏观上，这种疾病表现为儿童人群的大头畸形和前囟膨出，并推测这种轻度交通性脑积水与蛛网膜绒毛的延迟成熟有关[78]。

在临床实践中，产伤被认为是 CSDH 的一个原因[67]。有研究表明，从新生儿期开始出现相应症状或大头畸形的婴儿可能患有产伤性 CSDH[5]，甚至还有子宫内发生 CSDH 的病例[5,13,17]。除宫内损伤外，遗传性凝血功能障碍、颅内血管畸形和代谢紊乱也是新生儿慢性硬膜下血肿的病因[27, 47, 57, 79, 83]。

12.4 临床表现

临床上，儿科人群中 CSDH 的症状因患者的年龄和出血原因差异而表现不同[78]。急性期和慢性期患者的症状也存在不同，例如急性表现以呼吸暂停或癫痫发作为特征，而伴有呕吐、易怒、喂养不良或大头畸形病史的慢性表现在婴儿中很常见（表 12.2）。通常，对所有不明原因的 SDH 患儿来说仔细检查外伤体征以及视网膜出血是必要的，

表 12.2 按年龄组列出的 CSDH 患者的临床症状

儿童年龄分组	
婴儿组	年龄较大儿童组
窒息	头痛
癫痫	库欣三联征
呕吐	偏瘫
昏睡	感觉缺陷
易怒	反射不对称
巨颅	展神经麻痹
食欲不振	视乳头水肿
	语言障碍

Data in this table was taken from Emmahadi et al.[20] and Swift and McBride[78]

儿童 AHT 或 SBS 导致的急性创伤中一般均可发现视网膜损伤[90-91]。如果急性 SDH 通过 SDHy 或 SDHHy 已经转变为 CSDH，此时视网膜损伤症状通常已经消退[90-91]。

年龄较大的儿童通常会出现慢性头痛和 IICP 的体征[78]。头痛在年轻患者中比老年患者更常见[86]。其他症状则呈单侧病变，如偏瘫或反射不对称。值得注意的是，在年龄较大的儿童中 CSDH 通常发生在单侧，但婴儿年龄组中通常发生双侧 CSDH[1]。

临床上，CSDH 可能表现为轻微创伤后复发性出血，甚至在没有任何创伤的情况下自发性出血[82]。在一项调查慢性硬膜下血肿的文献调查中，一些病例报告中发现了不同的诱发因素[8, 25, 76, 87]。Shrestha 和 You 报告了 1 例 16 岁女性患者，头痛和头晕 2 个月；体格检查和血液检查正常，无外伤史[76]。在这个病例中，CT 扫描显示左额颞 CSDH 伴有颅中窝的 AC[76]。因此 AC 被认为是儿童年龄组脑损伤后发生 CSDH 的危险因素[20]。

之前的一项研究中，Basmaci 等报道了一名 2 岁的 CSDH 患者，已知患有急性髓系白血病，表现为癫痫、呕吐和躁动[8]。在这个病例中，血液检查结果提示血小板计数为 48 000/mm^3，且患者没有头部外伤史。Basmaci 等的研究中报道了肿瘤相关 SDH 的发生率为 0.5%~4%[8]。他们根据研究结果得出结论，头部创伤、凝血功能障碍和化疗药物增加了儿童人群[8]中颅内出血的风险。

2013 年，Wang 等报道了一位 14 岁的音乐系学生，在发现视物模糊和双侧视神经乳头水肿后头痛 2 周[87]。有趣的是，他们认为在没有任何诱发危险因素的情况下，Valsalva 动作可导致静脉压力升高，引发 SDH[87]。他们还补充了另一个类似的病例，一名 9 岁的男性患儿，有在学校玩躲避球史，导致了 CSDH 发生[86]。

最近，Glen 等描述了一位健康的 45 天大的女婴，由于从椅子上摔下而导致头部受伤，NECT 显示存在双侧额顶低密度积液[25]。他们对该病例进行了多次硬膜下积液手术，然而最后一次增强 MRI 提示在右额叶、枕叶和顶叶有多个不均匀的增强区[25]。令人惊讶的是，手术标本病理提示为有丝分裂活跃的高级别肉瘤性增生和肿瘤性增殖。因此 Glen 等得出结论，MRI 有助于区分 CSDH 和肉瘤[25]。

12.5 诊断

儿科人群的 CSDH 诊断首先应从临床评估开始，并从前囟进行经皮穿刺抽吸[63]。这种方法称为"硬膜下穿刺"，然而这可能导致出血在蛛网膜下腔和（或）硬膜下腔扩散，因此导致误诊。

CSDH 最好通过神经影像学技术如 CT 和 MRI 进行诊断。此外，神经影像学检查是从其他类型脑外积液中鉴别出 CSDH 的最佳方法[61]。NECT 是鉴别蛛网膜下腔出血与慢性硬膜下血肿的首选影像学检查方法[61]。在影像学中，CT 在区分急性和慢性 SDH 方面也很有价值[5]。在 MRI 中，CSDH 通常与 CSF 等信号[61]。

目前，MRI 是诊断 CSDH 的最佳影像学方法，其 T1 和 T2 加权液体衰减反转恢复（FLAIR）序列图像通常为高信号[61]，特别是使用 T1 加权序列可将 SDH 与蛛网膜下腔出血区分开来[78]。在 T1 和 T2 加权序列上，CSDH 与 CSF 呈等信号。复发性出血相较于 CSF 在 T1 上呈高信号，在 T2 上呈低信号[61]。在神经影像学上，CSDH 弥漫性分布于大脑半球凸面，伴有多个分隔和轴外脑膜的对比增强[61]。由于 MRI 能更好地显示不同时间的出血，因此对非意外创伤病例的评估尤其有用；此外，MRI 能更好地显示隔膜和血块[61]。

超声检查（USG）是评估婴儿 CSDH 的首选影像学方法，因为它简单且便宜。超声可显示 CSDH 内的间隔，但无法区分 SDH 和蛛网膜下腔出血[78]。

12.6 治疗

治疗儿童 CSDH 和大头畸形的目的是缓解 IICP，消除占位效应，并使头部正常生长[78]。多年来，各种外科手术方法出现，包括反复经皮硬膜下穿刺、硬膜下-腹膜分流术（SPS）、钻孔引流、麻花钻颅骨造口术、临时硬膜下外引流、开颅术和广泛切除血肿假膜[4, 6, 11-12, 26, 42, 53, 56, 59, 61, 70, 78, 80]。不幸的是，这些手术方式对 CSDH 患者的疗效均非常有限。

作为开颅手术的替代方法，各种侵入性手术在针对婴儿的治疗中被提出，如 Ingraham 和 Matson 首先提出的广泛切除硬膜内膜、上矢状窦下降术，以及广泛颅骨成形术，以减少婴儿的颅脑不称[29, 37, 58]。同时，用于控制 IICP 的微创治疗方法，如硬膜下穿刺、硬膜下引流和 SPS，已被广泛接受[4, 62]。McLaurin 等还提出了反复硬膜下穿刺治疗 IICP 的方法，疗效满意[54]。在 Aoki 的系列文献报道中，硬膜下穿刺主要针对血肿最厚区域，且 43% 的患者随后需要 SPS 治疗[1]。CSDH 和 SDHy 的最为广泛接受的治疗方法是将硬膜下分流器放置到腹膜腔中，称为 SPS。从技术上讲，尽管婴儿存在双侧血肿，但分流管通常是单侧放置的[13]。

目前，一些神经外科医生倾向于使用钻孔引流术治疗慢性硬膜下血肿，但应用该技术后血肿复发的发生率为 3%～33%[19]。Huang 等使用了各种药物如阿托伐他汀和低剂量地塞米松治疗了 4 例 CSDH 复发病例，他们认为这些药物对复发性 CSDH 患者有效[35]。

1998 年，Gruber 等引入了内镜冲洗作为 CSDH 儿童的另一种手术治疗方法[28]。他们认为在这些病例中使用内镜冲洗是安全的[28]。如今，相比于传统的开颅手术方法（如颅骨切开术和血肿膜切除术或矢状窦复位），包括内镜冲洗在内的微创技术更受外科医生们欢迎[29]。

另外，CSDH 合并 AC 的手术治疗存在争议[32]。一些学者主张仅钻孔引流[18, 77, 88]，而另一些学者建议通过开颅术去除 AC 膜[43, 74, 94]。然而 SDH 也可以仅通过临床随访进行保守治疗，特别是针对存在合并症的患者（图 12.4）。

12.7 结论

众所周知，婴儿和较大儿童的 CSDH 最常见发病因素是创伤。临床上，慢性硬膜下血肿很少表现为急性症状；然而如果 IICP 显著，则可能存在创伤后脑疝形成和永久性神经功能损伤的危险，并且其中的半数儿童可能发生发育迟缓、痉挛和癫痫发作的各种神经缺陷。因此，对于发生 CSDH 的儿童进行及时诊断和适当治疗是必要的，以尽量减少儿童人群的长期后遗症。根据目前的文献可以得出结论，CSDH 在这个年龄组的发病是非常罕见的，MRI 和 CT 等影像学方法是最广泛使用的诊断工具。如今，标准治疗方法是通过各种外科手术进行血肿引流，如麻花钻颅骨造口术、开颅术、钻孔引流、SPS 和内镜下清除儿科人群中的 CSDH。

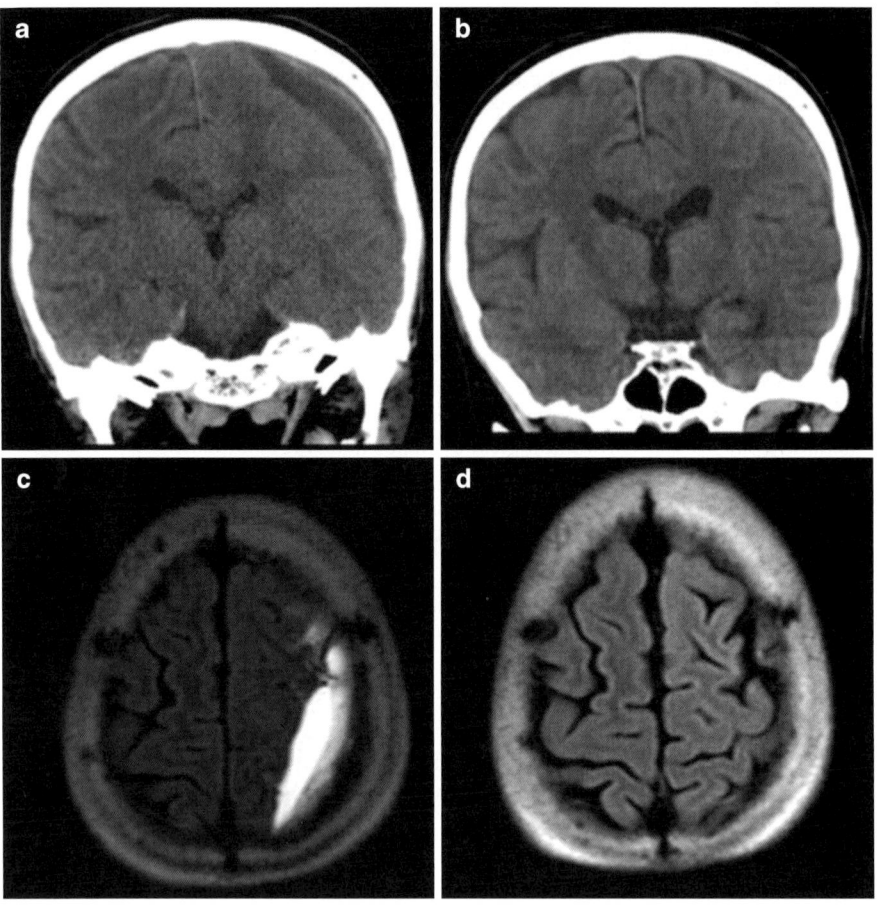

图 12.4　无临床症状的再生障碍性贫血患者偶然发现的左侧 CSDH。冠状面 NECT 切片（**a**）和轴向 MRI 切片（**c**）提示存在 CSDH。在随访 2 个月后，NECT 冠状面切片（**b**）和 MRI 轴向切片（**d**）显示血肿消退

参考文献

1. Aoki N, Masuzawa H. Bilateral chronic subdural hematomas without communication between the hematoma cavities: treatment with unilateral subdural-peritoneal shunt. Neurosurgery. 1988;22:911–3.
2. Aoki N, Masuzawa H. Subdural hematomas in abused children: report of six cases from Japan. Neurosurgery. 1986;18:475–7.
3. Aoki N, Mizutani H, Masuzawa H. Unilateral subdural-peritoneal shunting for bilateral chronic subdural hematomas in infancy. J Neurosurg. 1985;63:134–7.
4. Aoki N. Chronic subdural hematoma in infancy. Clinical analysis of 30 cases in the CT era. J Neurosurg. 1990;73:201–5.
5. Atluru V, Kumar I. Intrauterine chronic subdural hematoma with postoperative tension pneumocephalus. Pediatr Neurol. 1987;3(5):306–9.
6. Balser D, Rodgers SD, Johnson B, Shi C, Tabak E, Samadani U. Evolving management of symptomatic chronic subdural hematoma: experience of a single institution and review of the literature. Neurol Res. 2013;35:233–42.
7. Barlow KM, Minns RA. Annual incidence of shaken impact syndrome in young children. Lancet. 2000;356:1571–2.
8. Basmaci M, Hasturk AE. Chronic subdural hematoma in a child with acute myeloid leukemia after leukocytosis. Indian J Crit Care Med. 2012;16:222–4.
9. Borzone M, Capuzzo T, Perria C, Rivano C, Tercero E. Traumatic subdural hygromas: a report of 70 surgically treated cases. J Neurosurg Sci. 1983;27:161–5.
10. Caffey J. Multiple fractures in the long bones of infants suffering from chronic subdural hematoma. Am J Roentgenol. 1946;56:163–7.
11. Caldarelli M, Di Rocco C, Romani R. Surgical treatment of chronic subdural hygromas in infants and children. Acta Neurochir. 2002;144:581–8.
12. Camel M, Grubb RL Jr. Treatment of chronic subdural hematoma by twist-drill craniostomy

with continuous catheter drainage. J Neurosurg. 1986;65:183–7.
13. Capella L, Pierre-Karin A, Sainte Rose C, Renier D, Hoppe-Hirsch E, Hirsch JF. Treatment of chronic subdural collection in infants by subdural peritoneostomy. Neurochirurgie. 1989;35:404–6.
14. Christian CW, Block R, Committee on Child Abuse and Neglect, American Academy of Pediatrics. Abusive head trauma in infants and children. Pediatrics. 2009;123:1409–11.
15. Cohen I. Chronic subdural accumulation of cerebrospinal fluid after cranial trauma. Report of a case. Arch Neurol Psychiatry (Chicago). 1927;18:709–23.
16. Dandy WE. Chronic subdural hygroma and serous meningitis (pachymeningitis serosa; localized external hydrocephalus). In: Lewis D, editor. Practice of surgery. Hagerstown: W. F. Prior; 1952. p. 291–3.
17. Dias A, Taha S, Vinikoff L, Andriamamonjy C, Leriche B, Bintner M. Chronic subdural hematoma in utero. Case report with literature review. Neurochirurgie. 1998;44:124–6.
18. Domenicucci M, Russo N, Giugni E, Pierallini A. Relationship between supratentorial arachnoid cyst and chronic subdural hematoma: neuroradiological evidence and surgical treatment. J Neurosurg. 2009;110:1250–5.
19. Ducruet AF, Grobelny BT, Zacharia BE, Hickman ZL, DeRosa PL, Anersen KN, Sussman E, Carpenter A, Connolly ES Jr. The surgical management of chronic subdural hematoma. Neurosurg Rev. 2012;35:155–69.
20. Emmahadi M, Chadok SY, Alijani B, Behzadnia H, Rasoulian J, Andalib S. Chronic subdural hematoma in pediatrics: a case report and literature review of rare cases. Trauma Mon. 2016:38529.
21. Fanconi M, Lips U. Shaken baby syndrome in Switzerland: results of a prospective follow-up study, 2002-2007. Eur J Pediatr. 2010;169:1023–8.
22. Forman PM, Chipps BE, Meyer GA. Managing chronic subdural hematomas and effusions in infants: a continuing dilemma. Tex Med. 1974;70:62–6.
23. Friede RL. Hemorrhages in asphyxiated premature infants. In: Friede R, editor. Developmental neuropathology. Gottingen: Springer; 1989. p. 44–58.
24. Gelabert-Gonzalez M, Fernandez-Villa J, Cutrín-Prieto J, Allut AG, Martinez-Rumbo R. Arachnoid cyst rupture with subdural hygroma: report of three cases and literature review. Childs Nerv Syst. 2002;18:609–13.
25. Glenn CA, Fung KM, Tullos HJ, McNall-Knapp RY, Gunda D, Mapstone TB. Primary intracranial sarcoma presenting as chronic subdural fluid collections in a child. World Neurosurg. 2015;86(514):13–8.
26. Goodman JM, Mealey J Jr. Postmeningitic subdural effusions: the syndrome and its management. J Neurosurg. 1969;30:658–63.
27. Green PM. Idiopathic intracranial haemorrhage in the fetus. Fetal Diagn Ther. 1999;14:275–8.
28. Gruber DP, Crone KR. Endoscopic washout: a new tecnique for treatment chronic subdural hematomas in infants. Pediatr Neurosurg. 1997;27:292–5.
29. Gutierrez FA, McLone DG, Raimondi AJ. Physiopathology and a new treatment of chronic subdural hematoma in children. Childs Brain. 1976;5:216–32.
30. Haines DE, Harkey HL, al-Mefty O. The "subdural" space: a new look at an outdated concept. Neurosurgery. 1993;32:111–20.
31. Herrmann B. Epidemiologie, Klinik und Konzept des Schütteltrauma-Syndroms. Pädiatr Praxis. 2016;86:297–12.
32. Hobbs C, Childs AM, Wynne J, Livingston J, Seal A. Subdural haematoma and effusion in infancy: an epidemiological study. Arch Dis Child. 2005;90:952–5.
33. Hollenhorst RW, Stein HA, Keith HM, MacCarty LS. Subdural hematoma, subdural hygroma and subarachnoid hemorrage among infants and children. Neurosurgery. 1957;7:813–9.
34. Hoppe-Hirsch E, Sainte Rose C, Renier D, Hirsch JF. Pericerebral collections after shunting. Childs Nerv Syst. 1987;3:97–102.
35. Huang J, Li J, Zhang J, Gao C, Quan W, Tian Y, Sun J, Tian Q, Wang D, Dong J, Zhang J, Jiang R. Treatment of relapsed chronic subdural hematoma in four young children with atorvastatin and low-dose dexamethasone. Pharmacotherapy. 2019;39:783–9.
36. Hwang SK, Kim SL. Infantile head injury, with special reference to the development of chronic subdural hematoma. Childs Nerv Syst. 2000;16:590–4.
37. Ingraham FD, Matson DD. Subdural hematoma in infancy. J Pediatr. 1944;24:1–37.
38. Ito H, Yamamoto S, Komai T, Mizukoshi H. Role of local hyperfibrinolysis in the etiology of chronic subdural hematoma. J Neurosurg. 1976;45:26–31.
39. Jayawant S, Rawlinson A, Gibbon F, Price J, Schulte J, Sharples P, Sibert JR, Kemp

AM. Subdural haemorrhages in infants: population based study. BMJ. 1998;317:1558–61.
40. Keenan HT, Runyan DK, Marshall SW, Nocera MA, Merten DF, Sinal SH. A population-based study of inflicted traumatic brain injury in young children. JAMA. 2003;290:621–6.
41. Kobayashi M, Toshinami N, Maeda T, Ito K, Hisada K. Post-meningitis subdural hygroma in a child showing abnormal RI accumulation in 169Yb-DTPA RI cisternography (in Japan). Kaku Igaku. 1976;13:553–7.
42. Kolias AG, Chari A, Santarius T, Hutchinson PJ. Chronic subdural haematoma: modern management and emerging therapies. Nat Rev Neurol. 2014;10:570–8.
43. Kwak YS, Hwang SK, Park SH, Park JY. Chronic subdural hematoma associated with the middle fossa arachnoid cyst: pathogenesis and review of its management. Childs Nerv Syst. 2013;29:77–82.
44. Lee KS. The pathogenesis and clinical significance of traumatic sub-dural hygroma. Brain Inj. 1998;12:595–603.
45. Levy PA. Inborn errors of metabolism: part 1: specific disorders. Pediatr Rev. 2009;30:131–7.
46. Litofsky NS, Raffel C, McComb JG. Management of symptomatic chronic extra-axial fluid collections in pediatric patients. Neurosurgery. 1992;31:445–50.
47. Lutschg J, Vassella F. Neurological complications in hemophilia. Acta Paediatr Scand. 1981;70:235–41.
48. Markwalder TM. Chronic subdural hematomas: a review. J Neurosurg. 1981;54:637–45.
49. Matschke J, Herrmann B, Sperhake J, Körber F, Bajanowski T, Glatzel M. Shaken baby syndrome: a common variant of non-accidental head injury in infants. Dtsch Arztebl Int. 2009;106:211–7.
50. Matson DD. Neurosurgery of infancy and childhood. 2nd ed. Springfield: Charles C Thomas; 1969. p. 328–51.
51. Mayer S, Rowland L. Head injury. In: Merritt's neurology, Rowland L (Ed). Philadelphia: Lippincott Williams & Wilkins, 2000, pp. 401.
52. McLaurin RL, Crone RK. Subdural hematomas and effusions in children. In: Wilkins RH, Rengachary SS, editors. Neurosurgery. New York: McGraw-Hill; 1996. p. 3741–4.
53. McLaurin RL, Isaacs E, Lewis HP. Results of nonoperative treatment in 15 cases of infantile subdural hematoma. J Neurosurg. 1971;34:753–9.
54. McLaurin RL. Subdural hematomas and effusions in children. In: Wilkins RH, Rengachary SS, editors. Neurosurgery. New York: McGraw-Hill; 1985. p. 2211–4.
55. McLone DC, Cutierrir FA, Itaimondi A. Ultrastructure of subdural membranes in children. Concepts in pediatric neurosurgery, vol. 1. Basel: Karger; 1981. p. 174–37.
56. Mizoi K, Takaku A, Suzuki J. Subdural efusion following radical surgery for chiasmal region tumors in children. Childs Brain. 1981;8:307–15.
57. Morris AA. Glutaric aciduria and suspected child abuse. Arch Dis Child. 1999;80:404–5.
58. Nakamura N. Head injuries: its mechanism and diagnosis at the acute stage. Tokyo: Bunkodo; 1986. p. 723–33.
59. Njiokiktjien CJ, Valk J, Ponssen H. Subdural hygroma: results of treatment by ventriculo-abdominal shunt. Childs Brain. 1980;7:285–302.
60. Oka H, Motomochi M, Suzuki Y, Ando K. Subdural hygroma after head injury. A review of 26 cases. Acta Neurochir (Wien). 1972;26:265–73.
61. Osborn AG. Chronic subdural hematoma. In: Osborn AG, Jhaveri MD, Salzman KL, editors. Diagnostic imaging: brain. Philadelphia: Elsevier; 2016. p. 164–7.
62. Otake G. Experience in external drainage of traumatic infantile subdural effusion. Shoni No No Shinkei. 1983;8:67–78.
63. Parent AT. Pediatric subdural hematoma: a retrospective comparative analysis. Pediatr Neurosurg. 1992;18:266–71.
64. Parsch CS, Krass I, Hoffmann E, Meixensberger J, Roosen K. Arachnoid cysts associated with subdural hematomas and hygromas: analysis of in cases, long-term follow-up, and review of literature. Neurosurgery. 1997;40:432–90.
65. Payr E. Meningitis serosa bei un nach Schaedelwerletzungen (traumatica). Med Klin. 1916;12:841–6.
66. Pereira C, Monterio J, Santos E, Dias L. Subdural hematoma in childhood: considerations about twenty cases and review of the literature. Internet J Pediatr Neonatol. 2004;5:1.
67. Powers CJ, Fuchs HE, George TM. Chronic subdural hematoma of the neonate: report of two cases and literature review. Pediatr Neurosurg. 2007;43:25–8.
68. Proctor MB. Neurosurgical aspects of nonaccidental trauma in children. In: Loftus B, editor. Neurological surgery principles and practice. Philadelphia: Lippincott Williams & Wilkins;

2003. p. 1065.
69. Punt J. Mechanisms and management of subdural hemorrhage. In: Minns RA, Brown JK, editors. Shaking and other non-accidental head injuries in children. London: Mac Keith Press; 2005. p. 290–313.
70. Rabe EF. Subdural effusions in infants. Pediatr Clin North Am. 1967;14:831–50.
71. Rutty GN, Squier MVW. Subdural hematoma in children. Essentials of autopsy practice: current methods and modern trends. 2006;4:131–53.
72. Sajanti J, Majamaa K. High concentrations of procollagen propeptides in chronic subdural haematoma and effusion. J Neurol Neurosurg Psychiatry. 2003;74:522–4.
73. Saudubray JM. Clinical approach to inborn errors of metabolism in pediatrics. In: Saudubray JM, Berghe GB, Walter JH, editors. Inborn metabolic disease. Berlin, Heidelberg: Springer; 2012. p. 3–52.
74. Servadei F, Vergoni G, Frattarelli M, Pasini A, Arista A, Fagioli L. Arachnoid cyst of middle cranial fossa and ipsilateral subdural haematoma: diagnostic and therapeutic implications in three cases. Br J Neurosurg. 1993;7:249–53.
75. Sherwood D. Chronic subdural hematoma in infants. Am J Dis Child. 1930;39:980–1021.
76. Shrestha R, You C. Spontaneous chronic subdural hematoma associated with arachnoid cyst in children and young adults. Asian J Neurosurg. 2014;9:168–72.
77. Sun J, Wang W, Wang D, An S, Xue L, Wang Y, Zhu SG, Jiang RC, Yang XJ, Yue SY. Clinical analysis of 10 patients of chronic subdural hematoma associated with arachnoid cyst. Zhonghua Yi Xue Za Zhi. 2017;97:1502–4.
78. Swift DM, McBride L. Chronic subdural hematoma in children. Neurosurg Clin N Am. 2000;11:439–46.
79. Sychlowy A, Pyda E. Toxic diarrhea in a heterozygote with galactosemia complicated by chronic subdural hematoma. Pol Tyg Lek. 1971;26:349–51.
80. Tsubokawa T, Nakamura S, Satoh K. Effect of temporary subdural-peritoneal shunt on subdural effusion with subarachnoid effusion. Childs Brain. 1984;11:47–59.
81. Tzioumi D, Oates RK. Subdural hematomas in children under 2 years. Accidental or inflicted? A ill year experience. Child Abuse Negl. 1998;22:1105–12.
82. Uscinski R. Shaken baby syndrome: fundamental questions. Br J Neurosurg. 2002;16:217–9.
83. Vapalahti PM. Intracranial arterial aneurysm in a three-month-old infant. Case report. J Neurosurg. 1969;30:169–71.
84. Victor M, Ropper A. Craniocerebral trauma. In: Victor M, Ropper A, editors. Adams and Victor's principles of neurology. 7th ed. New York: McGraw-Hill; 2001. p. 925.
85. Vinchon M, Defoort-Dhellemmes S, Noule N, Duhem R, Dhellemmes P. Accidental or nonaccidental brain injury in infants. Prospective study of 88 cases. Presse Med. 2004;33:1174–9.
86. Wang HK, Chen HJ, Lu K, Liliang PC, Liang CL, Tsai YD, Wang KW. A pediatric chronic subdural hematoma after dodgeball head injury. Pediatr Emerg Care. 2010;26:667–8.
87. Wang HS, Kim SW, Kim SH. Spontaneous chronic subdural hematoma in an adolescent girl. J Korean Neurosurg Soc. 2013;53:201–3.
88. Wang KD, Zhao JZ, Li JS, Zhang Y. Clinical study of patients of arachnoid cyst associated with chronic subdural hematoma. Zhonghua Yi Xue Za Zhi. 2011;9:460–3.
89. Wittschieber D, Kinner S, Pfeiffer H, Karger B, Hahnemann ML. Forensic aspects of imaging procedures in shaken baby syndrome—methodology, findings, differential diagnoses (in German). Rechtsmedizin. 2018;28:486–94.
90. Wittschieber D, Karger B, Niederstadt T, Pfeiffer H, Hahnemann ML. Subdural hygromas in abusive head trauma: pathogenesis, diagnosis, and forensic implications. AJNR Am J Neuroradiol. 2015;36:432–9.
91. Wittschieber D, Karger B, Pfeiffer H, Hahnemann ML. Understanding subdural collections in pediatric abusive head trauma. AJNR Am J Neuroradiol. 2019;40:388–95.
92. Wu X, Li G, Zhao J, Zhu X, Zhang Y, Hou K. Arachnoid cyst-associated chronic subdural hematoma: report of 14 cases and a systematic literature review. World Neurosurg. 2017;109:118–30.
93. Yasunaga A, Mori K, Matsusaka T. Intracranial hemorrhage due to vitamin K deficiency and chronic subdural hemorrhage in infants (in Japan). Proceedings of the 17th Annual Meeting of the Japanese Society of Pediatric Neurosurgery, In: Hayakawa I (ed.). Tokyo: Neuron, 1989, pp. 28–29.
94. Zhang H, Zhang JM, Chen G. Chronic subdural hematoma associated with arachnoid cyst: report of two cases. Chin Med J. 2007;120:2339–40.

第 13 章 慢性硬膜下血肿的影像学表现

Ersen Ertekin，Tuna Sahin 和 Ahmet T. Turgut

译者：朱炳城

13.1 引言

慢性硬膜下血肿（CSDH）是一种以陈旧性积血积液在硬膜下异常积聚为特征的疾病。该病的发病率为 1.72/10 万人至 20.6/10 万人，且其发病率随着年龄增长而增加[23, 50-51]。

形成 CSDH 最重要的病因是脑部创伤，绝大多数患者发病前都有明显的轻型脑外伤史。有研究报道称，在自发性或因各种手术干预（包括脊髓麻醉和腰椎穿刺）出现的低颅压后，都会出现 CSDH。此外，在一些硬膜下积液中，由于毛细血管微出血而转化为 CSDH 的比例明显较高[13, 31, 46]。凝血功能障碍和使用抗凝血和抗血小板药物，即使在轻微的脑部创伤中也会引起继发性出血，从而促进 CSDH 的形成；特别是凝血因子Ⅷ的缺乏可引起无创伤的自发性 CSDH[4]。因此，在没有任何其他潜在致病因素的情况下却出现 CSDH，应评估患者是否存在凝血因子Ⅷ的缺乏。

一些和 CSDH 发生发展相关的危险因素已经被逐步发现。其中，高龄是公认的 CSDH 高危因素，老化脆弱的血管、增长的抗凝抗血小板药物使用率、潜在跌倒风险的增加均被认为是 CSDH 的主要致病因素[2, 21]。CSDH 在婴幼儿时期极为罕见，因此当出现双侧 CSDH 时，更倾向于认为是由非意外创伤或戊二酸血症Ⅰ型造成的[9, 36]。男性由于遭受创伤的可能性更高以及酗酒，因此也被认为是危险因素之一[2]。CSDH 的另一重要危险因素是抗凝或抗血小板治疗[2, 21, 40]。CSDH 一般表现为缓慢的临床过程，尽管临床表现从无症状到昏迷不尽相同，但最常见的症状是头痛、癫痫发作和精神状态改变。

可能观察到 CSDH 患者的临床症状包括恶心/呕吐、虚弱、构音障碍、步态障碍、感觉障碍、瘫痪和昏迷。这些临床症状通常是继发于颅内压增高或因现有血肿扩大而导致脑组织受压。3%～20% 的病例会出现昏迷，2% 的病例会出现脑疝。尽管大部分 CSDH 是无菌性积血积液，但也有存在潜在感染病灶的风险，因此更应警惕 CSDH 患者出现潜在临床感染可能[28, 41, 47]。

CSDH 的病理生理机制仍然不清楚。有许多假说被提出，其中最著名的理论是炎症反应和急性硬膜下血肿（SDH）的转变[13]。在 1847 年发表的病例报告中，Virchow 将硬脑膜表面的炎症反应解释为 CSDH 的根源，这种炎症波及脑膜而导致间质性脑膜炎出血[48]。另一方面，Trotter 认为 CSDH 由外伤导致的急性硬膜下出血转变而来[45]。此外，Holmes 等支持外伤理论，并指出反复发生的微创伤可引起桥接血管的重复破裂，而新生血管对破裂的抵抗能力较差，这可能导致 CSDH 的发生与发展[17]。相反，Gardner 和 Zollinger 认为，陈旧性的积血和血管之间的渗透压差是造成血肿生长的原因。然而，Weir 等的研究表明，血肿渗透压与脑脊液（CSF）或静脉血渗透压之间没有差异[15, 49, 53]。最近的研究认为，硬膜下积液（SDE）是形成 CSDH 的主要来源[14, 19, 24]，大约一半的 SDE 最终成为 CSDH。连接血管的破裂、新生毛细血管导致的积液壁出血、血管的高通透性、纤维蛋白溶解的增加以及积液中蛋白质含量的增加，对创伤性 SDE 转变为 CSDH 给出了部分解释[8, 11, 14]。我们可以将 CSDH 的临床进展分为三期。第一期为出血期，主要是由一次或多次微创伤所致。紧接着则是潜伏期，在这一时期由于新生血管继续破裂出血、血肿包膜的形成以及纤溶蛋白溶解活性的增加，血肿继续增大。当颅内代偿机制因血肿持续扩大而无法生效时，临床症状期开始。在这一时期，由于直接的占位效应和整体颅内压增高，从而出现一系列的相应症状[8, 11, 14, 19, 24]。

有症状的 CSDH 的治疗方法是手术，血肿的大小是影响手术方式选择的主要因素。对于体积较小的血肿，首选通过麻花钻钻孔或钻颅钻孔的方法，而对于体积较大的血肿和钻孔治疗效果不满意的情况，则采用开颅手术的方法。对于无症状的患者，除了提供对症治疗外，还必须纠正潜在的病理和药物引起的凝血功能障碍[1, 3, 38]。

关于 CSDH 的预后，据文献报道极少数病例会自然消退。虽然非手术治疗的治愈率约为 40%，但仍有 20% 的病例会出现血肿进展的情况，需要手术治疗[23, 50-51]，手术治疗的成功率接近 90%。虽然 CSDH 复发率很高（70%），但其中只有 10%～20% 的病例需要二次手术[30, 35]。CSDH 的位置、内部结构、患者的住院情况、高龄、饮酒、肝肾功能紊乱以及存在全身性疾病被认为是复发的危险因素[22, 42]。使用抗凝血或抗血小板药物在 CSDH 复发中的作用存在争议。同时，复发率也因治疗方法不同而不同。一般来说，钻孔血肿清除术的复发率比颅骨切除术的复发率高[6, 22, 42]。在非手术治疗的复发率方面，不同的研究之间存在差异，但总体来说非手术治疗比一般的手术治疗复发率要高一些。

13.2　CSDH 的放射成像：基本原则

计算机断层成像（CT）由于其应用的广泛性、快速的检测时间和非创伤性的特点，已经成为疑似 CSDH 患者首次检查中公认的标准检查方法。特别是多排 CT 设备可以快速扫描，同时由于双源、双能技术和交互式方法，显著减少了辐射暴露剂量，从而降低潜在风险。尽管磁共振成像（MRI）在急性硬膜下血肿的检查中作用有限，但它在揭示因硬膜肿瘤等导致的继发病因、评估脑实质或含有脑脊液的空腔病变等方面可以提供非常有用的信息[6]。

13.2.1　硬膜下血肿的一般影像特征

从形态上来说，硬膜下出血产生的血性沉积物呈覆盖大脑半球的新月形，但解剖屏障的存在决定了积聚在硬膜下的液体或血肿的整体外观。由于血肿倾向于通过硬脑膜和蛛网膜之间的潜在空间扩散，因此在不伴随蛛网膜下腔出血的情况下，它们不会延伸到脑沟和脑叶中。影响硬膜下血肿外观的另一个重要因素是积血存在的时间和现有血肿的发展阶段。由于 CSDH 一般由急性硬膜下血肿转化而来，因此有必要提及影像学研究中关于血肿存在时间的研究。CT 上病变以霍恩斯菲尔德单位（HU）表现其不同密度，以黑白深浅不同来显示。这是一种描述病变的标准方法，临床上可以通过测量其密度直接对组织类型有一个大致的了解。如果病变与参考组织相比密度较低，它们就会呈现更深的色调，被称为"低密度"。如果它们与参考组织的密度相等，则被认为是"等密度"，如果它们的密度高于参考组织，则被认为是"高密度"，并呈现更浅的色调。一般来说，对于颅内病变，选择脑灰质作为参考组织，急性期的 SDH 多表现为均匀的高密度。在随后的几天里，病变密度平均每天降低 1.5 HU，7～10 天后变为等密度。10～14 天之后，血肿通常变为低密度，无并发症的 CSDH 通常在 2 周后降至 CSF 密度[25]。表 13.1 总结了 SDH 的密度随时间的变化。

因为许多因素在磁共振成像（MRI）上的信号形成中起作用，所以 CSDH 的 MRI 表现比较复杂。决定血肿表现的主要因素是病灶内血红蛋白的结构及其氧化产物。当血液离开静脉时，红细胞中的氧合血红蛋白首先转变为脱氧血红蛋白，然后再转变为高铁血红蛋白。随后细胞裂解，细胞外的高铁血红蛋白最后成为铁蛋白和血色素。这也导致了超急性期（<24 h）、急性期（24～72 h）、早期亚急性期（3～7 天）、晚期亚急性期（7～14 天）和慢性期（>14 天）的积血的不同 MRI 表现。由于氧合血红蛋白和脱氧血红蛋白缺乏磁矩，硬膜下血肿在急性期和高急性期是等信号的，随着高铁血红蛋白的形成，SDH 变成高信号，在亚急性期是顺磁性的。在 T2 加权图像上，硬膜下的血肿块由于含水量高而呈高信号。然而，伴随着脱氧血红蛋白、细胞内高铁血红蛋白和血色素的磁感应效应，在急性期、亚急性晚期和慢性期会出现信号缺失，变成低信号。与 MRI 常规序列（T1 和 T2 加权图像）的这种复杂性表现相反，流

表 13.1　硬膜下血肿的 CT 表现

血肿阶段	时间	CT 表现
超急性期	<24 h	高密度
急性期	1～3 天	高密度
亚急性早期	3～7 天	高密度
亚急性晚期	7～14 天	等密度
慢性期	>14 天	低密度

体衰减反转恢复序列（FLAIR）图像在急性期、亚急性期和慢性期经常出现高信号。在梯度回波（GRE）T2*和磁感应强度加权图像（SWI）上，急性出血或慢性血色素边缘常出现低信号。这些磁感应强度序列（GRE、T2*和SWI）对检测陈旧性血肿产物（血色素和外周铁质沉着）极为敏感[6, 43]。表13.2总结了根据时间划分的硬膜下血肿的MRI表现特点。

在硬膜下血肿的自然病程中，尽管影像学特征明确，但在许多病例中，诊断血肿和确定其分期并不容易。最重要的原因是活动性出血的间断复发或持续进展。在许多情况下，由于同时存在不同阶段的血液成分，在病变内会观察到混杂的信号特征。此外，导致血肿自然演变中断的内源性和外源性因素可能使分期的确定变得困难。凝血功能障碍、抗凝药的使用、蛛网膜破裂导致的脑脊液漏至硬膜下腔、重度贫血导致的低血细胞比容（红细胞压积），或合并感染都会影响血肿的密度[10, 25, 43]。影像学在CSDH中的作用并不局限于诊断。除诊断外，评估可能的继发因素以及对CSDH治疗进行随访也是影像学检查的最常见的用途。

13.2.2 典型的慢性硬膜下血肿/积液表现

如前所述，CSDH是指在硬膜下间隙中已经存在至少2～3周的陈旧性积血积液。在因急性出血而形成的CSDH中，由于溶血机制和长期存在的炎症，急性出血导致的血肿会液化，同时周边有包膜形成。在这个阶段，CSDH的影像学表现与脑脊液相似。而外伤性蛛网膜撕裂或自发性低颅压、脱水或脑萎缩情况下的被动渗出导致的硬膜下积液是一种脑脊液的聚集。在这个阶段，通过CT不能将这两种病变区分开来，因为液化的CSDH和硬膜下积液在CT平扫上都呈现为均匀的低密度（图13.1）。在这些情况下，查看患者以往的影像学资料，可能有助于确定诊断。在以往的CT检查中有急性或亚急性出血的表现，那么就很容易做出CSDH的诊断。除此以外，由于重力引起的红细胞比容效应也有助于诊断CSDH（图13.2）。红细胞比容效应是指由于重力作用，密度不同的血液成分与脑脊液成分产生分层，这种现象在没有急性出血的硬膜下积液中不会出现。由于急性出血密度较高，所以急性出血也不会给慢性硬膜下血肿的诊断造成影响[5-6, 43]。

在MRI中，CSDH与硬膜下积液则很容易进行区分。由于慢性期的细胞外高铁血红蛋白的变性，血红蛋白降解产物开始形成。这些血色素的T1信号不如高铁血红蛋白的信号明显，导致血肿所呈现出的信号强度随时间推移而降低。然而，由于硬膜下血肿的蛋白质含量高于脑脊液，所以血肿的T1信号强度总是高于脑脊液的T1信号强度。

表13.2 不同时期血肿的MRI表现

硬膜下血肿时期	MRI序列		
	T1加权像	T2加权像	磁共振液体衰减反转恢复序列
超急性期	等信号	高信号	高信号
急性期	等信号	高信号	高信号
亚急性早期	高信号	高信号	高信号
亚急性晚期	高信号	高信号	高信号
慢性期	等信号	高信号	高信号

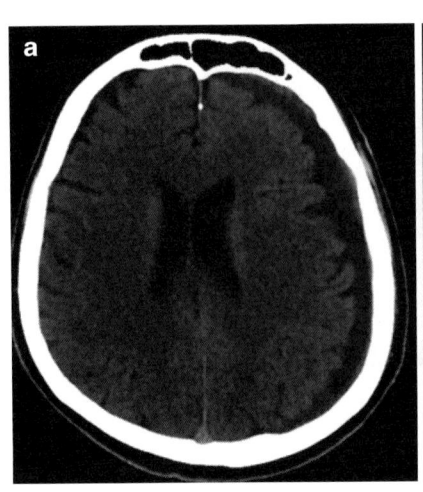 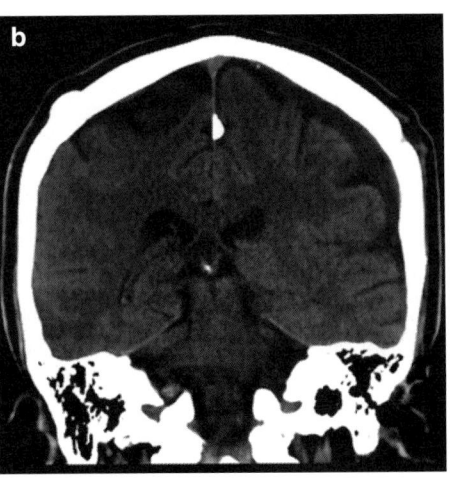

图13.1 一位60岁男性患者的轴位（a）和冠状位（b）CT图像。（a）观察到月牙形、轴外低密度集合（典型的慢性硬膜下血肿）。（b）观察到左侧额顶区有一新月形的轴外低密度集合（典型的慢性硬膜下血肿）

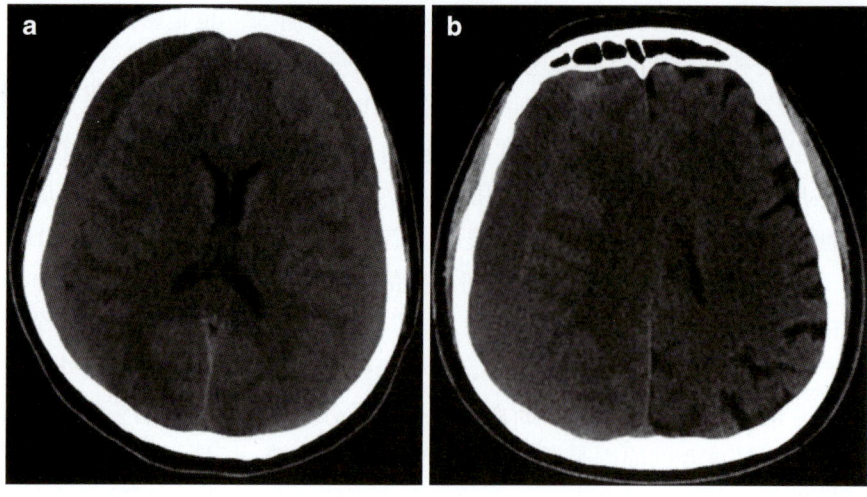

图 13.2 两个不同患者的轴向 CT 图像。(a) 双侧硬膜下出血的患者，在双侧额顶区观察到液体-液体分层。(b) 右侧额顶区慢性硬膜下血肿的患者，额部急性出血密度较高，后方继发有红细胞压积效应

由于磁敏感效应和高蛋白含量，T2 信号的强度随时间推移略有下降，但与脑灰质相比仍呈高强度，与脑脊液相比呈等密度。与脑实质血肿不同，含铁血黄素环在硬膜下血肿中较少见到，因为负责储存铁的巨噬细胞不能停留在轴突空间内。只有在 CSDH 中，外周铁素沉着环可以在对血液元素敏感的 GRE 和 SWI 序列中被识别为低信号。硬膜下积液不包含血色素，因此是低密度的，且观察到的信号强度与脑脊液相同。同时，正常的脑脊液信号在 FLAIR 序列中被抑制，但硬膜下血肿的信号仍然是高信号的，因此可以很容易地与硬膜下积液相区别（图 13.3）。均质性的 CSDH 不显示扩散受限，出现扩散受限应提示存在复发性出血或叠加感染可能[6, 43]。

在一些 CSDH 中可能会出现较厚的内部分隔膜。分隔膜和血肿包膜在 CT 上都显示为高密度，避免将这种高密度的内部分隔膜与活动性出血相混淆对临床诊疗工作是至关重要的。在长期存在的血肿中，硬膜偶尔会表现出弥漫性增厚的高信号，这是由于液化的血肿被吸收。这些厚的分隔膜和硬脑膜在增强的 CT 或 MRI 上显示出明显的增强（图 13.4）[5-6, 25, 43]。在部分存在时间较长的血肿中，增厚的硬膜会出现钙化。CT 检查能够更好地显示出这种钙化表现[6, 25, 43]。而 MRI 则无法区别钙化与出血的表现。因此，当怀疑 CSDH 出现钙化时，建议采用 CT 检查。

还需要对脑萎缩所导致的硬膜下腔扩大与 CSDH 和硬膜下积液进行鉴别诊断。由于在这些患者中没有观察到占位效应的表现，在诊断时应首选 MRI 而不是 CT。

13.2.3 慢性（混合型）硬膜下血肿的急性出血

CSDH 的发展过程是动态的。由于许多内源性和外源性因素导致的急性出血，包括连接血管和血肿包膜破裂导致的反复出血，均会使血肿的形态和

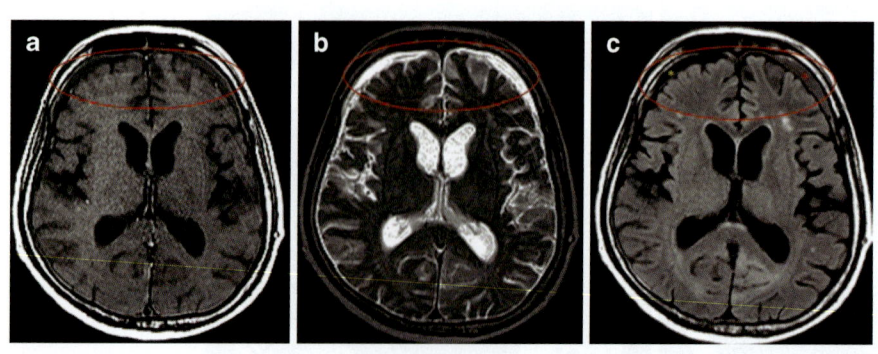

图 13.3 在一位 67 岁的男性患者的 MR 图像中观察到双额轴外积液，这些积液在 T1（a）上是低密度的，在 T2（b）上是高密度的，但是左侧积液的密度在 T1 上比 CSF 高。在 FLAIR 序列中（c），右侧的硬膜下积液信号被抑制，而左侧的信号由于其所含血液成分而未被抑制

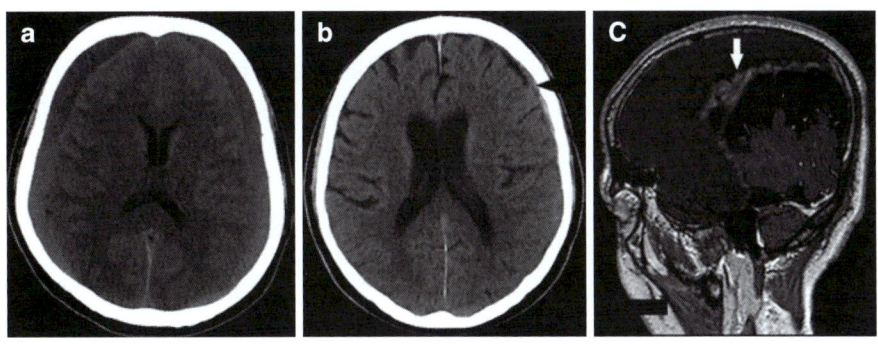

图 13.4　一位 56 岁的女性患者的轴向 CT（a）图像上可见双侧硬膜下血肿。3 个月后的随访 CT 图像（b）中，右侧的血肿完全消退。在左侧，虽然出血内容物已完全吸收，但由于硬脑膜增厚而出现了线性高密度。另一位 70 岁的女性患者的矢状面对比增强 T1 图（c）。值得注意的是，大型慢性硬膜下血肿伴有不规则的硬膜增厚（白色箭头）

构成产生差异。在同一个病灶中，各种出血的表现均可以被观察到。而在硬膜下积液的病例中，也会观察到新生血管出血的表现。所有这些情况都可能导致 CSDH 在 CT 和 MRI 上的复杂表现，从而给诊断带来困难。

在未增强的 CT 上，慢性硬膜下血肿的外观呈覆盖在大脑半球的新月形（图 13.5）。高密度的急性出血因重力作用而沉积，而液化的陈旧性出血则位于上层。特别是在有内部分隔的 CSDH 中，高密度的出血呈弥漫性分布[5]。可以看到高密度的血肿腔内包含的急性出血在多腔、多液平区域和局部聚集。

急性 CSDH 在 MRI 上的表现与 CT 上所见相似。混合型硬膜下血肿在 MRI 上的表现差异很大，主要是由于血红蛋白与其他血液成分的含量不同所导致的。CSDH 的 T1 和 T2 信号一般是不均匀的，而在 FLAIR 图像上信号一般是高信号的。在 GRE 和 SWI 上可以看到开花状伪影（图 13.5）。急性或亚急性血肿在 DWI 像上通常显示扩散受限。血肿包膜和内部分隔在增强后的 T1 加权像上则显示明

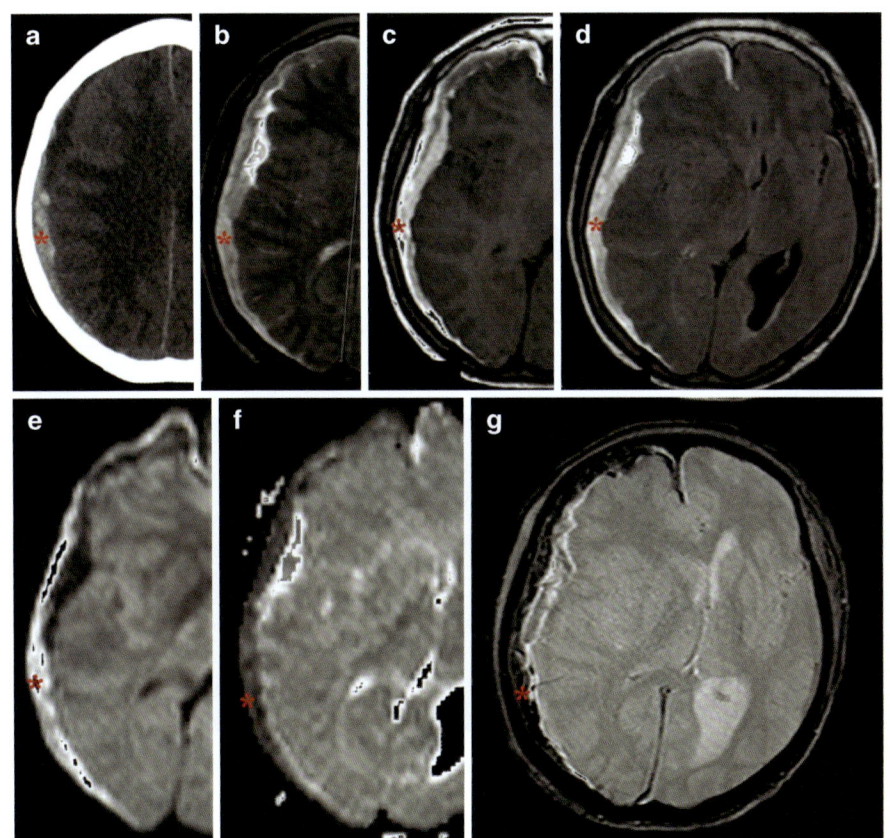

图 13.5　一位 58 岁男性患者的轴位脑 CT（a），观察到右侧额叶的急性或慢性出血引起的硬膜下血肿。在 2 天后的 MRI 检查中（b~g），观察到血肿体积增大。含有低等信号区域的 T2 图像（b），以及非对比度 T1 图像（c）中由于急性出血（红色星号）导致的高信号都很明显。在 FLAIR 图像（d）中，血肿被视为高信号。在扩散加权图像（e）中，由于急性出血区的扩散受限，观察到高信号影。在 ADC 图和梯度加权的 T2* 图像上则为低信号（f）

显的对比度增强[5]。

13.2.4 CSDH的继发性损伤

与检测硬膜下血肿同样重要的是确定可能危及生命的继发性损伤，并予以相应的对症治疗。造成继发性损伤的主要机制是血肿对大脑的占位效应。血肿产生占位可能压迫脑组织移位而产生脑疝，同时挤压血管出现脑缺血表现。

13.2.4.1 占位效应和中线移位

硬膜下血肿会压迫脑实质，从而产生占位效应。这在CT上表现为脑沟的消失。在血肿压迫较长时间后，由于血管外渗，脑实质开始出现脑水肿。脑水肿会造成皮质增厚，灰白质无法辨别等表现。在这个阶段，脑实质在CT上出现低密度，在T1序列上出现低信号，而在T2和FLAIR序列上出现高信号。随着占位效应的发展，开始出现侧脑室向中线的偏移（图13.6）。在这个阶段，当脑疝症状还未表现时，明确中线移位的程度对患者治疗是至关重要的。为了在CT或MRI上明确中线移位，首先必须标出中线位置。连接大脑镰与颅骨内层的前后两点之间直线即为大脑中线[6]。然后，用侧脑室之间的半球裂缝与中线的垂直距离来确定中线的位移程度。

13.2.4.2 脑疝综合征

随着占位效应强度的增加，可能出现脑疝综合征，即脑实质由于血肿压迫而产生移位的现象。

13.2.4.2.1 大脑镰下疝

大脑镰下疝为硬膜下血肿中最常见的脑疝类型，为大脑半球内侧面的扣带回及邻近的额回经大脑镰下缘向对侧移位疝出所致。位于半球间裂隙中的大脑前动脉（ACA）常常被疝出的脑实质压迫移位（图13.7），这常常导致ACA灌注区的梗死。在严重的大脑镰下疝的病例中，侧脑室所受的压力可能会增加，孟氏孔梗阻可能导致对侧脑积水。脑室扩张首先出现在对侧脑室的额角，其次是颞角[6, 29]。

13.2.4.2.2 小脑幕切迹下疝

部分CSDH病例中同样可以观察到小脑幕切迹下疝的存在。病变使幕上颅内压力增高，脑组织

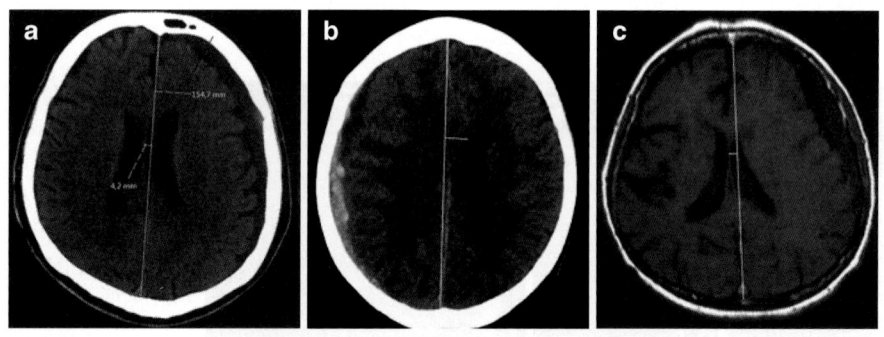

图13.6 在CT（a）和MRI（c）上观察到继发于血肿占位效应的中线移位以及慢性硬膜下出血中急性出血的CT（b）图像。在轴位CT上，在额部和枕部最突出的区域之间画一条线（中线）。这条线与脑室之间的距离显示了与中线的偏移程度。红色星号（b）表示由于肿块的影响，脑沟出现了渗出

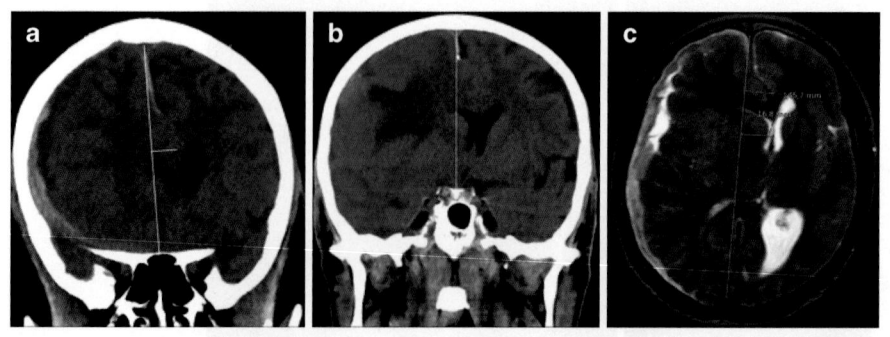

图13.7 在冠状面的CT（a，b）和轴向的MRI（c）上观察到不同患者的大脑镰下疝。在冠状位CT图像上（a，b），除了中线移位外，右侧扣带回也从大脑镰的游离缘下移至左侧（红色箭头）。在轴向T2磁共振成像（c）中，除了扣带回外，右脑前动脉也被观察到向左移动。在所有病例中，可以看到对侧侧脑室的扩大（脑积水）

经小脑幕切迹疝入幕下。表现为颞叶内侧结构经小脑幕切迹向下疝入同侧大脑脚池，中脑或脑干受压向对侧移位、旋转，可压迫同侧大脑后动脉及动眼神经、中脑导水管致内侧颞叶和枕叶梗死、瞳孔散大、偏瘫和脑积水（图13.8）。在更严重的情况下，由于脑干受压，可能会出现意识丧失、呼吸窘迫、脑神经病变，最终死亡。本例中，脑干两侧均受到压迫，出现双侧基底池闭塞。

在小脑幕切迹下疝中，大脑后动脉（PCA）的P2和P3段被压迫在小脑幕游离边缘和颞叶之间，导致PCA灌注区的梗死。因此，在这种类型的脑疝中，仔细评估同侧PCA区域的脑实质对于发现早期梗死非常重要[6, 29]。

另一个临床要点是，在严重的小脑幕切迹下疝中，对侧大脑脚（cerebral peduncle）可能与小脑幕切迹相互压迫。在这种情况下，可能出现同侧偏瘫。部分病例还会观察到下丘脑和基底神经节的梗死，这是由于Willis近端圆环的穿孔动脉被压迫。同时还存在脑桥腹侧和中脑的出血性梗死（称为Duret出血），多由基底穿孔动脉的压迫和闭塞所造成[6]。

13.2.4.2.3 上行性小脑幕疝

上行性小脑幕疝是最不常见的脑疝类型。与其他两种类型的脑疝不同，造成这种脑疝的占位效应的来源是颅后窝。尽管这种脑疝大多是由小脑梗死继发的脑水肿所造成，但是脑实质的出血和硬膜下血肿也可能导致类似的情况。由于占位性病变的肿块效应，小脑蚓部和小脑内侧半球向上移位。因此，向上移位的小脑结构会使中脑压迫脑室与基底池。由于中脑水管和第四脑室也受到压迫，患者可能会出现阻塞性脑积水的表现[6]。

13.2.4.2.4 后天性小脑扁桃体下疝

与上行性小脑幕疝相似，后天性小脑扁桃体下疝最常见的原因是颅后窝肿瘤和缺血性小脑梗死引起的脑水肿，但脑实质出血或硬膜下血肿也可能引起后天性小脑扁桃体下疝。目前临床工作中更倾向于采用矢状位CT或MRI来诊断。在轴状位的横断面图像中，小脑扁桃体完全填塞大孔是后天性小脑扁桃体下疝的一个标志（图13.9）[6, 29]。

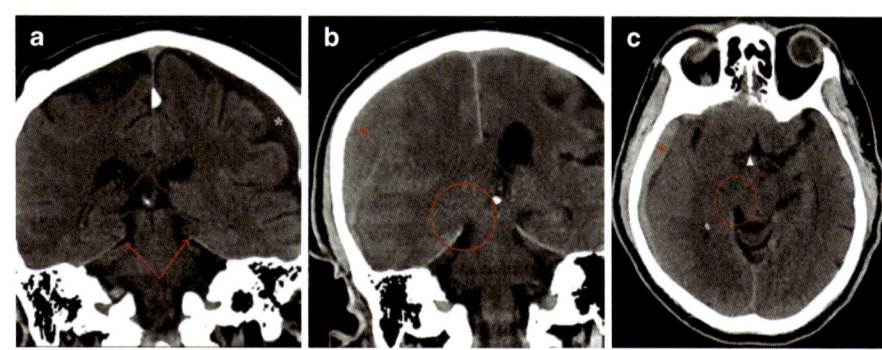

图13.8 （a）正常情况下，显示了小脑幕游离缘、周围结构和颞叶的关系（红色箭头）。（b）在右侧亚急性硬膜下血肿（红色星号）的案例中，继发于血肿占位效应，右侧颞叶内侧移至中线，使右侧脑室消失。（c）同一患者的轴位CT图像显示，由于硬膜下血肿的占位效应，右侧周围池（红色圆圈）和鞍上池（白色箭头）已经消失，右侧硬膜下血肿呈占位效应（红色星号）

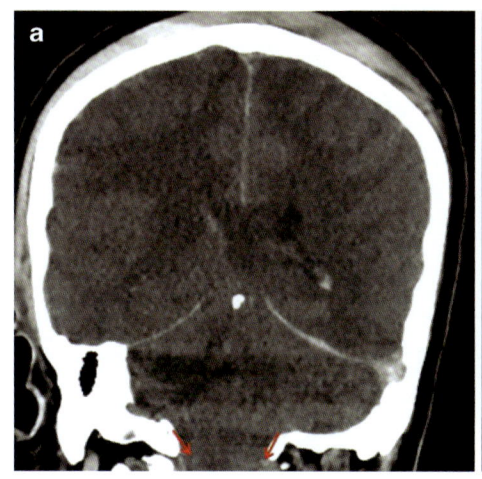
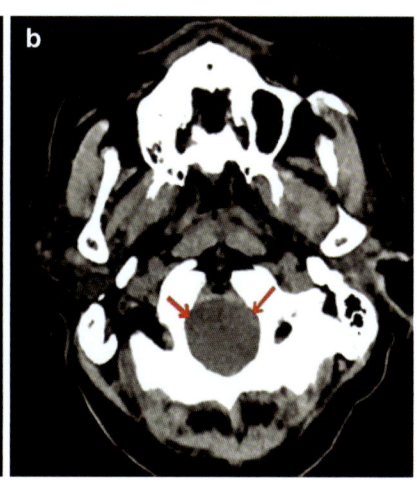

图13.9 在冠状位（a）和轴位（b）脑CT图像中，可见枕骨大孔较为饱满，同时压迫延髓

13.2.4.3 阻塞性脑积水

CSDH 引起的阻塞性脑积水一般继发于各种脑疝。最常见的形式是对侧脑室积水，主要是由于中线位移导致的。虽然整个对侧脑室都可能扩大，但以额角和颞角的扩大更为常见。小脑幕切迹下疝通常会导致双侧侧脑室出现脑积水，而小脑扁桃体下疝所导致的脑积水则会波及全部脑室。

侧脑室颞角的扩大是阻塞性脑积水的早期标志[6]。正常情况下，由于年轻人的脑容量正常，颞角完全不可见，或者只见一条细线。而在老年人群体中，由于脑实质萎缩或其他一些原因，颞角会扩大，这也使得脑积水的诊断变得困难。

13.2.5 鉴别诊断

同样有一些正常的解剖组织或其他疾病需要与 CSDH 进行鉴别。在这一部分我们将简要讨论这些鉴别点。

13.2.5.1 扩增的静脉窦和皮质静脉

一些静脉窦和皮质静脉由于血流缓慢或出现血栓时，可能与亚急性期和急性期硬膜下血肿相混淆。导致这种情况发生的最常见解剖结构是横窦，其次是蝶顶窦和皮质静脉。在无法确定的情况下，可以使用增强 CT 来进行鉴别。注射增强造影剂后，正常的静脉窦和皮质静脉将会显示明显的增强影像。在 MRI 图像上与横断面平行排列的血管结构，特别是流速较慢的静脉窦，在 T1 图像上显示高信号。通常来说，MRI 比 CT 更容易鉴别这种情况（图13.10）。在涉及静脉结构的情况下，可以通过使用增强磁共振静脉造影进行准确诊断[7, 26]。

13.2.5.2 正常脑实质的延伸

在轴状位图像中，额叶和小脑的后部延伸至颅中窝，可使人产生轴外病变的怀疑（图 13.11）[7, 32]。若怀疑病灶存在，可在矢状位或冠状位的 CT 或 MRI 扫描平片中证明脑组织的连续性，有助于进行相关鉴别诊断。

13.2.5.3 伪影

在 CT 扫描中，与硬膜下血肿最容易混淆的伪影是射线束硬化伪影。在这个伪影中，X 线在通过凹陷的骨面时可能会被散射，导致图像上出现线性的高密度。这种伪影多见于颅前窝和颅后窝，可以用各种过滤和校正软件将其降到最低。由于其呈现高密度，这种伪影可能被误认为是急性期的硬膜下血肿。在曝光时间较长的 MRI 中，患者的误动也可能造成这种伪影[7, 26]。

13.2.5.4 肿瘤

据既往文献报道，许多硬膜下血肿被误诊为脑部肿瘤。这种误诊的主要原因是血肿液成分混杂，增加了对可能疾病的考虑[44]。既往的恶性肿瘤病史是提示存在潜在肿瘤的最重要因素。病灶的扩大或随访影像学上的结节性表现可提示存在肿瘤的可能[26]。对于有恶性肿瘤病史的患者，在头部外伤后出现硬膜下积液时也应警惕颅内占位性病变的可能。大多数疑似硬膜下血肿的占位性病变多为转移性肿瘤、血液系统恶性肿瘤和脑膜瘤[34, 37]。

图 13.10 在继发于脑萎缩的硬膜下间隙增大的病例中，轴位脑 CT（a）中右侧横窦，冠状位脑 CT（b）中乙状窦被观察到高密度影

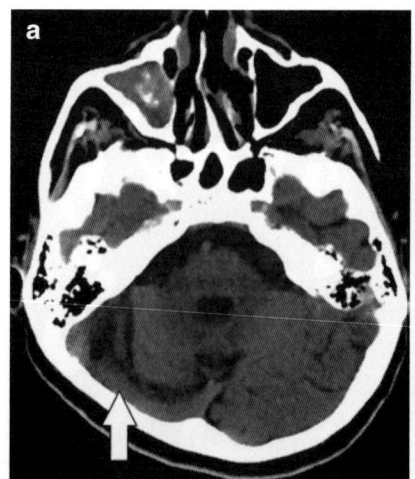
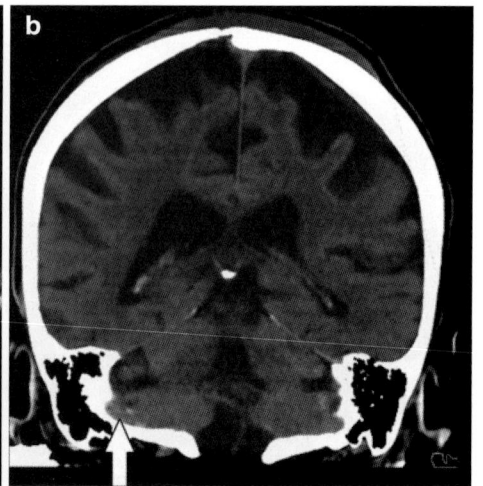

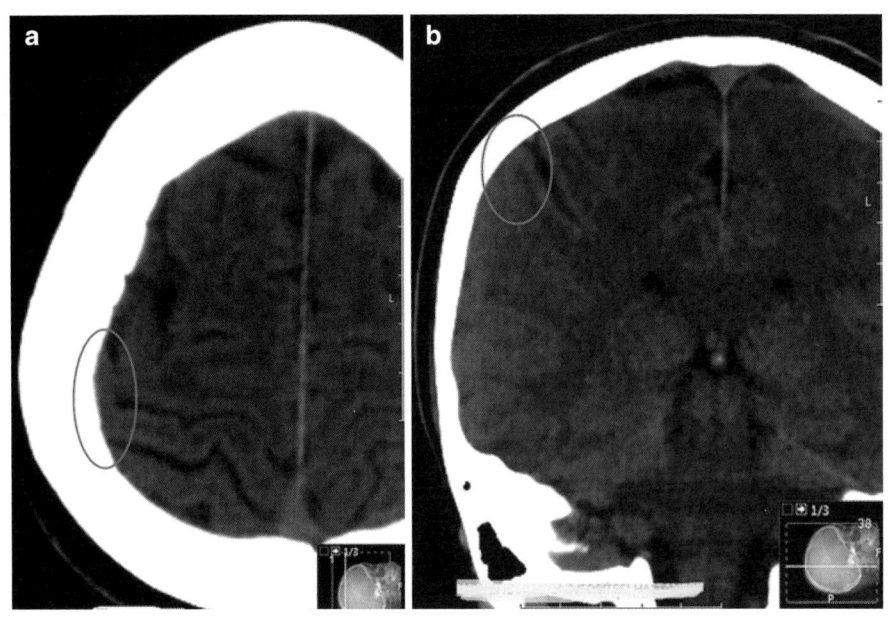

图 13.11 在轴位非对比脑 CT 中（a）的等密度影与慢性硬膜下血肿相似，但是由于在冠状位图像中显示其与邻近灰白质的连续性，因此并非慢性硬膜下血肿病变（b）

平扫 CT 是首选的检查方式，但一般不足以区分 CSDH 和颅内肿瘤。邻近的颅骨受累在 CSDH 中并不多见。若有骨质增生的存在，可能提示脑膜瘤。当骨质中出现侵蚀提示有转移性肿瘤的可能。也可以根据 CSDH 的外观与肿瘤进行相应的鉴别。CSDH 通常具有光滑的轮廓，而结节状或分叶状的轮廓提示有肿瘤的可能。同时，肿瘤存在于多灶性病变的可能性也更大。当硬膜下的沉积液含有不存在于正常血液中的异质性成分时，也提示肿瘤的可能性。硬膜下血肿附近的脑实质因占位效应可能出现脑水肿，但当颅内其他部位出现局灶性脑水肿时则应考虑颅内肿瘤的可能（图 13.12）[34, 37, 44]。

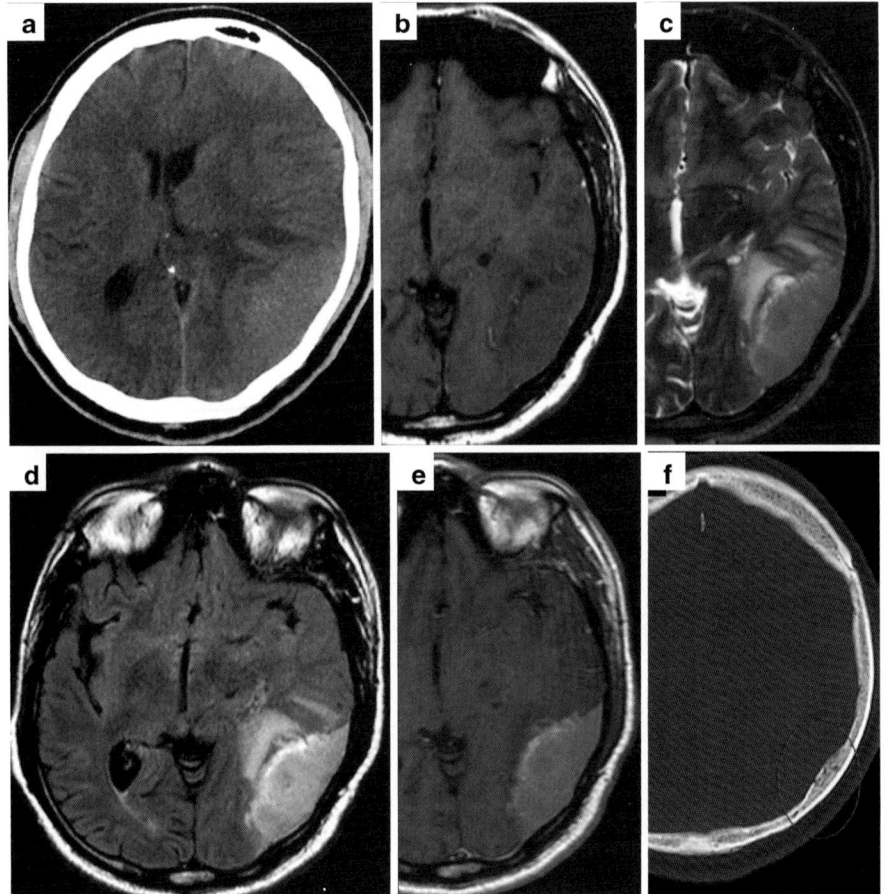

图 13.12 一位 55 岁男性脑膜瘤患者的颅脑 CT（a, f）和 MRI（b ～ e）图像。在轴位 CT 图像（a）中，在轴外有一个等密度（对灰质）的病变。该病变在 T1（b）上与灰质呈等信号，在 T2（c）上呈等高信号，在 FLAIR（d）上呈高信号。在造影剂增强的 T1 像（e）上，可以观察到病变有明显的均质强化。在骨窗轴位 CT 图像（f）中，由于骨质增生，邻近的骨质厚度增加

在怀疑有颅内肿瘤的情况下，推荐增强MRI作为首选检查。在急需手术而MRI不能立即进行的情况下，也可采取增强CT用于检查。在影像学扫描中，肿瘤性病变通常表现为均匀的明显强化，而CSDH则不显示强化。同样，若硬膜上出现增厚和均匀强化的病灶，则提示肿瘤可能存在硬膜转移[26]。在CSDH病例中，由于血肿液中的血液成分被吸收，同样可以观察到硬膜增厚和增强的表现。

13.2.5.5 缺氧缺血性脑损伤

脑实质的全面低灌注通常是由于心肌梗死而造成的。在这种情况下，由于脑实质弥漫性水肿导致在蛛网膜下腔/硬膜下腔出现的高密度信号被定义为假性蛛网膜下腔/硬膜下腔出血。这种缺氧缺血性损害多与急性硬膜下血肿相混淆，也可与完全吸收的CSDH中的增厚硬脑膜相混淆。在缺氧缺血性损害中常常出现弥散性低密度影、灰白质分界不清、脑沟模糊、蛛网膜下腔及脑池密度增高等表现，这有助于与CSDH相区别。MRI同样可以用于这两种疾病的鉴别[7, 26]。

13.2.5.6 肥厚性硬膜炎

肥厚性硬膜炎（HP）是一种以硬脑膜和（或）脊髓硬膜局限性或弥漫性纤维性增厚为特征的中枢神经系统罕见疾病。按发病部位可分为肥厚性硬脑膜炎和肥厚性硬脊膜炎。按病因肥厚性硬膜炎可分为特发性和继发性两种形式，前者更为多见。特发性肥厚性硬膜炎的诊断需排除潜在的病因，而继发性肥厚性硬膜炎病因多样，包括感染、自身免疫性疾病、肿瘤、外伤等[16]。详细的临床检查可发现全身累及性病变，对于鉴别该病非常重要。增厚的硬脑膜和增强的结节性特征病灶以及伴随的软脑膜增强有助于与CSDH鉴别诊断[26, 44]。

13.2.5.7 脑脓肿

硬膜下脓肿是一种危急的临床情况，其可以通过直接的毗邻入侵或通过血液途径发生。硬膜下脓肿常由鼻窦炎或中耳感染引起，但外伤、手术史和脑膜炎也是常见的致病因素[52]。硬膜下脓肿在CT上通常表现为硬膜下单侧等密度或低密度信号（图13.13）。

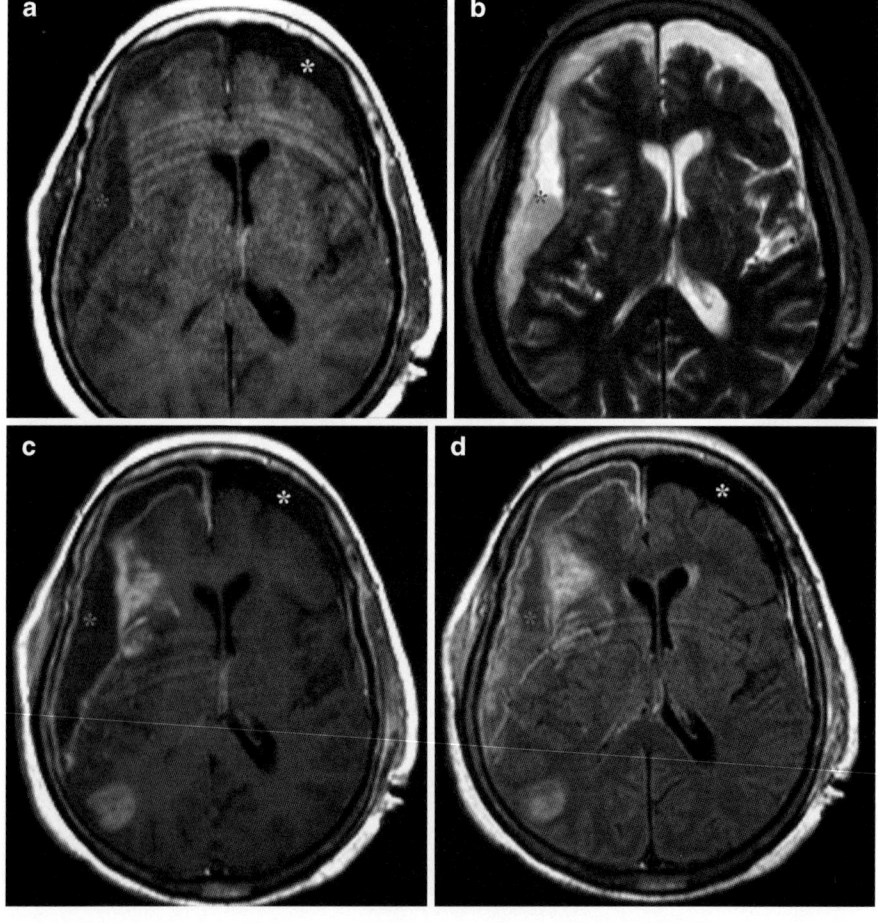

图13.13 一位61岁的男性患者在增强脑部MRI检查中观察到双侧硬膜下血肿。血肿在T1像上呈低信号（a），在T2像上呈高信号（b）。值得注意的是，由于血红蛋白的作用，右边的血肿信号更高，并呈现出液体-液体分层（星号）。在增强的T1像上（c），可以观察到硬脑膜有明显的增强。在对比后的FLAIR图像（d）上，可以观察到硬膜增厚，硬膜下血肿，脑脊液呈异质性高信号

脓肿通常由继发于慢性炎症的厚壁包裹，由于水肿，邻近脑实质的灰白质界限可能消失。在这种状态下，很难与 CSDH 相区别。若发现鼻窦炎或中耳炎等原发性感染灶，则将有助于诊断。在 MRI 上，大多数硬膜下脓肿在 T1 像上由于蛋白含量高而呈等信号，而在 T2 像上的信号强度低于脑脊液。硬膜下脓肿在增强的 T1 像上表现为硬膜增强。DWI 中的弥散限制对于区分硬膜下脓肿和 CSDH 很重要。在 MRI 上观察邻近结构的感染源也支持诊断[52]。

13.2.5.8 硬膜下积液

硬膜下积液（SH）是指脑脊液在硬膜下空间积聚。创伤性脑损伤、自发性颅内低血压均与 SH 相关。与 CSDH 不同，SH 不含陈旧性的积血。然而，正如在 CSDH 的病理生理学中提到的，由于硬膜下积聚的脑脊液不断增加，导致脆弱的新生血管形成破裂，可能会导致 SH 出血。一些研究表明，SH 是 CSDH 发生发展的病因之一[12]。在本例硬膜下出血中，在 CT 上 SH 和 CSDH 均为低密度，无法区分。在 MRI 上，由于血液降解产物在 T1 像上的信号比脑脊液高，所以 CSDH 在 T1 像上信号高于脑脊液，特别是在 FLAIR 序列图像上由于脑脊液信号受到抑制，CSDH 病灶处的高信号对于鉴别诊断十分具有价值（图 13.3）[6, 26]。SH 多见于双侧，但双侧性并不是鉴别 CSDH 和 SH 的充分证据。

13.2.6 血肿复发的影像学预测因素

手术是治疗有临床症状的 CSDH 的主要手段，但手术后血肿有一定的复发概率。影响复发的重要因素是患者的整体状况以及接受的手术方式。为此，应在术前确定是否存在血肿复发的可疑情况。在影像学方面，双侧血肿、中线移位超过 10 mm 和 CSDH 体积超过 150 ml 均被认为与复发相关。除此以外，还发现血肿的 CT 密度与复发之间存在相关性[42]。均匀的等密度或低密度的血肿，其复发率低于高密度或异质混合密度的血肿。同样有研究指出，层状型或分离型的血肿复发率要更高。术后存在颅内积气也会增加复发的风险[18, 27, 33, 39, 42]。

13.2.7 术后血肿的影像学表现

评估术后早期可能出现的并发症最常用的影像学方法是颅脑 CT[5-6, 26]。CT 可以准确地发现术后早期可能出现的新的出血、占位、脑疝及颅内积气。MRI 在检测术后早期的急性缺血或颅内感染方面具有很高的敏感性。然而，颅内积气及其他术后常见情况可能会在 MRI 上引起伪影。因此，应根据临床情况选择在术后是否使用 MRI。

13.3 结论

CSDH 是硬膜下积聚的陈旧性积血，它的发生发展是一个动态过程。CSDH 可以表现为无特异性的临床症状，也可以表现为危及生命的昏迷。影像学上，CSDH 可能是均匀的等密度或低密度的血肿，也可能是异质混合密度的血肿。在进行诊断时存在着一定的影像学误区，将血肿的发展阶段和影像学特征相对应将有助于进行鉴别诊断。

参考文献

1. Almenawer SA, Farrokhyar F, Hong C, Alhazzani W, Manoranjan B, Yarascavitch B, Arjmand P, Baronia B, Reddy K, Murty N, Singh S. Chronic subdural hematoma management: a systematic review and meta-analysis of 34,829 patients. Ann Surg. 2014;259(3):449–57.
2. Baechli H, Nordmann A, Bucher HC, Gratzl O. Demographics and prevalent risk factors of chronic subdural haematoma: results of a large single-center cohort study. Neurosurg Rev. 2004;27(4):263–6.
3. Blaauw J, Jacobs B, den Hertog HM, van der Gaag NA, Jellema K, Dammers R, Lingsma HF, van der Naalt J, Kho KH, Groen RJM. Neurosurgical and perioperative management of chronic subdural hematoma. Front Neurol. 2020;11:550.
4. Bosche B, Molcanyi M, Noll T, Kochanek M, Kraus B, Rieger B, El Majdoub F, Dohmen C, Löhr M, Goldbrunner R, Brinker G. Occurrence and recurrence of spontaneous chronic subdural haematoma is associated with a factor XIII deficiency. Clin Neurol Neurosurg. 2013;115(1):13–8.

5. Broder JS. Head computed tomography interpretation in trauma: a primer. Psychiatr Clin North Am. 2010;33(4):821–54.
6. Carroll JJ, Lavine SD, Meyers PM. Imaging of subdural hematomas. Neurosurg Clin N Am. 2017;28(2):179–203.
7. Catana D, Koziarz A, Cenic A, Nath S, Singh S, Almenawer SA, Kachur E. Subdural hematoma mimickers: a systematic review. World Neurosurg. 2016;93:73–80.
8. Cecchini G. Chronic subdural hematoma pathophysiology: a unifying theory for a dynamic process. J Neurosurg Sci. 2017;61(5):536–43.
9. Chiesa A, Duhaime AC. Abusive head trauma. Pediatr Clin North Am. 2009;56(2):317–31.
10. Duy L, Badeeb A, Duy W, Alqahtani E, Champion W, Kim DH, Martin D, Vartanians V, Coffin P, Small JE. CT attenuation of acute subdural hematomas in patients with anemia. J Neuroimaging. 2019;29(4):536–9.
11. Edlmann E, Giorgi-Coll S, Whitfield PC, Carpenter KLH, Hutchinson PJ. Pathophysiology of chronic subdural haematoma: inflammation, angiogenesis and implications for pharmacotherapy. J Neuroinflammation. 2017;14(1):108.
12. Fan G, Ding J, Wang H, Wang Y, Liu Y, Wang C, Li Z. Risk factors for the development of chronic subdural hematoma in patients with subdural hygroma. Br J Neurosurg. 2021;35(1):1–6.
13. Feghali J, Yang W, Huang J. Updates in chronic subdural hematoma: epidemiology, etiology, pathogenesis, treatment, and outcome. World Neurosurg. 2020;141:339–45.
14. Feng JF, Jiang JY, Bao YH, Liang YM, Pan YH. Traumatic subdural effusion evolves into chronic subdural hematoma: two stages of the same inflammatory reaction? Med Hypotheses. 2008;70:1147–9.
15. Gardner WJ. Traumatic subdural hematoma. Arch Neurpsych. 1932;27(4):847–58.
16. Hahn LD, Fulbright R, Baehring JM. Hypertrophic pachymeningitis. J Neurol Sci. 2016;367:278–83.
17. Holmes WH. Chronic subdural hematoma. Arch Neurpsych. 1928;20(1):162–70.
18. Huang YH, Lin WC, Lu CH, Chen WF. Volume of chronic subdural haematoma: is it one of the radiographic factors related to recurrence? Injury. 2014;45(9):1327–31.
19. Jafari N, Gesner L, Koziol JM, Rotoli G, Hubschmann OR. The pathogenesis of chronic subdural hematomas: a study on the formation of chronic subdural hematomas and analysis of computed tomography findings. World Neurosurg. 2017;107:376–81.
20. Ju MW, Kim SH, Kwon HJ, Choi SW, Koh HS, Youm JY, Song SH. Comparison between brain atrophy and subdural volume to predict chronic subdural hematoma: volumetric CT imaging analysis. Korean J Neurotrauma. 2015;11(2):87–92.
21. Kostić A, Kehayov I, Stojanović N, Nikolov V, Kitov B, Milošević P, Kostić E, Zhelyazkov H. Spontaneous chronic subdural hematoma in elderly people—arterial hypertension and other risk factors. J Chin Med Assoc. 2018;81(9):781–6.
22. Kung WM, Lin MS. CT-based quantitative analysis for pathological features associated with postoperative recurrence and potential application upon artificial intelligence: a narrative review with a focus on chronic subdural hematomas. Mol Imaging. 2020;19:1536012120914773.
23. Lee KS. History of chronic subdural hematoma. Korean J Neurotrauma. 2015;11(2):27–34.
24. Lee KS. Natural history of chronic subdural haematoma. Brain Inj. 2004;18(4):351–8.
25. Lee KS, Bae WK, Bae HG, et al. The computed tomographic attenuation and the age of subdural hematomas. J Korean Med Sci. 1997;12(4):353–9.
26. Lim M, Kheok SW, Lim KC, Venkatanarasimha N, Small JE, Chen RC. Subdural haematoma mimics. Clin Radiol. 2019;74(9):663–75.
27. Liu LX, Cao XD, Ren YM, Zhou LX, Yang CH. Risk factors for recurrence of chronic subdural hematoma: a single center experience. World Neurosurg. 2019;132:e506–13.
28. Májovský M, Netuka D. Chronic subdural hematoma—review article. Rozhl Chir. 2018;97(6):253–7.
29. Matsumoto H, Hanayama H, Okada T, Sakurai Y, Minami H, Masuda A, Tominaga S, Miyaji K, Yamaura I, Yoshida Y. Clinical investigation of chronic subdural hematoma with impending brain herniation on arrival. Neurosurg Rev. 2018;41(2):447–55.
30. Matsuoka K, Nakai E, Kawanishi Y, Kadota T, Fukuda H, Ueba T. Acute deterioration in a patient with bilateral chronic subdural hematomas associated with intracranial hypotension treated with an epidural blood patch. World Neurosurg. 2020;141:331–4.
31. Mcdonald RL. Pathophysiology of chronic subdural hematomas. In: Winn HR, editor. Youmans and Winn neurological surgery. 7th ed. Amsterdam: Elsevier; 2017. p. 304–9.
32. McKinney AM. Cerebellar flocculus pseudomass. In: Atlas of normal imaging variations of the brain, skull, and craniocervical vasculature. Cham: Springer; 2017. p. 13–8.

33. Miah IP, Tank Y, Rosendaal FR, Peul WC, Dammers R, Lingsma HF, den Hertog HM, Jellema K, van der Gaag NA, Dutch Chronic Subdural Hematoma Research Group. Radiological prognostic factors of chronic subdural hematoma recurrence: a systematic review and meta-analysis. Neuroradiology. 2021;63(1):27–40.
34. Miki K, Kai Y, Hiraki Y, Kamano H, Oka K, Natori Y. Malignant meningioma mimicking chronic subdural hematoma. World Neurosurg. 2019;124:71–8.
35. Nakaguchi H, Tanishima T, Yoshimasu N. Factors in the natural history of chronic subdural hematomas that influence their postoperative recurrence. J Neurosurg. 2001;95(2):256–62.
36. Orman G, Kralik SF, Meoded A, Desai N, Risen S, Huisman TAGM. MRI findings in pediatric abusive head trauma: a review. J Neuroimaging. 2020;30(1):15–27.
37. Patil S, Veron A, Hosseini P, Bates R, Brown B, Guthikonda B, DeSouza R. Metastatic prostate cancer mimicking chronic subdural hematoma: a case report and review of the literature. J La State Med Soc. 2010;162(4):203–5.
38. Ragland JT, Lee K. Chronic subdural hematoma ICU management. Neurosurg Clin N Am. 2017;28(2):239–46.
39. Ridwan S, Bohrer AM, Grote A, Simon M. Surgical treatment of chronic subdural hematoma: predicting recurrence and cure. World Neurosurg. 2019;128:e1010–23.
40. Rust T, Kiemer N, Erasmus A. Chronic subdural haematomas and anticoagulation or anti-thrombotic therapy. J Clin Neurosci. 2006;13(8):823–7.
41. Sahyouni R, Goshtasbi K, Mahmoodi A, Tran DK, Chen JW. Chronic subdural hematoma: a historical and clinical perspective. World Neurosurg. 2017;108:948–53.
42. Shimizu Y, Park C, Tokuda K. Gradation density hematoma is a predictor of chronic subdural hematoma recurrence associated with inflammation of the outer membrane. Clin Neurol Neurosurg. 2020;194:105839.
43. Sieswerda-Hoogendoorn T, Postema FAM, Verbaan D, Majoie CB, van Rijn RR. Age determination of subdural hematomas with CT and MRI: a systematic review. Eur J Radiol. 2014;83(7):1257–68.
44. Tan LQ, Loh DD, Qiu L, Ng YP, Hwang PYK. When hoofbeats mean zebras not horses: tumour mimics of subdural haematoma—case series and literature review. J Clin Neurosci. 2019;67:244–8.
45. Trotter W. Chronic subdural haemorrhage of traumatic origin, and its relation to pachymeningitis hemorrhagica interna. Br J Surg. 1914;2:271–91.
46. Uno M, Toi H, Hirai S. Chronic subdural hematoma in elderly patients: is this disease benign? Neurol Med Chir (Tokyo). 2017;57(8):402–9.
47. Vega RA, Valadka AB. Natural history of acute subdural hematoma. Neurosurg Clin N Am. 2017;28(2):247–55.
48. Virchow R. Das ha'matom der dura mater. Verh Phys Med Ges. 1857;7:134–42.
49. Weir B. The osmolality of subdural hematoma fluid. J Neurosurg. 1971;34(4):528–33.
50. Yadav YR, Parihar V, Namdev H, Bajaj J. Chronic subdural hematoma. Asian J Neurosurg. 2016;11(4):330–42.
51. Yang W, Huang J. Chronic subdural hematoma: epidemiology and natural history. Neurosurg Clin N Am. 2017;28(2):205–10.
52. Yuan X, Shi X, Xiao H, Sun G, Bai Y, Zhao H, Gao M. Intracranial subdural empyema mimicking chronic subdural hematoma. J Craniofac Surg. 2016;27(2):529–30.
53. Zollinger R, Gross RE. Traumatic subdural hematoma. JAMA. 1934;103(4):245–9.

第 14 章　机化的慢性硬膜下血肿

Mustafa Balevi，Ayşe M. Dumlu 和 Mehmet Turgut

译者：陈思畅

14.1　引言

慢性硬膜下血肿（CSDH）是一种常见的神经外科疾病，其特点是颅内硬膜下间隙进行性聚集血液及其降解产物[74]。在不同患者中，慢性硬膜下血肿可能呈现不同的结构，可出现多个血肿和分隔，血肿膜增厚和固态包裹的区域称为"机化"慢性硬膜下血肿[62, 80]。

Von Rokitansky 在 1841 年的一次尸检中首次报道了机化的慢性硬膜下血肿[89]。1930 年进行了第一例机化的慢性硬膜下血肿手术[26]。Feghali 等报道，慢性硬膜下血肿是一种复杂的疾病，每年发病率为（1.7～20.6）/10 万人，其中老年人发病率更高[21]。慢性硬膜下血肿的机化或钙化发生率仅为 0.3%～2.7%，随着时间的推移，其发生率逐渐增加，特别是在使用抗凝/抗血小板药物的老年人群中[9, 44, 59, 61]。慢性硬膜下血肿通常见于老年患者或 2 岁以下的儿童，年轻人的大脑由于顺应性较高，发生慢性硬膜下血肿的概率要低得多[83]。

14.2　机化的慢性硬膜下血肿的动态病理生理学

从病理生理学角度看，慢性硬膜下血肿的形成和扩张都与炎症事件（包括血管生成）导致的新的血肿膜的形成有关[21]。随后血肿导致纤维蛋白沉积，形成硬膜下膜，并在膜中形成脆弱的毛细血管[14, 19, 43]。有研究表明，慢性硬膜下血肿中纤溶酶原激活剂的存在增加了纤溶活性，引起止血失败，导致"外膜再出血"和硬膜下腔内"血浆渗出"[35, 39, 90]。需要注意的是，硬膜下腔积血的再吸收程度是慢性硬膜下血肿症状缓解或恶化的重要因素[14, 22, 39, 76]。此外，在接下来的 6～12 个月的时间里，各种凝血功能障碍在内外膜连接处的新膜和脆弱血管的形成中起到一定的作用，导致反复出血，最终形成内膜和外膜融合的固体纤维结构[24, 36, 62, 66, 70, 84, 93]。

部分慢性硬膜下血肿患者由于长期反复多次的腔内出血，可能在不同阶段的多个腔内出现液化血肿[19]。随后，慢性硬膜下血肿内可能发生钙化、化生或营养不良以及骨化，但其确切的发生机制尚不清楚[3, 5, 53-54]。钙化可能在出血后 6 个月至数年内发生[17, 33, 60, 94]。经过几年的钙化后，慢性硬膜下血肿可能发生骨化[47, 61]。

最近，该方面的专家及其同事报道了钙化或骨化的慢性硬膜下血肿这种罕见疾病的患者。该病患者可能多年无症状[87]。有研究表明，钙化或骨化的慢性硬膜下血肿的包膜可能附着于软脑膜和其下层的脑表面[44]，钙化或骨化的慢性硬膜下血肿的临床特征与非钙化或非骨化的血肿特征非常相似[18, 58]。

机化的慢性硬膜下血肿在儿童中很少见[85]。机化的慢性硬膜下血肿的患儿通常有在婴儿期行脑室-腹膜分流术或腹膜下分流术的病史[17, 59]。脑积水分流术、脑膜炎、脑炎和癫痫发作是机化的慢性硬膜下血肿发生的其他易感因素[17]。在非老年患者中，无症状的机化慢性硬膜下血肿患者应考虑手术，以防止因脑受压迫而可能造成的脑损伤[30, 44, 46, 55, 58, 63-64, 87]。

14.3　机化的慢性硬膜下血肿的临床表现

机化的慢性硬膜下血肿患者在临床上主要表现为：头痛、恶心呕吐、嗜睡、意识不清、神志淡漠、头晕、虚弱、行为改变、排尿功能障碍（表现为膀胱容量下降、逼尿肌过度活跃，而括约肌功能完好）、癫痫发作等[5, 28, 44, 58]。在一些患者中，机化的慢性硬膜下血肿可表现为痴呆症状。钙化或骨化的慢性硬膜下血肿可能多年无症状。机化的慢性硬膜下血肿通常发生在老年人中，也可能出现在年轻患者中，但很少见于婴儿。

14.4 机化的慢性硬膜下血肿的影像学表现

机化的慢性硬膜下血肿在 CT 上表现为混杂密度、多分隔、新发血肿、中线移位、内膜增厚或钙化的征象（图 14.1）[4, 6, 9-11, 13, 37, 44, 63, 82, 92]。在磁共振成像（MRI）上，机化的慢性硬膜下血肿在 T1 和 T2 加权图像上都呈高信号，但在某些患者中，它可能在 T1 像上呈低信号，在 T2 像上呈高信号。然而，机化的慢性硬膜下血肿可能在慢性硬膜下血肿的空腔内具有低信号的网状结构（图 14.2 和图 14.3）[9-11, 23, 29, 42, 79]。增强 MRI 可以显示结缔组织的存在，作为钙化或骨化慢性硬膜下血肿成熟的标志[5]。MRI 和 CT 均可见内膜增厚（图 14.1 和图 14.4）[63, 94]。如果初始 CT 证实慢性硬膜下血肿为多室、多层，则建议进行增强 MRI 检查[15]。钙化或骨化的慢性硬膜下血肿罕见，可能被误诊为颅骨肿块。注射造影剂增强成像对于确定是否存在相关的原发性或转移性硬脑膜疾病至关重要[16]。

14.5 机化的慢性硬膜下血肿形成的危险因素

包括年龄、饮酒、全身性合并症［如肝脏和（或）肾功能障碍］、凝血功能障碍或应用抗凝药物、长期使用阿司匹林或抗炎药物等在内的多种危险因素，都被认为是机化的慢性硬膜下血肿复发的原因[25]。

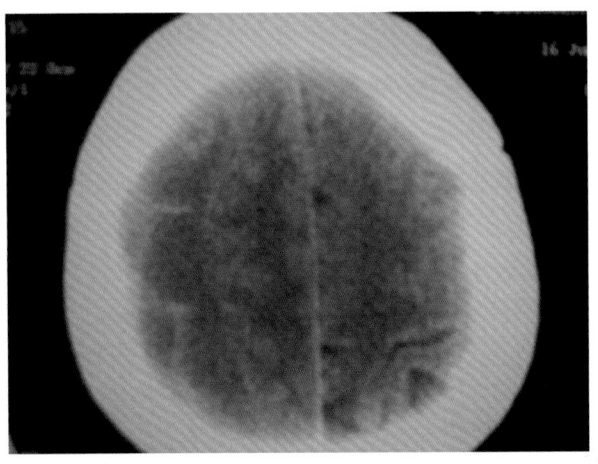

图 14.1 轴向计算机断层成像（CT）显示右侧混杂密度、多分隔的机化的慢性硬膜下血肿（CSDH），伴新发出血征象，内膜增厚，中线移位

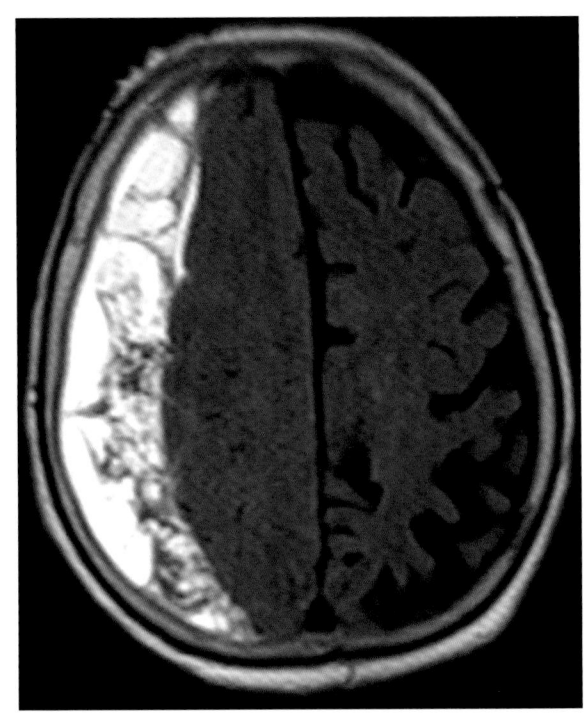

图 14.2 术前 T1 加权磁共振成像（MRI）显示慢性硬膜下血肿内多个空腔，在右脑半球机化的慢性硬膜下血肿内表现为低信号网状结构

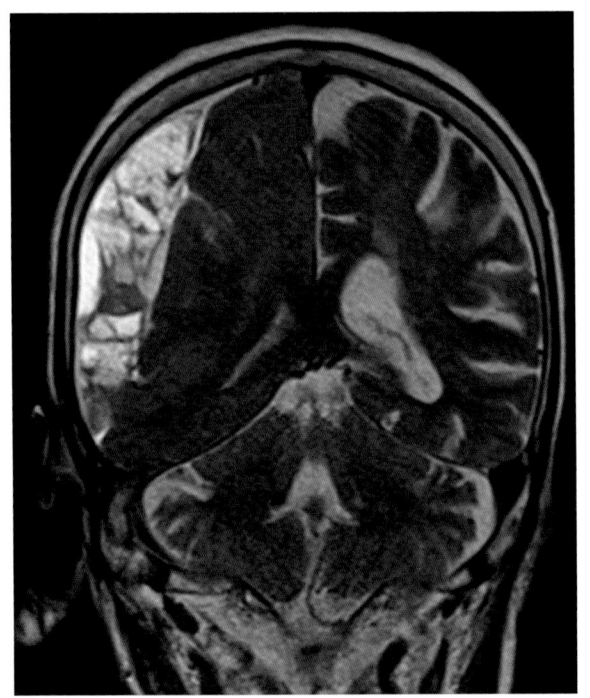

图 14.3 术前 T2 加权 MRI 图像显示右脑半球机化的慢性硬膜下血肿内多个血肿空腔，呈低信号网状结构

14.6 预防癫痫发作

虽然在慢性硬膜下血肿中预防癫痫发作的证据存在矛盾，但抗癫痫药物的应用可用于癫痫发作高

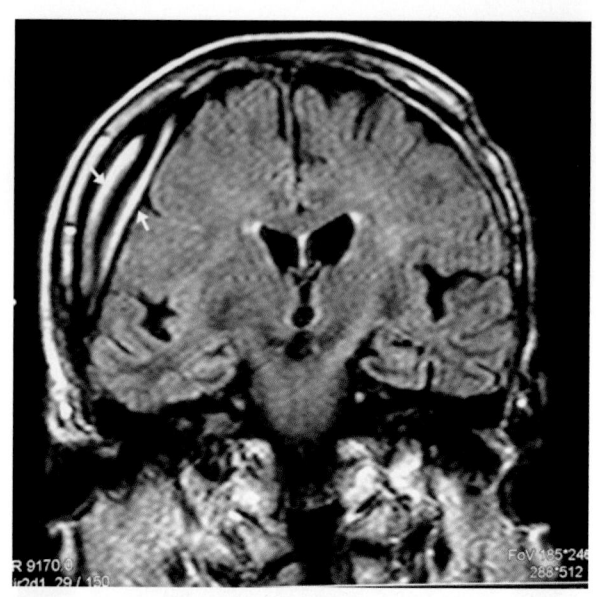

图 14.4 术前 T1 加权增强 MRI 图像显示右半球机化的慢性硬膜下血肿内、外膜增厚（白色箭头）

风险的患者[12]。由于术后癫痫患者死亡率高，因此高危患者应预防癫痫发作[12]。

14.7 治疗及并发症

对于慢性硬膜下血肿患者的治疗，已经提出了多种手术治疗方案，但对于慢性硬膜下血肿的最佳手术方式选择仍存在争议[45, 49]。从外科角度来看，钻孔冲洗或开颅伴或不伴血肿膜切除术是常见的治疗选择[88]。在临床实践中，大多数慢性硬膜下血肿患者普遍采用钻孔术加封闭系统引流，但部分患者可能无效[2, 20, 25, 86]。

即使在今天，术后硬膜下血肿复发的主要危险因素尚不清楚，慢性硬膜下血肿患者手术治疗的最佳方式也仍然存在争议。一些专家认为硬膜下血肿膜的发生发展可能成为术后患者脑复张和神经功能恢复的障碍，导致 70 岁及以上患者出现如复发等相关的术后并发症[7, 9, 45, 50]。

2003 年，Weigel 等报道，慢性硬膜下血肿的开颅手术应该是降低复发率的最差方式，因为开颅手术的复发率（12.3%）高于麻花钻开颅术（3%）和钻孔开颅术（3.8%）[91]。在一项类似的研究中，Callovini 等也报道过，只有复发性慢性硬膜下血肿或尝试钻孔引流后脑复张失败的患者才应开颅[15]。2011 年，Kim 等报道，与小开颅加部分膜切除术相比，采用大开颅加扩大膜切除术作为初始治疗可成

功降低慢性硬膜下血肿患者的再手术率[37]。这种手术方式可能对老年患者有用，因为急性硬膜下血肿（SDH）的形成或慢性硬膜下血肿的复发可能是由于血液从血肿膜切口线渗出[51, 80, 87-88]。

此外，Link 等认为脑膜中动脉栓塞是一种用于保守治疗失败或术后复发慢性硬膜下血肿的预防性治疗失败后的慢性硬膜下血肿微创治疗技术，尽管其确切作用尚不清楚[41, 95]。

最近，一些专家报道内镜下切除机化的慢性硬膜下血肿取得了良好的效果[48, 67, 78]。Ishikawa 等认为，多分隔性慢性硬膜下血肿患者可采用硬式内窥镜加小开颅抽吸管引流技术[33]。尽管开颅手术可能导致各种术后出血并发症和机化的慢性硬膜下血肿复发，但许多专家通常主张对机化的慢性硬膜下血肿进行手术治疗[5, 32, 34, 37, 50, 65, 73]。大开颅切除机化的慢性硬膜下血肿的厚膜或钙化膜可能在血肿手术清除后有助于大脑复张[5, 38, 40, 50, 76, 79]。老年、硬膜下积气和既往脑梗死史是术后脑再扩张不良的原因[52]。一些人认为脑顺应性是慢性硬膜下血肿排出后大脑再扩张的关键因素[45, 50]。可以确定的是，脑组织再扩张不良与慢性硬膜下血肿的复发有关。从这个角度来看，在手术过程中必须避免空气进入硬膜下间隙[52]。另外，针对机化的慢性硬膜下血肿进行扩大的血肿膜切除术存在较高风险损伤下层的蛛网膜表面，并可能引起新生毛细血管结构再出血[13, 54-55, 69]。同时，Acakpo-Satchivi 和 Luerssen 则认为，钙化或骨化的慢性硬膜下血肿患者部分内膜切除术可能会由于残存的内膜导致脑疝发生[1]。

理论上，手术干预后 3 个月内慢性硬膜下血肿再次出现被认为是"早期复发"，而术后 3 个月及以上慢性硬膜下血肿持续存在或扩大则是"晚期复发"[56]。机化的慢性硬膜下血肿经开颅联合膜切除术后早期复发率为 0～30%[32, 34, 40, 66, 79]。有研究表明，这些患者行大开颅手术后复发的主要原因是，内外膜交界处脆弱的毛细血管会导致反复多灶性出血[11]。据推测，复发是由于进入静脉窦（如上矢状窦）的桥静脉牵拉和破裂所致[37, 76]。

"颅腔积气"一词是指颅腔内存在空气（图 14.5）。它是慢性硬膜下血肿术后一种重要的危及生命的并发症，当颅内积气导致颅内压升高而引起神经功能恶化时，被称为"张力性气颅"（TP）[27, 31]。

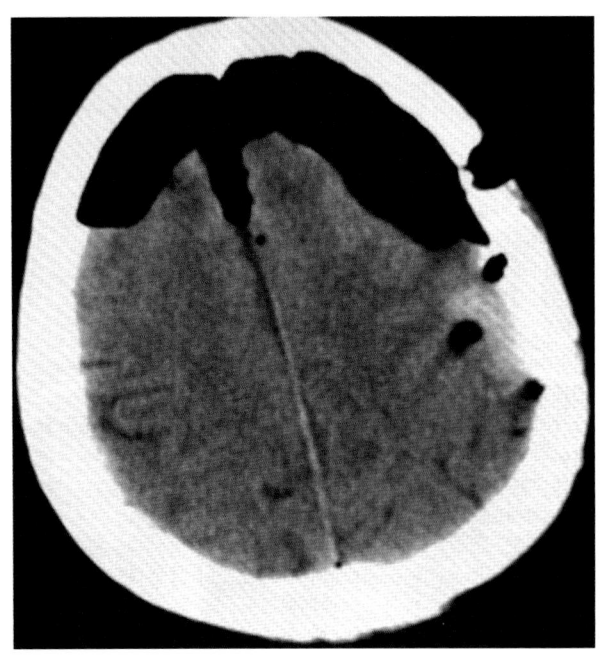

图 14.5　轴位 CT 扫描显示张力性气颅

本章的一位作者报道，大开颅联合膜切除术治疗 CSDH 后 TP 的发生率为 28.5%[11, 71-72, 77]，临床症状包括头痛、恶心、呕吐、眩晕、局灶性神经功能缺损及癫痫发作[72]。高张力的硬膜下积气容易分离和压迫双额叶，导致额叶受压，半球间隙变宽，在 CT 上显影形似富士山的轮廓，称为"富士山"标志[68]。慢性硬膜下血肿复发的主要机制是进入上矢状窦等静脉窦的静脉破裂[77]。气颅的另一个征象是在蛛网膜下腔存在多个小气泡，特别是在基底池。

对张力性气颅的治疗可通过密闭水封引流系统对患者进行控制性减压 2 天[8, 81]。TP 最合适的治疗方法是平卧、补液、吸 100% 纯氧[57]。

25% ～ 50% 的大开颅联合扩大膜切除术患者术后癫痫发作需要药物治疗[52]。

14.8　预后

机化的慢性硬膜下血肿患者的死亡率为 0 ～ 15.6%[75]。Callovini 等只报道了一例（3%）因脑室内和蛛网膜下腔出血而死亡的病例[15]。

14.9　结论

对于机化的慢性硬膜下血肿患者，尽管大开颅联合扩大膜切除术的并发症发生风险高，但仍应采取该术式作为主要手术方式。在机化的慢性硬膜下血肿患者中，手术前神经系统状况和患者年龄＞70 岁是影响预后的最重要因素[25]。张力性气颅和硬膜下血肿残留是老年患者常见的并发症。

参考文献

1. Acakpo-Satchivi L, Luerssen TG. Brain herniation through an internal subdural membrane. A rare complication seen with chronic subdural hematomas in children. Case report. J Neurosurg. 2007;107:485–8.
2. Adam D, Iftimie D, Moisescu C. Recurrence of chronic subdural hematomas requiring reoperation: could small trephination be a valid alternative to conventional approaches? Rom Neurosurg. 2018;32:187–204.
3. Afra D. Ossification of subdural hematoma. Report of two cases. J Neurosurg. 1961;18:393–7.
4. Al Whoaibi M, Russell N, Al Ferayan A. A baby with an armoured brain. CMAJ. 2003;169:46–7.
5. Altinel F, Altin C, Gezmis E, Altinors N. Cortical membranectomy in chronic subdural hematoma: report of two cases. Asian J Neurosurg. 2015;10:236–9.
6. Aoki N, Sakai T. Computed tomography features immediately after replacement of haematoma with oxygen through percutaneous subdural tapping for the treatment of chronic subdural haematoma in adults. Acta Neurochir (Wien). 1993;120:44–6.
7. Araújo Silva DO, Matis GK, Costa LF, Kitamura MA, de Carvalho Junior EV, de Moura Silva M, et al. Chronic subdural hematomas and the elderly: surgical results from a series of 125 cases: old "horses" are not to be shot! Surg Neurol Int. 2012;3:150.
8. Arbit E, Shah J, Bedford R, Carlon G. Tension pneumocephalus: treatment with controlled decompression via a closed water-seal drainage system. Case report. J Neurosurg. 1991;74:139–42.
9. Asghar M, Adhiyaman V, Greenway MW, Bhowmick BK, Bates A. Chronic subdural haematoma in the elderly—a North Wales experience. J R Soc Med. 2002;95:290–2.

10. Baek HG, Park SH. Craniotomy and membranectomy for treatment of organized chronic subdural hematoma. Korean J Neurotrauma. 2018;14:134–7.
11. Balevi M. Organized chronic subdural hematomas treated by large craniotomy with extended membranectomy as the initial treatment. Asian J Neurosurg. 2017;12:598–604.
12. Battaglia F, Lubrano V, Ribeiro-Filho T, Pradel V, Roche PH. Incidence and clinical impact of seizures after surgery for chronic subdural haematoma. Neurochirurgie. 2012;58:230–4.
13. Bremer AM, Nguyen TQ. Tension pneumocephalus after surgical treatment of chronic subdural hematoma: report of three cases. Neurosurgery. 1982;11:284–7.
14. Byrne P, Bartlett J. Chronic subdural haematoma: editorial. Br J Neurosurg. 1991;5:459–60.
15. Callovini GM, Bolognini A, Callovini G, Gammone V. Primary enlarged craniotomy in organized chronic subdural hematomas. Neurol Med Chir (Tokyo). 2015;54:349–56.
16. Cheng YK, Wang TC, Yang JT, Lee MH, Su CH. Dural metastasis from prostatic adenocarcinoma mimicking chronic subdural hematoma. J Clin Neurosci. 2009;16:1084–6.
17. Cho HR, Kim Y, Sim HB, Lyo IU. An organized chronic subdural hematoma with partial calcification in a child. J Korean Neurosurg Soc. 2005;37:386–8.
18. Dammers R, ter Laak-Poort MP, Maas AI. Neurological picture. Armoured brain: case report of a symptomatic calcified cchronic subdural haematoma. J Neurol Neurosurg Psychiatry. 2007;78:542–3.
19. Drapkin AJ. Chronic subdural haematoma: pathophysiological basis for treatment. Br J Neurosurg. 1991;5:467–73.
20. El-Kadi H, Miele VI, Kaufman HH. Prognosis of chronic subdural hematomas. Neurosurg Clin N Am. 2000;11:553–67.
21. Feghali J, Yang W, Huang J. Updates in chronic subdural hematoma: epidemiology, etiology, pathogenesis, treatment and outcome. World Neurosurg. 2020;141:339–45.
22. Firsching R, Muller W, Thun F, Boop F. Clinical correlates of erythropoiesis in chronic subdural hematoma. Surg Neurol. 1990;33:173–7.
23. Fobben ES, Grossman RI, Atlas SW, Hackney DB, Goldberg HI, Zimmerman RA, Bilaniuk LT. MR characteristics of subdural hematomas and hygromas at 1.5 T. AJR Am J Roentgenol. 1989;153:589–95.
24. Fujioka M, Okuchi K, Miyamoto S, Sakaki T, Tsunoda S, Iwasaki S. Bilateral organized chronic subdural haematomas: high field magnetic resonance images and histological considerations. Acta Neurochir (Wien). 1994;131:265–9.
25. Gelabert-Gonzalez M, Iglesias-Pais M, García-Allut A, Martínez-Rumbo R. Chronic subdural haematoma: surgical treatment and outcome in 1000 cases. Clin Neurol Neurosurg. 2005;107:223–9.
26. Goldhahn R. Uber ein gosses, perative entferntes, verkalktes, intrakranielles hamatoma. Dtsch Z Chir. 1930;224:323.
27. Goyal S, Batra AM, Rohatgi A, Acharya R, Sharma AG. Tension pneumocephalus: a neurosurgical emergency. J Assoc Physicians India. 2008;56:985.
28. Hirakawa T, Tanaka A, Yoshinaga S, Ohkawa M, Tomonaga M. Calcified chronic subdural hematoma with intracerebral rupture forming a subcortical hematoma. A case report. Surg Neurol. 1989;32:51–5.
29. Hosoda K, Tamaki N, Masumura M, Matsumoto S, Maeda F. Magnetic resonance images of chronic subdural hematomas. J Neurosurg. 1987;67:677–83.
30. Ide M, Jimbo M, Yamamoto M, Umebara Y, Hagiwara S. Asymptomatic calcified chronic subdural hematoma—report of three cases. Neurol Med Chir (Tokyo). 1993;33:559–63.
31. Ihab Z. Pneumocephalus after surgical evacuation of chronic subdural hematoma: is it a serious complication? Asian J Neurosurg. 2012;7:66–74.
32. Imaizumi S, Onuma T, Kameyama M, Naganuma H. Organized chronic subdural hematoma requiring craniotomy-five case reports. Neurol Med Chir (Tokyo). 2001;41:19–24.
33. Ishikawa T, Endo K, Endo Y, Sato N, Ohta M. Neuro-endoscopic surgery for multi-lobular chronic subdural hematoma (in Japan). No Shinkei Geka. 2017;45:667–75.
34. Isobe N, Sato H, Murakami T, Kurokawa Y, Seyama G, Oki S. Six cases of organized chronic subdural hematoma. No Shinkei Geka. 2008;36:1115–20.
35. Ito H, Komai T, Yamamoto S. Fibrinolytic enzyme in the lining walls of chronic subdural haematoma. J Neurosurg. 1978;48:197–200.
36. Kawano N, Endo M, Saito M, Nakayama K, Beppu T. Origin and pathological significance of smooth muscle cells and myofibroblasts in the subdural neomembrane (in Japan). Neurol Med Chir (Tokyo). 1986;26:361–8.
37. Kim JH, Kang DS, Kim JH, Kong MH, Song KY. Chronic subdural hematoma treated by small

or large craniotomy with membranectomy as the initial treatment. J Korean Neurosurg Soc. 2011;50:103–8.
38. Kondo S, Okada Y, Iseki H, Hori T, Takakura K, Kobayashi A, Nagata H. Thermological study of drilling bone tissue with a high-speed drill. Neurosurgery. 2000;46:1162–8.
39. Kwon TH, Park YK, Lim DJ, Cho TH, Chung YG, Chung HS, Suh JK. Chronic subdural hematoma: evaluation of the clinical significance of postoperative drainage volume. J Neurosurg. 2000;93:796–9.
40. Lee JY, Ebel H, Ernestus RI, Klug N. Various surgical treatments of chronic subdural hematoma and outcome in 172 patients: is membranectomy necessary? Surg Neurol. 2004;61:523–7.
41. Link TW, Boddu S, Paine SM, Kamel H, Knopman J. Middle meningeal artery embolization for chronic subdural hematoma: a series of 60 cases. Neurosurgery. 2019;85:801–7.
42. Liu W, Bakker NA, Groen RJ. Chronic subdural hematoma: a systematic review and meta-analysis of surgical procedures. J Neurosurg. 2014;121:665–73.
43. Maggio WW. Chronic subdural hematoma in adults. In: Apuzzo MCI, editor. Brain surgery, complication avoidance and management, vol. 2. New York: Churchill Livingstone; 1993. p. 1299–314.
44. Mahmoud B, Assiri A, Shaheen A. Excision of huge calcified chronic subdural hematoma: a case report and review of literature. Al-Azhar Assiut Med J. 2015;13:379.
45. Markwalder TM, Reulen HJ. Influence of neomembranous organisation, cortical expansion and subdural pressure on the post-operative course of chronic subdural haematoma-an analysis of 201 cases. Acta Neurochir (Wien). 1986;79:100–6.
46. Matsumura M, Nojiri K. Asymptomatic calcified chronic subdural hematoma in the elderly. Neurol Med Chir (Tokyo). 1984;24:504–6.
47. McLaurin RL, McLaurin KS. Calcified subdural hematomas in childhood. J Neurosurg. 1966;24:648–55.
48. Miki K, Oshiro S, Koga T, Inoue T. A case of organizing chronic subdural hematoma treated with endoscopic burr-hole surgery using a curettage and suction technique (in Japan). No Shinkei Geka. 2016;44:747–51.
49. Misra M, Salazar JL, Bloom DM. Subdural-peritoneal shunt: treatment for bilateral chronic subdural hematoma. Surg Neurol. 1996;46:378–83.
50. Mohamed EEH. Chronic subdural haematoma treated by craniotomy, durectomy, outer membranectomy and subgaleale suction drainage. Personal experience in 39 patients. Br J Neurosurg. 2003;17:244–7.
51. Moon KS, Lee JK, Kim TS, Jung S, Kim JH, Kim SH, et al. Contralateral acute subdural hematoma occurring after removal of calcified chronic subdural hematoma. J Clin Neurosci. 2007;14:283–6.
52. Mori K, Maeda M. Surgical treatment of chronic subdural hematoma in 500 consecutive cases: clinical characteristics, surgical outcome, complications, and recurrence rate. Neurol Med Chir. 2001;41:371–81.
53. Mori N, Nagao T, Nakahara A, Izawa M, Amano K, Kitamura K. A case of huge calcified subdural hematoma. No Shinkei Geka. 1982;10:1203–9.
54. Niwa J, Nakamura T, Fujishige M, Hashi K. Removal of a large asymptomatic calcified chronic subdural hematoma. Surg Neurol. 1988;30:135–9.
55. Oda S, Shimoda M, Hoshikawa K, Shiramizu H, Matsumae M. Organized chronic subdural haematoma with a thick calcified inner membrane successfully treated by surgery: a case report. Tokai J Exp Clin Med. 2010;35:85–8.
56. Oh HJ, Lee KS, Shim JJ, Yoon SM, Yun IG, Bae HG. Postoperative course and recurrence of chronic subdural hematoma. J Korean Neurosurg Soc. 2010;48:518–23.
57. Paiva WS, de Andrade AF, Figueiredo EG, Amorim RL, Prudente M, Teixeira MJ. Effects of hyperbaric oxygenation therapy on symptomatic pneumocephalus. Ther Clin Risk Manag. 2014;6:769–73.
58. Pappamikail L, Rato R, Novais G, Bernardo E. Chronic calcified subdural hematoma: case report and review of the literature. Surg Neurol Int. 2013;4:21.
59. Park J, Kwon TH, Park YK, Chung HS, Lee HK, Suh JK. Calcified chronic subdural hematoma: late sequelae of shunt operation in a child with hydrocephalus. J Korean Neurosurg Soc. 2000;29:968–72.
60. Park JS, Son EI, Kim DW, Kim SP. Calcified chronic subdural haematoma associated with intracerebral haematoma. J Korean Neurosurg. 2003;34:177–8.
61. Per H, Gümüş H, Tucer B, Akgün H, Kurtsoy A, Kumandaş S. Calcified chronic subdural hematoma mimicking calvarial mass: a case report. Brain Dev. 2006;28:607–9.

62. Prieto R, Pascual JM, Subhi-Issa I, Yus M. Acute epidural-like appearance of an encapsulated solid non-organized chronic subdural hematoma. Neurol Med Chir (Tokyo). 2010;50:990–9.
63. Rahman A, Haque M, Bhandari PB. Calcified chronic subdural haematoma. BMJ Case Rep. 2012;2012:5499.
64. Rao ZX, Li J, Yin H, You C. Huge calcified chronic subdural haematoma. Br J Neurosurg. 2010;24:722–3.
65. Richter HP, Klein HJ, Schäfer M. Chronic subdural haematomas treated by enlarged burr hole craniotomy and closed system drainage. Retrospective study of 120 patients. Acta Neurochir (Wien). 1984;71:179–88.
66. Rocchi G, Caroli E, Salvati M, Delfini R. Membranectomy in organized chronic subdural hematomas: indications and technical notes. Surg Neurol. 2007;67:374–80.
67. Rodziewicz GS, Chuang WC. Endoscopic removal of organized chronic subdural hematoma. Surg Neurol. 1995;43:569–72.
68. Sadeghian H. Mount Fuji sign in tension pneumocephalus. Arch Neurol. 2000;57:1366.
69. Sakamoto T, Hoshikawa Y, Hayashi T, Taguchi Y, Sekino H. Inner membrane preservation surgery for organized or calcified chronic subdural hematoma. Jpn J Neurosurg (Tokyo). 2000;9:541–6.
70. Sato S, Suzuki J. Ultrastructural observations of the capsule of chronic subdural hematoma in various clinical stages. J Neurosurg. 1975;43:569–78.
71. Schirmer CM, Heilman CB, Bhardwaj A. Pneumocephalus: case illustrations and review. Neurocrit Care. 2010;13:152–8.
72. Sharma BS, Tewari MK, Khosla VK, Pathak A, Kak VK. Tension pneumocephalus following evacuation of chronic subdural haematoma. Br J Neurosurg. 1989;3:381–7.
73. Shigeki I, Takehide O, Motonobu K, Hiroshi N. Organized chronic subdural hematoma requiring craniotomy-five case report. Neurol Med Chir. 2001;41:19–24.
74. Shim YS, Park CO, Hyun DK, Park HC, Yoon SH. What are the causative factors for a slow, progressive enlargement of a chronic subdural hematoma? Yonsei Med J. 2007;48:210–7.
75. Slater JP. Extramedullary hematopoiesis in chronic subdural hematoma. Case report. J Neurosurg. 1966;25:211–4.
76. Stroobandt G, Fransen P, Thauvoy C, Menard E. Pathogenetic factors in chronic subdural haematoma and causes of recurrence after drainage. Acta Neurochir (Wien). 1995;137:6–14.
77. Suda K, Sato M, Matsuda M, Handa J. Subdural tension pneumocephalus after trephination for chronic subdural hematoma. No To Shinkei. 1984;36:127–30.
78. Takahashi S, Yazaki T, Nitori N, Kano T, Yoshida K, Kawase T. Neuroendoscope-assisted removal of an organized chronic subdural hematoma in a patient on bevacizumab therapy—case report. Neurol Med Chir (Tokyo). 2011;51:515–8.
79. Tanikawa M, Mase M, Yamada K, Yamashita N, Matsumoto T, Banno T, Miyati T. Surgical treatment of chronic subdural hematoma based on intrahematomal membrane structure on MRI. Acta Neurochir (Wien). 2001;143:613–8.
80. Tatli M, Guzel A, Altinors N. Spontaneous acute subdural hematoma following contralatera calcified chronic subdural hematoma surgery: an unusual case. Pediatr Neurosurg. 2006;42:122–4.
81. Tommiska P, Lönnro K, Raj R, Luostarinen T, Kivisaari R. Transition of a clinical practice to use of subdural drains after burr hole evacuation of chronic subdural hematoma: the Helsinki experience. World Neurosurg. 2019;129:614–26.
82. Topsakal C, Yıldırım H, Erol FS, Akdemir I, Tiftikçi M. Mixed-density subdural hematoma on CT: case report and review of subdural hematoma classification. Turk Neurosurg. 2002;12:39–45.
83. Tsutsumi K. Chronic subdural hematoma (letter). J Neurosurg. 1998;88:937–8.
84. Tsutsumi K, Maeda K, Iijima A, Usui M, Okada Y, Kirino T. The relationship of preoperative magnetic resonance imaging findings and closed system drainage in the recurrence of chronic subdural hematoma. J Neurosurg. 1997;87:870–5.
85. Turgut M, Palaoglu S, Saglam S. Huge ossified crust-like subdural hematoma covering the hemisphere and causing acute signs of increased intracranial pressure. Childs Nerv Syst. 1997;13:415–7.
86. Turgut M, Akalan N, Saglam S. A fatal acute subdural hematoma occurring after evacuation of "contralateral" chronic subdural hematoma. J Neurosurg Sci. 1998;42:61–3.
87. Turgut M, Akhaddar A, Turgut AT. Calcified or ossified chronic subdural hematoma: a systematic review of 114 cases reported during last century with a demonstrative case report. World

Neurosurg. 2020;134:240–63.
88. Tyson G, Strachan WE, Newman P, Winn HR, Butler A, Jane J. The role of craniectomy in the treatment of chronic subdural hematomas. J Neurosurg. 1980;52:776–81.
89. Von Rokitansky C. Anatomie, vol. 2. Wien: Braunmuller und Seidel; 1884. p. 717.
90. Wang R, Gao L, Fu H, Shi W. Treatment of organized chronic subdural hematoma using urokinase. Int J Clin Exp Med. 2017;10:14834–40.
91. Weigel R, Schmiedek P, Krauss JK. Outcome of contemporary surgery for chronic subdural haematoma: evidence based review. Neurol Neurosurg Psychiatry. 2003;74:937–43.
92. Yamada K, Ohta T, Takatsuka H, Yamaguchi K. High-field magnetic resonance image of a huge calcified chronic subdural hematoma, so-called "armoured brain". Acta Neurochir (Wien). 1992;114:151–3.
93. Yamashima T. The inner membrane of chronic subdural hematomas: pathology and pathophysiology. Neurosurg Clin N Am. 2000;11:413–24.
94. Yang HZ, Tseng SH, Chen Y, Lin SM, Chen CJ. Calcified chronic subdural haematoma—case report. Tzu Chi Med J. 2004;16:261–5.
95. Yokoya S, Nishii S, Takezawa H, Katsumor HT. Organized chronic subdural hematoma treated with middle meningeal artery embolization and small craniotomy: two case reports. Asian J Neurosurg. 2020;15:421–5.

第 15 章 钙化或骨化的硬膜下血肿

Mehmet Turgut

译者：汤劼

15.1 引言

由于桥静脉破裂导致脑膜层（硬脑膜和蛛网膜）之间的血液聚集并覆盖大脑半球，这种情况导致的硬膜下血肿是临床中最常见的神经外科疾病之一[46]。然而慢性硬膜下血肿（CSDH）的钙化或骨化是非常罕见的，大多数病例都是在单个病例报告中报道的[30, 33, 49, 63, 83]。慢性硬膜下血肿常见于儿童和青少年而非成人[83]。尽管对慢性硬膜下血肿患者的治疗研究进展相对较小，但由于计算机断层成像（CT）和磁共振成像（MRI）等新的放射学手段的引入，其预后已得到改善[12]。不幸的是，目前还没有标准的手术或非手术治疗方法在随机对照试验中得到验证。即使在今天，关于钙化或骨化的慢性硬膜下血肿的临床治疗的争论仍在继续，尚未得出最终结论。

在本章中，详细讨论了钙化或骨化的慢性硬膜下血肿患者的临床特征、手术和组织病理学表现、并发症和预后。

15.2 研究历史

根据 Bull 报道，Prescott Hewitt 爵士于 1845 年报道了第一例双侧慢性硬膜下血肿病例[9]。1930 年，Goldhahn 首次进行了慢性硬膜下血肿的手术切除[23]，而 von Rokitansky 在 1884 年尸检后报道了第一例钙化/骨化的慢性硬膜下血肿患者[38-39, 64]。在对文献的系统回顾中，我们发现了 114 例以英语报道的此类慢性硬膜下血肿病例[70]。

15.3 发病机制

从病理上讲，慢性硬膜下血肿是一种进行性扩大的颅内病变，血肿具有内膜和外膜。血肿膜中有许多毛细血管，这是由于血管生成、炎症和纤维蛋白溶解导致的，此外还可能是因为血肿的延迟吸收[4-5, 33, 66-67, 79, 82]。除了乏氧诱导因子-1a 和环氧合酶-2 途径外，血管生成生长因子如血管内皮生长因子和碱性成纤维细胞生长因子、基质金属蛋白酶和各种炎症因子被认为是导致慢性硬膜下血肿扩大和复发的原因。血肿包块外膜微血管脆弱，通透性增加也是导致慢性硬膜下血肿扩大复发的原因[25, 27, 48, 79]。

尽管血肿通常会随着时间的推移而消退，但在某些病例中血肿的外膜可能首先会经历缓慢"透明化"，然后"钙化"，最后"骨化"的过程。需要注意的是，慢性硬膜下血肿的钙化或骨化很少会发展到覆盖整个大脑的程度，并且钙化或骨化的确切机制尚不清楚[2-3, 15, 19, 22, 24, 32-33, 40, 54, 57, 60-61, 63, 67-69, 71, 75, 80]。从宏观上来看，由于钙化或骨化的慢性硬膜下血肿的慢性压迫，会使同侧大脑半球萎缩[46]。在这些病例中，从最初的急性出血到发展为钙化或骨化的慢性硬膜下血肿的时间间隔为 3 个月至 46 年[1, 3, 7, 14, 34, 46]。

15.4 危险因素

慢性硬膜下血肿发生的危险因素包括长期饮酒，应用阿司匹林、抗炎药物、抗凝血药物，经常进行造成头部损伤的运动，蛛网膜囊肿，凝血功能降低的血液系统疾病和老年[45, 77, 79]。

15.5 病因学

虽然大多数钙化或骨化的慢性硬膜下血肿是由外伤性头部损伤引起的，但颅内低压（自发性、外伤性或医源性）和凝血障碍（凝血功能障碍、应用抗凝和抗血小板药物）也可能是主要原因。大多数钙化或骨化的慢性硬膜下血肿病例都有轻微的头部损伤，尤其儿童和青少年在玩耍时可能反复遭受过轻微的头部损伤[79]。脑积水分流术、腰椎穿刺、脊髓麻醉、脊柱手术或颅内病变突然减压后发生医源性颅内低压也应被视为慢性硬膜下血肿的潜在原因[79]。大量研究表明，钙化或骨化的慢性硬膜下血肿最常见的病因是外伤性损伤和脑室-腹膜（VP）或脑室-心房（VA）的分流[1-3, 6-7, 10, 14-15, 17, 19, 21-22, 24, 26, 29-33, 35, 38-40, 42, 51, 53-55, 57, 60, 63-64, 66, 68-69, 71, 75, 86]。

15.6 解剖位置

尽管慢性硬膜下血肿可以发生于颅内大脑表面的任何位置，但钙化或骨化的慢性硬膜下血肿发生的解剖位置通常在额顶叶和颞顶叶区域。与蛛网膜下腔相反，硬膜下腔桥静脉的脆弱性和蛛网膜小梁的缺乏被认为是这些区域易发生慢性硬膜下血肿的原因[79]。

15.7 临床表现

钙化或骨化的慢性硬膜下血肿的临床症状和体征通常与颅内压升高（IICP）有关，包括头痛、视乳头水肿、意识丧失、局部神经功能缺陷如偏瘫或感觉减退、视力和（或）记忆力丧失、发育迟缓和（或）癫痫，但钙化或骨化的慢性硬膜下血肿病例也可能无症状[46, 52, 82]。在某些情况下，这些患者的诊断可能很困难，因为他们的临床表现是缓慢进展和非特异性的[10, 14, 53, 55, 78]。

15.8 影像学表现

许多钙化或骨化的慢性硬膜下血肿患者都是通过 X 线检查、CT 和 MRI 等各种影像学手段偶然确诊的。在影像学上，巨大的钙化或骨化的慢性硬膜下血肿会累及整个大脑凸面，在 CT 中被称为"Matrioska 头"或"双颅骨"，其内、外层呈高密度，中间被低密度区隔开，这种特殊病变相关文献少有报道（图 15.1）[40, 61, 69-70, 73]。在某些病例中，钙化或骨化的慢性硬膜下血肿可表现为中线向对侧移位的占位性病变（图 15.1）[70, 73]。包括慢性硬膜下血肿在内的所有类型血肿体积的最简便估算方法是公式 2/3 Sh [最大轴向血肿切片面积（S）× 深度（h）乘以 2/3]，而不是公式 1/2abc[87]。在给予造影剂后，CT 和（或）MRI 对于鉴别原发性或转移性硬脑膜疾病与钙化或骨化的慢性硬膜下血肿至关重要[11]。在各种成像技术中，MRI 对于显示慢性硬膜下血肿的内部结构更为敏感，包括膜、分隔和网状结构，这些结构在 T1 和 T2 加权图像上都是呈高信号的[8]。最近，有研究表明，弥散加权成像和增强

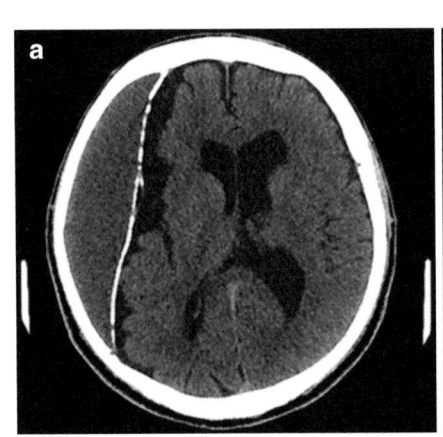
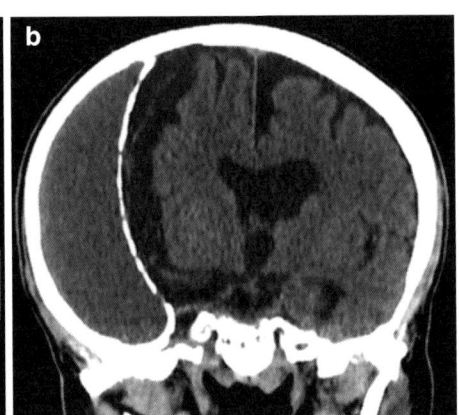
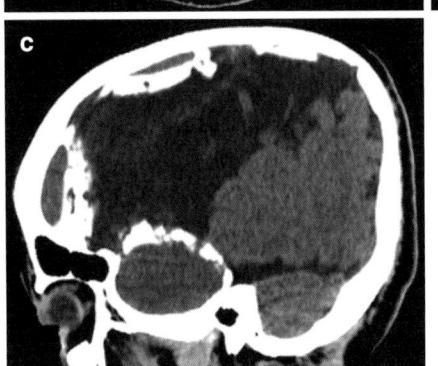

图 15.1 59 岁男性的轴位（a）、冠状位（b）和矢状位（c）CT 成像，患者约 4 年前头部外伤后有癫痫发作史，除左半感觉减退外，神经学检查显示一个巨大的骨化和钙化的慢性硬膜下血肿（CSDH）覆盖大脑半球，累及右侧额颞顶区并压迫侧脑室，被经显微手术完全切除后的组织病理学检查所证实[70, 73]

MRI 可用于检测新生膜和诊断感染性硬膜下血肿[79]。

15.9　鉴别诊断

CT 和（或）MRI 对于其他轴外病变的鉴别诊断是必要的，如硬膜外血肿钙化、蛛网膜囊肿钙化、颅凸硬脑膜钙化、钙化脓胸、良恶性肿瘤和各种转移性肿瘤[14, 34, 53, 55, 69, 81]。

15.10　外科手术

对于钙化或骨化的慢性硬膜下血肿，在没有进展性神经系统表现的情况下，加/不加皮质类固醇的保守治疗通常是足够的[18, 33, 41, 52, 85]。如今，对于伴有钙化或骨化的慢性硬膜下血肿的有进展性神经系统表现的婴儿、儿童和青少年，手术干预已成为必要[28, 33, 52, 82]。从技术角度看，全麻手术复发率低，并发症少[20, 29, 31, 33, 50, 71-72, 76]。与"小开颅联合部分膜切除术"相比，"大开颅联合扩大膜切除术"能显著降低钙化或骨化的慢性硬膜下血肿的复发率[36]。最近，一种称为"多重帐篷手术"的新技术也被报道用于消除钙化或骨化的慢性硬膜下血肿病例的死腔[31]。在显微外科解剖技术的帮助下，可以毫不费力地从大脑表面切除钙化或骨化的膜，在切除钙化或骨化的斑块后，可以观察到大脑透过内膜的搏动[33, 49-50]。然而需要注意的是，在手术干预过程中，由于颅底组织受到创伤性损伤，急性出血的风险很高[29, 44]。因为脑挫伤可能导致永久性神经功能缺损，许多神经外科医生选择不完全切除钙化膜，以降低对脑组织的损伤风险[1, 30, 44, 49, 53, 56, 63, 71, 80]。尽管手术技术取得了进步，但由于切除广泛的钙化或骨化的慢性硬膜下血肿后，萎缩的脑组织仍扩张不足，这些病例术后癫痫发作活动和（或）复发的风险仍然很高[46, 58-59]。对于脑积水分流术后的患儿，许多人还建议，除了直接手术切除钙化或骨化的慢性硬膜下血肿外，还应考虑再次手术[2-3, 6, 15, 17, 19, 21-22, 24, 26, 31-32, 40, 51, 54, 57, 60, 63-64, 66, 68, 75]。

15.11　并发症

慢性硬膜下血肿切除术后存在复发、感染、新颅内血肿、癫痫发作、脑水肿以及由于颅脑比例失调导致的脑扩张不足等潜在风险[16, 79]。慢性硬膜下血肿清除术后，在钙化或骨化的慢性硬膜下血肿患者中，约有 11% 的患者存在气颅或张力性气颅的潜在风险[13, 62, 65, 79]。特别是硬膜下空气的存在导致额叶被广泛压缩，称为"富士山"征，这类患者具有颅内压增高和（或）癫痫发作的病理特征[37, 74]。到目前为止，许多因素如手术时间延长、使用氧化亚氮和（或）渗透疗法、过度通气、脑脊液过度引流、脑膜层破裂等，被认为是这些病例中出现张力性气颅的原因[43]。因此，建议采用生理盐水替代、缓慢且同步的减压、使用抽吸引流、关颅时将钻孔点置于最高点、Valsalva 手法、角度为 30° 的 Trendelenburg 位来预防张力性气颅[79]。

15.12　病理学

在这些病例中，通过对切除组织的病理学检查，可以明确区分骨化和钙化。组织学上，在成纤维细胞、胶原纤维和新生毛细血管增生后，可观察到血肿膜依次发生透明化、钙化和骨化[47, 52]。此外，钙化或骨化的慢性硬膜下血肿患者还存在神经纤维扭曲、脑血流量减少和血管源性脑水肿[33, 84]。

15.13　预后

尽管绝大多数慢性硬膜下血肿病例通常被认为是相对良性的，但对于某些钙化或骨化的慢性硬膜下血肿病例，可能需要进行大开颅手术和扩大切除，这可能会导致高死亡率和发病率[65]。因此，如今一些学者建议只有在出现进行性神经症状或体征时才进行手术干预，从而提出了"无损伤不手术"的原则[50, 81]。据报道，钙化或骨化的慢性硬膜下血肿术后复发率为 5%～33%[65]。

15.14　结论

钙化或骨化的慢性硬膜下血肿是神经外科临床中很少报道的病例之一。从病因学的角度来看，颅脑外伤导致的慢性硬膜下血肿在成人患者中更为常见，而分流手术导致的慢性硬膜下血肿在儿童和青少年中更为常见。手术干预仅适用于出现钙化或骨化的慢性硬膜下血肿并伴有进行性症状的患者，但关于是否需要手术干预的争论仍在进行中，最终的决定应建立在个体化的基础上。术后，应高度警惕危及生命的张力性气颅的出现，及时诊断和正确治疗对出现术后并发症的患者至关重要。

参考文献

1. Afra D. Ossification of subdural hematoma. Report of two cases. J Neurosurg. 1961;18: 393–7.
2. Al Wohaibi M, Russell N, Al Ferayan A. A baby with armoured brain. CMAJ. 2003;169:46–7.
3. Amr R, Maraqa L, Choudry Q. 'Armoured brain'. A case report of a calcified chronic subdural haematoma. Pediatr Neurosurg. 2008;44:88–9.
4. Aoki N, Sakai T. Computed tomography features immediately after replacement of haematoma with oxygen through percutaneous subdural tapping for the treatment of chronic subdural haematoma in adults. Acta Neurochir (Wien). 1993;120:44–6.
5. Arbit E, Shah J, Bedford R, Carlon G. Tension pneumocephalus: treatment with controlled decompression via a closed water-seal drainage system. Case report. J Neurosurg. 1991;74:139–42.
6. Barmeir EP, Stern D, Harel S, Holtzman M, Krijie TJ. Calcified subdural hematomas associated with arrested hydrocephalus-late sequale of shunt operation in infancy. Eur J Radiol. 1985;3:186–9.
7. Boyd DA, Merrell P. Calcified subdural hematoma. J Nerv Ment Dis. 1943;98:609–17.
8. Bremer AM, Nguyen TQ. Tension pneumocephalus after surgical treatment of chronic subdural hematoma: report of three cases. Neurosurgery. 1982;11:284–7.
9. Bull JWD. The radiological diagnosis of chronic subdural haematoma. Proc R Soc Med. 1940;33:203–24.
10. Celik H, Karatay M, Erdem Y, Bayar MA. Ossified chronic subdural hematoma which is present with epilepsy. J Neurol Sci [Turk]. 2014;31:361–5.
11. Cheng YK, Wang TC, Yang JT, Lee MH, Su CH. Dural metastasis from prostatic adenocarcinoma mimicking chronic subdural hematoma. J Clin Neurosci. 2009;16:1084–6.
12. Cote DJ, Karhade AV, Larsen AM, Burke WT, Castlen JP, Smith TR. United States neurosurgery annual case type and complication trends between 2006 and 2013: an American College of Surgeons National Surgical Quality Improvement Program analysis. J Clin Neurosci. 2016;31:106–11.
13. Cummins A. Tension pneumocephalus is a complication of chronic subdural hematoma evacuation. J Hosp Med. 2009;4:E3–4.
14. Debois V, Lombaert A. Calcified chronic subdural hematoma. Surg Neurol. 1980;14:455–8.
15. Dimogerontas G, Rovlias A. Bilateral huge calcified chronic subdural hematomas (armoured brain) in an adult patient with a coexistent VA shunt infection. Br J Neurosurg. 2006;6:435–6.
16. Dinc C, Iplikcioglu AC, Bikmaz K, Navruz Y. Intracerebral haemorrhage occurring at remote site following evacuation of chronic subdural haematoma. Acta Neurochir (Wien). 2008;150:497–9.
17. Djoubairou BO, Gazzaz M, Dao I, Mostarchid BE. Chronic calcified extradural and subdural hematoma following a ventriculoperitoneal shunt placement. Neurol India. 2015;63:282–3.
18. Ducruet AF, Grobelny BT, Zacharia BE, Hickman ZL, Derosa PL, Anderson K, et al. The surgical management of chronic subdural hematoma. Neurosurg Rev. 2012;35:155–69.
19. Evans SJ. Armored brain. Neurology. 2007;68:1954.
20. Fang J, Liu Y, Jiang X. Ossified chronic subdural hematoma in children: case report and review of literature. World Neurosurg. 2019;126:613–5.
21. Gandolfi A, Matelli M, Cusmano F. Calcified chronic subdural hematoma following ventriculo-atrial shunting operation for infantile hydrocephalus. Acta Neurol (Napoli). 1983;2:130–7.
22. Garg K, Singh PK, Singla R, Chandra PS, Singh M, Satyarthee GD, et al. Armored brain-massive bilateral calcified chronic subdural hematoma in a patient with ventriculoperotoneal shunt. Neurol India. 2013;61:548–50.
23. Goldhahn R. Uber ein grobes, operativ entferntes, verkalktes, intrakranielles Hamatom. Dtsch Z Chir. 1930;224:323–31.
24. Gupta SK, Pandia MP. Anesthetic management of a case of armored brain. Saudi J Anaesth. 2015;9:89–90.

25. Hara M, Tamaki M, Aoyagi M, Ohno K. Possible role of cyclooxygenase-2 in developing chronic subdural hematoma. J Med Dent Sci. 2009;56:101–6.
26. He XS, Zhang X. Giant calcified chronic subdural hematoma: a long term complication of shunted hydrocephalus. J Neurol Neurosurg Psychiatry. 2005;76:367.
27. Hong HJ, Kim YJ, Yi HJ, Ko Y, Oh SJ, Kim JM. Role of angiogenic growth factors and inflammatory cytokine on recurrence of chronic subdural hematoma. Surg Neurol. 2009;71:161–5.
28. Ide M, Jimbo M, Yamamoto M, Umebara Y, Hagiwara S. Asymptomatic calcified chronic subdural hematoma-report of three cases. Neurol Med Chir (Tokyo). 1993;33:559–63.
29. Imaizumi S, Onuma T, Kameyama M, Naganuma H. Organized chronic subdural hematoma requiring craniotomy-five case reports. Neurol Med Chir (Tokyo). 2001;41:19–24.
30. Iplikcioglu AC, Akkas O, Sungur R. Ossified chronic subdural hematoma: case report. J Trauma. 1991;31:272–5.
31. Juan WS, Tai SH, Hung YC, Lee EJ. Multiple tenting techniques improve dead space obliteration in the surgical treatment for patients with giant calcified chronic subdural hematoma. Acta Neurochir (Wien). 2012;154:707–10.
32. Kanu OO, Igwilo AI, Daini O. Armoured brain: a case of bilateral calcified chronic subdural haematoma complicating infantile hydrocephalus. Rom Neurosurg. 2012;XIX:1.
33. Kaplan M, Akgün B, Seçer HI. Ossified chronic subdural hematoma with armored brain. Turk Neurosurg. 2008;18:420–4.
34. Kaspera W, Bierzynska-Macyszyn G, Majchrzak H. Chronic calcified subdural empyema occurring 46 years after surgery. Neuropathology. 2005;25:99–102.
35. Kavcic A, Meglic B, Meglic NP, Vodusek DB, Mesec A. Asymptomatic huge calcified subdural hematoma in a patient on oral anticoagulant therapy. Neurology. 2006;66:758.
36. Kim JH, Kang DS, Kim JH, Kong MH, Song KY. Chronic subdural hematoma treated by small or large craniotomy with membranectomy as the initial treatment. J Korean Neurosurg Soc. 2011;50:103–8.
37. Lega BC, Danish SF, Malhotra NR, Sonnad SS, Stein SC. Choosing the best operation for chronic subdural hematoma: a decision analysis. J Neurosurg. 2010;113:615–21.
38. Li H, Mao X, Tao XG, Li JS, Liu BY, Wu Z. A tortuous process of surgical treatment for a large calcified chronic subdural hematoma. World Neurosurg. 2017;108:996.e1–6.
39. Li X, Wan Y, Qian C, Yang S, Zhu X, Wang Y. Double-loculated calcification chronic subdural hematoma: case report and literature review. Neurosurg Q. 2015;25:167–73.
40. Ludwig B, Nix W, Lanksch W. Computed tomography of the armored brain. Neuroradiology. 1983;25:39–43.
41. Marcikić M, Hreckovski B, Samardzić J, Martinović M, Rotim K. Spontaneous resolution of post-traumatic chronic subdural hematoma: case report. Acta Clin Croat. 2010;49:331–4.
42. Matsumura M, Nojiri K. Asymptomatic calcified chronic subdural hematoma in the elderly. Neurol Med Chir (Tokyo). 1984;24:504–6.
43. Miranda LB, Braxton E, Hobbs J, Quigley MR. Chronic subdural hematoma in the elderly: not a benign disease. J Neurosurg. 2011;114:72–6.
44. Moon KS, Lee JK, Kim TS, Jung S, Kim JH, Kim SH, et al. Contralateral acute subdural hematoma occurring after removal of calcified chronic subdural hematoma. J Clin Neurosci. 2007;14:283–6.
45. Mori K, Yamamoto T, Horinaka N, Maeda M. Arachnoid cyst is a risk factor for chronic subdural hematoma in juveniles: twelve cases of chronic subdural hematoma associated with arachnoid cyst. J Neurotrauma. 2002;19:1017–27.
46. Mosberg WH Jr, Smith GW. Calcified solid subdural hematoma; review of literature and report of an unusual case. J Nerv Ment Dis. 1952;115:163–73.
47. Moskala M, Goscinski I, Kaluza J, Polak J, Krupa M, Adamek D, et al. Morphological aspects of the traumatic chronic subdural hematoma capsule: SEM studies. Microsc Microanal. 2007;13:211–9.
48. Nanko N, Tanikawa M, Mase M, Fujita M, Tateyama H, Miyati T, et al. Involvement of hypoxia-inducible factor-1a and vascular endothelial growth factor in the mechanism of development of chronic subdural hematoma. Neurol Med Chir (Tokyo). 2009;49:379–85.
49. Niwa J, Nakamura T, Fujishige M, Hashi K. Removal of a large asymptomatic calcified chronic subdural hematoma. Surg Neurol. 1988;30:135–9.
50. Oda S, Shimoda M, Hoshikawa K, Shiramizu H, Matsumae M. Organized chronic subdural haematoma with a thick calcified inner membrane successfully treated by surgery: a case report. Tokai J Exp Clin Med. 2010;35:85–8.
51. Papanikolaou PG, Paleologos TS, Triantafyllou TM, Chatzidakis EM. Shunt revision after

33 years in a patient with bilateral calcified chronic subdural hematomas. Case illustration. J Neurosurg. 2008;108:401.
52. Park JS, Son EI, Kim DW, Kim SP. Calcified chronic subdural hematoma associated with intracerebral hematoma: case report. J Korean Neurosurg Soc. 2003;34:177–8.
53. Per H, Gumus H, Tucer B, Akgun H, Kurtsoy A, Kumandas S. Calcified chronic subdural hematoma mimicking calvarial mass: a case report. Brain Dev. 2006;28:607–9.
54. Petraglia AL, Moravan MJ, Jahromi BS. Armored brain: a case report and review of the literature. Surg Neurol Int. 2011;2:120.
55. Rahman A, Haque M, Bhandari PB. Calcified chronic subdural haematoma. BMJ Case Rep. 2012;2012. pii: bcr0120125499.
56. Sakamoto T, Hoshikawa Y, Hayashi T, Taguchi Y, Sekino H. Inner membrane preservation surgery for organized or calcified chronic subdural hematoma. Jpn J Neurosurg (Tokyo). 2000;9:541–6.
57. Salunke P, Aggarwal A, Madhivanan K, Futane S. Armoured brain due to chronic subdural collections masking underlying hydrocephalus. Br J Neurosurg. 2013;27:524–5.
58. Sandhu K, Dash HH. Anesthesia related neurological complication. Indian J Anaesth. 2004;48:439–45.
59. Santarius T, Kirkpatrick PJ, Kolias AG, Hutchinson PJ. Working toward rational and evidence-based treatment of chronic subdural hematoma. Clin Neurosurg. 2010;57:112–22.
60. Satyarthee GD, Lalwani S. Armored brain associated with secondary craniostenosis development at 7-year following ventriculoperitoneal shunt surgery during infancy: extremely unusual association and review. Asian J Neurosurg. 2018;13:1175–8.
61. Sgaramella E, Sotgiu S, Miragliotta G, Fotios Kalfas Crotti FM. "Matrioska head". Case report of calcified chronic subdural hematoma. J Neurosurg Sci. 2002;46:28–31.
62. Shaikh N, Masood I, Hanssens Y, Louon A, Hafiz A. Tension pneumocephalus as complication of burr-hole drainage of chronic subdural hematoma: a case report. Surg Neurol Int. 2010;1:27.
63. Sharma RR, Mahapatra A, Pawar SJ, Sousa J, Athale SD. Symptomatic calcified subdural hematomas. Pediatr Neurosurg. 1999;31:150–4.
64. Siddiqui SA, Singh PK, Sawarkar D, Singh M, Sharma BS. Bilateral ossified chronic subdural hematoma presenting as diabetes insipidus-case report and literature review. World Neurosurg. 2017;98:520–4.
65. Sikahall-Meneses E, Salazar-Pérez N, Sandoval-Bonilla B. Chronic subdural hematoma. Surgical management in 100 patients. Cir Cir. 2008;76:199–203.
66. Spadaro A, Ambrosio D, Moraci A, Albanese V. Nontumoral aqueductal stenosis in children affected by von Recklinghausen's disease. Surg Neurol. 1986;26:487–95.
67. Spadaro R, Rotondo M, Di Celmo D, Simpatico S, Parlato C, Zotta DC, Albanese V. Bilateral calcified chronic subdural hematoma. Further pathogenetic and clinical consideration on the so-called armored brain. J Neurosurg Sci. 1987;2:49–52.
68. Taha MM. Armored brain in patients with hydrocephalus after shunt surgery: review of the literatures. Turk Neurosurg. 2012;22:407–10.
69. Tandon V, Garg K, Mahapatra AK. 'Double skull' appearance due to calcifications of chronic subdural hematoma and cephalhematoma: a report of two cases. Turk Neurosurg. 2013;23:815–7.
70. Turgut M, Akhaddar A, Turgut AT. Calcified or ossified chronic subdural hematoma: a systematic review of 114 cases reported during last century with a demonstrative case report. World Neurosurg. 2020;134:240–63.
71. Turgut M, Palaoglu S, Sağlam S. Huge ossified crust-like subdural hematoma covering the hemisphere and causing acute signs of increased intracranial pressure. Childs Nerv Syst. 1997;13:415–7.
72. Turgut M, Samancoğlu H, Ozsunar Y, Erkuş M. Ossified chronic subdural hematoma. Cent Eur Neurosurg. 2010;71:146–8.
73. Turgut M, Yay MO. A rare case of ossified chronic subdural hematoma complicated with tension pneumocephalus. J Neurol Surg Rep. 2019;80:e44–5.
74. Tyson G, Strachan WE, Newman P, Winn HR, Butler A, Jane J. The role of craniectomy in the treatment of chronic subdural hematomas. J Neurosurg. 1980;52:776–81.
75. Viozzi I, van Baarsen K, Grotenhuis A. Armored brain in a young girl with a syndromal hydrocephalus. Acta Neurochir (Wien). 2017;159:81–3.
76. Weigel R, Schmiedek P, Krauss JK. Outcome of contemporary surgery for chronic subdural haematoma: evidence based review. J Neurol Neurosurg Psychiatry. 2003;74:937–43.
77. Wester K, Helland CA. How often do chronic extra-cerebral haematomas occur in patients

with intracranial arachnoid cysts? J Neurol Neurosurg Psychiatry. 2008;79:72–5.
78. Xiao ZY, Chen XJ, Li KZ, Zhang ZP. Calcified chronic subdural hematoma: a case report and literature review. Transl Neurosci Clin. 2017;3:220–3.
79. Yadav YR, Parihar V, Namdev H, Bajaj J. Chronic subdural hematoma. Asian J Neurosurg. 2016;11:330–42.
80. Yamada K, Ohta T, Takatsuka H, Yamaguchi K. High-field magnetic resonance image of a huge calcified chronic subdural haematoma, so-called "armoured brain". Acta Neurochir (Wien). 1992;114:151–3.
81. Yan HJ, Lin KE, Lee ST, Tzaan WC. Calcified chronic subdural hematoma: case report. Changgeng Yi Xue Za Zhi. 1998;21:521–5.
82. Yang X, Qian Z, Qiu Y, Li X. Diagnosis and management of ossified chronic subdural hematoma. J Craniofac Surg. 2015;26:e550–1.
83. Yang HZ, Tseng SH, Chen Y, Lin SM, Chen CJ. Calcified chronic subdural haematoma—case report. Tzu Chi Med J. 2004;16:261–5.
84. Yokoyama K, Matsuki M, Shimano H, Sumioka S, Ikenaga T, Hanabusa K, et al. Diffusion tensor imaging in chronic subdural hematoma: correlation between clinical signs and fractional anisotropy in the pyramidal tract. AJNR Am J Neuroradiol. 2008;29:1159–63.
85. Zarkou S, Aguilar MI, Patel NP, Wellik KE, Wingerchuk DM, Demaerschalk BM. The role of corticosteroids in the management of chronic subdural hematomas: a critically appraised topic. Neurologist. 2009;15:299–302.
86. Zhang S, Wang X, Liu Y, Mao Q. Resection of a huge calcified chronic subdural haematoma: case report. Br J Neurosurg. 2018;14:1–3.
87. Zhao KJ, Zhang RY, Sun QF, Wang XQ, Gu XY, Qiang Q, et al. Comparisons of 2/3Sh estimation technique to computer-assisted planimetric analysis in epidural, subdural and intracerebral hematomas. Neurol Res. 2010;32:910–7.

第 16 章 颅脑创伤性硬膜下积液后的慢性硬膜下血肿

Ali Akhaddar

译者：吴量

16.1 引言

颅内慢性硬膜下血肿（CSDH）的病因是多样的。其中，创伤性硬膜下积液（SDHG）可能是 CSDH 的先兆表现（图 16.1）。虽然这两种疾病之间的关系是公认的，但转化的发病机制尚不完全清楚。

创伤性硬膜下积液定义为由于头部损伤后脑蛛网膜撕裂导致脑脊液在硬膜下聚集。Dandy 于 1932 年首次将其命名为 "subdural hydroma"，目前首选的表达是 "subdural hygroma"[1-3]。Hygroma 来自希腊语 "hygros"，字面意思是潮湿。文献中对相同疾病也使用了其他名称，如 "subdural fluid accumulation" "subdural fluid collection" 或 "subdural effusion"[4-9]。大多数 SDHG 通常与脑脊液成分的改变有关[5-6, 10-11]。继发于活瓣机制的积液可逐渐增大，产生对脑实质的占位效应和相应的神经系统表现。CSDH 和 SDHG 通常发生在创伤后的硬膜下腔；然而，CSDH 与硬膜下积液在许多方面不同，如硬膜下聚集液的成分、神经影像学特点和临床表现[5, 12-16]。在某些情况下，区分这两种疾病并不容易，因为 SDHG 的硬膜下内容物通常是血液和脑脊液的混合体[3, 7-8, 17-18]。

Yamada 等首次报道了三例创伤性 SDHG 发展为 CSDH 的病例[11]。自 1979 年首次发表以来，已有许多相关研究发表，特别是来自亚洲的研究[3-4, 6, 9-10, 12, 15-17, 19-26]。事实上，创伤性 SDHG 在 CSDH 发展中的作用似乎被忽视了，尤其是在西方国家。

本章全面概述了创伤性硬膜下积液在慢性硬膜下血肿发展中的作用。

16.2 创伤性硬膜下积液转化为 CSDH 的发生率

创伤性 SDHG 发展为 CSDH 的总发病率从 4% 到 48.8% 不等（表 16.1）。此外，4.7%～24.2% 的 CSDH 病例源于创伤性 SDHG（表 16.2）。所有发病率存在差异的原因尚不清楚。不同的病例系列在数据采集标准上也存在一定的不可预测性。例如，一些患者在头部损伤后出现 SDHG，而另一些患者在最初的脑成像时仅表现为 "硬膜下液体的聚集"。

在日本和韩国发表的研究中发病率相对较高，可能是由于患者年龄较大，以及这两个亚洲国家对头部损伤患者会进行常规的动态 CT 扫描和定期随访[9, 29-30, 34]。Ohno 等认为，在其他国家，如果没有详尽的神经影像学监测，这类患者可能会被忽

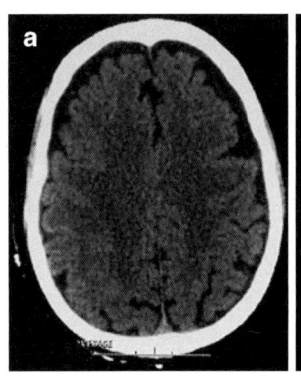 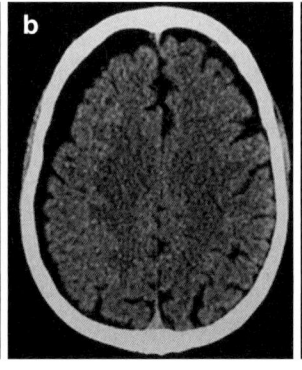 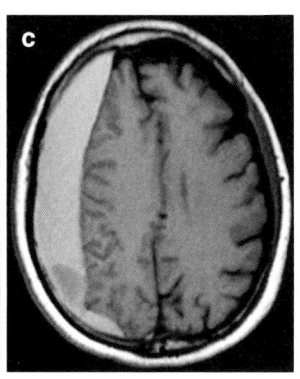

图 16.1 病例 1。一名经历右侧轻度头外伤的 64 岁男性患者的初始 CT 扫描（a）。6 周后，可见右侧少量硬膜下积液（b）。外伤后 3 个月，于 MRI 的 T1 像见明显慢性硬膜下血肿（c）

表 16.1 创伤性硬膜下积液中转化为慢性硬膜下血肿患者的文献回顾

作者[参考文献]	年份	国家	发病率（%）	结果
Yamada 等[27]	1980	日本	25	24 例创伤性 SDHG 含 6 例 CSDH
St John and Dila[28]	1981	美国	4	25 例创伤性 SDHG 含 1 例 CSDH
Ohno 等[29]	1987	日本	46.5	43 例创伤性 SDHG 含 20 例 CSDH
Koizumi 等[4]	1987	日本	1.8[a]	169 例开颅术后 SDHG 含 3 例 CSDH
Murata[8]	1993	日本	26.9	108 例创伤性 SDHG 含 29 例 CSDH
Lee 等[17]	1994	韩国	8.2	61 例创伤性 SDHG 含 5 例 CSDH
Parker 等[30]	1994	韩国	8.9	145 例创伤性 SDHG 含 13 例 CSDH
Lee 等[24]	2000	韩国	32.8	58 例创伤性 SDHG 含 19 例 CSDH
Kumar 等[22]	2008	印度	5[b]	20 例儿童创伤性 SDHG 含 1 例 CSDH
Liu 等[16]	2009	中国	22.7	192 例创伤性 SDHG 含 32 例 CSDH
Wang 等[26]	2015	中国	16.7	44 例创伤性 SDHG 含 10 例 CSDH
Ahn 等[19]	2016	韩国	44.4	45 例创伤性 SDHG 含 20 例 CSDH
Fan 等[20]	2020	中国	48.8	45 例创伤性 SDHG 含 22 例 CSDH

CSDH，慢性硬膜下血肿；SDHG，硬膜下积液。
[a] 开颅术后。
[b] 儿童患者。

表 16.2 初始影像学明确的创伤性硬膜下积液中进展为慢性硬膜下血肿患者的文献回顾

作者[参考文献]	年份	国家	发病率（%）	结果
Park 等[25]	2008	韩国	15	160 例 CSDH 含 24 例伤后 CT 证实的创伤性 SDHG
Akhaddar 等[31]	2009	摩洛哥	7.2	110 例 CSDH 含 8 例伤后 CT 证实的创伤性 SDHG[a]
Olivero 等[32]	2017	美国	18.9	37 例 CSDH 含 7 例伤后 CT 或 MRI 证实的创伤性 SDHG
Komiyama 等[21]	2019	日本	13.3	172 例 CSDH 含 23 例伤后 CT 证实的创伤性 SDHG
Akhaddar 等[b]	2020	摩洛哥	4.7	84 例 CSDH 含 4 例伤后 CT 或 MRI 证实的创伤性 SDHG
Chen 等[33]	2020	中国	24.2	70 例 CSDH 含 17 例伤后 CT 证实的创伤性 SDHG

CSDH，慢性硬膜下血肿；SDHG，硬膜下积液；CT，计算机断层成像；MRI，磁共振成像。
[a] 一名患者最初对对侧自发性脑内血肿进行了手术治疗。
[b] 未发表的个人研究（于 2013 年 10 月至 2020 年 10 月于作者所在科室收治的 84 例患者）。

视[9, 11, 29]。相反，与亚洲相比，来自西方国家的系列报道则很少[28, 32]。Park 和同事认为，西方神经外科医生报道的大多数急性 SDHG 病例可能都接受了手术治疗，而不是保守治疗[25, 30]。SDHG 是否会进展为 CSDH 仍未明确；其属罕见抑或报道不足有待厘清。为阐明二者关联与转化，仍需在欧洲与北美开展更多流行病学研究。在发展中国家，随着 CT 扫描在脑外伤患者中的广泛应用，根据我们的个人经验，肯定会发现更多继发于 SDHG 的 CSDH 病例（图 16.1 至图 16.5）。

16.3 演变机制与转化的危险因素

硬脑膜下积液被认为是创伤后硬脑膜/蛛网膜界面分离的结果；这看起来像是少量的硬膜下液体聚集。通常认为，蛛网膜的撕裂和活瓣作用是其致病机制[4, 35-41]。此外，充足的潜在硬膜下腔（特别是老年脑萎缩）是 SDHG 扩张至关重要的条件[3, 6, 17, 23, 36]。通常，脑萎缩主要发生在额叶，靠近额叶的脑脊液体积可增加约 11% 来弥补脑实质的丧失[28]。因此，大多数积液发生在额叶凸面和侧裂周围。

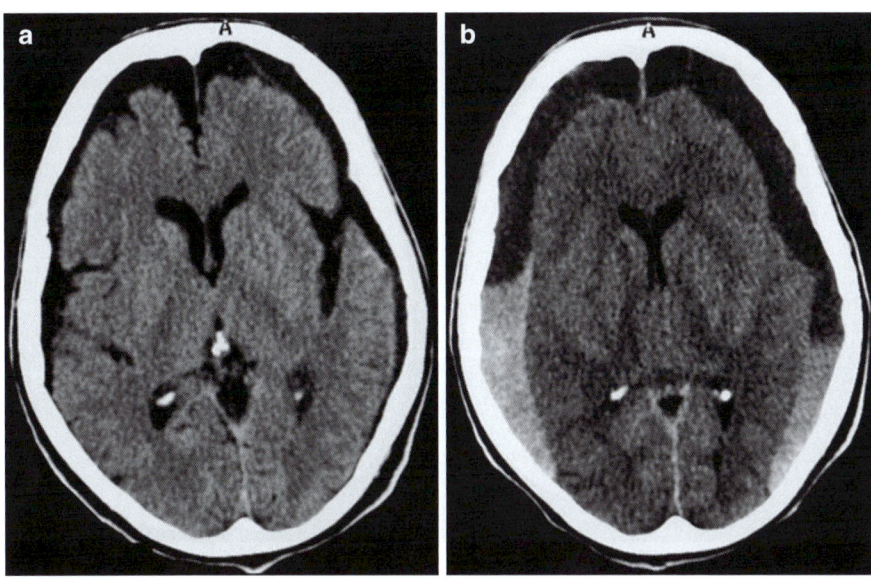

图16.2 病例2。一名有精神疾病史的60岁女性患者因跌倒就诊。伤后第三天的CT显示双额少量硬膜下积液（a）。2个月后患者神经功能恶化，复查头颅CT显示双侧慢性硬膜下血肿混杂急性出血（b）

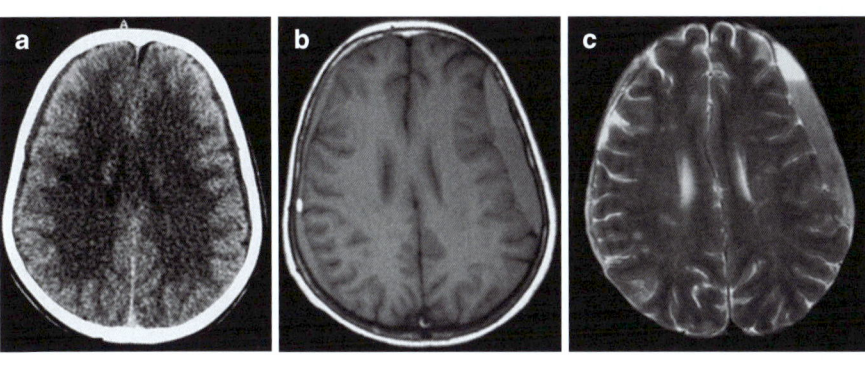

图16.3 病例3。一名48岁女性患者伤后2天的头颅CT，可见少量双侧硬膜下积液（a）。随访MRI的T1像（b）和T2像（c）显示左侧新发的慢性硬膜下血肿

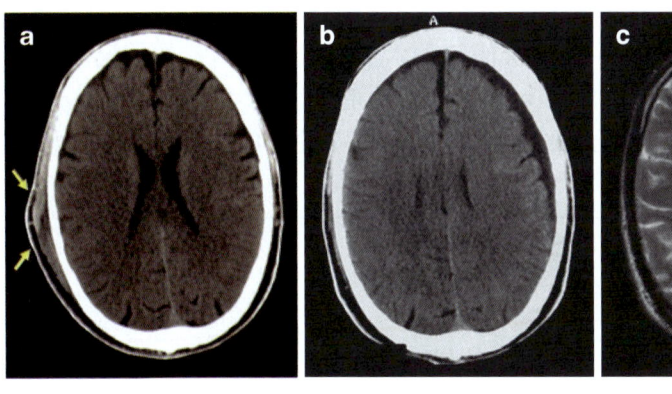

图16.4 病例4。一名44岁头部外伤的男性患者的CT扫描，未见颅内异常但右侧可见头皮挫伤（箭头）（a）。10天后，可见少量左侧（受伤对侧）硬膜下积液（b）。2个月后，在MRI的T2像上可见巨大慢性硬膜下血肿（初始受伤对侧）（c）

目前，已经提出了多种SDHG发展成CSDH的机制。一些作者提出，发病前的情况，如老年人脑萎缩（由于脑重量减少和硬膜下腔随着年龄的增长而增加）可能有助于SDHG向CSDH转化[3, 9, 17, 20, 25, 29, 42]。Park和其同事则不同意这个假设。在他们1994年发表的研究中，在13例患者中发现老年和CT显示的脑萎缩似乎并不是SDHG向CSDH转化的促进因素[30]。

对于SDHG转化为CSDH的其他机制也提出了假说：持续的硬膜下积液可能是新膜形成的来源，桥静脉破裂或囊壁微出血可能是积液增大的原因[3, 9, 22]。此外，过度的纤维蛋白溶解进入积液可能导致凝血功能障碍。众所周知，纤维蛋白原是再出血的标志物，凝血酶是凝血的指标，而组织型纤溶酶原激活物（tPA）和纤维蛋白降解产物（FDP）都是纤溶作用的指标[10, 13, 25, 43]。这种现象伴有炎症反应，可诱发CSDH[10, 12, 44-45]。另一种机制是混杂在积液中的蛋白或血液成分可以使SDHG演变为CSDH[9, 20, 44]。

许多作者认为，CT中能预测SDHG向CSDH

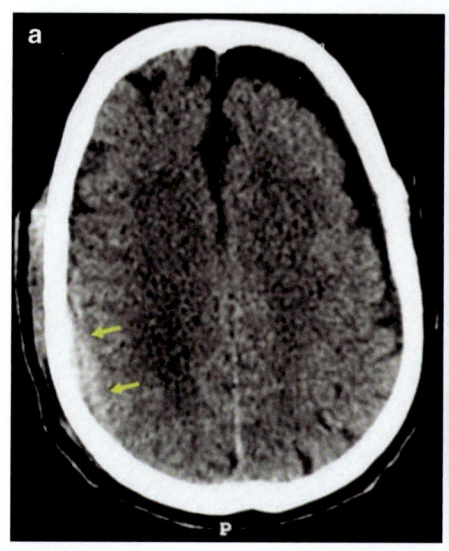
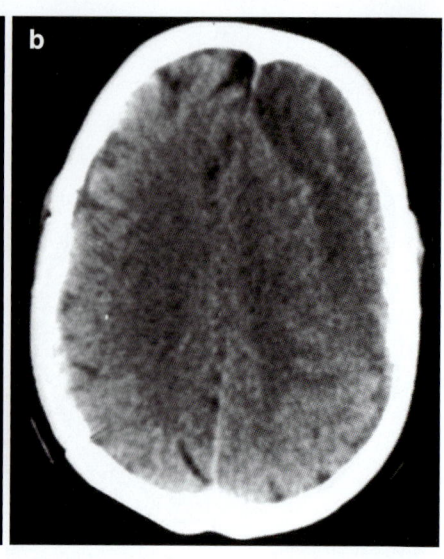

图 16.5 病例 5。一名 69 岁男性患者在交通事故后由创伤性硬膜下积液进展为慢性硬膜下血肿。伤后入院的 CT 显示在右侧（箭头）有一少量急性硬膜下血肿以及对侧的少量硬膜下积液（a）。10 周后，在复查颅脑 CT 上可见左侧不均匀慢性硬膜下血肿形成（初始受伤部位对侧）（b）

转变的表现是早期硬膜下液体增加，随后在后期积液的密度积累增加[25, 34]。

Ohno 和其他人表明创伤后 SDHG 最初倾向于发生在双侧。如果持续时间较长，任何一侧都可能发生 CSDH[9, 17, 25, 29]。本章中的两位患者也支持这一假设（图 16.4 和图 16.5）。Ahn 等认为，创伤性 SDHG 患者，尤其是双侧 SDHG 患者，应考虑其发展为 CSDH 的可能性[19]。最近，Fan 和同事进行的一项新研究发现，双侧 SDHG 和积液厚度是 SDHG 演变为 CSDH 的独立危险因素。有报道厚度大于 11.37 mm 的 SDHG 转化风险较高[20]。

先前的两项研究报道了一些创伤性 SDHG 患者在增强磁共振成像（MRI）中显示出脑膜增强[19, 37]。根据 Ahn 的经验，9 例脑膜增强患者中有 7 例发展为 CSDH[19]。Hasegawa 在 5 例脑膜增强患者的镜检中发现血管化的新膜，其中血管内皮显示大量的胞饮小泡和窗孔，表明伴有脑膜增强的 SDHG 有可能转变为 CSDH[37]。

男性优势在 SDHG 向 CSDH 转化中的作用已经被几位作者提出[19, 25, 30, 34]。很明显男性通常更容易暴露于创伤。在颅内出血或硬膜下出血的研究中，高血压被报道为 SDHG 转化为 CSDH 的危险因素。事实上，高血压可能会增加出血的风险[17, 23, 25, 30]。相反，也有人发现高血压、糖尿病和冠心病并不是 SDHG 转化的危险因素[20]。

16.4 临床特点及处理

如上所述，大多数由 SDHG 转化为 CSDH 的患者年龄较大。然而，年轻患者也不应该被忽视[18, 22, 26]。根据 Wang 的经验，32 例由 SDHG 发展为 CSDH 的患者中有 10 例年龄在 2 个月至 10 岁之间，并且 50% 的患者年龄在 40 岁以下[26]。

大多数患者从创伤后 SDHG 转化为 CSDH 的时间均在 1 个月以上。更准确地说，平均时间在 50～68 天[9, 12, 20, 25, 30-31]。一般情况下，所有患者均有与 CSDH 相关的体征和症状[46-48]。此外，手术治疗和结果与典型 CSDH 也没有任何不同。需要指出的是，根据许多研究报告和我们的个人经验，在不进行任何手术干预或药物治疗的情况下部分 CSDH 可能会自行消退[17, 23, 25, 30, 49]。然而，保守治疗的 CSDH 病例需要几个月的时间才能完全缓解。

16.5 未来展望

需要来自世界各地多个机构的神经放射学家和（或）神经外科医生进行进一步的前瞻性研究，以确定上述危险因素的作用。此外，期待更多来自亚洲以外的大样本流行病学研究。为了更好地了解创伤后 SDHG 向 CSDH 转化的机制，我们需要对 SDHG 的组织学变化进行更多研究。

16.6 结论

慢性硬膜下血肿可以作为创伤后 SDHG 的结果发生发展。当大脑无法扩张时，尤其是在人口老龄化的情况下，必须考虑到这种潜在的可能。头部损伤患者中高达 50% 的 SDHG 可能会发展为

CSDH，这在男性、双侧 SDHG 的老年人、积液厚度大于 11.37 mm 的患者，以及增强 MRI 显示脑膜强化的患者中更为常见。

所有创伤后 SDHG 患者都应由神经外科医生严密随访，以确定发生 CSDH 时的适当治疗方式。

今后还需进一步开展流行病学、神经影像学、组织病理学等方面的研究，以进一步了解 SDHG 转化为 CSDH 的机制。

参考文献

1. Dandy WE. Chronic subdural hydroma and serous meningitis (pachymeningitis serosa; localized external hydrocephalus). In: Lewis D, editor. Practice of surgery. Hagerstown: WF Prior Co.; 1932. p. 306–9.
2. Dandy WE. Chronic subdural hydroma and serous meningitis (pachymeningitis serosa; localized external hydrocephalus). In: Lewis D, editor. Practice of surgery. Hagerstown: WF Prior Co.; 1955. p. 291–3.
3. Lee KS. Chronic subdural hematoma in the aged, trauma or degeneration? J Korean Neurosurg Soc. 2016;59:1–5. https://doi.org/10.3340/jkns.2016.59.1.1.
4. Koizumi H, Fukamachi A, Nukui H. Postoperative subdural fluid collections in neurosurgery. Surg Neurol. 1987;27:147–53. https://doi.org/10.1016/0090-3019(87)90286-2.
5. Kristof RA, Grimm JM, Stoffel-Wagner B. Cerebrospinal fluid leakage into the subdural space: possible influence on the pathogenesis and recurrence frequency of chronic subdural hematoma and subdural hygroma. J Neurosurg. 2008;108:275–80. https://doi.org/10.3171/JNS/2008/108/2/0275.
6. Lee KS. The pathogenesis and clinical significance of traumatic subdural hygroma. Brain Inj. 1998;12:595–603. https://doi.org/10.1080/026990598122359.
7. McConnell AA. Traumatic subdural effusions. J Neurol Psychiatry. 1941;4:237–56. https://doi.org/10.1136/jnnp.4.3-4.237.
8. Murata K. Chronic subdural hematoma may be preceded by persistent traumatic subdural effusion. Neurol Med Chir (Tokyo). 1993;33:691–6. https://doi.org/10.2176/nmc.33.691.
9. Ohno K, Suzuki R, Masaoka H, Matsushima Y, Inaba Y, Monma S. Role of traumatic subdural fluid collection in developing process of chronic subdural hematoma. Bull Tokyo Med Dent Univ. 1986;33:99–106.
10. Tao Z, Lin Y, Hu M, Ding S, Li J, Qiu Y. Mechanism of subdural effusion evolves into chronic subdural hematoma: IL-8 inducing neutrophil oxidative burst. Med Hypotheses. 2016;86:43–6. https://doi.org/10.1016/j.mehy.2015.11.027.
11. Yamada H, Nihei H, Watanabe T, Shibui S, Murata S. Chronic subdural hematoma occurring consequently to the posttraumatic subdural hygroma—on the pathogenesis of the chronic subdural hematoma (author's transl). No To Shinkei. 1979;31:115–21.
12. Feng JF, Jiang JY, Bao YH, Liang YM, Pan YH. Traumatic subdural effusion evolves into chronic subdural hematoma: two stages of the same inflammatory reaction? Med Hypotheses. 2008;70:1147–9. https://doi.org/10.1016/j.mehy.2007.11.014.
13. Fujisawa H, Ito H, Saito K, Ikeda K, Nitta H, Yamashita J. Immunohistochemical localization of tissue-type plasminogen activator in the lining wall of chronic subdural hematoma. Surg Neurol. 1991;35(6):441–5. https://doi.org/10.1016/0090-3019(91)90177-b.
14. Fujisawa H, Nomura S, Kajiwara K, Kato S, Fujii M, Suzuki M. Various magnetic resonance imaging patterns of chronic subdural hematomas: indicators of the pathogenesis? Neurol Med Chir (Tokyo). 2006;46:333–8. https://doi.org/10.2176/nmc.46.333.
15. Liu Y, Zhu S, Jiang Y, Li G, Li X, Su W, et al. Clinical characteristics of chronic subdural hematoma evolving from traumatic subdural effusion. Zhonghua Wai Ke Za Zhi. 2002;40:360–2.
16. Liu Y, Gong J, Li F, Wang H, Zhu S, Wu C. Traumatic subdural hydroma: clinical characteristics and classification. Injury. 2009;40:968–72. https://doi.org/10.1016/j.injury.2009.01.006.
17. Lee KS, Bae WK, Park YT, Yun IG. The pathogenesis and fate of traumatic subdural hygroma. Br J Neurosurg. 1994;8:551–8. https://doi.org/10.3109/02688699409002947.
18. Nguyen VN, Wallace D, Ajmera S, Akinduro O, Smith LJ, Giles K, et al. Management of subdural hematohygromas in abusive head trauma. Neurosurgery. 2020;86:281–7. https://doi.org/10.1093/neuros/nyz076.
19. Ahn JH, Jun HS, Kim JH, Oh JK, Song JH, Chang IB. Analysis of risk factor for the develop-

ment of chronic subdural hematoma in patients with traumatic subdural hygroma. J Korean Neurosurg Soc. 2016;59:622–7. https://doi.org/10.3340/jkns.2016.59.6.622.
20. Fan G, Ding J, Wang H, Wang Y, Liu Y, Wang C, et al. Risk factors for the development of chronic subdural hematoma in patients with subdural hygroma. Br J Neurosurg. 2020;29:1–6. https://doi.org/10.1080/02688697.2020.1717444.
21. Komiyama K, Tosaka M, Shimauchi-Ohtaki H, Aihara M, Shimizu T, Yoshimoto Y. Computed tomography findings after head injury preceding chronic subdural hematoma. Neurosurg Focus. 2019;47:E12. https://doi.org/10.3171/2019.8.
22. Kumar R, Singhal N, Mahapatra AK. Traumatic subdural effusions in children following minor head injury. Childs Nerv Syst. 2008;24:1391–6. https://doi.org/10.1007/s00381-008-0645-1.
23. Lee KS, Bae WK, Doh JW, Bae HG, Yun IG. Origin of chronic subdural haematoma and relation to traumatic subdural lesions. Brain Inj. 1998;12:901–10. https://doi.org/10.1080/026990598121972.
24. Lee KS, Bae WK, Bae HG, Yun IG. The fate of traumatic subdural hygroma in serial computed tomographic scans. J Korean Med Sci. 2000;15:560–8. https://doi.org/10.3346/jkms.2000.15.5.560.
25. Park SH, Lee SH, Park J, Hwang JH, Hwang SK, Hamm IS. Chronic subdural hematoma preceded by traumatic subdural hygroma. J Clin Neurosci. 2008;15:868–72. https://doi.org/10.1016/j.jocn.2007.08.003.
26. Wang Y, Wang C, Liu Y. Chronic subdural haematoma evolving from traumatic subdural hydroma. Brain Inj. 2015;29:462–5. https://doi.org/10.3109/02699052.2014.990513.
27. Yamada H, Watanabe T, Murata S, Shibui S, Nihei H, Kohno T, et al. Developmental process of chronic subdural collections of fluid based on CT scan findings. Surg Neurol. 1980;13:441–8.
28. St John JN, Dila C. Traumatic subdural hygroma in adults. Neurosurgery. 1981;9:621–6. https://doi.org/10.1227/00006123-198112000-00002.
29. Ohno K, Suzuki R, Masaoka H, Matsushima Y, Inaba Y, Monma S. Chronic subdural haematoma preceded by persistent traumatic subdural fluid collection. J Neurol Neurosurg Psychiatry. 1987;50:1694–7. https://doi.org/10.1136/jnnp.50.12.1694.
30. Park CK, Choi KH, Kim MC, Kang JK, Choi CR. Spontaneous evolution of posttraumatic subdural hygroma into chronic subdural haematoma. Acta Neurochir. 1994;127:41–7. https://doi.org/10.1007/BF01808545.
31. Akhaddar A, Bensghir M, Abouqal R, Boucetta M. Influence of cranial morphology on the location of chronic subdural haematoma. Acta Neurochir. 2009;151:1235–40. https://doi.org/10.1007/s00701-009-0357-7.
32. Olivero WC, Wang H, Farahvar A, Kim TA, Wang F. Predictive (subtle or overlooked) initial head CT findings in patients who develop delayed chronic subdural hematoma. J Clin Neurosci. 2017;42:129–33. https://doi.org/10.1016/j.jocn.2017.03.005.
33. Chen S, Peng H, Shao X, Yao L, Liu J, Tian J, et al. Prediction of risk factors for the evolution of traumatic subdural effusion into chronic subdural hematoma. Neuropsychiatr Dis Treat. 2020;16:943–8. https://doi.org/10.2147/NDT.S245857.
34. Takahashi Y, Sato H, Inoue Y, Takeda S, Ohkawara S. CT findings and the evaluation of chronic subdural hematoma (Part I)–forecast of chronic subdural hematoma (author's transl). Neurol Med Chir (Tokyo). 1981;21:485–90.
35. Asano Y, Hasuo M, Takahashi I, Shimosawa S. Surgical outcome of 32 cases in traumatic subdural hygroma. No To Shinkei. 1992;44:1127–31.
36. Haines DE, Harkey HL, al-Mefty O. The "subdural" space: a new look at an outdated concept. Neurosurgery. 1993;32:111–20. https://doi.org/10.1227/00006123-199301000-00017.
37. Hasegawa M, Yamashima T, Yamashita J, Suzuki M, Shimada S. Traumatic subdural hygroma: pathology and meningeal enhancement on magnetic resonance imaging. Neurosurgery. 1992;31:580–5. https://doi.org/10.1227/00006123-199209000-00024.
38. Ishibashi A, Yokokura Y, Miyagi J. Clinical analysis of nineteen patients with traumatic subdural hygromas. Kurume Med J. 1994;41:81–5. https://doi.org/10.2739/kurumemedj.41.81.
39. Kamezaki T, Yanaka K, Fujita K, Nakamura K, Nagatomo Y, Nose T. Traumatic acute subdural hygroma mimicking acute subdural hematoma. J Clin Neurosci. 2004;11:311–3. https://doi.org/10.1016/j.jocn.2003.10.013.
40. So SK, Ogawa T, Gerberg E, Sakimura I, Wright W. Tracer accumulation in a subdural hygroma: case report. J Nucl Med. 1976;17:119–21.
41. Zanini MA, de Lima Resende LA, de Souza Faleiros AT, Gabarra RC. Traumatic subdural hygromas: proposed pathogenesis based classification. J Trauma. 2008;64:705–13. https://doi.

org/10.1097/TA.0b013e3180485cfc.
42. Cotton F, Euvrard T, Durand-Dubief F, Pachai C, Cucherat M, Ramirez Rozzi F, et al. Correlation between cranial vault size and brain size over time: preliminary MRI evaluation. J Neuroradiol. 2005;32:131–7. https://doi.org/10.1016/s0150-9861(05)83128-1.
43. Yamashita K, Sekino H, Hayashi T. Systemic and local activation of coagulofibrinolysis in the etiology of chronic subdural hematoma. Jpn J Neurosurg. 1994;3:390–7.
44. Suzuki M, Endo S, Inada K, Kudo A, Kitakami A, Kuroda K, et al. Inflammatory cytokines locally elevated in chronic subdural haematoma. Acta Neurochir (Wien). 1998;140:51–5. https://doi.org/10.1007/s007010050057.
45. Suzuki M, Kudo A, Kitakami A, Doi M, Kubo N, Kuroda K, et al. Local hypercoagulative activity precedes hyperfibrinolytic activity in the subdural space during development of chronic subdural haematoma from subdural effusion. Acta Neurochir. 1998;140:261–5. https://doi.org/10.1007/s007010050093.
46. Stanisic M, Lund-Johansen M, Mahesparan R. Treatment of chronic subdural hematoma by burr-hole craniostomy in adults: influence of some factors on postoperative recurrence. Acta Neurochir. 2005;147:1249–56. https://doi.org/10.1007/s00701-005-0616-1.
47. Su TM, Shih TY, Yen HL, Tsai YD. Contralateral acute subdural hematoma occurring after evacuation of subdural hygroma: case report. J Trauma. 2001;50:557–9. https://doi.org/10.1097/00005373-200103000-00025.
48. Sucu HK, Gökmen M, Bezircioglu H, Tektaş S. Contralateral development of chronic subdural hematoma after evacuation of chronic subdural hematoma. A case report. J Neurosurg Sci. 2006;50:71–4.
49. Zanini MA, Resende LA, Freitas CC, Yamashita S. Traumatic subdural hygroma: five cases with changed density and spontaneous resolution. Arq Neuropsiquiatr. 2007;65:68–72. https://doi.org/10.1590/s0004-282x2007000100015.

第17章 继发于脑脊液分流术和神经外科内镜手术的硬膜下出血

Alexander E. Braley 和 Walter A. Hall

译者：田润发

17.1 引言

脑脊液（CSF）分流术是大多数脑积水的主要治疗方法，该方法是在脑室系统和身体其他自然腔隙之间建立分流体系。脑室-腹腔分流术（VPS）是脑脊液分流最常见且成熟的一种分流术式，除此以外还有多种分流的方法，包括（顺序不分先后）从脑室分流至腹腔、胸膜腔、输尿管、膀胱、胆囊、全身静脉系统（或直接进入心房），甚至进入硬膜下或颞下间隙。从腰椎蛛网膜下腔分流脑脊液是另外一种分流方法，如腰大池-腹腔分流术。脑脊液分流术存在多种风险，包括直接脑实质损伤、卒中、引流过度/不足、出血和感染等。植入的引流管增加了感染风险，在感染过程中微生物会定植于引流管上，形成难以根除的生物膜，通常需要手术根除生物膜并更换引流管，治疗期间通过脑室外引流替代。

内镜下三脑室造瘘术（ETV）通常被认为不属于脑脊液分流术的一种，但确实创造了一条通路将脑脊液从三脑室经造瘘口引流至三脑室底的桥前池，该方法的优势在于不需要置入引流管。ETV因未植入引流管而不存在感染风险，减少了因手术感染需二次手术的风险[5]。同时在发生如脑膜炎等颅内感染时，也不需要更换或取出引流管。ETV与常规分流术的并发症总发生率相当，但也有报道指出ETV存在更多的围手术期并发症，更少的远期并发症[5]。

硬膜下积液，包括硬膜下血肿和硬膜下积水，是已知的脑脊液分流术后最常见的并发症[5]。这些积液可能无临床症状，也可能引起相关神经系统症状如头痛、肢体无力、麻木和癫痫，这些症状在很大程度上取决于积液的量。硬膜下积液可能由跌倒等创伤引起［在特发性正常压力脑积水（iNPH）患者人群中特别常见］，如果联合抗凝或抗血小板治疗，则风险会进一步增加[1, 15]。

17.2 脑脊液分流术后硬膜下积液的病因学

脑脊液分流术后的硬膜下积液被认为是由两个相互关联且常常并存的发病因素协同作用的结果，其协同发病因素分别为：①因脑室体积减小导致脑脊液聚集于硬脑膜下腔，②桥静脉破裂出血。硬膜下积液可发生在任何脑室扩大的患者中，这些患者扩大的脑室因为脑脊液引流而急剧缩小，导致硬脑膜下腔扩大。硬脑膜下腔扩大可能会导致出血，其机制类似于脑萎缩导致的出血：随着硬脑膜下腔扩大，桥静脉受到牵拉，这种情况下即使轻微脑创伤也可导致出血。这种出血可以表现为隐匿、多次的（在出现症状前不断累积），也可以表现为急性硬膜下出血，导致严重和突发的临床症状。

脑脊液过度引流是导致硬膜下积液形成的核心机制。这种过度引流可能继发于分流管设定压力过低，也可能是病情改善后未及时调整引流压力的结果。硬膜下积液与脑脊液过度引流的发生发展机制与脊髓脑脊液漏导致的低颅内压类似[2, 12]。这些病变通常有相似的临床表现如双侧硬膜下积液/血肿，患者症状将持续进展直到脑脊液漏口被修补或自发闭塞[2, 6, 9]。

17.3 硬膜下积液的管理

硬膜下积液的预防被认为是避免出现需要手术干预的硬膜下出血的关键，选择适当的分流阀压力和放置可调压分流阀是避免这一并发症[11]的关键因素。分流阀设定的压力可在术前或术中通过脑室或腰大池测压来估计，以指导初始或后续分流阀压力的设置[11]。

在分流阀压力选择这个问题上需要注意的是，即使在放置分流阀时设置了适当的压力，也会发生由于过度引流引起的硬膜下出血／积液，甚至在增加分流阀引流压力后也可能持续存在。这种情况可能是继发于虹吸效应[4, 13]。脑脊液分流阀可依靠相对简单的压力梯度来控制开启和关闭阀门，这一发现被应用于可调压的引流管阀门。当腹内压较低而颅内压较高时压力梯度达到临界点，设定该临界点压力为关闭阀门的引流压力。因此当患者体位转变为直立时，由于高度差腹内压远低于颅内压，引流阀门关闭预防过度引流。部分长期卧床的患者因为腹内压接近于颅内压，因引流量不足而导致脑脊液分流失败[3-4]。反之亦然，直立的患者可能会因过度引流出现相应的神经系统症状，并导致硬膜下积液和（或）出血，该状况与分流阀设定压力过低的患者相似[4]。这种情况特别难以治疗，因为单纯增加分流阀的设定压力是不足以解决该问题的。引入抗虹吸阀可以解决这一问题，部分文献报道放置抗虹吸阀的患者降低了因过度引流而产生并发症的概率[13]。这种抗虹吸装置可以安装在瓣膜组织中，也可以是瓣膜和远端导管之间的附加组件。

外科手术治疗仍是治疗硬膜下积液的主要方式，手术方法有钻孔引流、开颅清除术和硬膜下引流[15]。脑室持续引流脑脊液会进一步促进硬膜下出血和硬膜下积液扩大，因此应根据临床病情变化及时减少甚至停止脑脊液引流[15]。

硬膜下出血后减少脑脊液引流的方法受到放置的分流阀种类限制。若使用固定压力阀门仅有两种方法减少脑脊液引流：结扎引流管，或更换更高压力的阀门[8]。可调压分流阀的引入和日益普及为经皮改变脑脊液分流阀压力提供了一种新的非手术选择，并用于减少脑脊液分流量或暂时停止脑脊液分流[8]。这种可调节压力的非手术治疗方式已被证明可以用于以往主要采用手术治疗的硬膜下血肿／积液[8, 15]。使用可调压分流阀，可以调高脑脊液引流需要的压力，从而减少脑脊液的引流甚至停止引流[1, 7-8, 11]。该分流阀门可以维持于一个较高的引流压力，直到临床症状稳定或血肿消退，然后无创地将阀门压降低到满足日常脑脊液引流水平，以满足临床改变脑脊液引流量的需求。为了降低未来非创伤性硬膜下积液的风险，建议考虑使用较前稍高的引流压力。对这些患者应频繁随访，以便在出现临床症状之前尽早发现硬膜下积液，从而增加非手术治疗成功的机会。

虽然大多数分流术导致的硬膜下积液为亚临床状态或无手术指征，但在某些情况下部分症状需要通过手术干预治疗。这些症状包括难治性头痛、虚弱、麻木、癫痫、嗜睡、昏迷等。如果出现类似症状，最好以微创的方式完成引流手术。硬膜下抽吸系统（SEPS）是一种床旁操作的微创硬膜下引流方式，通常只需要局部麻醉或适度镇静，该床旁系统能进一步降低患者发生并发症的风险[10, 14]。该技术最适用于慢性硬膜下血肿或积液，同时也有数据证明其在亚急性甚至急性硬膜下出血中获得良好疗效[10]。血肿定位不准确会降低SEPS的成功率，但因为其风险小，患者避免了手术治疗，这种引流方法仍然值得尝试[10]。手术治疗方式包括单纯钻孔开颅术、双钻孔置管冲洗术或开颅血肿清除术。血肿清除效果随术中暴露的范围越大而越好，然而手术范围越大其并发症的发生率也越高[10, 14]。与SEPS相比，开放手术的额外风险还包括较大范围切开导致的伤口感染风险，以及需要后期颅骨修补等[10]。

17.4 结论

硬膜下积液包括出血或积水，是脑脊液分流术后的难治性并发症。硬膜下积液可表现为多种临床症状，从无症状的硬膜下积液／出血到危及生命导致脑疝发生的大量硬膜下出血。治疗硬膜下积液的主要目标是通过手术或非手术方法减少脑脊液分流，清除硬膜下出血。预防硬膜下积液的方法主要包括设置适当的引流阀门压力，使用抗虹吸分流阀等方法避免脑脊液过度引流。综上所述，仍然需要更多的实验和相关研究来寻找预防和治疗硬膜下积液这一并发症的最佳策略（图17.1至图17.3）。

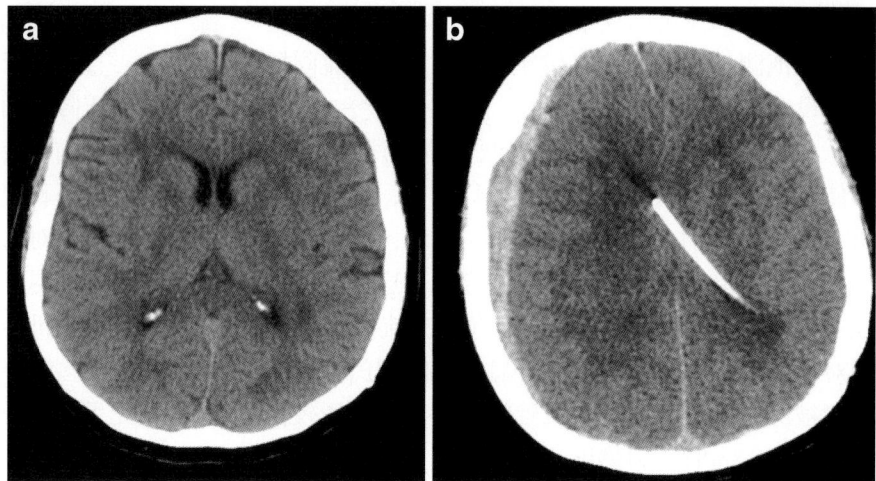

图 17.1 63 岁男性左顶叶分流术前的轴位平扫 CT 提示中等大小脑室（**a**）。脑脊液过度引流导致裂隙脑室后出现右侧急性硬膜下血肿（**b**）

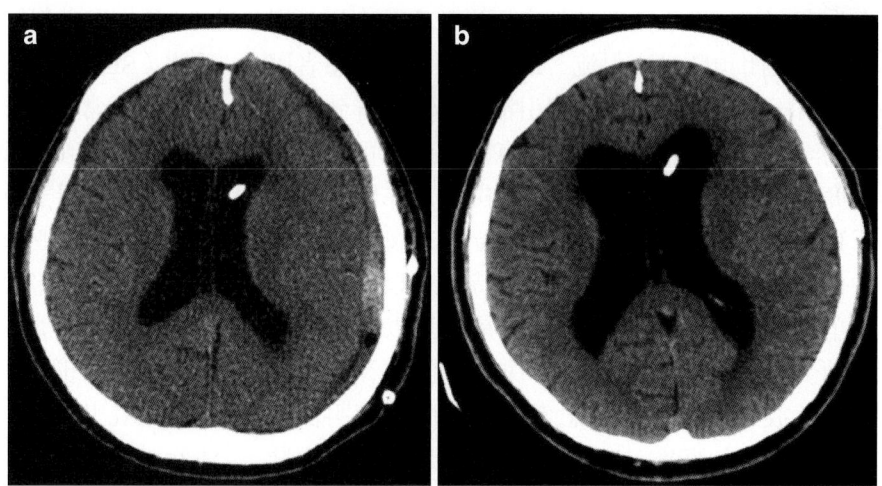

图 17.2 58 岁女性，正常压力性脑积水，采用可调压分流阀脑室-腹腔（VP）分流术治疗。（**a**）放置 VP 分流管后可见左侧急性或慢性硬膜下出血。（**b**）在 SEPS 引流和调节阀门至更高压力后，出血在 6 个月后的随访中消失。注意该患者脑室增大

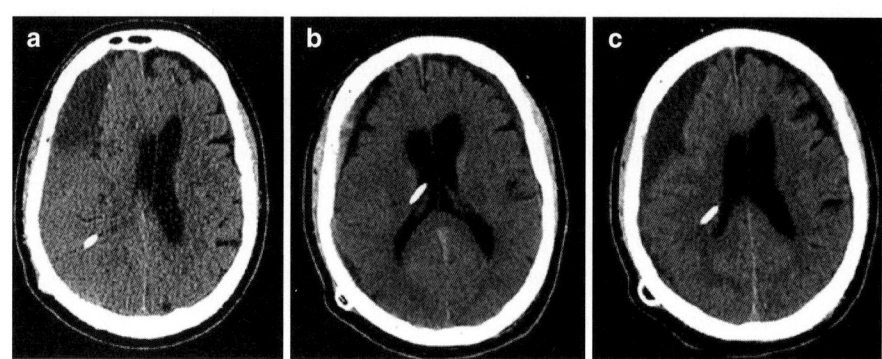

图 17.3 84 岁男性，正常压力性脑积水，在植入中等压力分流阀后出现了右侧混合密度硬膜下血肿（**a**）。在不改变分流阀压力的情况下，放置硬膜下引流孔系统后血肿缩小（**b**）。3 个月后，因为阀门压力没有改变，患者出现了无症状的硬膜下积液（**c**）

参考文献

1. Berger A, Constantini S, Ram Z, Roth J. Acute subdural hematomas in shunted normal-pressure hydrocephalus patients—management options and literature review: a case-based series. Surg Neurol Int. 2018;9:238.
2. Chan SM, Chodakiewitz YG, Maya MM, Schievink WI, Moser FG. Intracranial hypotension and cerebrospinal fluid leak. Neuroimaging Clin N Am. 2019;29:213–26.
3. Craven CL, Toma AK, Watkins LD. Persistent hydrocephalus due to postural activation of a ventricular shunt anti-gravity device. J Clin Neurosci. 2017;37:91–5.
4. Czosnyka Z, Czosnyka M, Richards HK, Pickard JD. Posture-related overdrainage: comparison of the performance of 10 hydrocephalus shunts in vitro. Neurosurgery. 1998;42(2):327–34.

5. Dewan MC, Lim J, Shannon CN, Wellons JC. The durability of endoscopic third ventriculostomy and ventriculoperitoneal shunts in children with hydrocephalus following posterior fossa tumor resection: a systematic review and time-to-failure analysis. J Neurosurg Pediatr. 2017;19:578–84.
6. Dillon WP. Challenges in the diagnosis and treatment of spontaneous intracranial hypotension. Radiology. 2018;289:773–4.
7. Feletti A, d'Avella D, Wikkelsø C, Klinge P, Hellström P, Tans J, et al. Ventriculoperitoneal shunt complications in the European idiopathic normal pressure hydrocephalus multicenter study. Oper Neurosurg. 2019;17:97–102.
8. Hayes J, Roguski M, Riesenburger RI. Rapid resolution of an acute subdural hematoma by increasing the shunt valve pressure in a 63-year-old man with normal-pressure hydrocephalus with a ventriculoperitoneal shunt: a case report and literature review. J Med Case Rep. 2012;6:393.
9. He F-F, Li L, Liu M-J, Zhong T-D, Zhang Q-W, Fang X-M. Targeted epidural blood patch treatment for refractory spontaneous intracranial hypotension in China. J Neurol Surg B Skull Base. 2018;79:217–23.
10. Hoffman H, Ziechmann R, Beutler T, Verhave B, Chin LS. First-line management of chronic subdural hematoma with the subdural evacuating port system: institutional experience and predictors of outcomes. J Clin Neurosci. 2018;50:221–5.
11. Kim KH, Yeo IS, Yi JS, Lee HJ, Yang JH, Lee IW. A pressure adjustment protocol for programmable valves. J Korean Neurosurg Soc. 2009;46:370–7.
12. Mokri B. Spontaneous CSF leaks. Neurol Clin. 2014;32:397–422.
13. Pereira RM, Suguimoto MT, de Oliveira MF, Tornai JB, Amaral RA, Teixeira MJ, et al. Efeito da válvula de pressão fixa com antisifão SPHERA® no tratamento da hidrocefalia de pressão normal e prevenção de hiperdrenagem. Arq Neuropsiquiatr. 2016;74:55–61.
14. Singla A, Jacobsen WP, Yusupov IR, Carter DA. Subdural evacuating port system (SEPS)—minimally invasive approach to the management of chronic/subacute subdural hematomas. Clin Neurol Neurosurg. 2013;115:425–31.
15. Sundstrom N, Lagebrant M, Eklund A, Koskinen L-O, Malm J. Subdural hematomas in 1846 patients with shunted idiopathic normal pressure hydrocephalus: treatment and long-term survival. J Neurosurg. 2018;129:797–804.

第 18 章 腰椎穿刺及椎管内麻醉后慢性硬膜下血肿

Hatim Belfquih，Hassan Baallal 和 Ali Akhaddar
译者：李姝

缩略语

CN（cranial nerve）	脑神经
CSDH（chronic subdural hematoma）	慢性硬膜下血肿
CSF（cerebrospinal fluid）	脑脊液
CT（computed tomography）	计算机断层成像
EBP（epidural blood patch）	硬膜外血补丁
ICHD-Ⅱ（International Classification of Headache Disorders-Ⅱ）	国际头痛疾病分类-Ⅱ
LP（lumbar puncture）	腰椎穿刺
MRI（magnetic resonance imaging）	磁共振成像
PDPH（postdural puncture headache）	硬膜穿刺后头痛

18.1 引言

椎管内麻醉被广泛用于产科、妇科、骨科和泌尿科手术。硬膜外麻醉是指将麻醉药剂注射到脊柱的硬膜外腔隙的麻醉方法[7]，它的优点是避免了全身麻醉，患者在手术过程中保持清醒。硬膜外麻醉过程中意外穿破硬脊膜的情况并不少见，发生率高达3.6%[18]。脊髓麻醉则是穿刺硬脊膜后在蛛网膜下腔注射麻醉药剂。脊髓麻醉具有与硬膜外麻醉相同的优点，并且起效时间更快[32]。

脊髓麻醉和硬膜外麻醉的安全性是广泛公认的，然而，麻醉操作偶尔也会导致并发症，包括腰背痛、硬膜穿刺后头痛（PDPH）、感染、血肿、神经损伤和颅内出血等。这些并发症的发生率大约为0.05%[5]。其中最常见的良性并发症是PDPH[49]，而慢性硬膜下血肿（CSDH）是罕见的、最严重的、可能致命的并发症之一，并且可能被误诊为PDPH[23]。提高临床医生对CSDH患者体征和症状的认识，及时处理出现的并发症，可以预防出现不必要的结果。

18.2 发生率

硬膜外麻醉导致的意外硬膜穿刺发生率在0.4%至6%之间[1-5]，大约1/3的硬膜穿刺患者均会出现PDPH[11, 22]。据估计，74%的产科患者出现PDPH但通常会自行消退[4]。

很少有关于脊髓麻醉引起的CSDH的数据。由于其症状常与PDPH相似，可能其中大部分患者并未确诊。根据文献记载，CSDH的发病率在1/500 000到1/1 000 000之间[31]。2004年在瑞典发表的一项回顾性研究历时十年（1990—1999年），确定了127例脊髓麻醉后发生神经系统并发症的病例。该研究报道脊髓麻醉后引起神经系统并发症风险为1/2000至1/30 000，其中报告了2例CSDH[29]。产科临床中使用硬膜外麻醉后CSDH的发生率估计为1:500 000。2019年加拿大发表的一项最新研究收集了22 130 815例椎管内麻醉后分娩数据，其中68 374例被确定为PDPH，总体发病率为每10万名女性中有309例；产后CSDH病例数为342例，发病率为每10万例分娩1.5例[30]。

最后，由于患者通常在没有进一步检查的情况下就接受治疗，硬膜穿刺或脊髓麻醉后CSDH的真实发生率可能比报道的要高。

18.3 病理生理

PDPH和穿刺后CSDH均是由CSF从硬膜破口漏出所导致的。

18.3.1 硬膜刺破的后果

硬膜穿刺有可能导致脑脊液过度渗漏。通过硬膜破孔丢失脑脊液速率为 0.084～4.5 ml/s，通常大于脑脊液产生速率 0.35 ml/min，特别是当穿刺针的尺寸大于 25G 时。脑脊液的过度丢失会导致颅内低压和脑脊液体积明显减少，成人蛛网膜下压会从 15 cmH$_2$O±5 cmH$_2$O 降至 4.0 cmH$_2$O 或以下[36]。

18.3.2 PDPH

虽然硬膜穿刺后脑脊液丢失和脑脊液压力降低没有争议，但导致 PDPH 的实际发病机制尚不清楚。存在两种可能的解释：①脑脊液压力的降低导致直立位的颅内结构受到牵拉，这些结构对疼痛敏感，导致典型的头痛。②脑脊液的丢失会产生代偿性静脉扩张，而颅内脑脊液和颅内血液的体积之和保持恒定，因此脑脊液容量减少的后果是通过静脉扩张导致血容量代偿性增加，从而导致头痛[37]。

18.3.3 CSDH

脊髓麻醉后出现 CSDH 的主要机制与 PDPH 相同，但有一些细微差别。蛛网膜撕裂处的脑脊液漏出可能会导致脊髓内压和颅内压降低，由此产生的脑脊液流量动态变化导致脑室相对塌陷和中枢神经系统向尾端移位，敏感的脑膜结构或脑膜疼痛感受器、脑神经和桥静脉受到牵拉。脑脊液容量的突然减少也可能激活腺苷受体，从而导致动静脉血管扩张，进而出现 PDPH 的临床症状。如果对桥静脉施加的牵引力很大，可能会导致其在硬膜下腔的最薄弱点破裂，从而形成慢性硬膜下血肿（图 18.1）[28]。

人体桥静脉的电子显微镜数据显示，桥静脉的血管壁厚度不同，其内胶原纤维呈圆周排列，并且缺乏蛛网膜小梁的外部强化支持。所有这些最终导致桥静脉的硬膜下部分比蛛网膜下部分更脆弱，这些特征解释了静脉撕裂和由此产生的血肿位于硬膜下位置，血肿可表现为急性或慢性[47]。

18.4 诱发因素

硬膜穿刺后头痛和 CSDH 的危险因素包括所用脊髓穿刺针的尺寸和设计、进行硬膜穿刺的人员的经验以及患者因素或临床状况。

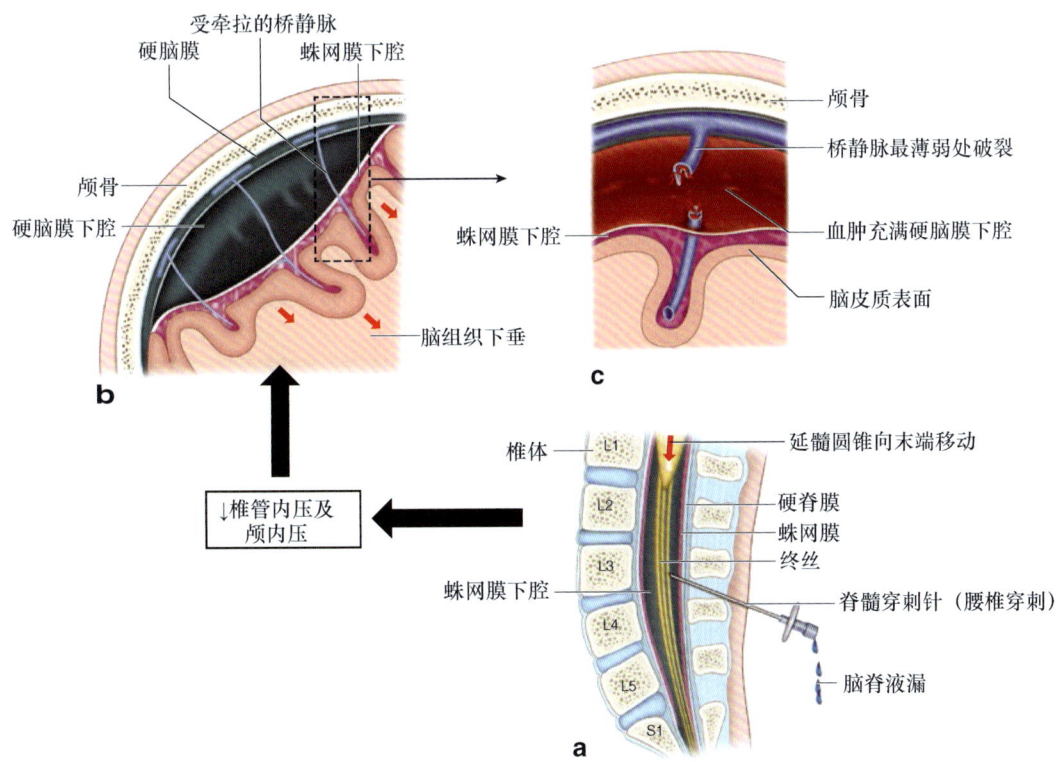

图 18.1 硬膜穿刺后发生 CSDH 的机制。脊髓处硬膜穿孔导致脑脊液渗漏（a）导致脊髓内压和颅内压下降，并导致大脑下垂（b）。这会给硬脑膜和蛛网膜之间的桥静脉带来张力（b）。如果桥静脉受到的牵引力较大，可能会导致桥静脉在硬膜下腔最薄弱处破裂，从而形成 CSDH（c）

18.4.1 脊髓穿刺针的大小及其设计

Zeidan 等学者[50]指出 CSDH 与 PDPH 一样，均是由于脑脊液从脊椎穿刺针产生的孔中渗漏而引发，因此穿刺针的大小和硬膜撕裂的程度与 PDPH 和 CSDH 有直接相关。如果使用大直径穿刺针操作并多次尝试进针，每天脑脊液的损失可能会超过 200 ml。

麻醉医生一直在积极尝试通过减小脊髓穿刺针的尺寸来降低 PDPH 的发生率。22G 针的 PDPH 发生率为 40%，25G 针为 25%[12]，26G Quincke 针为 2%±12%[13]，29G 针为 < 2%[16]。针头的改进，如 Whitacre、Sprotte 和 Atraucan 针，有望进一步减少 PDPH 的发生率（图 18.2）。

18.4.2 相关穿刺技术因素

有人提出，在置针时接触骨质结构以及反复穿刺可能会导致穿刺针尖变形，而损坏的针尖可能导致之后硬膜穿刺孔的变大。近期的活体研究表明，与同等尺寸的铅笔尖针相比，切割型的脊髓穿刺针在接触骨质结构后更容易变形。使用时，切割型针尖的切面（Quincke 型）应平行于纵向走行的蛛网膜纤维的方向插入。这样操作与垂直进针相比，可将 PDPH 风险降低 50%[20]。

有研究表明，穿刺孔保持开放状态可长达 18 周，而直径 0.6 mm 的孔口脑脊液外渗量可高达 240 ml/d，这将导致颅内压自动调节机制丧失，并为 PDPH 的长期发展提供了解释[36]。

18.4.3 患者状态相关因素

妊娠患者对硬膜穿刺后 CSDH 的易感性可能是由于分娩常使用硬膜外镇痛所致[3]。文献综述表明，在进行硬膜外阻滞期间，硬膜穿刺后意外发生 CSDH 的 22 例[43, 48]患者中有 20 例是产科患者。一些学者认为，与其他患者相比，由于凝血失衡、性别原因等导致的硬膜弹性以及颅骨形态差异，妊娠患者可能更容易发生 CSDH[2, 46]。剖宫产与 CSDH 的发生呈负相关，这可能是因为剖宫产时产妇不需要用力挤压子宫或剖宫产脊髓麻醉使用较小规格的脊髓穿刺针。此外，与没有头痛的产妇相比，椎管内麻醉后出现 PDPH 与发生 CSDH 风险小幅增加存在统计学意义相关性[2]。需要进一步的研究来确定两者的这一关联是否存在因果关系。

其他可能与脊髓麻醉无关但可能在 CSDH 的患者中并存的危险因素包括头部外伤、凝血功能障碍、颅内动脉瘤、动静脉畸形、肿瘤、脑萎缩、慢性酒精中毒、心血管疾病、脑膜血管性梅毒和糖尿病等。

性别被认为是硬膜穿刺后头痛发生的独立危险因素。一项系统性评价共检查了 18 项试验（包含 2163 名男性，1917 名女性），男性发生硬膜后穿刺头痛的概率明显低于非怀孕女性受试者（比值比 OR = 0.55）。此外，青春期开始后，相对于男性受试者，女性 PDPH 的发病率似乎有所增加[9, 21, 34]。雌激素已被证明可以调节脑动脉张力，并可能扩张软脑膜血管[14, 27]。

18.5 临床症状

CSDH 的临床表现取决于年龄、大小、部位、

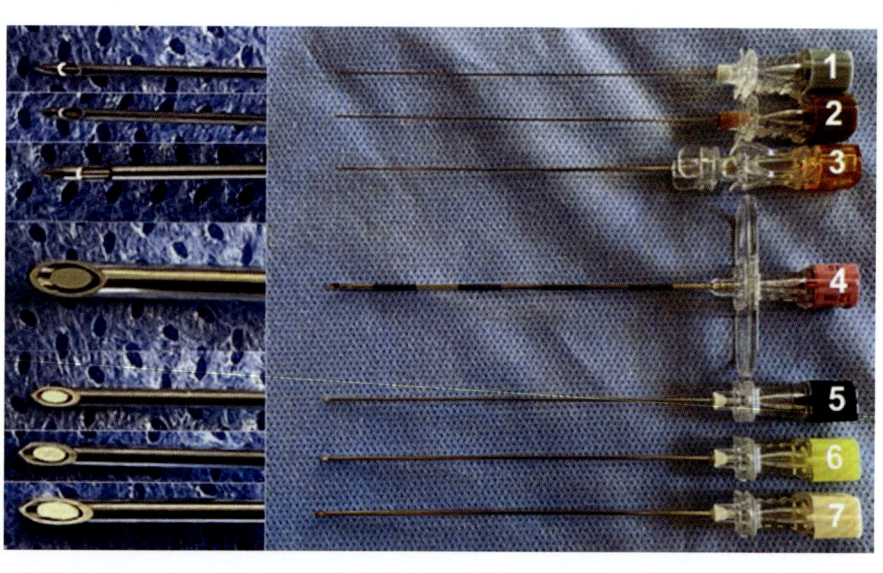

图 18.2 用于腰椎穿刺和脊髓麻醉的硬膜外穿刺针（图中 4 号针）和其他不同型号的脊髓穿刺针的针头外观图。1：27G Sprotte 型铅笔样针头；2：26G Sprotte 型铅笔样针头；3：25G Sprotte 型铅笔样针头；4：18G Tuohy 型硬膜外穿刺针；5：22G Quincke 型腰椎穿刺针；6：20G Quincke 型腰椎穿刺针；7：19G Quincke 型腰椎穿刺针

血肿形成的速度、颅内结构的受压情况以及患者的临床状况。根据症状，可能很难区分 CSDH 和 PDPH。PDPH 是脊髓麻醉最常见的良性并发症，如果使用镇痛药和卧床休息，几天内就会得到改善。

PDPH 表现为弥漫性头痛，通常被描述为搏动性和位置性头痛：站立时恶化，卧位时改善。增加颅内压的动作，如咳嗽或用力，可能会使症状恶化。

PDPH 的国际头痛疾病分类-Ⅱ（ICHD-Ⅱ）标准[41]规定必须满足以下所有条件：

1. 坐位或立位 15 min 内头痛加剧，卧位 15 min 内改善。
2. 头痛至少伴有下列症状之一：颈部僵硬、耳鸣、听力减退、畏光和（或）恶心。
3. 硬膜穿刺后 5 天内出现头痛。
4. 通常通过硬膜外血补丁（EBP）有效治疗脊髓液漏后，头痛在 1 周内或 48 h 内自行缓解。

PDPH 发生变化的特征包括非姿势性头痛症状以及局灶性神经功能异常，如意识障碍、恶心、呕吐、头晕、偏瘫、脑神经麻痹、视觉障碍、复视、畏光，癫痫发作少见[42]。如出现对常规治疗无效的头痛，应提高警惕，评估是否出现 CSDH [33, 35]。表 18.1 列出了诊断为硬脊膜穿刺导致的 CSDH 所报道的症状和体征[2, 6, 26]。

先前关于 CSDH 脑神经（CN）麻痹的报道表明，大脑的向下牵拉和 CN 的压迫导致神经功能缺损[25]。与其他脑神经相比，由于外展神经在颅内走行较长，外展神经麻痹是腰椎穿刺后 CSDH 中最常见的受影响 CN。外展神经麻痹通常发生在腰椎穿刺和脊髓麻醉后的 4～14 天，该神经功能障碍可以是单侧的亦可为双侧，通常与 PDPH 相关。也有报道心动过缓为相关症状之一，一般认为是由于大脑向尾端下移导致下丘脑受压而产生。这种对下丘脑的占位效应可导致自主神经信号改变[10]。

根据麻醉和症状出现之间的时间间隔，硬膜下血肿可能是急性和亚急性/慢性的。大多数报告的急性病例在最初 2 天内出现严重且持续的非体位性头痛，且镇痛药物无法缓解，并伴有急性神经功能恶化的症状，提示颅内压突然升高，如瞳孔不等大、偏瘫和意识水平改变。亚急性/慢性硬膜下出血可能会在数天或数周内发生，从而造成诊断困难。CSDH 可能与 PDPH 混淆，CSDH 可先出现直立性头痛，且镇痛药、卧床休息和补液有效。随着时间的推移，这些症状可能会经历改善和恶化的交替阶段，最终头痛与体位失去关联，且出现神经系统体征。根据一项已发表的研究，从硬膜穿刺到诊断 SDH 的时间范围从 4 小时到 29 周不等[11]。在一项病例系列中，37% 的病例在硬膜穿刺后 1 周内确诊，85% 在 1 个月内确诊[23]。

Nakanuno 等[31]研究了 69 例因麻醉、诊断或治疗目的的硬膜穿刺后发生颅内 CSDH 的病例。他们将这些与 CSDH 相关的、硬膜穿刺后 4 天内出现的头痛根据持续时间分为三种模式。第一种是疼痛一直持续到硬膜下出血发生。第二种是患者在硬膜穿刺后早期出现头痛，疼痛消失或暂时减轻，但又再次出现并加重，随后出现硬膜下出血。第三种是患者的头痛并非在硬膜穿刺后早期出现，而是随着硬膜下出血的发生而出现。在他们的研究中，第一种头痛模式占 47%（33 例），第二种头痛模式占 44%（30 例），第三种头痛模式占 6%（4 例）；另外 3%（2 例）未知。大多数病例在硬脊膜穿刺后早期都会出现头痛，第三种模式是急性发作且没有早期头痛，这种情况很罕见。

在 Cuypers 等的研究中[6]，56 例脊髓麻醉后 CSDH 的患者中，83% 的患者出现与 PDPH 不相符的头痛。即使仅出现 PDPH 症状，无其他严重的神经系统症状，也可能伴有临床隐匿的 CSDH。

18.6 CSDH 影像学

Grant 等使用磁共振成像（MRI）技术测量 20 例患者 LP 前及 LP 后 24 h 颅内脑脊液体积。进行脑脊液总量、脑室脑脊液体积、皮质沟脑脊液体积和颅后窝脑脊液体积测量。他们发现，颅内脑脊

表 18.1 硬脊膜穿刺引起 CSDH 的症状和体征[2, 6, 25]

症状/体征	发生率
头痛	74%～91%
恶心/呕吐	31%～41%
意识状态改变	31%～40%
局灶性运动功能障碍	23%～28%
复视/视力改变	14%～20%
失语/构音障碍	11%～13%

液体积变化较大的患者会出现头痛。这项研究还表明，腰椎穿刺后，颅内脑脊液总量几乎一直在降低，大部分是由于皮质脑沟脑脊液丢失导致。这一发现可以解释为什么 CSDH 会作为 LP 的并发症发生[17]。MRI 还可以检测由于脑脊液过多丢失而导致颅内压低的进一步经典体征，即侧脑室裂隙、垂体增大和无菌性硬脑膜炎[45]。

计算机断层成像（CT）是一种安全、简单且低成本的检测 CSDH 的方法。严重、长期或非典型头痛的患者必须首先接受 CT 扫描检查，以避免危及生命的结果[30]。

此前报道的大多数 CSDH 病例都是单侧的，然而少数病例为双侧硬膜下血肿，这可能是由于硬膜外麻醉中使用较大的针头导致脑脊液损失较多导致。Zeidan 和 Baraka[48] 对此问题做出了类似的讨论，因为在他们的综述中一些患者也出现了双侧血肿。

脊柱 MRI 或脊柱 CT 可以检测到脑脊液漏出区域。脊柱 MRI 通过 T1 和 T2 序列以及矢状面和冠状面的脂肪饱和度进行检查，可以检测导致脑脊液漏的瘘管，然而更多情况下，它仅用于检测硬膜外脑脊液汇集区域。在急性期，与脊柱 MRI 相比，脊柱 CT 具有更高的敏感性和特异性[8]。

18.7 治疗

腰椎穿刺或脊髓麻醉后 CSDH 的治疗包括保守治疗和手术清除，治疗方案主要取决于血肿的大小和患者的神经系统状态。

对于无精神状态变化、无癫痫发作、无颅内占位效应、血肿最大厚度 < 1 cm、中线移位 < 5 mm 的 CSDH 患者，建议采用保守治疗。这种方法需要卧床休息、镇痛（包括阿片类药物）、静脉补液以及密切的神经学和神经放射学随访，以尽早识别潜在的临床和影像学恶化征象[38]。此外，一些人主张使用 EBP 治疗由硬膜撕裂导致慢性脑脊液漏引起的 CSDH。采用正中入路在硬膜穿刺水平进行 EBP，并在透视下通过 Tuohy 针引入 15 ml 由患者自体血液和纤维蛋白胶组成的溶液，以形成血凝块来闭合硬脑膜瘘。手术后，患者需要平躺 2 h。PDPH 患者 EBP 的成功率为 60% ~ 90%[39]。然而，最近的研究表明，成功的可能性取决于打血补丁的时机。如果硬膜穿刺后 72 h 内进行 EBP，可以获得更好的结果[44]。对于小血肿，保守治疗无效后才考虑 EBP。在 Nakanuno 等的研究中，83% 的患者完全康复，而其余 17% 的患者死亡或出现永久性神经功能缺损。一些不良结果与诊断延迟有关[31]。尽管 EBP 有望封闭硬脑膜缺损并恢复 CSF 压力，但 CSDH 仍有可能扩大或复发，并可能需要进行血肿清除术[19]。

如果血肿厚度超过 10 mm、中线移位大于 5 mm 或出现神经功能恶化，则需要手术干预 CSDH。急性 SDH 通常会导致神经系统迅速恶化，有必要通过开颅手术或钻孔清除血肿，以降低颅内压并保留脑功能[15]。EBP 可在手术清除血肿的同时进行，特别是复发血肿患者。硬膜穿刺后 CSDH 的手术干预率从 9% 到 80% 不等[39, 51]，据报告死亡率为 7% ~ 10%[24]。

18.8 预防

预防 CSDH 包括对腰椎穿刺人员的操作进行详细的指导，如使用非切割（铅笔型）针头。卧床休息、补液和放置血补丁并不总能预防 CSDH 的发生。

根据文献数据，有一些方法可以潜在地减少 CSDH 的发生并进行早期诊断，特别是在硬膜外麻醉分娩后：

- 尽量使用小的、铅笔型脊髓穿刺针进入蛛网膜下腔[40]。
- 密切关注发生 PDPH 的患者。
- 对于保守治疗无效的 PDPH 患者及早提供 EBP 治疗，如硬膜穿刺口较大可重复 EBP 治疗[24]。
- 对于不符合 ICHD-Ⅱ PDPH 标准的产后头痛病例，预约头颅 CT 或 MRI 扫描[41]。

18.9 结论

作为腰椎穿刺或脊髓麻醉不可避免的并发症，我们必须意识到 CSDH 的严重性。长期和非体位性 PDPH、硬膜外血补丁治疗后临床状况仍然恶化以及出现神经系统症状应被视为 CSDH 的预警信号，需要及时进行诊断和治疗。

参考文献

1. Acharya R, Chhabra SS, Ratra M, Sehgal AD. Cranial subdural haematoma after spinal anaesthesia. Br J Anaesth. 2001;86:893–5. https://doi.org/10.1093/bja/86.6.893.
2. Amorim JA, Valença MM. Postdural puncture headache is a risk factor for new postdural puncture headache. Cephalalgia. 2008;28(1):5–8. https://doi.org/10.1111/j.1468-2982.2007.01454.x. Epub 2007 Oct 23.
3. Amorim JA, Remígio DS, Damázio Filho O, de Barros MA, Carvalho VN, Valença MM. Intracranial subdural hematoma post-spinal anesthesia: report of two cases and review of 33 cases in the literature. Rev Bras Anestesiol. 2010;60(6):620–9, 344–9. English, Portuguese, Spanish. https://doi.org/10.1016/S0034-7094(10)70077-5.
4. Angle P, Thompson D, Halpern S, Wilson DB. Second stage pushing correlates with headache after unintentional dural puncture in parturients. Can J Anaesth. 1999;46(9):861–6. https://doi.org/10.1007/BF03012976.
5. Cruvinel MG, Barbosa PR, Teixeira VC, Castro CH. Tampão peridural com dextran 40 na profilaxia da cefaléia pós-punção acidental da duramáter em paciente HIV positivo: relato de caso [Epidural patch with dextran 40 to prevent postdural puncture headache in an HIV patient: case report]. Rev Bras Anestesiol. 2002;52(6):712–8. Portuguese.
6. Cuypers V, Van de Velde M, Devroe S. Intracranial subdural haematoma following neuraxial anaesthesia in the obstetric population: a literature review with analysis of 56 reported cases. Int J Obstet Anesth. 2016;25:58–65. https://doi.org/10.1016/j.ijoa.2015.09.003.
7. de Lange JJ, Cuesta MA, Cuesta de Pedro A. Fidel Pagés Miravé (1886-1923). The pioneer of lumbar epidural anaesthesia. Anaesthesia. 1994;49(5):429–31. https://doi.org/10.1111/j.1365-2044.1994.tb03480.x.
8. De Lipsis L, Belmonte R, Cusano M, Giannetti MA, Muccio CF, Mancinelli M. Subdural hematoma as a consequence of labor epidural analgesia. Asian J Neurosurg. 2018;13(3):931–4.
9. Ebinger F, Kosel C, Pietz J, Rating D. Headache and backache after lumbar puncture in children and adolescents: a prospective study. Pediatrics. 2004;113(6):1588–92. https://doi.org/10.1542/peds.113.6.1588.
10. Evans RW. Complications of lumbar puncture. Neurol Clin. 1998;16(1):83–105. https://doi.org/10.1016/s0733-8619(05)70368-6.
11. Evans RW, Armon C, Frohman EM, Goodin DS. Assessment: prevention of post-lumbar puncture headaches: report of the therapeutics and technology assessment subcommittee of the american academy of neurology. Neurology. 2000;55(7):909–14. https://doi.org/10.1212/wnl.55.7.909.
12. Flaatten H, Rodt S, Rosland J, Vamnes J. Postoperative headache in young patients after spinal anaesthesia. Anaesthesia. 1987;42(2):202–5. https://doi.org/10.1111/j.1365-2044.1987.tb03001.x.
13. Flaatten H, Rodt SA, Vamnes J, Rosland J, Wisborg T, Koller ME. Postdural puncture headache. A comparison between 26- and 29-gauge needles in young patients. Anaesthesia. 1989;44(2):147–9. https://doi.org/10.1111/j.1365-2044.1989.tb11167.x.
14. Geary GG, Krause DN, Duckles SP. Estrogen reduces mouse cerebral artery tone through endothelial NOS- and cyclooxygenase-dependent mechanisms. Am J Physiol Heart Circ Physiol. 2000;279(2):H511–9. https://doi.org/10.1152/ajpheart.2000.279.2.H511.
15. Gerard C, Busl KM. Treatment of acute subdural hematoma. Curr Treat Options Neurol. 2014;16(1):275. https://doi.org/10.1007/s11940-013-0275-0.
16. Geurts JW, Haanschoten MC, van Wijk RM, Kraak H, Besse TC. Post-dural puncture headache in young patients. A comparative study between the use of 0.52 mm (25-gauge) and 0.33 mm (29-gauge) spinal needles. Acta Anaesthesiol Scand. 1990;34(5):350–3. https://doi.org/10.1111/j.1399-6576.1990.tb03101.x.
17. Grant R, Condon B, Hart I, Teasdale GM. Changes in intracranial CSF volume after lumbar puncture and their relationship to post-LP headache. J Neurol Neurosurg Psychiatry. 1991;54(5):440–2. https://doi.org/10.1136/jnnp.54.5.440.
18. Gurudatt CL. Unintentional dural puncture and postdural puncture headache-can this headache of the patient as well as the anaesthesiologist be prevented? Indian J Anaesth. 2014;58(4):385–7. https://doi.org/10.4103/0019-5049.138962.
19. Hashizume K, Watanabe K, Kawaguchi M, Fujiwara A, Furuya H. Evaluation on a clinical course of subdural hematoma in patients undergoing epidural blood patch for spontaneous cerebrospinal fluid leak. Clin Neurol Neurosurg. 2013;115(8):1403–6. https://doi.org/10.1016/j.

clineuro.2013.01.022.
20. Jokinen MJ, Pitkänen MT, Lehtonen E, Rosenberg PH. Deformed spinal needle tips and associated dural perforations examined by scanning electron microscopy. Acta Anaesthesiol Scand. 1996;40(6):687–90. https://doi.org/10.1111/j.1399-6576.1996.tb04511.x.
21. Karnik R, Valentin A, Winkler WB, Khaffaf N, Donath P, Slany J. Sex-related differences in acetazolamide-induced cerebral vasomotor reactivity. Stroke. 1996;27(1):56–8. https://doi.org/10.1161/01.str.27.1.56.
22. Kim EJ, Chang IY. Intracerebral hemorrhage after vesicolitholapaxy under spinal anesthesia. Korean J Anesthesiol. 2006;51:379–82.
23. Kuntz KM, Kokmen E, Stevens JC, Miller P, Offord KP, Ho MM. Post-lumbar puncture headaches: experience in 501 consecutive procedures. Neurology. 1992;42(10):1884–7. https://doi.org/10.1212/wnl.42.10.1884.
24. Landau R, Ciliberto CF, Goodman SR, Kim-Lo SH, Smiley RM. Complications with 25-gauge and 27-gauge Whitacre needles during combined spinal-epidural analgesia in labor. Int J Obstet Anesth. 2001;10(3):168–71. https://doi.org/10.1054/ijoa.2000.0834.
25. Liegl O. Neuroophthalmologische Komplikationen durch Liquor=leckage nach diagnostischen bzw. therapeutischen Eingriffen am Spinalkanal [Neuroophthalmological complications through liquor leakage after surgical operation on the spinal canal for diagnostic i.e. therapeutic purposes (author's transl)]. Klin Monbl Augenheilkd. 1977;171(4):526–30. German.
26. Lim G, Zorn JM, Dong YJ, DeRenzo JS, Waters JH. Subdural hematoma associated with labor epidural analgesia: a case series. Reg Anesth Pain Med. 2016;41(5):628–31. https://doi.org/10.1097/AAP.0000000000000455.
27. Littleton-Kearney MT, Agnew DM, Traystman RJ, Hurn PD. Effects of estrogen on cerebral blood flow and pial microvasculature in rabbits. Am J Physiol Heart Circ Physiol. 2000;279(3):H1208–14. https://doi.org/10.1152/ajpheart.2000.279.3.H1208.
28. Macon ME, Armstrong L, Brown EM. Subdural hematoma following spinal anesthesia. Anesthesiology. 1990;72(2):380–1.
29. Moen V, Dahlgren N, Irestedt L. Severe neurological complications after central neuraxial blockades in Sweden 1990-1999. Anesthesiology. 2004;101(4):950–9.
30. Moore AR, Wieczorek PM, Carvalho JCA. Association between post-dural puncture headache after neuraxial anesthesia in childbirth and intracranial subdural hematoma. JAMA Neurol. 2020;77(1):65–72. https://doi.org/10.1001/jamaneurol.2019.2995.
31. Nakanuno R, Kawamoto M, Yuge O. [Intracranial subdural hematoma following dural puncture]. Masui. 2007;56(4):395–403. Japanese.
32. Ng K, Parsons J, Cyna AM, Middleton P. Spinal versus epidural anaesthesia for caesarean section. Cochrane Database Syst Rev. 2004;(2):CD003765.
33. Nolte CH, Lehmann TN. Postpartum headache resulting from bilateral chronic subdural hematoma after dural puncture. Am J Emerg Med. 2004;22(3):241–2.
34. Oláh L, Valikovics A, Bereczki D, Fülesdi B, Munkácsy C, Csiba L. Gender-related differences in acetazolamide-induced cerebral vasodilatory response: a transcranial Doppler study. J Neuroimaging. 2000;10(3):151–6.
35. Ozdemir N, Ari MK, Gelal MF, Bezircioğlu H. Intracranial chronic subdural haematoma as a complication of epidural anesthesia. Turk Neurosurg. 2009;19(3):285–7.
36. Parker RK, White PF. A microscopic analysis of cut-bevel versus pencil-point spinal needles. Anesth Analg. 1997;85(5):1101–4.
37. Ready LB, Cuplin S, Haschke RH, Nessly M. Spinal needle determinants of rate of transdural fluid leak. Anesth Analg. 1989;69(4):457–60.
38. Rocchi R, Lombardi C, Marradi I, Di Paolo M, Cerase A. Intracranial and intraspinal hemorrhage following spinal anesthesia. Neurol Sci. 2009;30(5):393–6.
39. Safa-Tisseront V, Thormann F, Malassiné P, Henry M, Riou B, Coriat P, et al. Effectiveness of epidural blood patch in the management of post-dural puncture headache. Anesthesiology. 2001;95(2):334–9.
40. Santanen U, Rautoma P, Luurila H, Erkola O, Pere P. Comparison of 27-gauge (0.41-mm) Whitacre and Quincke spinal needles with respect to post-dural puncture headache and non-dural puncture headache. Acta Anaesthesiol Scand. 2004;48(4):474–9.
41. Silberstein SD, Olesen J, Bousser MG, Diener HC, Dodick D, First M, et al. The International Classification of Headache Disorders, 2nd Edition (ICHD-II)—revision of criteria for 8.2 Medication-overuse headache. Cephalalgia. 2005;25(6):460–5.
42. Suess O, Stendel R, Baur S, Schilling A, Brock M. Intracranial haemorrhage following lumbar myelography: case report and review of the literature. Neuroradiology. 2000;42(3):211–4.

43. Vaughan DJ, Stirrup CA, Robinson PN. Cranial subdural haematoma associated with dural puncture in labour. Br J Anaesth. 2000;84(4):518–20.
44. Verdu MT, Martínez-Lage JF, Alonso B, Sánchez-Ortega JL, Garcia-Candel A. Non-surgical management of intracranial subdural hematoma complicating spinal anesthesia. Neurocirugia (Astur). 2007;18(1):40–3.
45. Vien C, Marovic P, Ingram B. Epidural anesthesia complicated by subdural hygromas and a subdural hematoma. Case Rep Anesthesiol. 2016;2016:5789504.
46. Wu CL, Rowlingson AJ, Cohen SR, Michaels RK, Courpas GE, Joe EM, et al. Gender and post-dural puncture headache. Anesthesiology. 2006;105(3):613–8.
47. Yamashima T, Friede RL. Why do bridging veins rupture into the virtual subdural space? J Neurol Neurosurg Psychiatry. 1984;47(2):121–7.
48. Zeidan A, Baraka A. Is bilateral cerebral subdural hematoma more frequent after epidural anesthesia than spinal anesthesia? Anesthesiology. 2006;105(6):1277–8; author reply 1278.
49. Zeidan A, Chaaban M, Farhat O, Baraka A. Cerebral rebleeding by spinal anesthesia in a patient with undiagnosed chronic subdural hematoma. Anesthesiology. 2006;104(3):613–4.
50. Zeidan A, Farhat O, Maaliki H, Baraka A. Does postdural puncture headache left untreated lead to subdural hematoma? Case report and review of the literature. Int J Obstet Anesth. 2006;15(1):50–8.
51. Zhang J, Jin D, Pan KH. Epidural blood patch for spontaneous intracranial hypotension with chronic subdural haematoma: a case report and literature review. J Int Med Res. 2016;44(4):976–81.

第 19 章 低颅内压

Justin Oh，Timothy Beutler 和 Satish Krishnamurthy

译者：田润发

19.1 引言

低颅内压（IH）是慢性硬膜下血肿（CSDH）的一种罕见病因。最常见的临床表现是头痛且随体位变化，于直立时加重。根据国际头痛疾病分类（ICHD-3），IH 的诊断需要头痛与低脑脊液（CSF）压力之间的时间联系[16]，所以应评估患者是否有低脑脊液压力以及影像学上是否有脊髓液漏的证据。

与 IH 相关的病因包括颅脑外伤、医源性和自发性。外伤性、退行性和医源性通常可以明确脊髓液漏的病因，而自发性 IH 则需要更多的检查用于判断。自发性 IH 是罕见的，通常在小型回顾性研究和文献综述中被提及。据准确估计，自发性 IH 的年发病率为 5/10 万人[40]。

因为 IH 最常见的症状是头痛，因此无论何种病因 IH 的诊断均是困难的。同时在临床和影像学上，还有其他几种疾病的病理表现相似，也可能会混淆诊断。本章的重点是临床症状表现为 CSDH 或硬膜下积液的 IH。IH 是区分 CSDH 的一个重要病因，因为它的治疗方法不同于其他硬膜下积液。通常 CSDH 可以通过手术治疗清除血肿，但如果同时存在 IH 手术则可能导致症状恶化。

本章中，我们将回顾在 IH 的病理环境下，硬膜下血肿（SDH）/积液的发病机制、临床表现、影像学表现和治疗方法。

19.2 发病机制

虽然 IH 本质上是自发的，但据文献报道很多病例继发于手术后。常见的医源性病因包括腰椎穿刺、脊柱手术中的硬脊膜切开、椎管内手术和颅内手术[11, 22-23, 53]。任何打开或破坏硬脑膜的手术或操作导致脑脊液持续漏出，最终结果都可能导致 IH。外伤性 IH 的病因也可以是继发于硬脑膜损伤，一些外伤性 IH 的病例与隐匿性创伤有关[39]。同时，也存在退行性脊柱病变并发硬脑膜缺损导致 IH 的病例报道[6, 46, 49]。

另外，自发性 IH 病例被认为是继发于硬脑膜的薄弱部位，从而导致脑脊液漏。自发性 IH 病例与结缔组织病有关，但它们与这些特定的疾病发生发展过程没有直接联系。自发性病因也与脑脊膜憩室相关，脑脊膜憩室是神经根鞘与硬脑膜的连接处，该部位易破裂和损伤。然而，值得注意的是，最近的一项回顾性研究显示，IH 患者与非 IH 患者在憩室的存在和数量上没有差异[20]。

无论何种病因，低颅内压的发生机制都是脑脊液漏，发病结局是出现硬膜下积液或血肿。关于 IH 患者硬膜下积液发生率的数据仅局限于回顾性研究，其发病率为 19.8%～50%[5, 10, 22, 39, 45, 50]。

在 IH 情况下硬膜下积血或血肿形成的机制尚不清楚。一种假设是颅内压力和浮力的相对损失导致桥静脉被牵拉，使桥静脉易受剪切力的影响破裂[22]。另一种理论认为，IH 导致硬脑膜内的血管发育不良，容易破裂。6 例弥漫性强化的硬脑膜样本脑膜活检显示，硬脑膜下侧小而薄的血管位于疏松不规则的成纤维细胞基质中[22, 32]。CSDH 也被包膜包裹和分隔，包膜中存在新生血管，这与硬膜下积液再出血和体积扩张相关[17-18, 51]。

19.3 临床表现

IH 最常见的表现是头痛，有时头痛可与体位性因素相关，当患者直立时头痛可能加重。然而，当患者因 IH 出现硬膜下积液时，会有其他各种可能的症状出现（表 19.1），这些症状从轻度局灶性神经功能缺损到重度精神状态改变不等。患者可能出现其他的症状包括但不限于颈项强直、头晕、眩晕、局灶性神经功能缺损（如无力或感觉异常）、视野缺损、复视、听力障碍、耳鸣和意识水平下降等[25, 41, 45]。在极少数情况下，IH 可能出现类似神

表 19.1　低颅内压的症状

头疼（体位性或非体位性）
颈项强直
头晕或眩晕
局灶性无力或感觉异常
视觉障碍（如复视）
听觉障碍（如耳鸣）
意识水平下降

经退行性疾病的表现，如痴呆、帕金森病和记忆缺陷[3]。

IH 的症状通常是非特异性的。因此，完整的临床病史对临床鉴别诊断有着重要作用。一些与自发性 IH 相关的临床病史包括举重、紧张、剧烈打喷嚏或咳嗽、腹内压升高和推拿等[37-38]。有文献报道，高达 50% 因 IH 而出现 SDH 的患者存在既往腰椎穿刺史[22]，也有一些关于脊柱或颅后窝术后发生 IH 的报道[23, 49, 53]。

最近的一项回顾性研究表明，与继发于其他病因的 SDH 相比，因 IH 而出现 SDH 的患者往往会合并更少的并发症，然而会合并更多的影像学特征，如脑膜增强和少量的硬膜下出血[19]。年龄作为一项人口统计学因素，已被研究认为是 SDH 的一项危险因素，但对于 IH 导致的 SDH 来说，更年轻还是更年长的患者风险更高尚存争议[19, 50]。

有文献报道了一种罕见的 IH，其临床症状为自发性脑静脉血栓形成。虽然静脉窦血栓形成本身罕见，但几例病例报告均将其病因归因于 IH[35, 52, 54]。在 CSDH 存在的情况下，治疗继发于 IH 的静脉窦血栓可能变得很困难。其病理生理学尚不清楚，有一种理论认为是颅内压降低增加了脑血容量，导致静脉系统淤滞[52]。标准的静脉窦血栓治疗需要全身抗凝，然而在 IH 和硬膜下出血的情况下，全身性抗凝治疗可能会增加患者出现并发症的风险。在 IH 背景下治疗脑静脉血栓需要找出并治疗 IH 的潜在病因[54]。

19.4　影像学表现

影像学在诊断 IH 和明确病因方面起着重要作用。由于该病起病隐匿，颅脑影像学检查在明确诊断中起重要作用。如果临床病史未提示 IH 的明显病因，则可能还需要对脊柱进行的影像学检查以确定诊断。

19.4.1　颅脑影像学检查

颅脑计算机断层成像（CT）通常是在出现神经系统症状或缺陷的患者中首选的影像学检查。在 IH 中，CT 扫描结果通常都为阴性，但可以发现存在硬膜下积液，最常见的表现是继发于 IH 的低密度的硬膜下积液。它们通常表现为双侧积液，外观类似于慢性硬膜下血肿或积液（图 19.1）。在 CT 成像中，如果病灶很小或与大脑呈等密度，则很难发现阳性结果。有时病灶呈亚急性，密度混杂，呈包房状。CT 有时也能发现脑组织向下移位，可见小脑扁桃体移位至枕骨大孔周围，脑池或脑干腹侧面受到挤压。这些表现可能会被误诊为 Chiari 畸形。

IH 情况下的脑磁共振成像（MRI）经常可发现典型的、共性的表现。T1 增强序列可显示弥漫性硬脊膜或硬脑膜强化（图 19.2），这一发现被认为是特征性的 IH 表现。在一些回顾性研究中，95% 被诊断为 IH 的患者发现了这一结果[1, 25, 31, 50]。硬脑膜造影增强的原因尚不清楚，但也可见于部分分流术后的患者[7]。

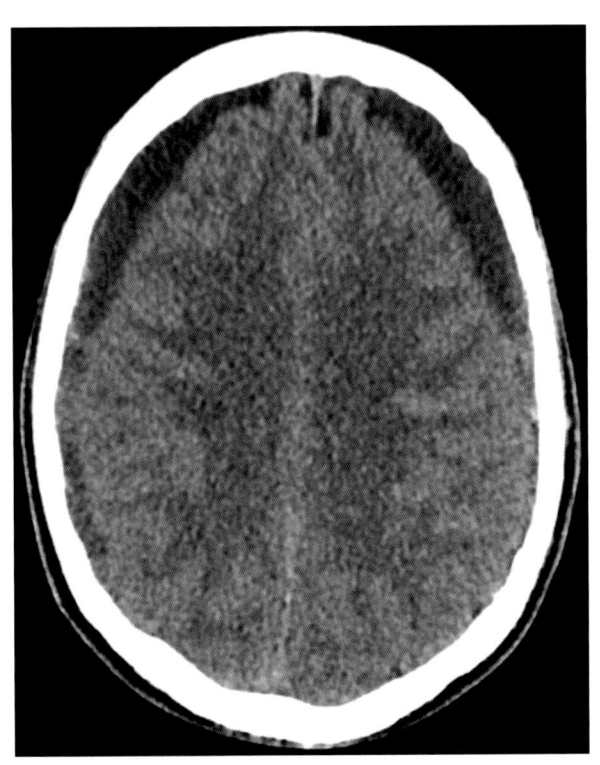

图 19.1　继发于低颅内压的双侧慢性硬膜下血肿的轴位头部 CT

图 19.2 低颅内压的冠状位 MRI 表现。（a）FLAIR 成像显示双侧慢性硬膜下血肿伴额叶受压。（b）T1 对比加权成像，弥漫性硬脑膜强化

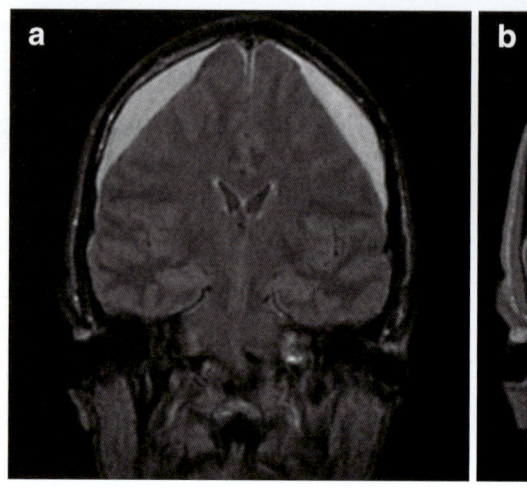
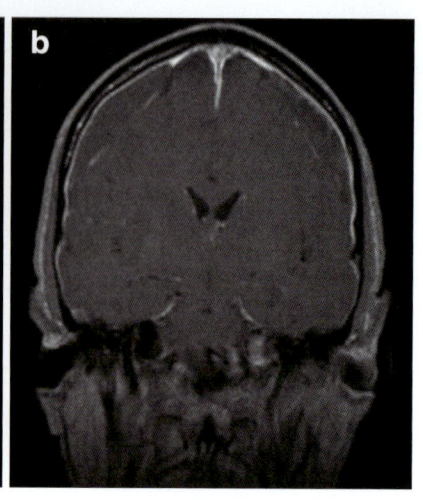

部分 IH 患者在 MRI 上也可能存在小的硬膜下积液或血肿，但在 CT 上不明显。这些积液通常是双侧的，但也可以表现为单侧的硬膜下积液或血肿[15, 34]。这些积液可以是硬膜下积液或脑脊液积液，也可以是慢性出血。在一组 40 例患者的队列研究中，Schievenk 等报道了 50% 的患者有异常的硬膜下积液，其中 60% 的患者有硬膜下积液，40% 的患者有 SDH[41]。一部分患者发生血肿而另一部分患者发生积液的基本机制则尚不清楚。

MRI 检测 IH 的特征性病变比 CT 更加敏感，同时可检测出多种特异的影像学表现（图 19.3）。典型的脑桥变平可被量化为脑桥中脑角小于 50°或乳突与脑桥距离小于 5.5 mm。基底池受压迫，并在乳头体水平处存在一个小于 40°的脚间角。小脑扁桃体下移和顶盖下降到小脑幕以下也提示 IH。

IH 是一种由脑脊液容量减少导致的颅内低压状态，有学者认为充血代偿机制导致了静脉充血[10]。

Kim 等报道了硬脑膜直窦和硬脑膜横窦扩大和充血可用于检测 IH[19]。静脉窦血栓形成也被认为是 IH 的并发症之一，并可以在这些病例中观察到[35-36, 54]。最后，MRI 增强序列显示垂体明显充血和增强，这进一步为低颅内压下大脑充血的相关理论提供了证据[11, 25, 31]。

19.4.2 脊柱成像

一旦确诊为 IH，如果患者的病史中没有明确的病因，则还需要进行额外脊髓成像用于明确病因。脑脊液漏可有隐匿性表现，可能表现为间歇性、低流量或高流量的脑脊液漏，而成像模式的选择会影响漏口的显示和定位[21]。CT 脊髓造影、放射性核素脑池造影、数字减影脊髓造影、磁共振成像（带或不带脊髓造影）都是用于检测脑脊液漏来源的方法。除了 T2 加权脂肪饱和度 MRI 外，所有这些成像方式都需要鞘内注射造影剂。脑脊液漏有

图 19.3 低颅内压的相关其他 MRI 表现。（a）在乳头体水平的 T1 轴位成像可以显示脚间角 < 40°（橙色星号）。（b）直窦静脉充血（白色箭头），顶盖移位至小脑幕水平以下（绿色箭头），小脑扁桃体下降（蓝色箭头），垂体增大（红色箭头），脑桥变平，脑桥中脑角 < 50°，乳突与脑桥距离 < 5.5 mm（黄色星号）

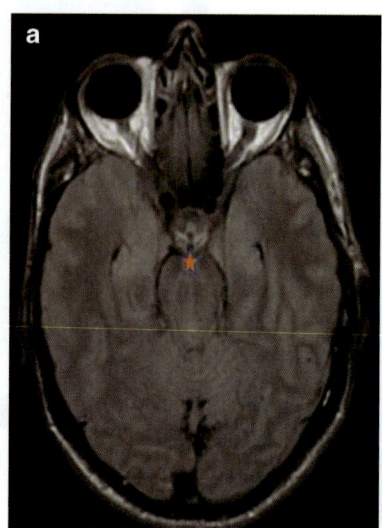
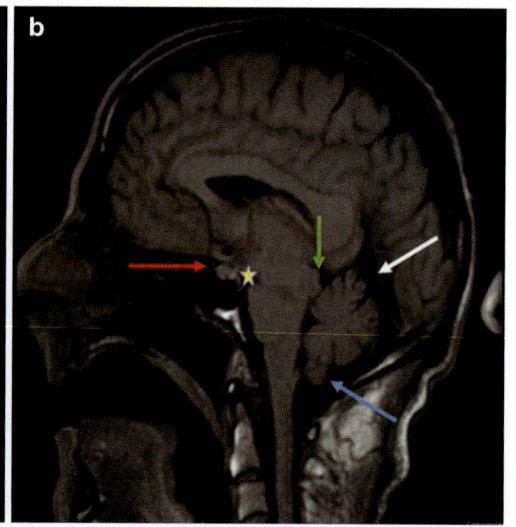

多种表现形式，如硬膜外积液、神经根周围积液或椎旁积液。

CT 脊髓造影因其使用广泛、技术成熟，被认为是识别脑脊液漏的传统检测方法[21]。其操作流程为通过腰椎穿刺将碘化造影剂注入鞘囊，随后或同时对脊柱进行 CT 成像。脑脊液泄漏率是可变的，高流量渗漏可表现为广泛的造影剂从鞘囊外渗，并且难以定位渗漏点。在这种情况下，可以使用动态 CT 脊髓造影。使用该技术可以在注射造影剂期间和之后获得脊柱的连续 CT 扫描，从而观察到造影剂的早期外渗[27]。

脊柱 MRI 在最近的文献报道中被描述为一种与 CT 脊髓造影相媲美的方法，用于鉴别脊髓脑脊液漏。由于脑脊液和脂肪在 T2 加权像上均呈高信号，因此脂肪抑制的 T2 加权像可用于鉴别脑脊液渗漏。脊柱 MRI 识别高流量脑脊液漏的表现为异常液体（T2 高信号）于硬膜外或神经根旁聚积[44]。此外，也有一些证据支持 MRI 与 CT 脊髓造影在识别脑脊液漏上的效果相当。Starling 等报道，91.7% 的 CT 脊髓造影证实有脑脊液漏的患者在 MRI 上也发现有脑脊液漏[44]。Wang 等的研究结果也证实了两种方法之间具有高度一致性[47]。鞘内注射钆的 MRI 脊髓造影也有报道，然而鞘内注射钆被 FDA 认为是超指南使用[4]。

最后，放射性核素脑池造影和数字减影脊髓造影在识别脑脊液漏中不常用。数字减影脊髓造影可用于实时检测，但定位脑脊液漏口需要耗费大量时间和资源。由于 CT 和 MRI 成像具有更高的分辨率，放射性核素脑池造影作为检测脊髓脑脊液漏的成像方式似乎已经不再适用[21]。

虽然脊柱影像学检查可用于识别出脑脊液漏口，对漏口进行针对性的治疗，但有时也无法检测出微小的漏口。与自发性 IH 相关的一种病理因素是周围神经囊肿（图 19.4）。这些发生在神经根鞘的脊髓硬脊膜憩室被认为是硬脊膜的薄弱部分，容易受到颅内压升高或剪切力的影响而造成损伤。

19.5 治疗

IH 的主要治疗目标是定位并修复脑脊液漏口。由于 IH 是一种罕见的疾病，且硬脑膜下积液只发生在小部分患者中，治疗相关的文献较少，但是有一些回顾性研究探讨了治疗策略及其有效性。

19.5.1 保守治疗

IH 的保守治疗包括卧床休息和充分补水。床头应常保持水平状态，同时患者应尽量避免用力过猛，患者躁动时可使用镇静药物。Takahashi 等在对 55 例 IH 硬膜下血肿患者的回顾性分析中研究发现，23.6% 的患者通过保守治疗成功治愈[45]。

19.5.2 硬膜外血补丁疗法

硬膜外血补丁是治疗 IH 的有效方法。硬膜外血补丁可在 X 线透视下进行，将自体血注入硬膜外腔。该操作可特异性针对在影像学上发现散发的渗漏或异常。大量回顾性研究表明，硬膜外血补丁疗法不仅能有效缓解 IH 产生的症状，同时还能改善影像学后续结果。文献报道硬膜外血补丁的成功率为 46.8% ~ 100%，该数据包括需多次或重复血补丁注射的患者[13-14, 26, 30]。

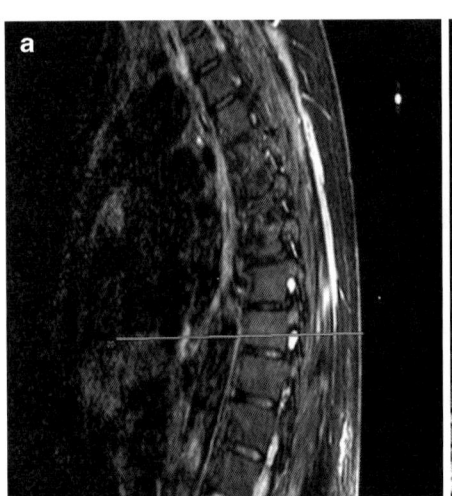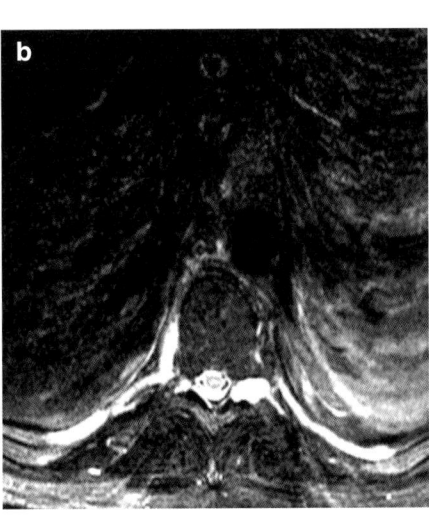

图 19.4 脊柱的 T2 加权像。矢状位（a）和轴位（b）成像显示周围神经囊肿

然而，并非所有被确诊为 IH 的患者都会检测出具体脑脊液漏口[41-42, 45]。硬膜外血补丁疗法可作为"靶向"或"盲法"操作进行。既可在确定的脑脊液漏口位置精确地进行自体血注射，也可在腰椎水平进行"盲法"注射[2, 28]。靶向硬膜外血补丁与盲法硬膜外血补丁的疗效尚未经过充分研究，但据报道两组的疗效均较为满意。He 等证实，在确定的脑脊液漏口以下 1 或 2 个椎体水平进行第一次血补丁疗法后，87.9% 的患者症状得到缓解[14]。Levi 等的研究也证明，包括接受重复血补丁疗法在内 89.1% 的患者在盲法治疗后症状缓解[24]。

19.5.3 纤维蛋白胶

据文献报道，纤维蛋白胶硬膜外注射可成为硬膜外血补丁的替代或辅助疗法。已有报道称纤维蛋白胶与自体血混合、单独使用纤维蛋白胶或硬膜外血补丁治疗失败后使用纤维蛋白胶来治疗 IH 成功的病例[8, 29, 43]。然而，关于纤维蛋白胶使用的文献较少，需要进一步的研究来评估其疗效和安全性。

19.5.4 开放性手术修补

虽然保守治疗和硬膜外血补丁治疗是有效的治疗方案，但对于难治性脑脊液漏的患者，如果可以确认具体的漏口仍需手术切开修补。文献中关于 IH 脑脊液漏开放性修补手术的报道很少，具体的修补方法因漏的位置而异[12, 15, 46, 49]。在病例报告中，开放性手术修补的方法也作为多次硬膜外血补丁治疗失败或出现急性神经功能减退症状患者的最终治疗方式。此外，大多数病例涉及脊柱腹侧退行性病变，如椎间盘骨赘复合体。脊柱的前路和后路入路均有报道，一些手术方式甚至需要切除部分椎体，以达到硬脑膜缺损的一期或二期修复。

19.5.5 硬膜下血肿清除术

在 IH 的原发病因被治疗后，CSDH 和积液在影像学上的表现可有所改善。这些积液无需手术清除即可自愈[9]，然而一些由 IH 引起的 CSDH 可扩大致中线移位、意识水平改变和脑疝出现。在这些病例中，如果患者出现神经系统危象，则需行硬膜下血肿清除术。然而硬膜下血肿清除术不解决原发病因其收益并不客观，甚至可能会导致症状恶化。Schievenk 等和 Ferrante 等报道了仅接受硬膜下血肿清除术的患者，这些患者的症状在接受清除术后没有得到改善或有显著的神经功能减退[9, 15, 41]。幸运的是，这些研究中的大多数患者在 IH 的原发病因得到治疗后神经系统功能得到恢复。

在 IH 情况下，如何管理重型 CSDH 患者尚无共识或指南。Takahashi 等和 Yoon 等报道了他们的临床经验，并建议采用盲法或靶向硬膜外血补丁治疗结合 SDH 血肿清除术的方法治疗重型 CSDH[45, 52]。关于 SDH 血肿清除术应该在 IH 原发病得到治愈的之前或之后进行，目前还没有相关研究。极端的 IH 病例可能会出现下疝综合征。当怀疑出现 IH 下疝综合征时，应立即采取相应措施抢救患者。患者应采取头低俯卧位，扩大血容量。两份病例报告也报道了鞘囊内灌注生理盐水对于有下疝迹象的患者是一种有效的抢救措施，待患者病情平稳后应立刻处理原发病[33, 48]。

19.6 结论

CSDH 是常见于神经外科领域的疾病之一。由 IH 引起的 CSDH 是一种罕见疾病，正确鉴别诊断该病以便为患者提供恰当的治疗是极其重要的。因为 IH 在临床中很少见，因此诊断常常会出现延误。临床病史在确诊 IH 时常起到重要作用，同时辅助以多模态头颅和脊髓影像学检查有助于确诊 IH。绝大多数硬膜下血肿可以在解决 IH 的病因后得到治愈。除了表现出神经系统危象且检查可迅速完成的患者外，在确定和治愈脑脊液漏口之前应谨慎进行脑血肿清除术，对继发于 IH 的 SHD 患者进行手术干预可能导致神经功能症状恶化。

参考文献

1. Barahona ML, Mora-Encinas JP, Gonzalez-Montano VM, Pozo-Zamorano T, Fernandez-Gil MA. [Intracranial hypotension syndrome: a review of the magnetic resonance findings]. Rev Neurol. 2011;52:676–80.
2. Berroir S, Loisel B, Ducros A, Boukobza M, Tzourio C, Valade D, et al. Early epidural blood

patch in spontaneous intracranial hypotension. Neurology. 2004;63:1950–1.
3. Capizzano AA, Lai L, Kim J, Rizzo M, Gray L, Smoot MK, et al. Atypical presentations of intracranial hypotension: comparison with classic spontaneous intracranial hypotension. Am J Neuroradiol. 2016;37:1256–61.
4. Chazen JL, Talbott JF, Lantos JE, Dillon WP. MR myelography for identification of spinal CSF leak in spontaneous intracranial hypotension. Am J Neuroradiol. 2014;35:2007–12.
5. Chen YC, Wang YF, Li JY, Chen SP, Lirng JF, Hseu SS, et al. Treatment and prognosis of subdural hematoma in patients with spontaneous intracranial hypotension. Cephalalgia. 2016;36:225–31.
6. Cornips E, Grouls M, Bekelaar K. Transdural thoracic disk herniation with longitudinal slitlike dural defect causing intracranial hypotension: report of 2 cases. World Neurosurg. 2020;140:e311–9.
7. Gupta M, Patidar Y, Khwaja GA, Chowdhury D, Batra A, Dasgupta A. Intracranial hypotension due to shunt overdrainage presenting as reversible dorsal midbrain syndrome. Neurology Asia. 2014;19(1):107–110.
8. Elwood J, Dewan M, Smith J, Mokri B, Mauck W, Eldrige J. Efficacy of epidural blood patch with fibrin glue additive in refractory headache due to intracranial hypotension: preliminary report. Springerplus. 2016;5:317.
9. Ferrante E, Rubino F, Beretta F, Regna-Gladin C, Ferrante MM. Treatment and outcome of subdural hematoma in patients with spontaneous intracranial hypotension: a report of 35 cases. Acta Neurol Belg. 2018;118:61–70.
10. Ferrante E, Savino A, Sances G, Nappi G. Spontaneous intracranial hypotension syndrome: report of twelve cases. Headache. 2004;44:615–22.
11. Gilmour GS, Scott J, Couillard P. Leaking the diagnosis: a case of convulsive status epilepticus due to intracranial hypotension. Neurocrit Care. 2019;31:562–6.
12. Hasiloglu ZI, Abuzayed B, Imal AE, Cagil E, Albayram S. Spontaneous intracranial hypotension due to intradural thoracic osteophyte with superimposed disc herniation: report of two cases. Eur Spine J. 2012;21(Suppl 4):383.
13. Hazama A, Loree J, Braley A, Awawdeh F, Swarnkar A, Chin L, et al. Spontaneous Intracranial Hypotension and the durability of Epidural Blood Patch. World Neurosurg. 2019;66(1):90. https://doi.org/10.1093/neuros/nyz310_353.
14. He FF, Li L, Liu MJ, Zhong TD, Zhang QW, Fang XM. Targeted epidural blood patch treatment for refractory spontaneous intracranial hypotension in China. J Neurol Surg B Skull Base. 2018;79:217–23. Thieme Medical Publishers, Inc.
15. Inamasu J, Moriya S, Shibata J, Kumai T, Hirose Y. Spontaneous intracranial hypotension manifesting as a unilateral subdural hematoma with a marked midline shift. Case Rep Neurol. 2015;7:71–7.
16. International Classification of Headache Disorders. 3rd ed. Headache attributed to non-vascular intracranial disorder. 2019. https://ichd-3.org/7-headache-attributed-to-non-vascular-intracranial-disorder/7-2-headache-attributed-to-low-cerebrospinal-fluid-pressure/7-2-3-headache-attributed-to-spontaneous-intracranial-hypotension/. Accessed 14 Jan 2021.
17. Ito H, Komai T, Yamamoto S. Fibrinolytic enzyme in the lining walls of chronic subdural hematoma. J Neurosurg. 1978;48:197–200.
18. Killeffer JA, Killeffer FA, Schochet SS. The outer neomembrane of chronic subdural hematoma. Neurosurg Clin N Am. 2000;11:407–12.
19. Kim JH, Roh H, Yoon WK, Kwon TH, Chong K, Hwang SY, et al. Clinical features of patients with spontaneous intracranial hypotension complicated with bilateral subdural fluid collections. Headache. 2019;59:775–86.
20. Kranz PG, Stinnett SS, Huang KT, Gray L. Spinal meningeal diverticula in spontaneous intracranial hypotension: analysis of prevalence and myelographic appearance. Am J Neuroradiol. 2013;34:1284–9.
21. Kranz PG, Luetmer PH, Diehn FE, Amrhein TJ, Tanpitukpongse TP, Gray L. Myelographic techniques for the detection of spinal CSF leaks in spontaneous intracranial hypotension. Am J Roentgenol. 2016;206:8–19.
22. Lai TH, Fuh JL, Lirng JF, Tsai PH, Wang SJ. Subdural haematoma in patients with spontaneous intracranial hypotension. Cephalalgia. 2007;27:133–8.
23. Lau D, Lin J, Park P. Cranial nerve III palsy resulting from intracranial hypotension caused by cerebrospinal fluid leak after paraspinal tumor resection: etiology and treatment options. Spine J. 2011;11:e10–3.
24. Levi V, Di Laurenzio NE, Franzini A, Tramacere I, Erbetta A, Chiapparini L, et al. Lumbar

epidural blood patch: effectiveness on orthostatic headache and MRI predictive factors in 101 consecutive patients affected by spontaneous intracranial hypotension. J Neurosurg. 2020;132:809–17.
25. Li C, Raza HK, Chansysouphanthong T, Zu J, Cui G. A clinical analysis on 40 cases of spontaneous intracranial hypotension syndrome. Somatosens Mot Res. 2019;36:24–30.
26. Loya JJ, Mindea SA, Yu H, Venkatasubramanian C, Chang SD, Burns TC. Intracranial hypotension producing reversible coma: a systematic review, including three new cases. A review. J Neurosurg. 2012;117:615–28.
27. Luetmer PH, Schwartz KM, Eckel LJ, Hunt CH, Carter RE, Diehn FE. When should i do dynamic CT myelography? Predicting fast spinal CSF leaks in patients with spontaneous intracranial hypotension. Am J Neuroradiol. 2012;33:690–4.
28. Madsen SA, Fomsgaard JS, Jensen R. Epidural blood patch for refractory low CSF pressure headache: a pilot study. J Headache Pain. 2011;12:453–7.
29. Mammis A, Agarwal N, Mogilner AY. Alternative treatment of intracranial hypotension presenting as postdural puncture headaches using epidural fibrin glue patches: two case reports. Int J Neurosci. 2014;124:863–6.
30. Martin R, Louy C, Babu V, Jiang Y, Far A, Schievink W. A two-level large-volume epidural blood patch protocol for spontaneous intracranial hypotension: retrospective analysis of risk and benefit. Reg Anesth Pain Med. 2020;45:32–7.
31. Michali-Stolarska M, Bladowska J, Stolarski M, Sąsiadek MJ. Diagnostic imaging and clinical features of intracranial hypotension—review of literature. Pol J Radiol. 2017;82:842–9.
32. Mokri B, Parisi JE, Scheithauer BW, Piepgras DG, Miller GM. Meningeal biopsy in intracranial hypotension: meningeal enhancement on MRI. Neurology. 1995;45:1801–7.
33. Muram S, Yavin D, DuPlessis S. Intrathecal saline infusion as an effective temporizing measure in the management of spontaneous intracranial hypotension. World Neurosurg. 2019;125:37–41.
34. Osada Y, Shibahara I, Nakagawa A, Sakata H, Niizuma K, Saito R, et al. Unilateral chronic subdural hematoma due to spontaneous intracranial hypotension: a report of four cases. Br J Neurosurg. 2020;34:632–7.
35. Paris D, Rousset D, Bonneville F, Fabre N, Faguer S, Huguet-Rigal F, et al. Cerebral venous thrombosis and subdural collection in a comatose patient: do not forget intracranial hypotension. A case report. Headache. 2020;60:2583–8.
36. Perry A, Graffeo CS, Brinjikji W, Copeland WR, Rabinstein AA, Link MJ. Spontaneous occult intracranial hypotension precipitating life-threatening cerebral venous thrombosis: case report. J Neurosurg Spine. 2018;28:669–78.
37. Pettyjohn EW, Donlan RM, Breck J, Clugston JR. Intracranial hypotension in the setting of post-concussion headache: a case series. Cureus. 2020;12:e10526.
38. Sarrafzadeh AS, Hopf SA, Gautschi OP, Narata AP, Schaller K. Intracranial hypotension after trauma. Springerplus. 2014;3:1–7.
39. Schievink WI. Spontaneous spinal cerebrospinal fluid leaks and intracranial hypotension. J Am Med Assoc. 2006;295:2286–96.
40. Schievink WI, Maya MM, Moser F, Tourje J, Torbati S. Frequency of spontaneous intracranial hypotension in the emergency department. J Headache Pain. 2007;8:325–8.
41. Schievink WI, Meyer FB, Atkinson JLD, Mokri B. Spontaneous spinal cerebrospinal fluid leaks and intracranial hypotension. J Neurosurg. 1996;84:598–605.
42. Schievink WI, Morreale VM, Atkinson JLD, Meyer FB, Piepgras DG, Ebersold MJ. Surgical treatment of spontaneous spinal cerebrospinal fluid leaks. J Neurosurg. 1998;88:243–6.
43. Schievink WI, Maya MM, Moser FM. Treatment of spontaneous intracranial hypotension with percutaneous placement of a fibrin sealant. Report of four cases. J Neurosurg. 2004;100:1098–100.
44. Starling A, Hernandez F, Hoxworth JM, Trentman T, Halker R, Vargas BB, et al. Sensitivity of MRI of the spine compared with CT myelography in orthostatic headache with CSF leak. Neurology. 2013;81:1789–92.
45. Takahashi K, Mima T, Akiba Y. Chronic subdural hematoma associated with spontaneous intracranial hypotension: therapeutic strategies and outcomes of 55 cases. Neurol Med Chir (Tokyo). 2016;56:69–76.
46. Veeravagu A, Gupta G, Jiang B, Berta SC, Mindea SA, Chang SD. Spontaneous intracranial hypotension secondary to anterior thoracic osteophyte: resolution after primary dural repair via posterior approach. Int J Surg Case Rep. 2013;4:26–9.
47. Wang YF, Lirng JF, Fuh JL, Hseu SS, Wang SJ. Heavily T2-weighted MR myelography vs CT

myelography in spontaneous intracranial hypotension. Neurology. 2009;73:1892–8.
48. Watanabe A, Takai H, Ogino S, Ohki T, Ohki I. Intracranial subdural hematoma after resection of a thoracic spinal cord tumor. J Spinal Disord Tech. 2002;15:533–6.
49. Witiw CD, Fallah A, Muller PJ, Ginsberg HJ. Surgical treatment of spontaneous intracranial hypotension secondary to degenerative cervical spine pathology: a case report and literature review. Eur Spine J. 2012;21(Suppl 4):S422–7.
50. Xia P, Hu X-Y, Wang J, Hu B-B, Xu Q-L, Zhou Z-J, et al. Risk factors for subdural haematoma in patients with spontaneous intracranial hypotension. PLoS One. 2015;10:e0123616.
51. Yamashima T, Yamamoto S. How do vessels proliferate in the capsule of a chronic subdural hematoma? Neurosurgery. 1984;15:672–8.
52. Yoon KW, Cho MK, Kim YJ, Lee SK. Sinus thrombosis in a patient with intracranial hypotension: a suggested hypothesis of venous stasis. A case report. Interv Neuroradiol. 2011;17:248–51.
53. Zakaria AF, Tsuji M. Intracranial subdural hematoma after lumbar spine surgery: a case report. Malays Orthop J. 2019;13:85–7.
54. Zhang D, Wang J, Zhang Q, He F, Hu X. Cerebral venous thrombosis in spontaneous intracranial hypotension: a report on 4 cases and a review of the literature. Headache. 2018;58:1244–55.

第20章 电休克疗法后的慢性硬膜下血肿：一种罕见但严重的并发症

Anil Kalyoncu，Ali Saffet Gonul 和 Mehmet Turgut

译者：田润发

20.1 引言

电休克疗法（ECT）是一种被广泛应用的治疗方法，它基于通过颅骨的电传导来诱导治疗癫痫发作。ECT是治疗各种精神疾病的常用方法，包括抑郁症、躁狂症、紧张症和精神分裂症。ECT通常应用于对药物治疗无效的患者或有严重症状的患者，如自杀倾向和认知功能障碍。美国食品和药物管理局（FDA）对ECT的使用进行了规范，全球每年约有100万患者接受ECT治疗，美国每年有10万患者接受治疗[2, 20]。治疗方式随着电极置入位置的变化而变化，电极可单侧或双侧置入。单侧ECT最常应用于通常是非优势半球的右侧大脑，双侧ECT电极放置在管理左、右颞叶前部的双额或双颞[22]。

尽管ECT具体的作用机制尚未明确，但其具有的神经电生理效应能够在癫痫发作期间增加脑血流量和提高血脑屏障通透性。除了改变脑血流量外，ECT还能增加海马体积并提高脑源性神经营养因子水平，在疾病治疗中发挥积极作用[17-18, 23]。

20.2 ECT的副作用

现今，ECT是一种公认的安全治疗方法，并且没有绝对的禁忌证[1]。在ECT治疗的第一天，患者死亡率为2.4/10万例，但在14天内患者死亡率上升到18/10万例[11]。从全球角度看，其死亡风险几乎与使用短效巴比妥类麻醉药的风险相同[13]。文献记载ECT有各种并发症，按其来源可分为癫痫引起的并发症和全身麻醉引起的并发症两大类[3]。ECT常见的并发症包括头痛、口干、恶心、精神错乱和肌痛等，这些并发症通常是轻微的和一过性的。使用全身麻醉还会出现其他并发症，如持续性呼吸暂停、恶性高热和高钾血症。心血管系统并发症可能也与ECT有关，ECT可导致高血压、心肌梗死和心肌病等[9]。ECT神经系统并发症从常见的如记忆丧失和认知障碍等到脑血管事件等罕见的并发症[3]。

20.3 ECT和慢性硬膜下血肿

慢性硬膜下血肿（CSDH）被认为是ECT的主要神经系统并发症。这种并发症非常罕见，已知文献报道中只有5例ECT治疗后的CSDH（表20.1）[6, 10, 13, 21, 27]。文献报道的患者年龄在38～76岁。在这些病例中，2例患者被诊断为双相障碍，3例患者患有难治性抑郁症，2例患者治疗前正在进行抗凝或抗血小板治疗，其他患者未提供具体相关信息。然而可获得的已知信息表明，华法林在ECT治疗中是安全的[8, 16]，因此目前尚无明确证据表明接受ECT治疗的患者发生CSDH是由抗凝治疗引起的。在硬膜下血肿（SDH）被确诊之前，ECT治疗的次数在1次到12次不等。在2例病例中，ECT治疗前神经影像学结果未提示出血，因此硬膜下出血可能是在ECT治疗期间形成的新发病变，或ECT治疗可能导致先前存在的病变引发出血。1例患者在ECT治疗前被诊断为左侧CSDH，由于CSDH的存在该患者仅接受了右侧ECT治疗。2例患者在接受双颞ECT后均被确诊为SDH，且出现相关临床症状。在老年人群中，因为SDH往往是无症状的，因此ECT后发生SDH的数量可能比已发表报道中所记录的要多[10, 26]。除1例患者外，其余患者均接受了手术治疗清除血肿。未接受手术治疗的患者出现了大小约6 mm的左侧SDH且无中线位移，该患者仅接受药物治疗。药物治疗后该患者CT提示SDH未扩大，但该患者仍在

表 20.1 迄今英文文献报道的 5 例 ECT 治疗后慢性硬膜下血肿的总结

作者，年代[参考文献]	性别	年龄	精神病学诊断	抗凝/抗血小板药物	ECT 方式	初始 ECT 剂量	ECT 次数	ECT 前影像学资料	神经系统症状/GCS	ECT 后影像学资料	中线位移	SDH 治疗方式	结局
Wijeratne 等，1999[27]	男	76 岁	持续性抑郁症	未注明	右侧/单侧	378 mC	6	左侧慢性硬膜下出血	意识水平降低	左顶叶慢性硬膜下出血	否	药物治疗	28 天内死亡
Awasthy 等，2005[6]	男	63 岁	双相情感障碍	未注明	未注明	未注明	10	未注明	E3V3M6	左额顶慢性硬膜下出血	是	手术钻孔治疗	治愈
Saha 等，2012[21]	女	38 岁	双相情感障碍	未注明	未注明	未注明	12	未注明	右侧偏瘫	左颞顶慢性硬膜下出血	是	手术治疗	未注明
Kulkarni 等，2012[13]	男	42 岁	持续性抑郁症	否	双颞	120 mC	1	无脑皮质萎缩	E2V4M2	右额顶、左顶叶（双侧）急性硬膜下出血	是	手术钻孔治疗	未注明
Dauleac 等，2019[10]	女	64 岁	持续性抑郁症	否	双颞	176 mC	4	脑皮质萎缩	E1V2M4	右额顶慢性硬膜下出血	是	手术钻孔治疗	治愈

ECT 治疗后的第 28 天死亡。另有 2 例患者恢复良好，无神经系统后遗症。

20.4　ECT 后 SDH 的处理

有脑萎缩史和抗凝/抗血小板治疗史的患者应被列入 ECT 危险组，因此 ECT 治疗前应通过影像学检查查看是否患有 SDH 以确定这些患者是否存在治疗风险[10]。ECT 治疗引起的并发症可能与脑血管意外的症状相混淆，包括恶心、术后意识模糊和 Todd 麻痹[14, 24]。当患者出现意识水平持续改变、局灶性神经系统体征、反复癫痫性惊厥、顽固性呕吐和失禁等脑血管事件体征时应进行神经影像学检查[13]。脑血管意外与 ECT 之间的关系可能是由于癫痫发作时血压和血脑屏障渗透性短暂升高导致颅内压（ICP）升高[4]。因此，颅内压升高可以诱发 SDH 或扩大现有 SDH 的体积[27]。尽管 ECT 的治疗机制包括改变颅内压，但仍有 CSDH 患者在 SDH 大小未改变的情况下成功获得治疗[5, 15, 27]。在 ECT 治疗前，过度通气可降低脑脊液压力进而降低颅内压。因此，过度通气有助于预防 ECT 治疗中 SDH 的发生发展[7, 13]。导致 ECT 治疗副作用的其他重要因素是电极的放置位置和 ECT 治疗剂量。电极之间的宽度决定了激活区域癫痫的发作程度，电极放置距离越宽受影响的大脑区域越大。长期以来比较单侧和双侧电极放置的研究表明，单侧电极置入的治疗效果不如双侧电极置入，但副作用更少[19, 25]。电流刺激剂量是影响副作用和疗效的另一个重要因素，电流量越大神经元去极化程度越高，癫痫发作程度则越强[22]。Wijeratne 和 Shome 建议对已诊断患有 SDH 的患者进行对侧 ECT 治疗[27]，但有研究报道单侧 ECT 治疗不能作用于大脑下层皮质[12]。考虑到单侧电休克治疗（ECT）的疗效低于双侧电休克治疗，且所需剂量更高，因此在严重精神疾病病例中可以采用双侧电休克治疗，而不会产生不良后果[27]。既往 CSDH 病史并非 ECT 的绝对禁忌证，但是治疗期间建议神经外科专科随访。CSDH 是一种已知且罕见的 ECT 并发症，其发生发展在临床中不易预测，因此早期发现和治疗 CSDH 对于防止进一步的神经损伤至关重要。

20.5　结论

ECT 是针对特定精神疾病患者的常规治疗方法，已经安全使用了 80 多年。该疗法虽然被认为是安全的，但仍可能会发生多种并发症。SDH 是文献报道过的并发症之一，虽然在 ECT 治疗的患者中 SDH 是非常罕见的并发症，但在高危人群特别是在 ECT 治疗后几天出现相关临床症状的患者更需格外小心。因此，为了确定 ECT 治疗后是否会出现并发症，治疗前对患者进行相关评估是必不可少的。

参考文献

1. American Psychiatric Association. The practice of electroconvulsive therapy: recommendations for treatment, training, and privileging. Washington, DC: APA Press; 1990.
2. American Psychiatric Association. The practice of electroconvulsive therapy. Recommendations for treatment, training, and privileging: a task force report of APA. Washington, DC: American Psychiatric Association; 2002.
3. Andrade C, Arumugham SS, Thirthalli J. Adverse effects of electroconvulsive therapy. Psychiatr Clin North Am. 2016;39:513–30.
4. Andrade C, Bolwig TG. Electroconvulsive therapy, hypertensive surge, blood-brain barrier breach, and amnesia: exploring the evidence for a connection. J ECT. 2014;30:160–4.
5. Anwar N, Brakoulias V. Safety of electroconvulsivetherapy after subdural hemorrhage. Aust N Z J Psychiatry. 2010;44:294.
6. Awasthy N, Chand K. Subdural hematoma: as complication of electroconvulsive therapy. Pak J Med Sci. 2005;21:491–3.
7. Bryson EO, Kellner CH. Chronic subdural hematoma following electroconvulsive therapy. Indian J Psychol Med. 2013;35:220.
8. Bleich S, Degner D, Scheschonka A, Ruther E, Kropp S. Electroconvulsive therapy and anticoagulation [letter]. Can J Psychiatry. 2000;45:87–8.
9. Cristancho MA, Alici Y, Augoustides JG, O'Reardon JP. Uncommon but serious complications

associated with electroconvulsive therapy: recognition and management for the clinician. Curr Psychiatry Rep. 2008;10:474–80.
10. Dauleac C, Vinckier F, Bourdillon P. Subdural hematoma and electroconvulsive therapy: a case report and review of the literature. Neurochirurgie. 2019;65:40–2.
11. Dennis NM, Dennis PA, Shafer A, Weiner RD, Husain MM. Electroconvulsive therapy and all-cause mortality in Texas, 1998-2013. J ECT. 2017;33:22–5.
12. Hsiao JK, Evans DL. ECT in a depressed patient after craniotomy. Am J Psychiatry. 1984;141:442–4.
13. Kulkarni RR, Melkundi S. Subdural hematoma: an adverse event of electroconvulsive therapy case report and literature review. Case Rep Psychiatry. 2012;2012:585303.
14. Liff JM, Bryson EO, Maloutas E, Garruto K, Pasculli RM, Briggs MC, Kellner CH. Transient hemiparesis (Todd's paralysis) after electroconvulsive therapy (ECT) in a patient with major depressive disorder. J ECT. 2013;29:247–8.
15. Malek-Ahmadi P, Beceiro JR, McNeil BW, Weddige RL. Electroconvulsive therapy and chronic subdural hematoma. Convuls Ther. 1990;6:38–41.
16. Mehta V, Mueller PS, Gonzalez-Arriaza HL, Pankratz VS, Rummans TA. Safety of electroconvulsive therapy in patients receiving long-term warfarin therapy. Mayo Clin Proc. 2004;79:1396–401.
17. Nordanskog P, Dahlstrand U, Larsson MR, Larsson EM, Knutsson L, Johanson A. Increase in hippocampal volume after electroconvulsive therapy in patients with depression: a volumetric magnetic resonance imaging study. J ECT. 2010;26:62–7.
18. Rocha RB, Dondossola ER, Grande AJ, Colonetti T, Ceretta LB, Passos IC, Quevedo J, da Rosa MI. Increased BDNF levels after electroconvulsive therapy in patients with major depressive disorder: a meta-analysis study. J Psychiatr Res. 2016;83:47–53.
19. Sackeim HA, Prudic J, Devanand DP, Kiersky JE, Fitzsimons L, Moody BJ, McElhiney MC, Coleman EA, Settembrino JM. Effects of stimulus intensity and electrode placement on the efficacy and cognitive effects of electroconvulsive therapy. N Engl J Med. 1993;328:839–46.
20. Sadock, Sadock VA. Kaplan & Sadock's comprehensive textbook of psychiatry. Philadelphia: Lippincott Williams & Wilkins; 2009.
21. Saha D, Bisui B, Thakurta RG, Ghoshmaulik S, Singh OP. Chronic subdural hematoma following electroconvulsive therapy. Indian J Psychol Med. 2012;34:181–3.
22. Swartz CM, Nelson AI. Rational electroconvulsive therapy electrode placement. Psychiatry (Edgmont). 2005;2:37–43.
23. Taylor S. Electroconvulsive therapy: a review of history, patient selection, technique, and medication management. South Med J. 2007;100:494–8.
24. Tzabazis A, Schmitt HJ, Ihmsen H, Schmidtlein M, Zimmermann R, Wielopolski J, Münster T. Postictal agitation after electroconvulsive therapy: incidence, severity, and propofol as a treatment option. J ECT. 2013;29:189–95.
25. UK ECT Review Group. Efficacy and safety of electroconvulsive therapy in depressive disorders: a systematic review and meta-analysis. Lancet. 2003;361:799–808.
26. Uno M, Toi H, Hirai S. Chronic subdural hematoma in elderly patients: is this disease benign? Neurol Med Chir (Tokyo). 2017;57:402–9.
27. Wijeratne C, Shome S. Electroconvulsive therapy and subdural hemorrhage. J ECT. 1999;15:275–9.

第 21 章 血液病导致的慢性硬膜下血肿

Alican Tahta, Yaşar B. Turgut 和 Gökhan Pektaş

译者：张烁

21.1 引言

慢性硬膜下血肿（chronic subdural hematoma，CSDH）在美国人群中的总发病率为 5/10 万人[51]，在 70 岁以上的人群中升至 58/10 万人[50]。随着老年人口数量日益增加，CSDH 的发病率在未来可能进一步上升[15]。以往研究表明，头部创伤是 CSDH 最常见的原因；然而随着人口平均年龄增长、癌症患病率上升及抗栓药物应用，因头部创伤而引发 CSDH 的患者比例逐渐降低[17, 33, 50, 62]。脑萎缩在老年人中很常见，萎缩的脑组织导致桥静脉受到的牵拉增强，出血的可能性升高[8]。目前公认的 CSDH 病理生理理论基础是血肿腔反复吸收和复发性出血[37]。钻单孔/双孔同时放置/不放置外引流装置是目前治疗 CSDH 的主要外科手术方法。CSDH 患者的再手术率为 2.3%～38.7%[63]。血肿复发率与患者预后有显著相关性，预后随着 CSDH 复发率的增加而变差[38]。老年患者复发的风险较高[5]。此外，老年患者使用抗栓药物的比例较高，这也是 CSDH 复发的又一个危险因素。

21.2 抗血栓药物

由于患有慢性病的老年患者普遍服用抗血栓药物，因此随访这些药物对 CSDH 的影响以及探讨术后患者应采取的预防措施非常重要。目前已有多项针对抗血栓药物与 CSDH 复发的关系研究，但结果并不一致[1, 13, 16]。根据 Nathan 等于 2017 年发表的综述，共有 4 篇文章探讨了抗凝和抗血小板药物联合使用对 CSDH 复发的影响[41]。其中 3 项研究表明，联合用药不是 CSDH 复发的显著危险因素[5-6, 20]。然而另一项研究认为联合用药是 CSDH 复发的重要因素[24]。Wang 等于 2019 年进行的 meta 分析认为，联合使用抗血小板和抗凝药物的患者 CSDH 复发风险较高（OR：1.30，95% CI：1.11～1.52，$P = 0.001$），但联合使用并未增加 CSDH 患者的死亡率[63]。此外，Motoie 等也指出，急性硬膜外血肿和急性硬膜下血肿出现严重并发症与入院时抗血栓药物的使用有关，但它们不会增加这些患者的复发率[39]。

21.3 抗凝药物

维生素 K 环氧化还原酶复合物 1（VKORC1）是一种体内维生素 K 的激活酶，而华法林可通过抑制 VKORC1，从而消耗维生素 K 储备，继而减少活性凝血因子的合成[45]。神经外科医生在接诊华法林治疗的老年患者时应考虑诊断 CSDH（图 21.1）。

术前必须将活化凝血酶原时间（APTT）和国际标准化比值（INR）调整到正常范围内，以防止

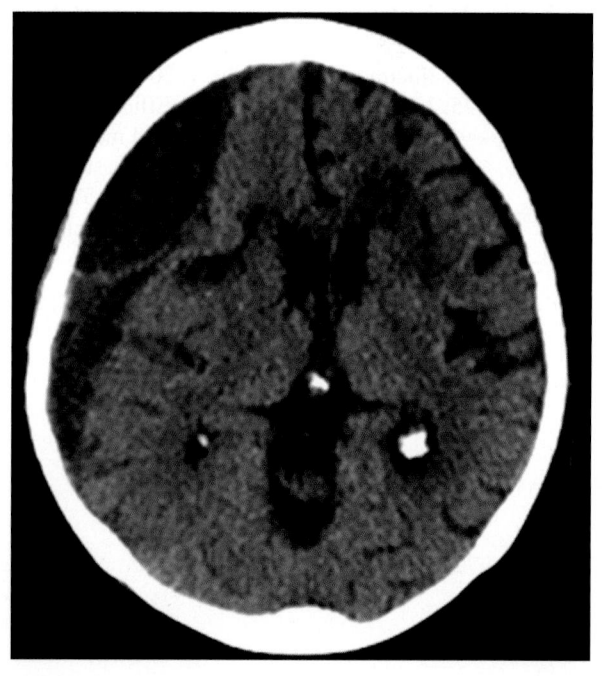

图 21.1 86 岁女性患者，服用华法林，轴位 CT 平扫提示右脑额顶叶慢性硬膜下血肿（CSDH）

并发症发生，特别是血肿复发[37]。如果患者需要急诊手术治疗，可以通过给予包括凝血因子2、7、9、10在内的凝血酶原复合物将INR降低到正常值。新鲜冷冻血浆（FFP）含有所有凝血因子，但根据因子浓度不同，只能部分逆转华法林的抗凝效果，且由于静脉容量有限，导致逆转华法林的作用需要较长时间[22, 30]。凝血酶原复合物浓缩物（PCC）因含有较多的凝血因子通常是首选的药物，其目的是提高凝血因子浓度进行凝血。此外，还可以静脉注射维生素K用以刺激辅助因子的合成。维生素K通常作为PCC和（或）FFP的辅助治疗[21]。华法林应在择期手术前至少停用5天，且应在手术当天复查INR值。

普通肝素和低分子量肝素（LMWH）都能增强抗凝血酶-Ⅲ的活性，从而抑制凝血酶的形成。两种类型的肝素在使用时都应监测APTT水平，其作用可用鱼精蛋白逆转。然而，低分子量肝素不能被完全逆转。因此，神经外科医生应注意低分子量肝素治疗的患者存在的持续性凝血功能障碍。

新型口服抗凝药（NOAC）的靶点是Xa因子或凝血酶[55]。由于NOAC缺乏逆转剂，可能为手术带来困难。PraxBind是达比加群的逆转剂，药物可在11 h内使凝血相关检查结果恢复正常[66]。尽管PCC/FFP可以在手术前使用，但尚未发现这些药物可以改善预后[40]。利伐沙班在32 h可代谢完全，阿哌沙班在28 h可代谢完全，达比加群在56 h可代谢完全[61]。由于缺乏有效的逆转剂，NOAC应在病情允许的情况下停用一段时间。然而Motoie等发现在21例服用NOAC的患者中CSDH复发率没有增加[39]。但Arai等进行的一项研究表明，上述药物会增加复发率[4]。

Ohba等和Chon等发现CSDH患者的复发率增加[13, 42]，但只有Chon等的发现具有统计学意义[13]。此外，Wang等[63]的meta分析显示，抗凝药物的使用会增加复发的风险，然而没有证据表明它会增加死亡风险[63]。

21.4 抗血小板药物

乙酰水杨酸（ASA，阿司匹林）是最常用的抗血小板药物。ASA在低剂量使用时不可逆地抑制环氧合酶-2（COX2），导致血小板功能障碍[58]。

在临床实践中，每一位神经外科医生都应注意抗血小板治疗的CSDH患者（图21.2）。血小板的平均寿命是5～7天。因此，服用ASA药物的患者应在手术前5～7天停药，紧急情况下输注血小板也是可行的。Taylor等的研究表明，输注血小板是针对服用ASA患者的有效治疗方法[57]。氯吡格雷、普拉格雷、替格瑞洛、噻氯匹定和坎格雷洛是P2Y12受体的抑制剂[37]，通过结合或阻断血小板腺苷二磷酸（ADP）受体引起血小板功能障碍，然而这些药物没有逆转剂。除了替格瑞洛，其他药物的作用都是不可逆的。替格瑞洛可在28 h内从血液循环中清除。择期手术建议在停药后等待5～10天后进行，涉及其他药物的紧急手术可于术中进行血小板输注[37]。

Ohba等发现使用抗血小板药物组患者CSDH复发率为15.2%[42]，未使用抗血小板药物组患者复发率为10.4%，两组比较差异无统计学意义[42]。Chon等发现使用抗血小板药物和不使用抗血小板药物的患者再出血率之间没有显著差异[13]。Wang等进行的meta分析显示，抗血小板药物的使用可增加CSDH的复发率[63]。然而，大多数研究表明使用抗血小板药物不会增加CSDH的复发[7, 16, 36, 59]。

21.5 重启抗血栓治疗的时机

停用华法林后7天内缺血性并发症发生率为2.6%～4.8%[65]。Guha等比较了接受抗血栓治疗和未接受抗血栓治疗的CSDH患者手术后血栓栓塞的发生率[20]。所有具有抗血栓药物服用史的患者在围手术期抗血栓药物均停用，约有一半患者在神经外科手术后52天内恢复服用，结果发现在接受抗血栓治疗的患者中血栓栓塞并发症的发生率有增加的趋势（2.6% vs. 0.8%）[20]。Amano等发现，与未接受抗血栓治疗的CSDH患者相比，接受抗血栓治疗的CSDH患者血栓栓塞并发症发生率显著增加（9.1% vs. 0.9%）[3]。Phan等发表的一项meta分析显示，恢复抗血栓治疗的患者血栓栓塞并发症发生率低于未恢复抗栓治疗的患者（2.9% vs. 15.3%）[46]。根据这些结果，血栓栓塞是接受抗血小板治疗的CSDH患者术后重要的并发症。

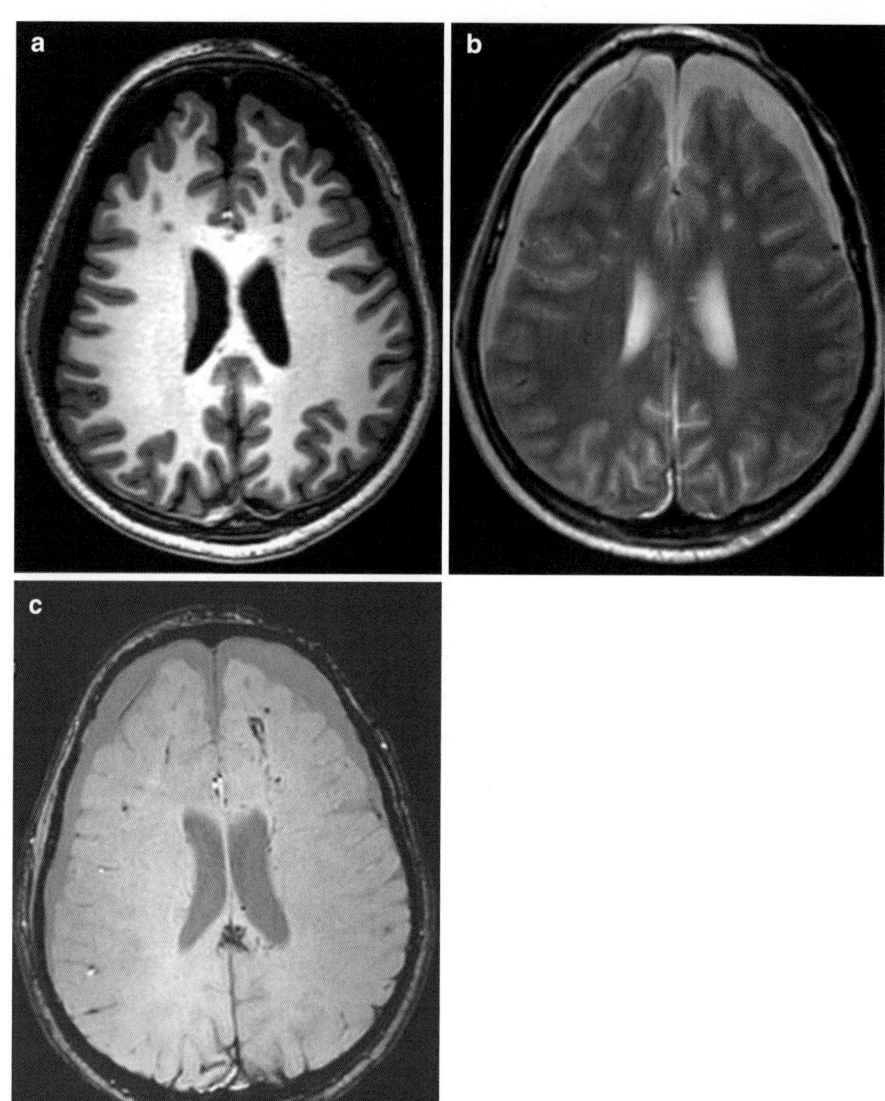

图 21.2 74 岁接受抗血小板治疗男性患者轴位 T1WI（a）、轴位 T2WI（b）和轴位 SWI（c）提示双侧 CSDH

到目前为止，CSDH 患者手术后重新开始使用抗血栓药物的时机仍不清楚。大多数研究表明，CSDH 复发于手术后的第一个月[11]。Phan 等建议在这段时间后再重新使用抗血栓药物[46]。Amano 等指出在确认 CSDH 术后出血并发症风险消失后，必须尽快恢复抗血栓治疗用药[3]。因此，他们建议在手术治疗后的第二天恢复使用抗血栓药物[3]。然而，没有关于重新使用抗血栓药物最佳时间的随机对照试验。因此未来的研究应集中于明确重新开始抗血栓治疗在不同时期的效果。决定何时重新开始抗血栓药物是困难且复杂的，所以恢复抗血栓药物应基于个体化的建议。

21.6 血液系统恶性肿瘤

与 SDH 相比，血液系统恶性肿瘤患者更容易发生脑实质内脑出血（intracerebral hemorrhage，ICH）和蛛网膜下腔出血。然而，随着新的治疗方案的出现，白血病和淋巴瘤患者的预期寿命随之增加，这些患者更容易发生 CSDH[9-10, 29]。造血干细胞移植、诊断治疗性腰椎穿刺、化疗给药、凝血功能障碍、血小板功能障碍均是该患者组 CSDH 发生及治疗后复发的危险因素[25, 43, 60]。与其他血液系统恶性肿瘤相比，急性髓系白血病（AML）患者发生脑出血的风险增加[12]。其他恶性肿瘤如原发性中枢神经系统（CNS）淋巴瘤、血管内淋巴瘤和骨髓瘤也可导致脑出血风险增加[12]。与 ICH 相比，SDH 更常在老年患者中出现[12]。此外，SDH 患者的临床症状出现时间比 ICH 患者更晚。

与创伤或使用抗血栓药物引起的 SDH 相比，血液系统恶性肿瘤引起的 SDH 的复发率、手术致残率和死亡率更高[29]。血液系统恶性肿瘤患者的手术风险高。术前缩短出血时间，适当输血纠正凝血功能障碍是必要的，但这种术前干预的作用通常只是暂时的。血液系统恶性肿瘤患者通常年龄较大，同时也患有其他的临床疾病，因此手术治疗方案很难选择，需经多学科讨论。在 Reichman 等发表的一项研究中，32% 的血液系统恶性肿瘤合并 SDH 的患者接受了手术治疗[48]。在 Owattanapanich 等的队列研究中 10% 的患者接受了手术治疗，结果显示接受手术治疗的患者生存率高于未接受手术治疗的患者[44]。Wright 等发现，血液系统恶性肿瘤患者中 SDH 患者的预后较 ICH 患者好[64]。然而，无论是何种治疗方案，患者的中位生存期仍小于 5 个月[64]，手术患者的复发率为 9%～30%[34, 52]。血红蛋白和血小板水平低、凝血酶原时间延长和高龄均与死亡率增加相关[12, 64]。

临床密切关注老年患者的神经症状和体征是很重要的。如果怀疑相关神经系统症状或体征是 SDH 引起的，应迅速进行神经影像学检查并进一步诊断。老年患者的预期寿命通常不到 5 个月，因此血液科医生、肿瘤科医生、神经外科医生和患者家属应该共同讨论是否有必要对预期寿命有限的患者进行手术[64]。

21.7　难治性血小板减少

CSDH 清除术不属于神经外科重大手术。即使在局部麻醉下也可以进行手术，手术过程中预计不会大量失血[2]。建议在手术前血小板计数应达到 100 000/μl[35]。如果血小板计数低于此值，术后急性出血的风险增加。在急诊手术中，建议血小板计数不低于 80 000/μl[2]。Abdelfatah 等对 41 例 CSDH 合并难治性血小板减少症患者进行了评估[2]。所有患者入院时血小板计数均少于 60 000/μl。尽管采用了异体血小板输注，但所有患者血小板总值也无法高于 80 000/μl。手术采用双点钻孔方法进行 SDH 清除并在术中留置硬脑膜下引流管，所有患者临床症状均有改善且术后早期未发现急性 SDH。只有 2 例患者在 1 个月内出现 CSDH 复发，并再次进行了引流手术。尽管尚无充分研究证实顽固性血小板减少症对 CSDH 患者的影响，但采用异体血小板输注将血小板计数提升至 50 000/μl 以上，似乎足以满足手术需求。

21.8　造血干细胞移植（hematopoietic stem cell transplantation，HSCT）

HSCT 后的 CSDH 是一种罕见但严重且危及生命的并发症[14, 47]。因为 HSCT 后的 CSDH 有时并不表现出典型的临床症状和体征，因此该病诊断比较困难。在非霍奇金淋巴瘤患者中，有 5%～9% 可检测到软脑膜浸润或实质肿块[32]，特别是当造血干细胞移植再生期出现血小板减少时，发生 CSDH 的风险相当高。虽然只有少数病例报告提到 HSCT 后并发 CSDH，但当患者在 HSCT 后出现头痛、偏瘫、吞咽困难或意识改变时，应考虑与 CSDH 进行鉴别诊断。HSCT 后的 CSDH 诊断和治疗应与包括血液科和神经外科在内的专家进行多学科会诊[23, 26]。

21.9　特发性血小板减少性紫癜（idiopathic thrombocytopenic purpura，ITP）

特发性血小板减少性紫癜是一种自身免疫性疾病，主要病因为抗体结合的血小板被免疫系统破坏[27]。颅内出血是一种罕见的出血来源，发生在 1% 的 ITP 患者中[18]。出血通常表现为实质内或蛛网膜下腔出血，但 CSDH 很少见。在目前的文献中，仅病例报告报道了少数患者出现 CSDH[28, 53-54, 56]。

CSDH 患者通常存在外伤病史，然而创伤在合并 ITP 的 CSDH 患者病史中并不常见[54]。合并 ITP 的 CSDH 患者临床表现为头痛、偏瘫、意识改变，常伴有皮肤黏膜出血[49]，相关神经症状和体征在 20 岁以下的患者中更为常见。手术清除 SDH 应在纠正患者血液疾病后进行。对于无神经功能缺损或血肿大小未增大的患者可考虑保守治疗。皮质类固醇、丙种球蛋白静脉注射和脾切除术可改善患者的血液学状况[54]。Lee 和 Kim 的一项研究表明，脾切除术对 3 例伴有 CSDH 的 ITP 患者中的 2 例是有益的[31]。此外，研究表明皮质类固醇和丙种球蛋白静脉注射有助于提高大多数患者的血小板水平，皮质类固醇具有预防 CSDH 进展的作用[49]。手术治疗需在患者神经功能缺损进行性加重或血肿增大时立刻进行。

21.10 结论

关于抗血栓药物与 CSDH 复发的关系已有多项研究，然而结果并不一致。抗凝药的使用增加了 CSDH 的复发风险。使用抗血小板和抗凝药物的患者有较高的 CSDH 复发风险，然而联合用药并未增加 CSDH 患者的死亡风险。随着白血病和淋巴瘤患者的预期寿命随着新的治疗方案诞生而增加，这些患者更有可能发展为 CSDH 而不是 ICH。此外，ITP、血小板减少症和 HSCT 都是发生 CSDH 的危险因素。

参考文献

1. Abboud T, Dhrsen L, Gibbert C, Westphal M, Martens T. Influence of antithrombotic agents on recurrence rate and clinical outcome in patients operated for chronic subdural hematoma. Neurocirugía (English Edition). 2018;29:86–92.
2. Abdelfatah M. Management of chronic subdural hematoma in patients with intractable thrombocytopenia. Turk Neurosurg. 2018;28:400–4.
3. Amano T, Takahara K, Maehara N, Shimogawa T, Mukae N, Sayama T, Arihiro S, Arakawa S, Morioka T, Haga S. Optimal perioperative management of antithrombotic agents in patients with chronic subdural hematoma. Clin Neurol Neurosurg. 2016;151:43–50.
4. Arai N, Mine Y, Kagami H, Maruyama M, Daikoh A, Inaba M. Safe burr hole surgery for chronic subdural hematoma using dabigatran with idarucizumab. World Neurosurg. 2018;109:432–5.
5. Aspegren OP, Åstrand R, Lundgren MI, Romner B. Anticoagulation therapy a risk factor for the development of chronic subdural hematoma. Clin Neurol Neurosurg. 2013;115:981–4.
6. Baraniskin A, Steffens C, Harders A, Schmiegel W, Schroers R, Spangenberg P. Impact of prehospital antithrombotic medication on the outcome of chronic and acute subdural hematoma. J Neurol Surg A Cent Eur Neurosurg. 2014;75:031–6.
7. Bartek J, Sjåvik K, Kristiansson H, Ståhl F, Fornebo I, Förander P, Jakola AS. Predictors of recurrence and complications after chronic subdural hematoma surgery: a population-based study. World Neurosurg. 2017;106:609–14.
8. Beck J, Gralla J, Fung C, Ulrich CT, Schucht P, Fichtner J, Andereggen L, Gosau M, Hattingen E, Gutbrod K. Spinal cerebrospinal fluid leak as the cause of chronic subdural hematomas in nongeriatric patients. J Neurosurg. 2014;121:1380–7.
9. Bower H, Björkholm M, Dickman PW, Höglund M, Lambert PC, Andersson TM-L. Life expectancy of patients with chronic myeloid leukemia approaches the life expectancy of the general population. J Clin Oncol. 2016;34:2851–7.
10. Bureau UC. An aging nation: projected number of children and older adults. In: The United States Census Bureau. https://www.census.gov/library/visualizations/2018/comm/historic-first.html. Accessed 3 July 2020.
11. Chari A, Clemente Morgado T, Rigamonti D. Recommencement of anticoagulation in chronic subdural haematoma: a systematic review and meta-analysis. Br J Neurosurg. 2014;28:2–7.
12. Chen CY, Tai CH, Cheng A, Wu HC, Tsay W, Liu JH, Chen PY, Huang SY, Yao M, Tang JL, Tien HF. Intracranial hemorrhage in adult patients with hematological malignancies. BMC Med. 2012;10:97.
13. Chon K-H, Lee J-M, Koh E-J, Choi H-Y. Independent predictors for recurrence of chronic subdural hematoma. Acta Neurochir. 2012;154:1541–8.
14. Colosimo M, McCarthy N, Jayasinghe R, Morton J, Taylor K, Durrant S. Diagnosis and management of subdural haematoma complicating bone marrow transplantation. Bone Marrow Transplant. 2000;25:549–52.
15. Ducruet AF, Grobelny BT, Zacharia BE, Hickman ZL, DeRosa PL, Anderson K, Sussman E, Carpenter A, Connolly ES. The surgical management of chronic subdural hematoma. Neurosurg Rev. 2012;35:155–69.
16. Fornebo I, Sjåvik K, Alibeck M, Kristiansson H, Ståhl F, Förander P, Jakola AS, Bartek J. Role of antithrombotic therapy in the risk of hematoma recurrence and thromboembolism after chronic subdural hematoma evacuation: a population-based consecutive cohort study. Acta Neurochir (Wien). 2017;159:2045–52.
17. Forster M, Mathé A, Senft C, Scharrer I, Seifert V, Gerlach R. The influence of preoperative anticoagulation on outcome and quality of life after surgical treatment of chronic subdural

hematoma. J Clin Neurosci. 2010;17:975–9.
18. George JN, Woolf SH, Raskob GE, Wasser JS, Aledort LM, Ballem PJ, Blanchette VS, Bussel JB, Cines DB, Kelton JG, Lichtin AE, McMillan R, Okerbloom JA, Regan DH, Warrier I. Idiopathic thrombocytopenic purpura: a practice guideline developed by explicit methods for the American Society of Hematology. Blood. 1996;88:3–40.
19. Gray E, Hogwood J, Mulloy B. The anticoagulant and antithrombotic mechanisms of heparin. Handb Exp Pharmacol. 2012;207:43–61.
20. Guha D, Coyne S, Macdonald RL. Timing of the resumption of antithrombotic agents following surgical evacuation of chronic subdural hematomas: a retrospective cohort study. J Neurosurg. 2016;124:750–9.
21. Hanley JP. Warfarin reversal. J Clin Pathol. 2004;57:1132–9.
22. Harrison NE, Gottlieb M. Comparison of fresh frozen plasma with prothrombin complex concentrate for warfarin reversal. Ann Emerg Med. 2017;69:777–9.
23. Hilgendorf I, Wilhelm S, Prall F, Junghanss C, Steiner B, Wolff D, Freund M, Casper J. Headache after hematopoietic stem cell transplantation: being aware of chronic bilateral subdural hematoma. Leuk Lymphoma. 2006;47:2247–9.
24. Honda Y, Sorimachi T, Momose H, Takizawa K, Inokuchi S, Matsumae M. Chronic subdural haematoma associated with disturbance of consciousness: significance of acute-on-chronic subdural haematoma. Neurol Res. 2015;37:985–92.
25. Jourdan E, Dombret H, Glaisner S, Micléa JM, Castaigne S, Degos L. Unexpected high incidence of intracranial subdural haematoma during intensive chemotherapy for acute myeloid leukaemia with a monoblastic component. Br J Haematol. 1995;89:527–30.
26. Kannan K, Koh LP, Linn YC. Subdural hematoma in two hematopoietic stem cell transplant patients with post-dural puncture headache and initially normal CT brain scan. Ann Hematol. 2002;81:540–2.
27. Karpatkin S. Autoimmune thrombocytopenic purpura. Semin Hematol. 1985;22:260–88.
28. Kolluri VR, Reddy DR, Reddy PK, Naidu MR, Kumari CS. Subdural hematoma secondary to immune thrombocytopenic purpura: case report. Neurosurgery. 1986;19:635–6.
29. Krok-Schoen JL, Fisher JL, Stephens JA, Mims A, Ayyappan S, Woyach JA, Rosko AE. Incidence and survival of hematological cancers among adults ages ≥75 years. Cancer Med. 2018;7(7):3425–33. https://doi.org/10.1002/cam4.1461.
30. Le Roux P, Pollack CV, Milan M, Schaefer A. Race against the clock: overcoming challenges in the management of anticoagulant-associated intracerebral hemorrhage. J Neurosurg. 2014;121(Suppl):1–20.
31. Lee MS, Kim WC. Intracranial hemorrhage associated with idiopathic thrombocytopenic purpura: report of seven patients and a meta-analysis. Neurology. 1998;50:1160–3.
32. Levitt LJ, Dawson DM, Rosenthal DS, Moloney WC. CNS involvement in the non-Hodgkin's lymphomas. Cancer. 1980;45:545–52.
33. Lindvall P, Koskinen L-OD. Anticoagulants and antiplatelet agents and the risk of development and recurrence of chronic subdural haematomas. J Clin Neurosci. 2009;16:1287–90.
34. Liu W, Bakker NA, Groen RJM. Chronic subdural hematoma: a systematic review and meta-analysis of surgical procedures. J Neurosurg. 2014;121:665–73.
35. Liumbruno G, Bennardello F, Lattanzio A, Piccoli P, Rossetti G, Italian Society of Transfusion Medicine and Immunohaematology (SIMTI) Work Group. Recommendations for the transfusion of plasma and platelets. Blood Transfus. 2009;7:132–50.
36. Matsumoto H, Hanayama H, Okada T, Sakurai Y, Minami H, Masuda A, Tominaga S, Miyaji K, Yamaura I, Yoshida Y, Yoshida K. Clinical investigation of refractory chronic subdural hematoma: a comparison of clinical factors between single and repeated recurrences. World Neurosurg. 2017;107:706–15.
37. Mehta V, Harward SC, Sankey EW, Nayar G, Codd PJ. Evidence based diagnosis and management of chronic subdural hematoma: a review of the literature. J Clin Neurosci. 2018;50:7–15.
38. Motiei-Langroudi R, Stippler M, Shi S, Adeeb N, Gupta R, Griessenauer CJ, Papavassiliou E, Kasper EM, Arle J, Alterman RL. Factors predicting reoperation of chronic subdural hematoma following primary surgical evacuation. J Neurosurg. 2017;129:1143–50.
39. Motoie R, Karashima S, Otsuji R, Ren N, Nagaoka S, Maeda K, Ikai Y, Uno J, Gi H. Recurrence in 787 patients with chronic subdural hematoma: retrospective cohort investigation of associated factors including direct oral anticoagulant use. World Neurosurg. 2018;118:e87–91.
40. Nagalla S, Thomson L, Oppong Y, Bachman B, Chervoneva I, Kraft WK. Reversibility of apixaban anticoagulation with a four-factor prothrombin complex concentrate in healthy vol-

unteers. Clin Transl Sci. 2016;9:176–80.
41. Nathan S, Goodarzi Z, Jette N, Gallagher C, Holroyd-Leduc J. Anticoagulant and antiplatelet use in seniors with chronic subdural hematoma: systematic review. Neurology. 2017;88:1889–93.
42. Ohba S, Kinoshita Y, Nakagawa T, Murakami H. The risk factors for recurrence of chronic subdural hematoma. Neurosurg Rev. 2013;36:145–9.
43. Openshaw H, Ressler JA, Snyder DS. Lumbar puncture and subdural hygroma and hematomas in hematopoietic cell transplant patients. Bone Marrow Transplant. 2008;41:791–5.
44. Owattanapanich W, Auewarakul CU. Intracranial hemorrhage in patients with hematologic disorders: prevalence and predictive factors. J Med Assoc Thai. 2016;99:15–24.
45. Patel S, Singh R, Preuss CV, Patel N. Warfarin. StatPearls; 2020.
46. Phan K, Abi-Hanna D, Kerferd J, Lu VM, Dmytriw AA, Ho Y-T, Fairhall J, Reddy R, Wilson P. Resumption of antithrombotic agents in chronic subdural hematoma: a systematic review and meta-analysis. World Neurosurg. 2018;109:e792–9.
47. Pomeranz S, Naparstek E, Ashkenazi E, Nagler A, Lossos A, Slavin S, Or R. Intracranial haematomas following bone marrow transplantation. J Neurol. 1994;241:252–6.
48. Reichman J, Singer S, Navi B, Reiner A, Panageas K, Gutin PH, Deangelis LM. Subdural hematoma in patients with cancer. Neurosurgery. 2012;71:74–9.
49. Rodeghiero F. Idiopathic thrombocytopenic purpura: an old disease revisited in the era of evidence-based medicine. Haematologica. 2003;88:1081–7.
50. Rust T, Kiemer N, Erasmus A. Chronic subdural haematomas and anticoagulation or antithrombotic therapy. J Clin Neurosci. 2006;13:823–7.
51. Santarius T, Hutchinson P. Chronic subdural haematoma: time to rationalize treatment? Br J Neurosurg. 2004;18:328–32.
52. Schwarz F, Loos F, Dünisch P, Sakr Y, Safatli DA, Kalff R, Ewald C. Risk factors for reoperation after initial burr hole trephination in chronic subdural hematomas. Clin Neurol Neurosurg. 2015;138:66–71.
53. Sebe A, Ohshima T, Ebisudani D, Oka H, Matsumoto K, Yoshizima S. A case of chronic subdural hematoma associated with idiopathic thrombocytopenic purpura (ITP) (in Japan). No Shinkei Geka. 1990;18:761–5.
54. Seçkin H, Kazanci A, Yigitkanli K, Simsek S, Kars HZ. Chronic subdural hematoma in patients with idiopathic thrombocytopenic purpura: a case report and review of the literature. Surg Neurol. 2006;66:411–4.
55. da Silva RMFL. Novel oral anticoagulants in non-valvular atrial fibrillation. Cardiovasc Hematol Agents Med Chem. 2014;12:3–8.
56. Sreedharan PS, Rakesh S, Sajeev S, Pavithran K, Thomas M. Subdural haematoma with spontaneous resolution—rare manifestation of idiopathic thrombocytopenic purpura. J Assoc Physicians India. 2000;48:432–4.
57. Taylor G, Osinski D, Thevenin A, Devys J-M. Is platelet transfusion efficient to restore platelet reactivity in patients who are responders to aspirin and/or clopidogrel before emergency surgery? J Trauma Acute Care Surg. 2013;74:1367–9.
58. Tohgi H, Konno S, Tamura K, Kimura B, Kawano K. Effects of low-to-high doses of aspirin on platelet aggregability and metabolites of thromboxane A2 and prostacyclin. Stroke. 1992;23:1400–3.
59. Toi H, Kinoshita K, Hirai S, Takai H, Hara K, Matsushita N, Matsubara S, Otani M, Muramatsu K, Matsuda S, Fushimi K, Uno M. Present epidemiology of chronic subdural hematoma in Japan: analysis of 63,358 cases recorded in a national administrative database. J Neurosurg. 2018;128:222–8.
60. Ureshino H, Nishioka A, Kojima K, Kizuka H, Sano H, Shindo T, Kubota Y, Ando T, Kimura S. Subdural hematoma associated with dasatinib and intrathecal methotrexate treatment in Philadelphia Chromosome-positive Acute Lymphoblastic Leukemia. Intern Med. 2016;55:2703–6.
61. Vílchez JA, Gallego P, Lip GYH. Safety of new oral anticoagulant drugs: a perspective. Ther Adv Drug Saf. 2014;5:8–20.
62. Wada M, Yamakami I, Higuchi Y, Tanaka M, Suda S, Ono J, Saeki N. Influence of antiplatelet therapy on postoperative recurrence of chronic subdural hematoma: a multicenter retrospective study in 719 patients. Clin Neurol Neurosurg. 2014;120:49–54.
63. Wang H, Zhang M, Zheng H, Xia X, Luo K, Guo F, Qian C. The effects of antithrombotic drugs on the recurrence and mortality in patients with chronic subdural hematoma: a metaanalysis. Medicine (Baltimore). 2019;98:e13972.

64. Wright CH, Wright J, Alonso A, Raghavan A, Momotaz H, Burant C, Zhou X, Selman W, Sajatovic M, Hoffer A. Subdural hematoma in patients with hematologic malignancies: an outcome analysis and examination of risk factors of operative and nonoperative management. World Neurosurg. 2019;130:e1061–9.
65. Yeon JY, Kong D-S, Hong S-C. Safety of early warfarin resumption following burr hole drainage for warfarin-associated subacute or chronic subdural hemorrhage. J Neurotrauma. 2012;29:1334–41.
66. Yogaratnam D, Ditch K, Medeiros K, Doyno C, Fong JJ. Idarucizumab for reversal of dabigatran-associated anticoagulation. Ann Pharmacother. 2016;50:847–54.

第 22 章 合并颅内血管畸形的急性和慢性硬膜下血肿

Haydn Hoffman 和 Grahame C. Gould

译者：张烁

22.1 引言

硬膜下血肿（subdural hematoma，SDH）的最常见病因是外伤，但是一部分自发性 SDH 是由血管畸形引起的，颅内血管畸形包括动静脉畸形（arteriovenous malformations，AVM）和海绵状血管畸形（cavernous malformations，CM）。AVM 是动脉与静脉之间的异常连接，中间没有毛细血管的存在，大致表现为扩张的血管团。AVM 破裂通常会导致脑实质出血（intraparenchymal hemorrhage，IPH）伴或不伴蛛网膜下腔出血（subarachnoid hemorrhage，SAH）或脑室内出血（intraventricular hemorrhage，IVH），但 SDH 也有可能发生。CM 是脑实质内扩张的异常血管团，占颅内血管畸形的 10%～20%，它们的破裂通常导致局部 IPH，然而 SDH 也可能发生于表浅的 CM。虽然不是真正的畸形，但硬脑膜动静脉瘘（dAVF）经常被认为是其他颅内血管畸形的一类而归在本章中讨论。dAVF 被认为是后天形成的，是硬脑膜动脉和静脉之间的瘘性连接，占颅内血管畸形的 10%～15%。dAVF 存在特异性的临床症状，包括头痛、眼部症状、耳鸣和非出血性神经功能缺损（non-hemorrhagic neurologic deficits，NHND）。dAVF 破裂可能导致 IPH 和 SAH，SDH 则较少见。在 Lasjaunias 对 191 例 dAVF 的回顾中，41 例出血中的 5 例（12.2%）导致了 SDH[9]。在最近的一系列研究中，在发生 dAVF 相关出血的患者中，有 18% 发生了 SDH[5]。

22.2 流行病学

临床中 AVM 罕见，因此缺乏基于人群的流行病数据，但据估计发病率为每年（0.55～1.21）/10 万[18]。AVM 在男性中稍多见，平均发病年龄为 33 岁，与 Osler-Weber-Rendu 综合征（遗传性出血性毛细血管扩张症）相关。CM 存在于 0.02%～0.16% 的人群中，其发病特点是散发性或遗传性的，后者经常出现多发性病变。CM 发病无性别差异。dAVF 通常在五六十岁时被发现，并且发病无性别差异[15]。

22.3 自然史

AVM 的自然史是存在争议的。经常被引用的 4% 的年出血率来源于一项针对有症状 AVM 患者的经血管造影结果证实的大型前瞻性研究[13]。考虑到纳入的是症状性人群，4% 的出血率可能是被高估的，并不适用于所有的动静脉畸形。最近的研究发现，AVM 的年出血率接近 2%～3%[6, 8]。AVM 破裂的危险因素包括既往出血史、深静脉引流、相关动脉瘤（约 7% 的 AVM 患者存在）和引流静脉狭窄。

偶然发现的非脑干部位的 CM 年出血率很低（0.3%），脑干部位的 CM 年出血率为 2.8%[20]。与 AVM 类似，存在既往出血史的 CM 未来出血的风险也大大增加。此外，CM 的出血可能表现出一种时间聚集现象，即在初次出血后不久就容易再次出现出血[2]。

dAVF 的自然史是由皮质静脉引流（CVD）的存在或缺失决定的。无 CVD 的 dAVF 被认为是良性病变，无出血风险。CVD 的存在预示着高出血风险，出血概率从 1.5% 到 8%[15]。在那些合并 CVD 的患者中，既往出血史或 NHND 会增加其血管破裂出血的风险。

22.4 解剖学

硬脑膜主要由脑膜前动脉（AMA）、脑膜中动脉（MMA）和脑膜后动脉（PMA）供血。对脑膜血液供应贡献最大的是 MMA，它是上颌内动脉的近端分支。慢性 SDH 患者的 MMA 可能是增粗的，如图 22.1 所示。大多数 dAVF 患者的病变部位的供血来自于 MMA 的分支动脉，该动脉容易栓塞是因为它相对较直且易于导航。MMA 栓塞疗法是一种越来越流行的治疗慢性 SDH 的方法，慢性 SDH 由于其脆弱的血管膜在血管造影中有特征性表现。图 22.2 显示慢性 SDH 膜内的造影剂滞留和来自 MMA 的供血。PMA 通常是椎动脉 V3 段的一个分支，供应颅后窝硬脑膜。颅后窝硬脑膜也有来自枕动脉、咽升动脉和耳后动脉的供血，在岩鳞部区域与 MMA 血供达到血流动力学平衡。颅后窝 dAVF 可能来自多支血管供血。AMA 起源于筛动脉（眼动脉的分支），并在上矢状窦壁内行进，供应额突硬脑膜。脑膜下干是颈内动脉海绵窦段的一个分支，分别经小脑幕动脉（Bernasconi 和 Cassinari）和脑膜背动脉供应小脑幕和斜坡硬膜。

22.5 分类

AVM 通常根据 Spetzler-Martin 进行分级，该量表根据病灶大小（1：< 3 cm；2：3 ~ 6 cm；3：> 6 cm），有无深静脉引流（0：无；1：有）和是

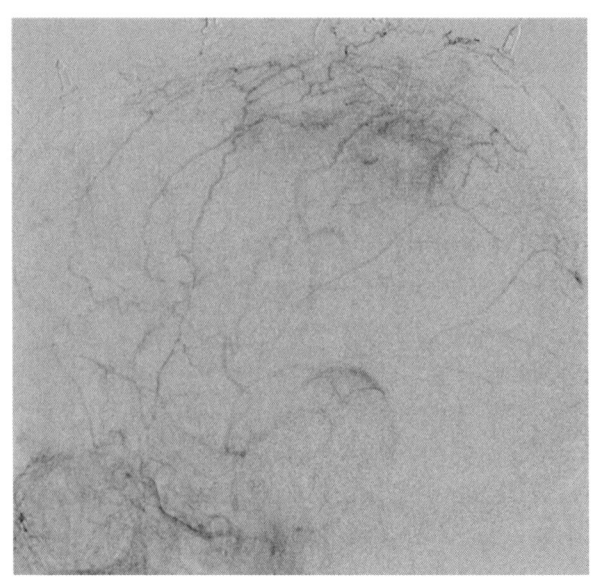

图 22.2 如图 22.1 所示，同一例患者左侧颈外动脉毛细血管期注射造影剂，提示慢性硬膜下血肿内出现高浓度造影剂

否为功能区（0：非功能区；1：功能区）进行分级。分级从 1 到 5 级，与手术发病率和死亡率成正比。Spetzler 和 Ponce 根据 Spetzler-Martin 分级将 AVM 归纳为三类，并提出了治疗建议。1 级和 2 级合并（A 类），建议手术切除，3 级（B 类）认为最适合多模态治疗，4 级和 5 级合并（C 类）建议观察[17]。最后，Lawton 和 Young 补充了现有的 Spetzler-Martin 评分方案，加入了年龄（1：< 20 岁；2：20 ~ 40 岁；3：> 40 岁），未破裂 AVM（0：破裂；1：未破裂）和弥散形态（0：紧密型；1：弥散型）[10]。当这些因素被添加到 Spetzler-Martin 分级中并以 6 分为阈值后（1 ~ 6：中低风险；> 6：高风险），该评分能够比单独的 Spetzler-Martin 量表更加准确地预测手术效果[10]。

目前尚不存在具有广泛临床应用价值的 CM 分类，但已经提出了一种基于 MRI 表现与出血风险相关的影像学分类。Zabramski 等描述：1 型病变在 T1 像上呈高信号，在 T2 像上呈高或低信号；2 型病变呈典型的"爆米花"状，核心呈网状；3 型病变在 T1 和 T2 像上呈等信号，提示慢性出血；4 型病变以点状低信号为特征，仅在 GRE 序列上可见[21]。4 型病变通常见于家族型。1 型和 2 型 CM 的出血率高于 3 型和 4 型[12]。

dAVF 最常用的分类方案是 Borden 和 Cognard 量表。静脉引流方式是 dAVF 出血倾向的最重要决定因素，上述两种量表评分都受静脉引流方式

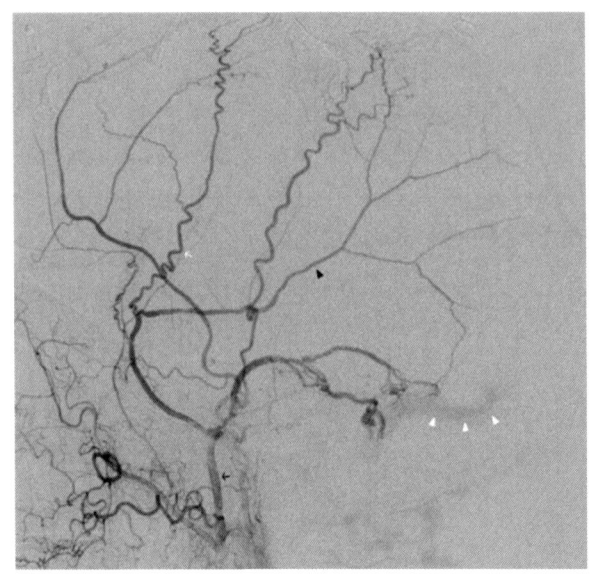

图 22.1 一例复发性 CSDH 患者行右侧颈外动脉动脉期栓塞治疗，表现为脑膜中动脉（MMA）栓塞，横窦、乙状窦交界处出现早期逆行性阴影来源于 MMA 岩部分支的扩大。（黑色箭号：MMA 主干近端；白色箭号：MMA 额支；黑色三角箭头：MMA 顶支；白色三角箭头：横窦早期阴影）

的影响。Borden 分类包括 1 型：顺行引流至硬脑膜窦或脑膜静脉；2 型：顺行引流至硬脑膜窦并逆行皮质静脉引流；3 型：孤立的逆行皮质静脉直接引流至皮质静脉[3]。Cognard 分类包括 1 型：顺行引流至硬脑膜窦；2a 型：逆行引流至硬脑膜窦；2b 型：顺行引流至硬脑膜窦伴皮质静脉回流；2a+b 型：逆行引流至硬脑膜窦伴皮质静脉回流；3 型：直接皮质静脉引流；4 型：直接皮质静脉引流伴静脉扩张；5 型：引流至脊髓髓周静脉[4]。

22.6　诊断

当患者在没有外伤的情况下出现急性 SDH 时，进行血管成像是必要的。无其他原因的 SDH 血肿量延迟增加也应警惕血管畸形的可能[14]。老年患者出现慢性 SDH 可能是由于其远期轻微创伤无法回忆。此类情况通常无需进行血管成像，除非存在其他提示潜在结构性血管病因的发现。

当需要对颅内血管系统进行检查时，通常首先进行无创成像，如 CT 血管造影（CTA）或 MR 血管造影（MRA）。AVM 表现为血管的团簇状异常连接，有供血动脉和引流静脉分别进入和离开畸形血管团。CM 在血管造影上是隐匿的，在 CT、CTA 或 MRA 上不能很好地显示，但可以检测到异常的静脉发育。CM 的首选成像方式是 MRI。它们在 MRI 上的典型表现是不同出血时期的血液成分被含铁血黄素环包围，通常被描述为"爆米花"外观，尽管这仅适用于 Zabramski 2 型病变。磁敏感性加权成像序列对血液成分高度敏感，非常适合检测 CM。大多数 dAVF 用 CTA 和 MRA 评估不理想，但可能表现为扩张的供血动脉或扩张的引流静脉，伴或不伴静脉充血。时间飞跃法磁共振血管成像可用于早期静脉引流的检测。当无创成像怀疑存在 AVM 或 dAVF 诊断时，要进行数字减影血管造影（DSA）以确认诊断，获得其血管结构的更多细节，并计划择期治疗。DSA 是评估这些病变的金标准，而 DSA 不适用于 CM。

22.7　治疗

急性 SDH 引起的占位效应和神经功能障碍需要尽快解除，然后才能确定相关的血管病因。慢性 SDH 如果出现严重的中线移位和神经功能障碍，也需要紧急手术清除。等患者病情稳定后，如有需要可进行出血病因检查。

AVM 通常可采用手术切除、介入栓塞、立体定向放射治疗或几种方式联合治疗。主要是 Spetzler 和 Ponce 记载的 Spetzler-Martin 分级中 Ⅰ 级 Ⅱ 级的 AVM 病灶，如果术后致残率相对较低，手术切除是最佳的治愈办法[17]。Spetzler-Martin Ⅲ 级 AVM 具有更大的手术风险，通常在术前进行栓塞或放疗联合栓塞治疗。在放疗联合栓塞治疗 2～3 年后 AVM 血管才能完全闭塞，这限制了其在已破裂病例中的应用。Spetzler-Martin Ⅳ 级和 Ⅴ 级 AVM 的任何治疗方法都是高风险的，除非出现症状，否则通常不应积极干预。与 Ⅲ 级 AVM 一样，治疗通常采取多方案联合。

CM 病变如果合并出血并在手术可以达到的位置，应当手术切除。在 SDH 的情况下，CM 可能部位比较浅表，可以在血肿清除时一并切除。在一项研究中提到 CM 可能附着在硬脑膜上，可于 SDH 清除时一并切除[19]。放射手术已被认作为 CM 的一种治疗选择，但并不能确认可有效改变其疾病自然史。

dAVF 常用血管内治疗，但某些部位适合应用显微手术来阻断瘘间连接。包括前颅底、小脑幕和枕骨大孔 dAVF。相关文献综述报道，dAVF 引起孤立性 SDH 病变均匀分布于颅前窝、颅中窝以及额、颞、顶枕部[11]。

22.8　预后

AVM 破裂后的预后取决于出血的多少和位置、是否存在 IVH、是否存在相关动脉瘤和患者年龄[1,7]。在颅后窝和功能区 AVM 的患者预后较差[1]。总体而言，AVM 出血后的死亡率约 20%，只有 35% 的患者能完全恢复[7]。手术预后与 Spetzler-Martin 分级密切相关，不良预后的发生率从 Ⅰ 级病变的 4% 增加到 Ⅴ 级病变的 37%[16]。CM 出血后的预后与病变位置有关，功能区和脑干 CM 预后较差，并且可能遗留永久神经功能障碍。脑干 CM 的手术治疗往往会导致神经功能症状的短暂恶化，但患者最终结局会得到改善。破裂的 dAVF 预后总体较好，超过 2/3 的患者恢复后症状很轻微或没有症状[5]。

22.9 结论

血管畸形是 SDH 发生的罕见原因，当没有外伤史出现 SDH 时应对其予以警惕。在巨大 SDH 引起脑疝的情况下，评估血管畸形之前应将血肿及时清除，防止神经系统症状进一步加重。引起 SDH 的 CM 通常是表面性或外生性的，可以在血肿清除时一并切除。AVM 和 dAVF 需要 DSA 来确定其形态并制订治疗策略。血管畸形的成功治疗需要对其自然史、血管结构、病理特征和治疗方式有透彻的了解。

参考文献

1. Abla AA, Nelson J, Rutledge WC, Young WL, Kim H, Lawton MT. The natural history of AVM hemorrhage in the posterior fossa: comparison of hematoma volumes and neurological outcomes in patients with ruptured infra- and supratentorial AVMs. Neurosurg Focus. 2014;37:E6.
2. Barker FG 2nd, Amin-Hanjani S, Butler WE, Lyson S, Ojemann RG, Chapman PH, et al. Temporal clustering of hemorrhages from untreated cavernous malformations of the central nervous system. Neurosurgery. 2001;49:15–24.
3. Borden JA, Wu JK, Schucart WA. A proposed classification for spinal and cranial dural arteriovenous fistulous malformations and implications for treatment. J Neurosurg. 1995;82:166–79.
4. Cognard C, Gobin YP, Pierot L, Bailly AL, Houdart E, Casasco A, et al. Cerebral dural arteriovenous fistulas: clinical and angiographic correlation with a revised classification of venous drainage. Radiology. 1995;194:671–80.
5. Daniels DJ, Vellimana AK, Zipfel GJ, Lanzino G. Intracranial hemorrhage from dural arteriovenous fistulas: clinical features and outcome. Neurosurg Focus. 2013;34:E15.
6. Gross BA, Du R. Natural history of cerebral arteriovenous malformations: a meta-analysis. J Neurosurg. 2013;118:437–43.
7. Karlsson B, Jokura H, Yang H, Yamamoto M, Martinez R, Kawagishi J, et al. Clinical outcome following cerebral AVM hemorrhage. Acta Neurochir (Wien). 2020;162:1759–66.
8. Kim H, Salman RA, McCulloch CE, Stapf C, Young WL. Untreated brain arteriovenous malformation: patient-level meta-analysis of hemorrhage predictors. Neurology. 2014;83:590–7.
9. Lasjaunias P, Chiu M, ter Brugge K, Tolia A, Hurth A, Bernstein M. Neurological manifestations of intracranial dural arteriovenous malformations. J Neurosurg. 1986;64:724–30.
10. Lawton MT, Kim H, McCulloch CE, Mikhak B, Young WL. A supplementary grading scale for selecting patients with brain arteriovenous malformations for surgery. Neurosurgery. 2010;66:702–13.
11. Li G, Zhang Y, Zhao J, Zhu X, Yu J, Hou K. Isolated subdural hematoma secondary to dural arteriovenous fistula: a case report and literature review. BMC Neurol. 2019;19:43.
12. Nikoubashman O, Rocco D, Davagnanam I, Mankad K, Zerah M, Wiesmann M. Prospective hemorrhage rates of cerebral cavernous malformations in children and adolescents based on MRI appearance. AJNR Am J Neuroradiol. 2015;36:2177–83.
13. Ondra SL, Troupp H, George ED, Schwab K. The natural history of symptomatic arteriovenous malformations of the brain: a 24-year follow-up assessment. J Neurosurg. 1990;73:387–91.
14. Parr M, Patel N, Kauffmann J, Al-Mufti F, Roychowdhury S, Narayan V, et al. Arteriovenous malformation presenting as traumatic subdural hematoma: a case report. Surg Neurol Int. 2020;11:203.
15. Reynolds MR, Lanzino G, Zipfel GJ. Intracranial dural arteriovenous fistulae. Stroke. 2017;48:1424–31.
16. Spetzler RF, Martin NA. A proposed grading system for arteriovenous malformations. J Neurosurg. 1986;65:476–83.
17. Spetzler RF, Ponce FA. A 3-tier classification of cerebral arteriovenous malformations. Clinical article. J Neurosurg. 2011;114:842–9.
18. Stapf C, Mohr JP, Pile-Spellman J, Solomon RA, Sacco RL, Connolly ES. Epidemiology and natural history of arteriovenous malformations. Neurosurg Focus. 2001;11:1–5.

19. Suzuki K, Kamezaki T, Tsuboi K, Kobayashi E. Dural cavernous angioma causing acute subdural hemorrhage—case report. Neurol Med Chir (Tokyo). 1996;36:580–2.
20. Taslimi S, Modabbernia A, Amin-Hanjani S, Barker FG 2nd, Macdonald RL. Natural history of cavernous malformation: systematic review and meta-analysis of 25 studies. Neurology. 2016;86:1984–91.
21. Zabramski JM, Wascher TM, Spetzler RF, Johnson B, Golfinos J, Drayer BP, et al. The natural history of familial cavernous malformations: results of an ongoing study. J Neurosurg. 1994;80:422–32.

第 23 章 慢性硬膜下血肿与颅内蛛网膜囊肿

Nevin Aydın，Ceren Kızmazoğlu，Hasan Emre Aydın 和 Ali Arslantaş

译者：张烁

23.1 引言

慢性硬膜下血肿（CSDH）多与创伤有关，极少数情况下与蛛网膜囊肿（arachnoid cyst，AC）破裂有关。CSDH 和 AC 都是神经外科领域的常见疾病，然而 CSDH 和 AC 同时出现则非常罕见。AC 相关 CSDH 常发生在青年人，除了自发性破裂及其相关出血外，还包括由运动引起的轻微头部创伤。尽管其病因尚不清楚，但已经提出有关其形成机制的假说。临床和影像学的随访观察对其治疗非常重要。对于临床表现有进展的病例，可根据病情采取钻孔或开颅等手术方法进行血肿引流，在确定手术方法时应考虑其发病率和死亡率。

23.2 慢性硬膜下血肿

CSDH 是自发性或外伤后发生在硬脑（脊）膜或蛛网膜层与脑实质表面之间的颅内出血。CSDH 可能是独立发生的，也可由于老年人脑萎缩和静脉脆性增加所致，通常发生在最初出血后的 2～3 周，预后一般较差。CSDH 是一种发病率和死亡率（经有效治疗后）极低的疾病，其病因和病理生理改变可由渗透理论或纤维溶解理论解释。人群中 CSDH 的发病率为（8.2～17.6）/10 万。由于全球老年人口的增加，CSDH 患病率有所增加[2]。创伤是 CSDH 的病因中重要的因素之一。由于创伤原因，CSDH 在男性中更为常见[31]。硬膜下血肿是由于脑实质的突然减速和加速导致桥静脉撕裂而发生的，更常发生于酗酒者和出现脑组织萎缩的老年患者[32]。

23.2.1 诊断

CT（计算机断层成像）常用于 CSDH 的诊断和术后随访。根据 Lanksch 等的分类（图 23.1），与脑实质相比，CSDH 密度可分为低密度、等密度、高密度或混合密度。急性出血合并包膜形成可引起高密度血肿。应在术后第 1 天和第 7 天行颅脑 CT 检查，对患者病情进行临床随访和影像学分析。此外，磁共振成像（MRI）可提供硬膜下血肿的更多信息如血肿所处时期、血肿大小和形成时间，用于临床决策。在等密度或双侧病变的情况下，更适合进行颅脑 MRI 检查[10]。在高达 2.7% 的病例中慢性硬膜下血肿存在钙化现象，其原因尚不完全清楚。大面积钙化的 CSDH 病例被称为"装甲脑"[19]。Von Rokitansky 首次在尸检中发现伴钙化的 CSDH，Goldhahn 报道了第一例手术切除血肿的 CSDH 病例[12, 30]。

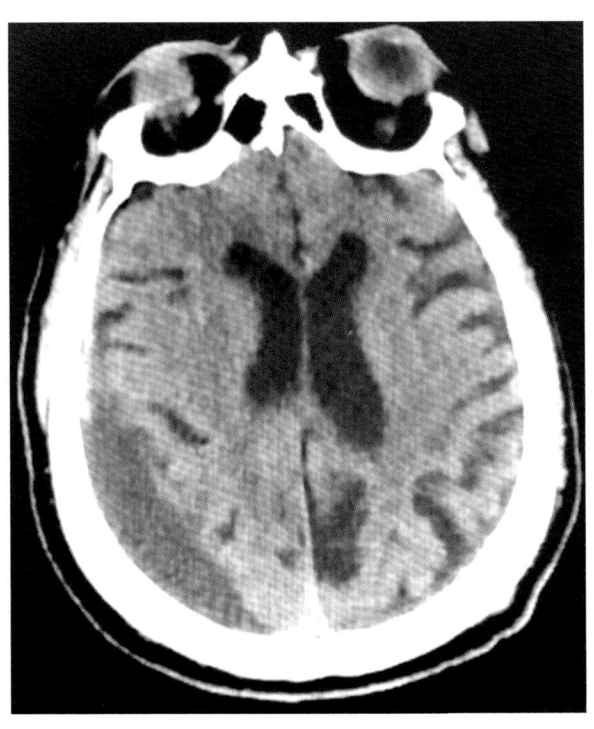

图 23.1 右侧慢性硬膜下血肿。注意低密度的血肿

23.2.2　临床表现

头痛、癫痫发作、偏瘫或行为改变都是 CSDH 可能的临床症状。虽然单侧 CSDH 中神经功能障碍更为常见如行为改变和思维变慢等感觉障碍，行走障碍等症状也很突出[16]。虽然头痛不具有特异性，但也是神经系统疾病常见的症状之一[28]。术前、术后临床分级可采用格拉斯哥昏迷量表（GCS）、KPS 评分和 CSDH 神经学分级系统[21]。虽然 CSDH 通常处于无症状阶段，但也可能出现非特异性的临床表现，如头痛、癫痫发作、偏瘫[6]。早期诊断和治疗可显著降低发病率和死亡率。

23.2.3　治疗

CSDH 的治疗方法有开颅手术、内镜手术或保守治疗。开颅手术治疗方法为单、双钻孔开颅同时生理盐水冲洗。据报道，CSDH 保守治疗的成功率达到 18%，临床症状较轻的老年人或偶然发现出血的患者可定期随访观察[17]。尽管目前 CSDH 的治疗仍有争议，但主流治疗方式仍是手术治疗。手摇钻开颅、钻孔开颅术和开颅血肿清除术是最常用的手术方法。采用钻孔引流术治疗脑出血可显著降低死亡率。与钻孔开颅术相比，扭钻开颅术对血肿引流更为有利。这种治疗方法也用于其他类型的血肿，如多发血肿和分散性血肿，而神经内镜技术在处理其他类型血肿时很少运用。钻孔引流术可专门用于未形成分隔且大部分已液化的 CSDH[25, 34]。

23.2.4　并发症

CSDH 的复发是一项重要的术后挑战，文献报道 CSDH 术后复发率高达 31%。脑组织由于长期处于压力下导致复张能力下降被认为是血肿复发的最重要因素[31]。患者入院时的神经系统状况是 CSDH 复发重要的危险因素之一，当神经系统临床状态较差时手术成功率降低，复发风险也增加。颅内积气和癫痫是潜在的并发症。硬脑膜下积气最常发生在手术后，并且会限制大脑的复张。研究建议在 CSDH 诊断后 6 个月内使用预防性抗癫痫药物。有研究报道，手术后并发症的发生率在小骨窗开颅组为 6.7%，钻孔组为 22.8%。因此，开颅被认为是一种更好的手术选择[20]。脑萎缩、脑扩张不足和围手术期血肿体积已被认为是 CSDH 术后复发的危险因素。

创伤后 CSDH 发生钙化的风险高于其他原因导致的钙化[15]。有学者研究了从受伤到手术之间的时间和预后的关系，发现从受伤到接受手术在 60 天以内的患者死亡率和发病率较高，预后较差。

23.3　颅内蛛网膜囊肿

蛛网膜囊肿（arachnoid cysts，AC）是非肿瘤性的轴外病变。AC 在颅内占位性病变中的发生率为 1%，男性的发生率是女性的 3 倍。AC 被定义为先天性或儿童时期获得性病变。先天性病变的 AC 是由于蛛网膜在发育过程中脑脊液通路发生变异，AC 随着脑脊液的流动形成网膜状结构，网膜在胚胎期的蛛网膜下腔形成后形成网膜囊[3]。获得性 AC 主要因为外部因素，大多是由于瘢痕组织内的脑脊液聚集，特别是继发于创伤、出血或肿瘤病变[4]。

23.3.1　临床表现

颅内 AC 通常无症状，偶然于检查时发现。尽管颅内 AC 的临床表现随病变部位的不同而变化，但它们通常的临床症状并不典型，可能表现为头痛、呕吐或癫痫发作。

23.3.2　诊断

AC 常用放射学方法如 CT 和 MRI 进行诊断。AC 在 CT 成像上表现为局限、低密度、无增强的蛛网膜下腔病变（图 23.2）。CSDH 的鉴别诊断很重要，仅仅依靠 CT 检查可能不够。弥散磁共振成像和磁共振光谱可做出更明确的诊断。在脑 MRI 上，AC 与脑脊液信号相似，在所有序列中外观相同（图 23.3）。如果需要确切的影像学成像进行病情评估，则可以使用稳态构成干扰（CISS）序列，明确 MRI 中神经结构与脑脊液之间的 T2 比值和病理结构，以监测 AC 的发生发展[1]。

23.3.3　发病部位

颅内 AC 最常发生于颅中窝，其次发生于颅后窝。1982 年 Galassi 等定义的 Galassi 分类法将 AC 分为 3 种不同类型（表 23.1）。此分类用于评估颅中窝囊肿的大小、对颅压的改变。1 型蛛网膜囊肿很小，位于颅中窝前部；2 型蛛网膜囊肿位于外侧

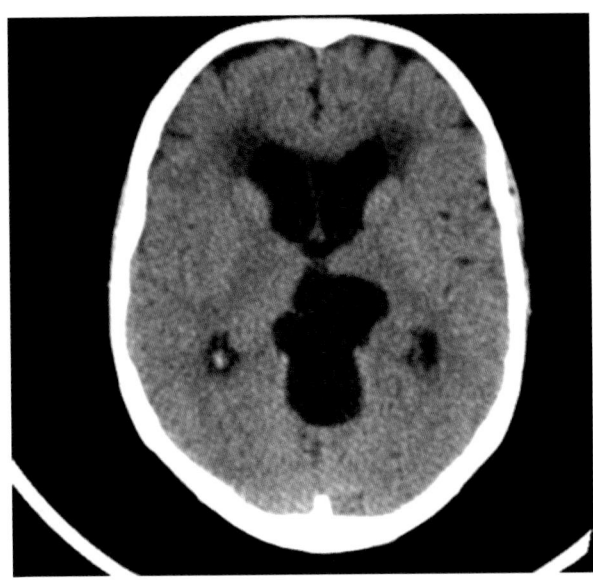

图 23.2 四叠体部的蛛网膜囊肿合并脑积水

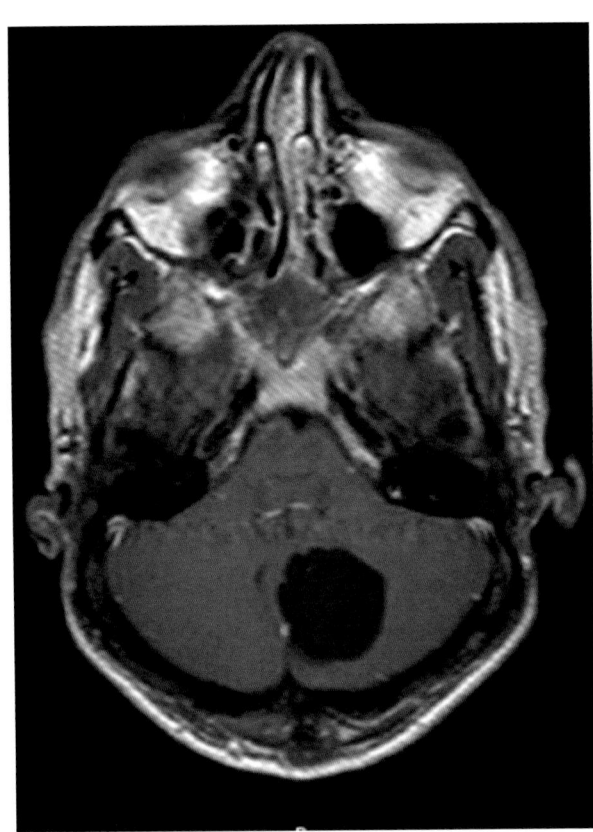

图 23.3 左侧小脑半球蛛网膜囊肿

裂,对颞叶存在压迫;3 型蛛网膜囊肿可压迫顶叶和额叶,并填满整个颅中窝,造成大脑移位。该分类系统可以很好地评价 AC 的临床和影像学表现,便于做出诊断[9]。

23.3.4 治疗

尽管 AC 的治疗方法仍存在争议,但对于影像

表 23.1 Galassi 分类法 [a]

- I 型
  - 体积小,梭形
  - 局限于颅中窝前部,位于蝶骨嵴平面以下
  - 与蛛网膜下腔存在沟通
- II 型
  - 沿外侧裂向上延伸
  - 与蛛网膜下腔联系欠通畅
- III 型
  - 体积大
  - 占据颅中窝全部
  - 不仅累及颞叶,同时累及额顶叶
  - 常造成中线移位
  - 与周围脑池无联系

[a]:表格摘自 Galassi 等学者研究结果[9]。

学检查无进展并且没有临床症状的病变定期影像学随访很重要[5]。当病变范围增大,且在随访期间观察到持续存在的临床表现时,可考虑手术治疗。具体的手术指征是颅内压升高、进展性脑积水、脑实质受压和脑电图证实的药物抵抗性癫痫。手术治疗可用于治疗囊肿或因囊肿占位效应引起的脑积水。手术治疗方法可以考虑囊肿腹腔分流术、脑室腹腔分流术、内镜下囊肿开窗脑室/枕大池引流。临床评估对决定手术方式非常重要。由于表现为头痛等颅内压升高的临床症状通常不具有特异性,因此在排除其他原因后,应确认所出现的临床表现是由于 AC 引起后再决定手术[13]。

23.3.5 并发症

接受手术治疗的患者术后常出现硬膜下血肿和积液等并发症。放置膀胱-腹腔或脑室-腹腔分流器后可能发生排异反应和脑膜炎[7]。合并脑积水的病例手术治疗总体并发症较少,手术成功率高。

23.4 慢性硬脑膜下血肿合并蛛网膜囊肿

研究发现运动时头部外伤或类似情况下发生的 CSDH 与 AC 有关。先天性 AC 引起同侧 CSDH 的风险很高,尤其是在年轻患者中。与自发性 CSDH 不同,AC 相关性 CSDH 主要影响青少年男性和存在运动相关损伤的青年患者。虽然撞击伤造成头部创伤的风险尚不清楚,但当颅内存在 AC 时 CSDH 形成的可能性增加[21]。从文献资料来看,CSDH

与 AC 的形成与足球以及跆拳道运动相关[22]。位于颞窝的 AC 同时出现 CSDH 的风险更高[11]。临床表现一般为颅内压增高，同时可伴有头痛、呕吐、偏瘫等非特异性症状[27]。

钻孔引流通常用于治疗出现临床症状的病例。手术方式的决定应综合考虑慢性硬膜下血肿和颅内蛛网膜囊肿的关系以及两者的病变特点[13]。无症状 AC 患者术中不应追求蛛网膜囊肿膜的全切[33]。

AC 是一种透明、无色、充满液体的囊肿，通过蛛网膜分化形成，在大脑发育过程中出现。CSDH 通常是存在于硬脑膜和蛛网膜之间的完全液化的陈旧性出血。除了自发形成外，创伤也是形成 CSDH 的一个重要原因。

AC 和 CSDH 的关系以及疾病的自然史尚未完全明确。AC 通常无症状，当囊肿生长和囊肿破裂后可出现临床症状，囊肿破裂可能与硬膜下积液或硬膜下出血有关。合并蛛网膜囊肿的硬膜下出血的年轻患者多由运动相关的头部创伤所致，自发性出血相当罕见。囊肿内或囊肿壁上薄弱的软脑膜和桥静脉撕裂会引起硬膜下出血，严重的膜粘连和脑顺应性降低则是硬膜下出血出现的诱因[14]。

当受到轻型颅脑创伤时，蛛网膜囊肿破裂后硬膜下远隔部位可能会出现自发性硬膜下出血。由于单向阀门机制，囊肿内流出的液体不能回流到囊肿内而在硬膜下远隔部位聚集[11]。另一种假说认为颅脑创伤后脑脊液从远处的蛛网膜下腔进入蛛网膜囊肿，蛛网膜囊肿内压力增加撕裂囊肿壁，囊内积液流入远处的硬膜下。既往有自发性或创伤后破裂的 AC 液体流至远隔部位硬膜下的报道。临床症状是决定等待水肿自行消退或进行手术引流的重要依据[13]。

AC 可能自发破裂。囊肿壁与凸面的硬脑膜连接相对薄弱，头部外伤时产生的机械力会导致囊肿壁与硬脑膜剥离引发出血。顶叶囊肿膜覆盖了侧裂静脉引起出血的区域，并形成了进入蝶骨嵴后硬脑膜窦的桥接结构。即使是对壁膜的适度操作也可能造成静脉损伤，导致硬膜下出血[8,10]。

大部分 AC 相关性 CSDH 均应接受手术治疗，AC 破裂可能导致突发危及生命的临床症状。因此应慎重考虑囊肿破裂的风险，特别是出现任何新发的临床症状[10]。根据 AC 出现的并发症，CSDH 及囊内出血的治疗方法不尽相同。对于这些并发症，通常首选手术治疗。也有文献报道，外伤或自发性破裂后的囊肿和出血可在保守治疗后愈合[13]。

AC 相关的 CSDH 可采取多种治疗方法。Parsch 等对 16 例 AC 继发性 CSDH 和 13 例积液患者进行了治疗，在未对囊肿进行任何处理的情况下于远端硬膜下对积液引流，并对先前无症状的 AC 进行了影像学随访[26]。血肿排出后行 AC 切除，清除蛛网膜下腔膜与囊肿壁之间的粘连是目前最常用的治疗方法。另一种治疗方法是采用手术分流。James 等指出，分流术不仅手术创伤小，且可以使囊肿收缩的同时实现脑实质组织扩张[18]。Lesoin 等对 7 例脑外伤 AC 患者中的 5 例进行了分流术[23]。Kulali 和 von Wild 通过硬膜下腹腔分流术治疗了 1 例 1 个月前有头部外伤史，具有头痛、恶心和呕吐症状的患者[21]。与硬膜下腹腔分流术相比，AC 切开引流术的死亡率和并发症发生率（发病率为 10%～15%）较高，但二次手术率低于腹腔分流术[13,24,29]。

虽然 AC 和 CSDH 在解剖上是独立的两种疾病，但影像学表现相似。当 CSDH 渗透到 AC 中，可以观察到细微的液体成分变化。这一机制可能解释了术后血肿再吸收区脑脊液积聚的原因。由于开颅手术的并发症比钻孔引流更高，因此钻孔引流术应作为 CSDH 合并 AC 的首选治疗方法[7]。

23.5 结论

尽管 CSDH 常见于老年人群，但合并 AC 的情况更多见于年轻人。CT 对蛛网膜囊肿和 CSDH 诊断十分重要。虽然 AC 相关的 CSDH 发病机制尚未明确，但它被认为与远端硬膜下脑脊液回流有关。合并 AC 的 CSDH 临床表现根据出血和囊肿部位而异，主要由 CT 结果确诊。MRI 可用于患者术后随访。如果患者已出现临床症状，一般治疗方法是钻孔引流血肿。因此，临床症状和手术治疗方式主要取决于患者是否出现 CSDH，病因并非首要考虑因素。

参考文献

1. Aleman J, Jokura H, Higano S, Akabane A, Shirane R, Yoshimoto T. Value of constructive interference in steady-state three-dimensional, Fourier transformation magnetic resonance imaging for the neuroendoscopic treatment of hydrocephalus and intracranial cysts. Neurosurgery. 2001;48:1291–5.
2. Bostantjopoulou S, Katsarou Z, Michael M, Petridis A. Reversible parkinsonism due to chronic bilateral subdural hematomas. J Clin Neurosci. 2009;16(3):458–60.
3. Brackett CE, Rengachary SS. Arachnoid cysts. Youmans JR (ed), Neurological surgery, Philadelphia: WB Saunders, 1982;3(2)1436–1446.
4. Cagnoni G, Fonda C, Pancani S, Pampaloni A, Mugnaini L. Intracranial arachnoid cysts in pediatric age. Pediatr Med Chir. 1996;18:85–90.
5. Cokluk C, Senel A, Celik F, Ergur H. Spontaneous disappearance of two asymptomatic arachnoid cysts in two different locations. Minim Invasive Neurosurg. 2003;46(2):110–2.
6. Dammers R, ter Laak-Poort MP, Maas AI. Neurological picture. Armoured brain: case report of a symptomatic calcified chronic subdural haematoma. J Neurol Neurosurg Psychiatry. 2007;78:542–3.
7. Duz B, Kaya S, Daneyemez M, Gonul E. Surgical management strategies of intracranial arachnoid cysts: a single institution experience of 75 cases. Turk Neurosurg. 2012;22:591–8.
8. Fewel ME, Levy ML, McComb JG. Surgical treatment of 95 children with 102 intracranial arachnoid cysts. Pediatr Neurosurg. 1996;25:165–73.
9. Galassi E, Tognetti F, Gaist G, et al. CT scan and metrizamide CT cisternography in arachnoid cysts of the middle cranial fossa: classification and pathophysiological aspects. Surg Neurol. 1982;17(5):363–9.
10. Gelabert-González M, Iglesias-Pais M, García-Allut A, Martínez-Rumbo R. Chronic subdural haematoma: surgical treatment and outcome in 1000 cases. Clin Neurol Neurosurg. 2005;107:223–9. https://doi.org/10.1016/j.clineuro.2004.09.015.
11. Gelabert-González M, Castro-Bouzas D, Arcos-Algaba A, Santín-Amo JM, Díaz-Cabanas L, Serramito-García R, Arán-Echabe E, Prieto-González A, García-Allut A. Hematoma subdural crónico asociado a quiste aracnoideo. Presentación de 12 casos [Chronic subdural hematoma associated with arachnoid cyst. Report of 12 cases]. Neurocirugia (Astur). 2010;21(3):222–7.
12. Goldhahn R. Uber ein grosso-es, operativ entferntes, verkaklktes, intra-kranielles Hamatom. Dtsch Z Chir. 1930;224:323–31.
13. Gregori F, Colistra D, Mancarella C, Chiarella V, Marotta N, Domenicucci M. Arachnoid cyst in young soccer players complicated by chronic subdural hematoma: personal experience and review of the literature. Acta Neurol Belg. 2020;120(2):235–46. https://doi.org/10.1007/s13760-019-01224-1.
14. Harding BN, Copp AJ. Malformations. In: Graham DI, Lantos PL, editors. Greenfield's neuropathology. 7th ed. New York: Oxford University Press; 2002. p. 451–2.
15. He XS, Zhang X. Giant calcified chronic subdural hematoma: a long term complication of shunt hydrocephalus. J Neurol Neurosurg Psychiatry. 2005;76:367.
16. Huang KT, Bi WL, Abd-El-Barr M, et al. The neurocritical and neurosurgical care of subdural hematomas. Neurocrit Care. 2016;24:294–307. https://doi.org/10.1007/s12028-015-0194-x.
17. Iorio-Morin C, Touchette C, Lévesque M, et al. Chronic subdural hematoma: toward a new management paradigm for an increasingly complex population. J Neurotrauma. 2018;35:1882–5. https://doi.org/10.1089/neu.2018.5872.
18. James HE. Encephalocele, dermoid sinus and arachnoid cyst. Pediatr Neurosurg. 1989:97–106.
19. Kavcic A, Meglic B, Meglic NP, Vodusek DB, Mesec A. Asymptomatic huge calcified subdural hematoma in a patient on oral anticoagulant therapy. Neurology. 2006;66:758.
20. Kertmen H, Gürer B, Yilmaz ER, Sekerci Z. Chronic subdural hematoma associated with an arachnoid cyst in a juvenile taekwondo athlete: a case report and review of the literature. Pediatr Neurosurg. 2012;48(1):55–8. https://doi.org/10.1159/000339354. Epub 2012 Jul 21. PMID: 22832284.
21. Kulali A, von Wild K. Post-traumatic subdural hygroma as a complication of arachnoid cysts of the middle fossa. Neurosurg Rev. 1989;12(Suppl):508–13.
22. Lee JK, Choi JH, Kim CH, Lee HK, Moon JG. Chronic subdural hematomas: a comparative study of three types of operative procedures. J Korean Neurosurg Soc. 2009;46:210–4. https://doi.org/10.3340/jkns.2009.46.3.210.

23. Lesoin F, Dhellemmes P, Rousseaux M, Jomin M. Arachnoid cysts and head injury. Acta Neurochir (Wien). 1983;69:43–51.
24. Markwalder TM. Chronic subdural haematomas: a review. J Neurosurg. 1981;54:637–45.
25. Okada Y, Akai T, Okamoto K, Iida T, Takata H, Iizuka H. A comparative study of the treatment of chronic subdural hematoma—burr hole drainage versus burr hole irrigation. Surg Neurol. 2002;57:405–9. https://doi.org/10.1016/S0090-3019(02)00720-6.
26. Parsch CS, Krauss J, Hofmann E, Meixensberger J, Roosen K. Arachnoid cysts associated with subdural hematomas and hygromas: analysis of 16 cases, long-term follow-up, and review of the literature. Neurosurgery. 1997;40:483–90. PubMed: 9055286.
27. Prabhu VC, Bailes JE. Chronic subdural hematoma complicating arachnoid cyst secondary to soccer-related head injury: case report. Neurosurgery. 2002;50(1):195–7; discussion 197–8. https://doi.org/10.1097/00006123-200201000-00029. PMID: 11844251.
28. Stanisic M, Lund-Johansen M, Mahesparan R. Treatment of chronic subdural hematoma by burr-hole craniostomy in adults: influence of some factors on postoperative recurrence. Acta Neurochir (Wien). 2005;147(12):1249–56; discussion 1256–7. https://doi.org/10.1007/s00701-005-0616-1. Epub 2005 Aug 29. PMID: 16133770.
29. Tabaddor K, Shulmon K. Definitive treatment of chronic subdural hematoma by twist-drill craniostomy and closed-system drainage. J Neurosurg. 1977;46:220–6. https://doi.org/10.3171/jns.1977.46.2.0220.
30. von Rokitansky C. Handbuch der pathologischen anatomie. Cilt:2 Vienna: Braunmuller and Scidel; 1844. p. 717.
31. Wright DW, Merck LH. Head trauma in adults and children. In: Tintinalli JE, Stapczynski JS, Ma OJ, Cline DM, Cydulka RK, Meckler GD, editors. Tintinalli's emergency medicine, vol. 7. New York: McGraw Hill; 2011. p. 1692–708.
32. Wu X, Li G, Zhao J, Zhu X, Zhang Y, Hou K. Arachnoid cyst-associated chronic subdural hematoma: report of 14 cases and a systematic literature review. World Neurosurg. 2018;109:118–30. https://doi.org/10.1016/j.wneu.2017.09.115. Epub 2017 Sep 28. PMID: 28962953.
33. Yang W, Huang J. Chronic subdural hematoma epidemiology and natural history. Neurosurg Clin N Am. 2017;28:205–10. https://doi.org/10.1016/j.nec.2016;11:002.
34. Yoshimoto Y, Kwak S. Frontal small craniostomy and irrigation for treatment of chronic subdural haematoma. Br J Neurosurg. 1997;11:150–1. https://doi.org/10.1080/02688699746519.

第 24 章 慢性硬膜下血肿的罕见颅内部位

Kossi Kouma Félix Segbedgi，Gbetoho Fortuné Gankpe 和 Mohammed Benzagmout

译者：李云飞

24.1 引言

慢性硬膜下血肿（CSDH）是指包裹在硬脑膜和蛛网膜之间的血液和液体的聚集。积液的形成需要 3 周或更长时间。血肿包膜被确定为液体渗出和持续出血的来源。事实上，血管生成会刺激血肿膜壁内脆弱血管的形成，而纤溶过程则会防止凝块形成[9, 30]。在血肿包膜和硬膜下血肿液中发现了大量的炎症细胞和血清标志物[2, 9-10]。它们可能有助于传播炎症反应，从而进一步刺激膜生长和液体积聚。

CSDH 通常位于幕上、皮质凸面上方[39]。然而，也有不常见的位置被报道，特别是在颅后窝、半球间间隙，甚至在椎管内。本章重点关注这些罕见颅内部位 CSDH 的临床和放射学特征，并讨论其适当的治疗方法。

24.2 颅后窝硬膜下血肿

24.2.1 病因

颅后窝 CSDH（pCSH）极为罕见[6, 22, 28]。pCSH 的发病机制尚不清楚[7]。患者通常没有明显外伤史[14]。然而，枕骨、乙状窦和横窦壁损伤；小脑静脉或一些较大的导静脉损伤；凝血功能障碍、抗凝 / 抗血小板治疗；颅后窝手术、蛛网膜囊肿、颅内低压等都是该特定部位血肿的病理生理学提示[7, 32, 40-41]。

24.2.2 临床表现

由于临床表现多种多样，pCSH 的临床诊断具有挑战性[7]。它们包括头痛、恶心、呕吐、头晕、意识改变、肢体共济失调和步态障碍[42]。在某些情况下，出现的相应症状可能提示颅后窝病变，特别是小脑症状、脑神经功能障碍、眩晕和眼球震颤[17, 29, 40]。

值得注意的是，相关部位脑积水可能突然导致患者神经状态恶化，导致在做出正确诊断之前患者因脑干受压而死亡[7, 18, 40]。

24.2.3 影像特征

CT 扫描通常显示颅后窝硬膜下间隙有一个从低到高的密度区域。然而，由于骨伪影的干扰，这种成像方式不适合对颅后窝占位性病变进行放射学探查，从而难以评估硬膜下血肿及其可能的根本原因[6-7, 18, 32, 40]。

磁共振成像（MRI）是首选的检查方法。本研究结果显示硬膜下积液在 T1 加权像上为低信号至高信号，在 T2 加权像上为高信号（图 24.1）。Izumihara 等[18] 在文献中报道了第一例经 MRI 诊断的 pCSH。术前脑血管造影术不是必需的，但它在评估静脉窦、导静脉和其他潜在的血管结构方面可有重要贡献。

24.2.4 治疗

有症状的患者通常需要手术治疗。手术方法

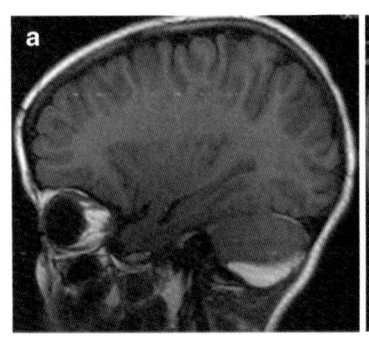 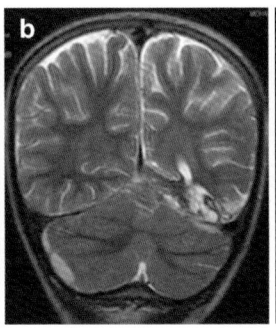 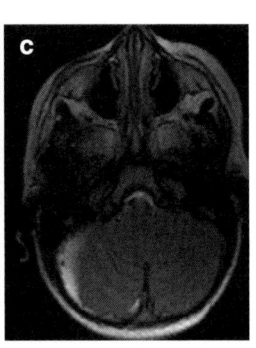

图 24.1 头颅 MRI 矢状位平扫 T1（a）、冠状位 T2（b）和灌注轴位序列（c）显示右侧小脑半球颅后窝 CSDH

包括硬膜下外侧开颅术、小骨瓣开颅术和钻孔开颅术。患者一般在局部或全身麻醉下以俯卧位进行手术[14]。

由于大多数 pCSH 患者存在凝血功能障碍，即使是双侧 CSDH，也建议行局部麻醉下的微创钻孔手术[14]。然而，通过一个简单的钻孔将很难处理术中窦损伤引起的过多出血[14]，因此必须考虑是否需要行颅骨切除术，使手术野足够大以解决任何可能的出血问题[42]。术中可放置硬膜下引流管，并在术后 48 h 内取出[42, 44]。

双侧 pCSH 可通过枕下中线入路（俯卧位）用两个钻孔（每侧一个）排出[22, 32, 40]。然而，Inoue 等建议，由于血肿两侧存在连接，建议在横窦-乙状窦交界处附近单个钻孔以清除双侧 pCSH[14]。

与梗阻性脑积水相关的颅后窝慢性硬膜下血肿仍然是危及生命的紧急病情，因此强烈建议早期治疗[14]。血肿清除后相关脑积水也会消失[3-4, 14, 40]，否则需要进行脑室分流[23, 32]。

对于没有相关脑积水的无症状或轻微症状的 pCSH 患者，保守治疗可以获得良好的临床预后[18, 23, 41]。此外，对于那些凝血功能障碍的患者，保守治疗可能是一种合理的治疗选择[41]。在抗凝治疗和血小板减少的情况下进行手术具有较高的围手术期风险，在这种情况下输注血小板和停用抗凝药被认为是有效的，至少在短期内有效；血肿在 2 周到 2 个月内会自行消失，患者表现出良好的神经功能恢复[41]。

24.3 纵裂慢性硬膜下血肿

24.3.1 病因

在纵裂位置的 CSDH 并不常见。首次由 Aring 和 Evans[3] 报道的大脑纵裂 CSDH（ICSH）极为罕见，约占所有慢性硬膜下血肿的 0.4%[36]。在大多数情况下，ICSH 通常是单侧的，主要原因是头部创伤[5]。ICSH 的其他原因包括凝血功能障碍、动脉瘤破裂和自发性高血压性脑出血，导致慢性血肿增厚[16, 25]。ICSH 的起源是多种多样的，包括大脑半球间裂的桥静脉、胼胝体周围动脉的分支或大脑半球间裂伤[43]。

24.3.2 临床表现

神经系统症状取决于多种因素，包括疾病的临床病程、患者的年龄、大脑纵裂的厚度和病变的解剖位置[33]。一般来说，ICSH 的临床表现以头痛、癫痫发作为特征，并伴有典型的 falx 综合征，定义为对侧偏瘫，最突出的症状是下肢偏瘫[5, 24, 31]。

24.3.3 影像学特征

CT 扫描是诊断 ICSDH 的首选神经影像学方法。靠近大脑皮质表面的低密度轴外聚集的经典描述也适用于 ICSH（图 24.2）。此外，CT 扫描还可以确定血肿的大小、厚度、前后位置以及是否有其他相关病变。在某些情况下，MRI 有助于术前精准定位桥静脉，为选择开颅手术的最佳入路提供指导[34]。

ICSH 位于上矢状窦下方的大脑半球间沟内。由

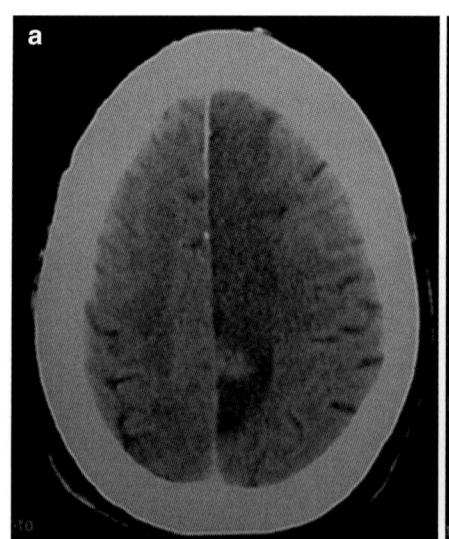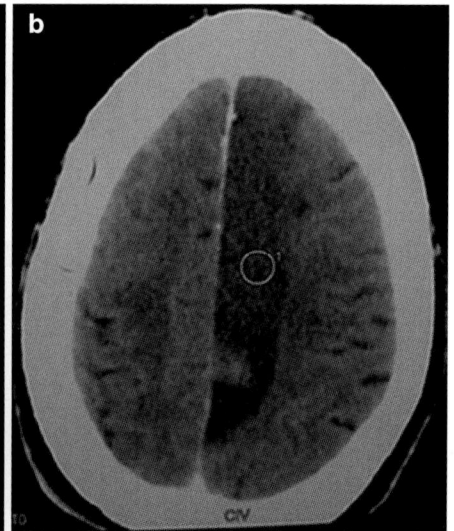

图 24.2 （a）和（b）增强前后轴位 CT 扫描显示左侧大脑半球间 CSDH

于重力作用，在大脑镰后部比前部更常见[1]。ICSH可以被分离[21, 34, 37]或与凸形CSDH[13, 26, 34]相汇合。这种汇合多发生在血肿液化和迁移之后，可以被认为是ICSH的吸收方式[11, 13, 15, 31]。

血肿通常位于纵裂的一侧[34]。然而，也有报告报道了双侧ICSH[8, 19, 46]。纵裂血肿的形状具有突出的外侧和笔直的内侧边缘[46]。

24.3.4 治疗

ICSH的治疗选择有矢状面旁开颅、单侧小骨瓣开颅或环钻、钻孔冲洗引流、麻花钻开颅术和非手术治疗[34]。

临床上有症状的ICSH多局限于半球间裂，需要手术治疗[34]。ICSH可以通过在纵裂间隙上方或附近钻孔来治疗[12]。然而，上矢状窦正下方的解剖位置使得如钻孔或麻花钻颅骨造口术等手术入路变得短而直接，具有潜在的危险。

此外，ICSH的手术清除可以通过开颅手术进行[20, 33, 38]。在全身麻醉下行旁正中骨瓣或骨环钻术。开颅术的内侧边缘必须接近中线，以便在大脑皮质内表面最小程度受损的情况下方便地探查半球间区。可使用柔性导管用生理盐水冲洗纵裂血肿[34]。如果血肿内有明显的膜和小叶，可能需要进行扩大的前后开颅手术。此外，内窥镜检查可能是一种合适的手术技术[34]，它允许在血肿腔内切割不同的间隔，打开内部膜，并最终凝固新生血管[27, 45]。

值得注意的是，有报道称当ICSH伴有凸面血肿时，凸面钻孔冲洗术可间接减压[13]。

对于没有感觉障碍或明显运动障碍的患者，推荐保守治疗，这些患者在密切观察下可保持病情稳定。这一策略已经被用于一些半球间性CSDH的病例，并取得了良好的临床预后[21, 35]。

24.4 结论

颅内CSDH通常位于幕上间隙，位于皮质凸面之上。CSDH在大脑半球间和颅后窝位置极为罕见。CSDH的临床表现多种多样，诊断多采用头颅CT和MRI检查。目前，对这些不常见的CSDH部位的最佳治疗仍然存在争议，因为病例相对较少，而且缺乏指南指导。对无症状或临床症状稳定且有密切随访的患者，我们建议保守治疗。然而，对于出现明显的神经功能损害或神经功能恶化的患者，尤其是意识状况较差的患者，应及早手术减压。

参考文献

1. Ahn JM, Lee KS, Shim JH, Oh JS, Shim JJ, Yoon SM. Clinical features of interhemispheric subdural hematomas. Korean J Neurotrauma. 2017;13:103–7.
2. Aoyama M, Osuka K, Usuda N, Watanabe Y, Kawaguchi R, Nakura T, Takayasu M. Expression of mitogen-activated protein kinases in chronic subdural hematoma outer membranes. J Neurotrauma. 2015;32:1064–70.
3. Aring C, Evans JP. Aberrant location of subdural hematoma. Arch Neurol Psychiatr (Chicago). 1940;4:1296–306.
4. Ashkenazi E, Pomeranz S. Nystagmus as the presentation of tentorial incisure subdural haematoma. J Neurol Neurosurg Psychiatry. 1994;57:830–1.
5. Bartels RH, Verhagen WI, Prick MJ, Dalman JE. Interhemispheric subdural hematoma in adults: case reports and a review of the literature. Neurosurgery. 1995;36:1210–4.
6. Berhouma M, Houissa S, Jemel H, Khaldi M. Spontaneous chronic subdural hematoma of the posterior fossa. J Neuroradiol. 2007;34:213–5.
7. Costa LB Jr, de Andrade A, Valadão GF. Chronic subdural hematoma of the posterior fossa associated with cerebellar hemorrhage: report of rare disease with MRI findings. Arq Neuropsiquiatr. 2004;62:170–2.
8. Cronin TG, Shippey DU. Bilateral interhemispheric subdural hematoma: a case report. Am J Neuroradiol. 1987;8:909–10.
9. Edlmann E, Giorgi-Coll S, Whitfield PC, Carpenter KLH, Hutchinson PJ. Pathophysiology of chronic subdural haematoma: inflammation, angiogenesis and implications for pharmacotherapy. J Neuroinflammation. 2017;14:108.
10. Fedorko S, Walter J, Younsi A, Zweckberger K, Unterberg AW, Beynon C. Intraoperative point-of-care assessment of an inflammatory biomarker in chronic subdural hematomas: technical note. Clin Neurol Neurosurg. 2019;183:105396.

11. Fruin AH, Juhl GL, Taylon C. Interhemispheric subdural hematoma. Case report. J Neurosurg. 1984;60:1300–2.
12. Ho SU, Spehlmann R, Ho HT. CT scan in interhemispheric subdural hematoma. Clinical and pathological correlation. Neurology. 1977;27:1097–8.
13. Houtteville JP, Toumi K, Theron J, Derlon JM, Benazza A, Hubert P. Interhemispheric subdural haematomas: seven cases and review of the literature. Br J Neurosurg. 1988;2:357–67.
14. Inoue T, Hirai H, Shima A, Suzuki F, Matsuda M. Bilateral chronic subdural hematoma in the posterior fossa treated with a burr hole irrigation: a case report and review of the literature. Case Rep Neurol. 2019;11:87–93.
15. Iplikçioğlu AC, Bayar MA, Kökes F, Doğanay S, Gökçek C. Interhemispheric subdural hematomas. Br J Neurosurg. 1994;8:627–31.
16. Ishikawa E, Sugimoto K, Yanaka K, et al. Interhemispheric subdural hematoma caused by a ruptured internal carotid artery aneurysm: case report. Surg Neurol. 2000;54:82–6.
17. Isla A, Alvarez F, Manrique M, Castro A, Amaya C, Blázquez MG. Posterior fossa subdural hematoma. J Neurosurg Sci. 1987;31:67–9.
18. Izumihara A, Orita T, Kajiwara K, Tsurutani T. Simultaneous supra-and infratentorial chronic subdural hematoma. Eur J Radiol. 1993;16:183–5.
19. Kasdon DL, Magruder MR, Stevens EA, Paullus WS Jr. Bilateral interhemispheric subdural hematomas. Neurosurgery. 1979;5:57–9.
20. Koyama S, Nishimura T. A case of bilateral interhemispheric subdural hematoma. No Shinkei Geka. 1990;18:289–94.
21. Kuk-Jin L, Eun-Jeong K, Ha-Young C. Interhemispheric chronic subdural hematoma showing falx syndrome—case report. J Korean Neurosurg Soc. 2002;32:268–71.
22. Kurisu K, Kawabori M, Niiya Y, Ohta Y, Mabuchi S, Houkin K. Bilateral chronic subdural hematomas of the posterior fossa. Neurol Med Chir. 2012;52:822–5.
23. Lagares A, Domínguez J, Lobato RD, González P. Bilateral posterior fossa subdural hematomas secondary to anticoagulant therapy. Acta Neurochir. 1998;140:1097–8.
24. Lang EW, Hohenstein C, Nabavi A, Mehdorn HM. Interhemispheric subdural hematoma. Nervenarzt. 1998;69:342–5.
25. Marinelli L, Parodi RC, Renzetti P, Bandini F. Interhemispheric subdural haematoma from ruptured aneurysm: a case report. J Neurol. 2005;252:364–6.
26. Minami M, Hanakita J, Suwa H, Suzui H, Fujita K, Nakamura T. Interhemispheric chronic subdural hematoma-case report. Neurol Med Chir. 1997;37:177–80.
27. Mobbs R, Khong P. Endoscopic-assisted evacuation of subdural collections. J Clin Neurosci. 2009;16:701–4.
28. Mochizuki Y, Kobayashi T, Kawashima A, Funatsu T, Kawamata T. Chronic subdural hematoma of the posterior fossa treated by suboccipital craniotomy. Surg Neurol Int. 2018;9:20.
29. Murthy VS, Deshpande DH, Narayana-Reddy GN. Chronic subdural hematoma in the cerebellopontine angle. Surg Neurol. 1980;14:227–9.
30. Nomura S, Kashiwagi S, Fujisawa H, Ito H, Nakamura K. Characterization of local hyperfibrinolysis in chronic subdural hematomas by SDS-PAGE and immunoblot. J Neurosurg. 1994;81:910–3.
31. Ogsbury JS, Schneck SA, Lehman RA. Aspects of interhemispheric subdural haematoma, including the falx syndrome. J Neurol Neurosurg Psychiatry. 1978;41:72–5.
32. Pollo C, Meuli R, Porchet F. Spontaneous bilateral subdural hematomas in the posterior cranial fossa revealed by MRI. Neuroradiology. 2003;45:550–2.
33. Requejo PR, Vaitsman RP, Paiva MS, Machado AL, Barroso MV, Salame JM, Louzada PR. Interhemispheric chronic subdural haematoma: case report and brief review of the literature. Brain Inj. 2010;24:1039–43.
34. Sadrolhefazi A, Bloomfield SM. Interhemispheric and bilateral chronic subdural hematoma. Neurosurg Clin N Am. 2000;11:455–63.
35. Sakashita Y, Kuzuhara S, Fuse S, Yamanouchi H, Toyokura Y. Interhemispheric subdural hematoma complicated by chronic neurologic diseases: report of two cases diagnosed by CT scan. Rinsho Shinkeigaku. 1987;27:31–7.
36. Sambasivan M. An overview of chronic subdural hematoma: experience with 2300 cases. Surg Neurol. 1997;47:418–22.
37. Shankar A, Joseph M, Chandy MJ. Interhemispheric subdural hematoma: an uncommon sequel of trauma. Neurol India. 2003;51:63–4.
38. Sibayan RQ, Gurdjian ES, Thomas LM. Interhemispheric chronic subdural hematoma. Report

of a case. Neurology. 1970;20:1215–8.
39. Sikahall-Meneses E, Salazar-Pérez N, Sandoval-Bonilla B. Chronic subdural hematoma: surgical management in 100 patients. Cir Cir. 2008;76:199–203.
40. Stendel R, Schulte T, Pietilä TA, Suess O, Brock M. Spontaneous bilateral chronic subdural haematoma of the posterior fossa. Case report and review of the literature. Acta Neurochir. 2002;144:497–500.
41. Takami H, Oshiro N, Hiraoka F, Murao M, Ide T. Rapid resolution of a spontaneous large chronic subdural hematoma in the posterior fossa under conservative treatment with platelet administration to aplastic anemia. Clin Neurol Neurosurg. 2013;115:2236–9.
42. Takemoto Y, Matsumoto J, Ohta K, Hasegawa S, Miura M, Kuratsu J. Bilateral posterior fossa chronic subdural hematoma treated with craniectomy: case report and review of the literature. Surg Neurol Int. 2016;7:S255–8.
43. Wang Y, Wang C, Cai S, Dong J, Yang L, Chen L, Maas A. Surgical management of traumatic interhemispheric subdural hematoma. Turk Neurosurg. 2014;24:228–33.
44. Weigel R, Krauss JK, Schmiedek P. Concepts of neurosurgical management of chronic subdural haematoma: historical perspectives. Br J Neurosurg. 2004;18:8–18.
45. Yan K, Gao H, Wang Q, et al. Endoscopic surgery to chronic subdural hematoma with neovessel septation: technical notes and literature review. Neurol Res. 2016;38:467–76.
46. Zimmerman RD, Russell EJ, Yurberg E, Leeds NE. Falx and interhemispheric fissure on axial CT: II. Recognition and differentiation of interhemispheric subarachnoid and subdural hemorrhage. Am J Neuroradiol. 1982;3:635–42.

第 25 章 运动性头部损伤相关慢性硬膜下血肿

Hassan Baallal，Hatim Belfquih 和 Ali Akhaddar

译者：李云飞

25.1 引言

体育运动因其有益于健康，且一些运动的广泛流行，其在现代社会中已经变得非常重要，并拥有大量的爱好者。运动损伤是西方社会最常见的损伤之一[55]，运动相关的慢性硬膜下血肿多是由于球类运动、自行车运动、单板滑雪、竞走和过山车等造成的，所有这些运动都会导致与头部创伤相关的慢性硬膜下血肿（chronic subdural hematoma，CSDH）。颅内出血是一种罕见但具有潜在破坏性的疾病，会对运动员造成严重影响。上肢和下肢的损伤是运动中最常见的损伤，但头部损伤可能会产生毁灭性的后果，可能致命。硬膜下血肿可在撞击后的几个小时或几天内发展，是运动员死亡和发病的主要原因[11]。据报道，如果不及时发现和治疗，硬膜下血肿的死亡率高达90%[69]。在与运动相关的头部损伤中，硬膜下血肿（subdural hematoma，SDH）是最常见的死亡和严重致残原因[40, 50]。

总体来说，硬膜下血肿是根据从最初的头部创伤到症状首次出现的时间推移来分类的，如发生在 48~72 h 内，则为急性硬膜下血肿；如发生在初始创伤后 3~20 天，则为亚急性血肿；如发生在初始创伤后 3 周或更长时间，则为慢性血肿。随着患者年龄的增长，出现首发症状的时间间隔也会随之增加，由于脑萎缩的缘故，血肿不断累积直到出现明显症状。

CSDH 是神经外科实践中常见的疾病，它被定义为血液聚集并覆盖于大脑表面，在头颅成像上被诊断为 CT 上硬膜下间隙的主要低密度或等密度集合[68]。

本章回顾了 52 项研究，分析了 66 例与运动相关的 CSDH 的临床特征，以为未来提供定量的分析。

25.2 文献综述

对 PubMed/MEDLINE、谷歌 EMBASE 和 Cochrane 从 1950 年到 2020 年 3 月 1 日的数据库进行了全面的搜索，内容包括所有报道运动员发生 CSDH 病例的病例报告、病例系列、图像或图片、论著、技术说明、会议记录以及编辑来信。我们的搜索策略包括以下关键词：运动中的慢性硬膜下血肿，运动后轻度创伤性脑损伤，以及它们的主题相关同义词，以检索所有可能讨论运动与慢性硬膜下血肿的文献。

本研究的目的是总结所有与运动相关的慢性硬膜下血肿病例，并提供量化分析。对于每个病例，我们分析了年龄、性别、从事的体育活动、体育活动与诊断之间的延迟、症状、颅脑成像、所进行的治疗、结果和演变，所有数据汇总于表 25.1 中。

25.3 流行病学

当首次出血持续 3 周或更长时间而没有出现临床体征或症状时，硬膜下血肿被归类为慢性。

慢性硬膜下血肿通常被认为发生在老年患者，偶尔发生在有某些诱因的儿科或年轻患者中。它在普通人群中的总发病率约为每年 5/10 万[68]，在 70 岁以上人口中的发病率至少为每年 8.2/10 万[1]。在我们的研究中，我们分析了从 1950 年开始的 52 项研究中发现的 66 例病例，其中 53 例（80.3%）为男性，13 例（19.7%）为女性，年龄 6~75 岁，平均 24.51 岁。最具代表性的体育项目是足球，发病例数为 16 例（24.2%）。其他体育活动包括坐过山车、一般运动/体育锻炼/活动和骑自行车各 6 例（9%），篮球和武术各 4 例（7.5%）。据报道，其他病例出现在下列体育活动中：滑水、橄榄球、

第 25 章 运动性头部损伤相关慢性硬膜下血肿

表 25.1 66 例分析数据汇总

第一作者[参考文献]	发表年份	年龄(岁)/性别	既往史	运动	从创伤到诊断的时间间隔	症状	影像学表现	治疗	结局
Oliver[52]	1958	21/男	无	足球	12 周	头痛、呕吐和复视	脑电图提示左顶叶有病变，但脑室造影显示脑室向左移位	开颅手术	完全恢复
Weinberg[83]	1973	20/男	未报道	武术	未报道	头痛	左侧颈动脉造影：凸面存在硬膜下血肿	钻孔引流；开颅手术	未报道
Lacour[38]	1978	13/女	无	滑水	2 个月	双额部头痛伴呕吐	CT 扫描：右侧等密度硬膜下血肿	钻孔引流	完全恢复
Varma[81]	1981	17/男	无	橄榄球	5 周	额部头痛	颈动脉造影显示右侧脑外积液的证据	颞叶开颅手术	完全恢复
Hara[27]	1984	13/男	无	自行车	几周	头痛伴恶心	CT 扫描：右侧额颞区有大面积的低密度区域	额颞开颅手术	完全恢复
McNeil[46]	1987	17/男	无	篮球，霹雳舞	3 个月	头痛	等密度硬膜下血肿	颞叶开颅手术	完全恢复
Page[53]	1987	57/男	无	马术	未报道	头痛、恶心	CT 扫描：左侧等密度硬膜下血肿	开颅手术	未报道
Yokoyama[86]	1989	17/男	蛛网膜囊肿	柔道	2 个月	头痛伴恶心	CT 扫描：低密度硬膜下血肿	双孔钻孔引流	未报道
Rogers[66]	1990	11/男	无	自行车	1 个月	头痛、复视、呕吐	CT 扫描：右侧低密度硬膜下血肿	双孔钻孔引流	未报道
Rogers[66]	1990	10/女	蛛网膜囊肿	篮球	3 周	头痛、复视	CT 扫描：左侧低密度硬膜下血肿	双孔钻孔引流	未报道
Maeda[42]	1993	14/男	无	足球	2 个月	头痛	CT 扫描：左侧等密度硬膜下血肿	颞叶开颅手术	临床症状恢复
Fernandes[21]	1994	26/男	无	坐过山车	未报道	头痛伴呕吐	CT 扫描：双侧慢性硬膜下血肿	双孔钻孔引流	未报道
Ochi[51]	1995	11/男	蛛网膜囊肿	体能训练	3 个月	头痛伴呕吐	凸面血肿	未报道	未报道
Bo-abbass[6]	1995	64/男	无	坐过山车	10 周	头痛	CT 扫描：左侧硬膜下血肿	未报道	完全恢复
Jacome[31]	1989	65/男	无	举重	2 个月	头痛伴灼热性感觉迟钝	CT 扫描：右侧大面积等密度硬膜下血肿	双孔钻孔引流	完全恢复
Keller[35]	1998	43/男	无	篮球	3 周	双额搏动性头痛	CT 扫描：双侧额顶叶硬膜下血肿	开颅手术	完全恢复
Kawanishi[34]	1999	11/男	蛛网膜囊肿	足球	7 周	头痛伴呕吐	凸面血肿	双孔钻孔引流	完全恢复
Kawanishi[34]	1999	14/男	无	足球	2 个月	头痛	未报道	双孔钻孔引流	完全恢复
Fukutake[23]	2000	26/女	无	坐过山车	未报道	头痛	CT 扫描：双侧硬膜下血肿	未报道	完全恢复
Fukutake[23]	2000	64/男	无	坐过山车	未报道	头痛	CT 扫描：左侧慢性硬膜下血肿	未报道	完全恢复

（续表）

第一作者[参考文献]	发表年份	年龄（岁）/性别	既往史	运动	从创伤到诊断的时间间隔	症状	影像学表现	治疗	结局
Chillala[14]	2001	21/男	无	足球	3周	头痛伴呕吐	CT扫描：双侧低密度慢性硬膜下血肿	手术，无确切手术名称	完全恢复
Fukutake[23]	2000	73/男	无	坐过山车	未报道	头痛	CT扫描：左侧硬膜下血肿	未报道	13天后死亡
Mori[50]	2002	14/男	无	体能训练	1个月	头痛伴右侧肢体偏瘫	CT扫描：左侧高密度硬膜下血肿	双孔钻孔引流	完全恢复
Prabhu[60]	2002	15/女	无	足球	2个月	头痛	MRI：左侧额颞叶凸面硬膜下血肿	颞叶开颅手术	完全恢复
Ulmer[80]	2002	44，男	无	未报道	4周	头痛	未报道	开颅手术	完全恢复
Prabhu[60]	2002	16/女	无	足球	1个月	枕部头痛伴右侧肢体及面部麻木	CT扫描：等密度硬膜下血肿	双孔钻孔引流	临床症状恢复满意
Tsuzuki[79]	2003	16/女	无	篮球	几周	顽固性头痛	MRI：左侧额颞叶凸面慢性硬膜下血肿	双孔钻孔引流	未报道
Carmont[13]	2002	65/男	无	竞走	几周	头痛伴左脚下垂，左臂无力	CT扫描：右侧硬膜下血肿	双孔钻孔引流	完全恢复
Demetriades[16]	2004	24/男	无	足球	6周	进行性头痛，呕吐伴轻度右侧肢体无力	CT扫描：大面积硬膜下血肿	双孔钻孔引流	临床症状满意
Miele[47]	2004	24/女	无	拳击	12个月	头痛伴早上恶心加重	CT扫描：左侧异质性硬膜下血肿	额颞顶开颅手术	未报道
Pretorius[61]	2005	11/男	无	旅途中的活动	几周	头痛及恶心进行性加重	MRI：右侧凸面的硬膜下血肿	双孔钻孔引流	完全恢复
Alaraj[2]	2005	24/男	无	举重	几周	头痛加重	CT扫描：左侧额顶叶硬膜下血肿	双孔钻孔引流	未报道
Miele[48]	2006	31/男	无	拳击	几周	头痛伴记忆丧失	MRI：两个小的硬膜下血肿，没有引起占位效应或中线偏移	开颅手术	临床症状恢复满意
Robles[64]	2006	20/男	无	拳击	1个月	头痛伴呕吐	具有占位效应的左侧等密度慢性硬膜下血肿	开颅手术	完全恢复
Roldan-Valadez[67]	2006	13/女	无	坐过山车	3周	头痛伴右侧肢体偏瘫	MRI：左侧凸面亚急性硬膜下血肿	未报道	完全恢复

(续表)

第一作者[参考文献]	发表年份	年龄(岁)/性别	既往史	运动	从创伤到诊断的时间间隔	症状	影像学表现	治疗	结局
Zhang[88]	2007	21/男	无	游泳/水上运动	未报道	头痛伴呕吐	CT扫描：左额叶-顶叶-颞叶慢性硬膜下血肿	开颅手术	完全恢复
Zhang[88]	2007	9/女	无	跑步	3周	头痛伴呕吐	CT扫描：左侧额叶-顶叶-颞叶硬膜下血肿	开颅手术	完全恢复
Türkoğlu[78]	2008	25/男	无	武术	6个月	头痛	CT扫描：左侧硬膜下区域密度低	双孔钻孔引流	完全恢复
Tsitsopoulos[76]	2008	15/男	无	体育赛事	3周	头痛伴恶心和间歇性呕吐	CT扫描：右侧额颞区亚急性硬膜下血肿	双孔钻孔引流	完全恢复
Domenicucci[18]	2009	7/男	无	足球	未报道	未报道	CT扫描：左侧额颞叶硬膜下血肿	双孔钻孔引流	完全恢复
Domenicucci[18]	2009	41/男	无	自行车	未报道	未报道	CT扫描：右侧额颞叶硬膜下血肿	双孔钻孔引流	完全恢复
Pillai[57]	2009	23/男	蛛网膜囊肿	自行车	1周	头痛伴恶心、呕吐	CT扫描：双侧混合密度硬膜下血肿	钻孔引流+开颅手术	完全恢复
Pillai[57]	2009	41/男	无	未报道	12周	头痛伴恶心	CT扫描：左侧额颞叶低密度硬膜下血肿	双孔钻孔引流	完全恢复
Hamada[26]	2010	15/男	无	排球	几周	头痛伴呕吐	MRI：左外侧凸面硬膜下血肿	开颅手术	临床症状恢复满意
Zeng[87]	2011	14/男	无	跳高训练	3周	头痛伴喷射性呕吐	CT扫描：左侧额叶-顶叶低密度颞部硬膜下血肿	开颅手术	完全恢复
Zeng[87]	2011	16/男	蛛网膜囊肿	足球	4周	头痛及恶心进行性加重	CT扫描：颞叶-额叶-顶叶低密度硬膜下血肿	双孔钻孔引流	完全恢复
Işik[30]	2010	13/男	无	足球	几周	头痛	CT扫描：等密度硬膜下血肿	未报道	未报道
Kertmen[36]	2012	12/男	无	跆拳道训练	3周	进行性头痛	CT扫描：额顶叶等密度硬膜下血肿	双孔钻孔引流	完全恢复
Park[54]	2013	75/男	高血压、糖尿病、肾功能不全和痛风	重量训练	3周	头痛	CT扫描：双侧等密度硬膜下血肿	双孔钻孔引流	完全恢复
Blereau[5]	2013	7/女	未报道	自行车	未报道	未报道	未报道	双孔钻孔引流	完全恢复
Maher[43]	2013	16/男	未报道	足球	3周	头痛	未报道	未手术	完全恢复
Maher[43]	2013	12/女	未报道	足球	3周	头痛、呕吐	未报道	未手术	完全恢复

(续表)

第一作者[参考文献]	发表年份	年龄(岁)/性别	既往史	运动	从创伤到诊断的时间间隔	症状	影像学表现	治疗	结局
Cress[15]	2013	45/男	无	足球	2个月	头痛伴记忆丧失	CT扫描：凸面血肿	开颅手术	未报道
Zheng[90]	2013	16/男	无	运动相关（无指定）	7周	头痛伴恶心	CT扫描：等密度硬膜下血肿	未报道	完全恢复
Edmondson[19]	2014	14/男	无	足球	未报道	头痛	CT扫描：高密度左侧额叶-颞叶-顶叶硬膜下血肿	双孔钻孔引流	未报道
Hou[29]	2014	17/男	无	篮球	未报道	进行性头痛伴恶心	CT扫描：凸面血肿	双孔钻孔引流	临床症状恢复满意
Takizawa[74]	2015	15/男	无	足球	8周	头痛伴记忆问题	CT扫描：左侧等密度硬膜下血肿	开颅手术	完全恢复
Takizawa[74]	2015	13/男	无	自行车	7周	头痛	CT扫描：左侧低密度硬膜下血肿	双孔钻孔引流	未报道
Takizawa[74]	2015	31/男	无	武术	4周	头痛	CT扫描：右侧等密度硬膜下血肿	双孔钻孔引流	未报道
Takizawa[74]	2015	35/女	无	滑雪/单板滑雪	20周	头痛，GCS8分	CT扫描：左侧低密度硬膜下血肿	双孔钻孔引流	未报道
Takizawa[74]	2015	32/男	无	滑雪/单板滑雪	16周	头痛	CT扫描：左侧低密度硬膜下血肿	开颅手术	未报道
Pascoe[56]	2015	43/男	蛛网膜囊肿	足球	3周	恶心，呕吐，头痛	CT扫描：右侧等密度硬膜下血肿	开颅手术	未报道
Yaldiz[85]	2016	16/男	蛛网膜囊肿	足球	3周	进行性头痛	CT扫描：右侧等密度硬膜下血肿	开颅手术	完全恢复
Gregori[25]	2019	18/男	无	足球	1个月	头痛和恶心	MRI：左额叶-颞顶叶高信号硬膜下血肿	双孔钻孔引流	完全恢复
Gregori[25]	2019	6/男	无	足球	3周	头痛和恶心	CT扫描：高密度左侧额叶-颞叶-顶叶硬膜下血肿	额颞开颅术	完全恢复

足球、柔道、跆拳道、霹雳舞和排球。所有数据已汇总于表25.2。

在我们的研究中，男性和女性的比例为10∶1.91，这表明在年轻的CSDH患者中男性占优势是一个明显的趋势。H. Baallal等报道的66例病例中有13例是踢足球的年轻男性。在我们的研究中，66名患者中有38名年龄在18岁以下。Fabrizio Gregori[25]报道的研究数据中，33名患者年龄在18岁或以下，其中包括13名踢足球患者。这一发现明确地提出了一个问题：根据最近的苏黎世指导方针建议，18岁以下的运动员在脑震荡后不应重返同一场比赛，该建议是否也应该扩大到18岁以上的运动员。

由于参与足球的人数众多，而且频繁参与可能会导致脑震荡的发病率升高（10年比赛发病率为50%），可能是时候考虑使用足球头盔了[34]。在足球运动员中，大约每1000名运动员暴露于0.15次脑震荡[3, 7]。最近一项对高中十项运动的分析报告显示，女性足球是导致脑震荡的第三大常见原因。Master等[44]最近报道指出，27%的业余足球运动员经历过一次与足球相关的脑震荡，23%的人在他们的业余生涯中经历过多次脑震荡。

25.4 病理生理学与二次冲击综合征

直接头部创伤是硬膜下血肿最常见的原因，它是通过将外力传递到大脑而发生的；由于平移（线性）加速或旋转加速，会导致脑损伤发生，即静态或动态能量传递到头骨。在非接触性头部创伤的情况下，脑损伤可以通过头部的平移、旋转或角运动来解释，从而导致大脑的加速和减速。这种能量有时会非常剧烈，以至于导致非常严重的脑出血和移位性颅骨骨折，偶尔也只是轻微的静脉拉伸。这些拉伸力可能导致蛛网膜或桥静脉撕裂。离心力对大脑实质的影响比对大脑表面的影响更明显，它干扰了神经纤维束和脑内血管。

除了硬脑膜下血肿占位效应造成的损伤外，由于多次（有时是数百次）打击，通常还会对大脑内部造成明显的相关损害（挫伤或水肿）。"二次冲击综合征"（SIS）是决定脑震荡后运动员是否能重返赛场的主要因素。SIS的定义是当运动员遭受了初始的头部损伤（最常见的是脑震荡），在第一次相关的症状未完全消除之前，又遭受了第二次头部损伤[9, 12]。

从历史上看，SIS的第一例临床报道是1881年

表25.2 纳入的66例病例中的体育活动

运动类型	第一作者和年份	例数（%）
足球	Gregori 2019（2例）/Yaldiz 2016 Takizawa 2015/Edmondson 2014/Maher 2013/Işik 2011/Domenicucci 2009/Demetriades 2004/Prabhu 2002（2例）/Chillala 2001/Kawanishi 1999（2例）/Maeda 1993/Oliver 1958	16（24.2%）
自行车	Takizawa 2015/Blereau 2013/Domenicucci 2009/Pillai 2009/Rogers 1990/Hara 1984	6（9%）
坐过山车	Roldan-Valadez 2006/Fukutake 2000（3例）/Bo-abbass 1995/Fernandes 1994	6（9%）
体能/重量训练	Park 2013/Zeng 2011/Tsitsopoulos 2008/Zhang 2007/Carmont 2002/Mori 2002	6（9%）
篮球	Hou 2014/Tsuzuki 2003/Rogers1990/Keller 1998/McNeil 1987	5（7.5%）
武术	Takizawa 2015/Kertmen 2012/Türkoğlu 2008/Yokoyama 1989/Weinberg 1973	5（7.5%）
足球	Pascoe 2015/Maher 2013/Cress 2013/	4（6%）
游泳/水上运动	Zhang 2007/Mori 1995/Rogers 1990	3（4.5%）
拳击	Roldan-Valadez 2006/Fukutake 2000（3例）/Bo-abbass 1995/Fernandes 1994	3（4.5%）
滑雪/单板滑雪	Takizawa 2015/Rogers 1990/Lacour 1978	3（4.5%）
排球	Hamada 2010	1（1.5%）
橄榄球	Varma 1981	1（1.5%）
跳舞	McNeil 1987	1（1.5%）
马术	Page 1987	1（1.5%）
举重	Jacome 1989	1（1.5%）

由 Otto Bollinger 提出的，他使用了"创伤性卒中"一词[9]。当一个人在第一次脑损伤的症状消失之前遭受第二次脑损伤时，就会发生 SIS[9, 12]。发生严重的脑水肿是由脑血管自身调节失衡引起的，并导致明显的神经功能障碍[9, 84]。SIS 是一种罕见的疾病，主要发生在青少年和年轻人中。SIS 通常会出现严重的神经功能缺陷和死亡[9, 12]。关于 SIS 的流行病学数据很少，因此确切的发病率尚不清楚，危险因素尚未确定。十多年前，这种综合征的存在仍在受到质疑，从那时起其他学者也开始对潜在的类似病变提出关注[4, 8]。

二次撞击综合征的病理生理学被认为与大脑血液供应的自我调节丧失有关，大脑血液供应的自我调节指于血压变化期间，大脑循环能够将血液流量维持在相对恒定的水平。颅脑手术、创伤甚至药物都会干扰大脑血液的自动调节，但其与颅脑损伤严重程度或患者结局并不相关[8]。在没有外伤和任何易感条件的情况下，硬膜下出血可能是由于静脉压力突然增加而引起的，这可能发生在患者强行呼气时。有人提出，举重训练可能会因为在"挺举"过程中产生 Valsalva 动作而导致硬膜下血肿。在"挺举"过程中，运动员首先下蹲并吸气，然后将重物从地面抬到胸部。然后，当重量被移到他们头顶上方的位置时，他们进行腹式呼吸腹内压上升（Valsalva 动作）。颅内低血压也可继发于脱水引起的全身性低血压。然而，运动时发生急性和短暂性脱水也有可能导致颅内低血压和硬膜下血肿，马拉松运动员在比赛中平均损失 5% 的体重和 6.5% 的血浆量[45]。

在坚硬的颅骨内，脑、脑脊液和颅内血液的总容量保持不变。因此，其中一个成分的减少会导致其余两个成分中的一个或两个的相互增加[49]。脑脊液压力低导致脑向下移位，可造成硬脑膜边界细胞层的桥静脉撕裂，导致这些静脉破裂。在举重进行 Valsalva 动作时，硬脑膜桥静脉破裂可引起出血。运动后可发生颅内低血压，这是自发性硬膜下出血的另一个危险因素，因为单次极限负荷运动可导致全身性血管低血压[17]。一项研究发现，运动后 10 min 收缩压降低 20 mmHg[35, 41]。

25.5 硬膜下血肿的部位

单侧血肿 43 例（65.2%），双侧血肿 5 例（7.6%）。33 例（50%）患者患侧在左侧，10 例（15.2%）患者患侧在右侧。最后，18 例（27.3%）患者未明确患侧。有趣的是，我们发现 80.3%（53/66）的慢性硬膜下血肿患者有蛛网膜囊肿（AC）。

25.6 临床表现

慢性硬膜下血肿（CSDH）的定义是创伤后 3 周或 3 周以上出现血肿。CSDH 的发病机制之一是外伤导致硬膜下腔出血。最初的出血可能是少量的，不能产生明显的脑组织压迫。然而，可能会有持续的出血或渗血进入硬膜下间隙[33]。

创伤与临床症状出现的时间间隔随年龄增长而延长，这是由于老年人脑萎缩，使得血肿需增长至更大体积才会出现明显症状。重要的是要了解，运动员的慢性硬膜下血肿与老年人和许多非运动员创伤受害者的常见慢性硬膜下血肿不同。运动员通常没有老年患者所具有的大的潜在硬膜下空间，因此占位效应和颅内压升高可以更快地发生。除了硬脑膜下血液的占位效应造成的损伤外，通常还伴有明显的脑实质损伤（挫伤或水肿）。在本系列中，患者最常见的症状是头痛。这在年轻患者中更为常见，因为他们往往患有由慢性硬膜下血肿引起的颅内压升高。

根据我们的回顾研究发现，96% 的患者出现头痛，近 40% 的患者出现呕吐和（或）恶心，10% 的患者出现复视。在我们的调查中，年轻的 CSDH 患者在寻求治疗前症状持续时间较短，这是由于老年患者合并脑萎缩而导致颅内代偿空间较大（表 25.1）。持续时间较长可以解释为 CSDH 患者症状的隐匿性发作，这与颅内成分减少导致蛛网膜下腔容纳血肿的能力升高有关。

老年患者在出现临床症状前，在硬膜下腔往往已经积累了大量的积血，症状延缓出现与老年患者合并脑萎缩有关。正如我们在 Fogelholm 等[22]学者的综述中发现，老年慢性硬膜下血肿患者更容易出现偏瘫和精神恶化，而年轻患者在体检时更容易出现头痛和乳头水肿。老年患者在出现临床表现前，可能已在硬膜下腔积累了大量的积血。

我们有理由假设，体育运动员与典型非意外创伤（NAT）患者之间发生的 CSDH 的影像学具有相似性。这两种类型的受害者都可能遭受了反复的头部损伤。有研究表明，与意外头部损伤相比，发生 NAT 的婴儿和儿童的缺氧缺血性脑损伤的发生率更高。也有动物研究证据表明，年轻的大脑更容易受到反复的轻度创伤性脑损伤[62]。

25.7 影像学表现

硬膜下血肿的发生形式可为急性或慢性。硬膜下血肿通常是由高速损伤引起的，头部受到剪切力或大脑挫伤，导致大脑表面的桥静脉渗出的血液不断积聚。诊断的首选影像学检查是 CT 扫描，主要是因为它比 MRI 更快、更经济，而且还可以用于有金属植入物和心脏起搏器的患者。

慢性硬膜下血肿在 CT 上具有多种影像学特征，相对于脑实质的低、中或高密度，其中等密度是最常见的密度类型[70]。也有报道称低密度是 CT 扫描中最常见的慢性硬膜下血肿类型，然而等密度慢性硬膜下血肿常被报道为比低密度病变更常见[89]。这可能取决于患者群体、CT 扫描分辨率和密度分类方法。本组病例中，等密度 17 例（25.8%），低密度 17 例（25.8%），混合型 3 例（4.5%），未明确密度 29 例（43.9%）。

CSDH 通常呈凹凸状，急性硬膜外血肿很少出现类似的影像学表现。MRI 在确定 CSDH 的大小和内部结构（如多部位和血肿膜）方面比 CT 更敏感。在 MRI 上也可观察到新鲜出血、溶血和血红蛋白变化。DTI 成像可以检测慢性硬膜下血肿导致锥体束的移位变化[89]。

25.8 治疗

治疗的主要目标应该是通过去除硬膜下腔的纤维蛋白降解产物来中断纤维蛋白再生和溶解的恶性循环。慢性硬膜下血肿的手术方式是一个有争议的话题，有多种手术方式可用于血肿的清除，从经皮硬膜下穿刺[20]到大开颅去除血肿膜[73,79]，其中钻孔开颅和封闭系统引流是最为广泛接受的血肿引流方法[82]。许多其他手术方式已被报道，如麻花钻开颅术、开颅切除硬膜下膜、血肿分流伴持续冲洗引流、经皮针穿刺和开放系统引流反复盐水冲洗等。

64 例与运动损伤相关的慢性硬膜下血肿患者在进行脑成像后因其临床情况接受了手术。29 例（43.9%）采用钻孔手术，24 例（36.4%）采用开颅手术。在 8 例（12.1%）患者中，作者选择了钻孔和开颅术的组合。有 3 例（4.5%）患者所采用的手术方式没有明确记录。

25.9 预后

46 例患者（69.6%）术前临床症状在术后 48 h 内完全缓解，临床预后良好，19 例患者（28.78%）术后临床随访未见复发。遗憾的是，Fukutake 等报道的一名 73 岁的患者在 13 天后死亡，其死亡情况没有详细描述[23]。

在医学文献中，很少有关于运动员在发生慢性硬膜下血肿后重返运动的指导。需要指出的是，个体情况以及基础疾病、创伤甚至衰老对不同的运动员造成的影响是不同的。"内生能力"是指身体和心理的能力，而"功能能力"是指进行活动的能力。由于环境和（或）使用辅助设备存在增加内生能力的可能，其可以涉及人与事务的互动、规则与程序的制定、节奏和目标、内容、分工与分层等多种内生能力[28]。

我们需要在症状缓解和认知恢复的基础上，前瞻性地评估重返赛场的方法，并确定这种方法的结果对相关运动员是安全的，并且适合所其从事的运动[10]。在进行此类研究之前，研究人员应遵循大多数团队医生的指导，结合丰富的知识和临床判断安全地治疗这些运动员。人们普遍认为，为了避免过早回归比赛的潜在危险后果，球员在重返比赛之前应该完全康复。

目前关键的问题是我们如何预防脑肿胀的发生，我们能否预测哪些儿童或运动员有患这种疾病的风险，并积极治疗以降低脑肿胀的发病率和死亡率。到目前为止，我们还没有这些问题的答案。为了成功地治疗头部损伤，球员和教练都需要了解多发性头部损伤的风险，以及如何正确指导回归比赛的方法。球员经常在头部受伤后决定返回比赛，而不寻求医疗治疗，出现这种行为有时是因为对教练组和其他球员态度的担忧。此外，运动员往往不知道在没有适当医学治疗的情况下重返比赛可能带来的危及生命的后果[24]。虽然这些重返赛场的运动员没有出现颅内出血的复发，但对他们受伤后的远期影响知之甚少。

25.10 结论

随着几乎所有国家体育运动参与度的提高，运动性损伤的患者发展为硬膜下血肿的病例数量也有所增加。运动性损伤并发慢性硬膜下血肿的真实发生率尚不清楚。这项研究将引起所有神经外科医生和其他治疗与运动损伤相关慢性硬膜下血肿患者的医生的关注。在参与接触或碰撞运动的人群中，蛛网膜囊肿的存在被认为是参与相关运动的相对禁忌证，因为有出血并进入囊肿腔的风险。因此，我们应该告知这些患者及其家属出现慢性硬膜下血肿并发症的可能性，并建议无论囊肿的大小和位置如何，都要注意避免运动中头部受伤。

参考文献

1. Adhiyaman V, Asghar M, Ganeshram K, Bhowmick B. Chronic subdural haematoma in the elderly. Postgrad Med J. 2002;78:71–5.
2. Alaraj AM, Chamoun RB, Dahdaleh NS, Haddad GF, Comair YG. Spontaneous subdural haematoma in anabolic steroids dependent weight lifters: reports of two cases and review of literature. Acta Neurochir. 2005;147:85–7.
3. Barnes B, Cooper L, Kirkendall D, McDermott T, Jordan B, Garrett W. Concussion history in elite male and female soccer players. Am J Sports Med. 1998;26:433–8.
4. Bey T, Ostick B. Second impact syndrome. West J Emerg Med. 2009;10:6–10.
5. Blereau RP, Haley TJ. Arachnoid cyst. Consultant. 2013;53:540–1.
6. Bo-abbass Y, Bolton CF. Roller coaster headache. N Engl J Med. 1995;332:1585.
7. Boden B, Kirkendall D, Garrett W. Concussion incidence in elite college soccer players. Am J Sports Med. 1998;26:238–41.
8. Byard R, Vink R. The second impact syndrome. Forensic Sci Med Pathol. 2009;5:36–8.
9. Cantu R. Second-impact syndrome. Clin Sports Med. 1998;17:37–44.
10. Cantu R. Athletic concussion: current understanding as of 2007. Neurosurgery. 2007;60:963–4.
11. Cantu R, Mueller F. Brain injury-related fatalities in American football, 1945–1999. Neurosurgery. 2003;52:846–52.
12. Cantu R, Gean A. Second-impact syndrome and a small subdural hematoma: an uncommon catastrophic result of repetitive head injury with a characteristic imaging appearance. J Neurotrauma. 2010;27:1557–64.
13. Carmont M, Mahattanakul W, Pigott T. Acquisition of a chronic subdural haematoma during training for competitive race walking. Br J Sports Med. 2002;36:306–7.
14. Chillala S, Read C, Evans PA. An unusual case of subdural haematoma presenting to the accident and emergency department. Emerg Med J. 2001;18:308–9.
15. Cress M, Kestle JRW, Holubkov R, Riva-Cambrin J. Risk factors for pediatric arachnoid cyst rupture/hemorrhage: a case control study. Neurosurgery. 2013;72:716–22.
16. Demetriades AK, McEvoy AW, Kitchen ND. Subdural haematoma associated with an arachnoid cyst after repetitive minor heading injury in ball games. Br J Sports Med. 2004;38:E8.
17. Denoronha R, Sharrack B, Hadjivassiliou M, Romanowski C. Subdural haematoma: a potentially serious consequence of spontaneous intracranial hypotension. J Neurol Neurosurg Psychiatry. 2003;74:752–5.
18. Domenicucci M, Russo N, Giugni E, Pierallini A. Relationship between supratentorial arachnoid cyst and chronic subdural hematoma: neuroradiological evidence and surgical treatment. J Neurosurg. 2009;110:1250–5.
19. Edmondson L, Upshaw J, Tuuri R. A 14-year-old male with a 10-week history of headaches. Pediatr Ann. 2014;43:220–3.
20. Ernestus R, Beldzinski P, Lanfermann H, Klug N. Chronic subdural hematoma: surgical treatment and outcome in 104 patients. Surg Neurol. 1997;48:220–5.
21. Fernandes CMB, Daya MR. A roller-coaster headache: case report. J Trauma. 1994;37:1007–10.
22. Fogelholm R, Heiskanen O, Waltimo O. Chronic subdural hematoma in adults. Influence of patient's age on symptoms, signs, and thickness of hematoma. J Neurosurg. 1975;42:43–6.
23. Fukutake T, Mine S, Yamakami I. Roller coaster headache and subdural hematoma. Neurology. 2000;54:264.
24. Gerberich SG, Priest JD, Boen JR, Straub CP, Maxwell RE. Concussion incidences and sever-

ity in secondary school varsity football players. Am J Public Health. 1983;73:1370–5.
25. Gregori F, Colistra D, Mancarella C, Chiarella V, Marotta N, Domenicucci M. Arachnoid cyst in young soccer players complicated by chronic subdural hematoma: personal experience and review of the literature. Acta Neurol Belg. 2020;120:235–46.
26. Hamada H, Hayashi N, Umemura K. Middle cranial fossa arachnoid cyst presenting with subdural effusion and endoscopic detection of tear of the cyst. Neurol Med Chir (Tokyo). 2010;50:512–4.
27. Hara H, Inoue T, Matsuo K. Unusual computed tomographic findings in a case of arachnoid cyst in the middle cranial fossa. Surg Neurol. 1984;22:79–82.
28. Hilleshein E, Souza L, Lautert L, Paz A, Catalan VM, Teixeira M, et al. Capacidade para o trabalho de enfermeiros de umhospitaluniversitário. Rev Gaúcha Enf. 2011;32:509–15.
29. Hou K, Li CG, Zhang Y, Zhu BX. The surgical treatment of three young chronic subdural hematoma patients with different causes. J Korean Neurosurg Soc. 2014;55:218–21.
30. Işik SH, Yildiz O, Ceylan Y. Chronic subdural hematoma caused by soccer ball trauma associated with arachnoid cyst in childhood: case report. Neurol Sci Neurophysiol. 2011;28:398–401.
31. Jacome DE, Yanez GF. Subdural haematoma upon straining. J Neurol Neurosurg Psychiatry. 1989;52:134.
32. Jones N, Blumbergs P, North J. Acute subdural haematomas: aetiology, pathology and outcome. Aust N Z J Surg. 1986;56:907–13.
33. Kaste M, Waltimo O, Heiskanen O. Chronic bilateral subdural haematoma in adults. Acta Neurochir (Wien). 1979;48:231–6.
34. Kawanishi A, Nakayama M, Kadota K. Heading injury precipitating subdural hematoma associated with arachnoid cysts: two case reports. Neurol Med Chir (Tokyo). 1999;39:231–3.
35. Keller T, Holland M. Chronic subdural haematoma: an unusual injury from playing basketball. Br J Sports Med. 1998;32:338–9.
36. Kersey RD. Acute subdural hematoma after a reported mild concussion: a case report. J Athl Train. 1998;33:264–8.
37. Kertmen H, Gürer B, Yilmaz ER, Sekerci Z. Chronic subdural hematoma associated with an arachnoid cyst in a juvenile taekwondo athlete: a case report and review of the literature. Pediatr Neurosurg. 2012;48:55–8.
38. Lacour F, Trevor R, Carey M. Arachnoid cyst and associated subdural hematoma. Observations on conventional roentgenographic and computerized tomographic diagnosis. Arch Neurol. 1978;35:84–9.
39. Lindsay KW, McLatchie G, Jennett B. Serious head injury in sport. BMJ. 1980;281:789–91.
40. Logan S, Bell G, Leonard J. Acute subdural hematoma in a high school football player after 2 unreported episodes of head trauma: a case report. J Athl Train. 2001;36:433–6.
41. MacDonald JR, MacDougall JD, Interisano SA, Smith KM, McCartney N, Moroz JS, et al. Hypotension following mild bouts of resistance exercise and submaximal dynamic exercise. Eur J Appl Physiol Occup Physiol. 1999;79:148–54.
42. Maeda M, Kawamura Y, Handa Y. Value of MR imaging in middle fossa arachnoid cyst with intracystic and subdural hematoma. Eur J Radiol. 1993;17:145–7.
43. Maher CO, Garton HJ, Al-Holou WN, Trobe JD, Muraszko KM, Jackson EM. Management of subdural hygromas associated with arachnoid cysts. J Neurosurg Pediatr. 2013;12:434–43.
44. Matser E, Kessels A, Lefak M, Jordan B, Troost J. Neuropsychological impairment in amateur soccer players. JAMA. 1999;282:971–3.
45. Maughan R, Whiting P, Davidson R. Estimation of plasma volume changes during marathon running. Br J Sports Med. 1985;19:138–41.
46. McNeil SL, Austin Spruill W, Langley RL. Multiple subdural hematomas associated with breakdancing. Ann Emerg Med. 1987;16:114–6.
47. Miele VJ, Carson L, Carr A. Acute on chronic subdural hematoma in a female boxer: a case report. Med Sci Sports Exerc. 2004;36:1852–5.
48. Miele VJ, Bailes JE, Cantu RC, Rabb CH. Subdural hematomas in boxing: the spectrum of consequences. Neurosurg Focus. 2006;21:E10.
49. Mokri B. The Monro-Kellie hypothesis: applications in CSF volume depletion. Neurology. 2001;56:1746–8.
50. Mori T, Katayama Y, Kawamata T. Acute hemispheric swelling associated with thin subdural hematomas: pathophysiology of repetitive head injury in sports. Acta Neurochir Suppl. 2006;96:40–3.
51. Ochi M, Morikawa M, Ogino A. Supratentorial arachnoid cyst and associated subdural hematoma: neuroradiologic studies. Eur Radiol. 1996;6:640–4.

52. Oliver LC. Primary arachnoid cysts: report of two cases. BMJ. 1958;1:1147–9.
53. Page A, Paxton RM, Mohan D. A reappraisal of the relationship between arachnoid cysts of the middle fossa and chronic subdural haematoma. J Neurol Neurosurg Psychiatry. 1987;50:1001–7.
54. Park HR, Lee KS, Bae HG. Chronic subdural hematoma after eccentric exercise using a vibrating belt machine. J Korean Neurosurg Soc. 2013;54:265–7.
55. Parkkari J, Kujala M, Kannus P. Is it possible to prevent sports injuries? Sports Med. 2001;31:985–95.
56. Pascoe HM, Phal PM, King JA. Progressive post traumatic tearing of an arachnoid cyst membrane resulting in intracystic and subdural haemorrhage. J Clin Neurosci. 2015;22:897–9.
57. Pillai P, Menon SK, Manjooran RP, Kariyattil R, Pillai AB, Panikar D. Temporal fossa arachnoid cyst presenting with bilateral subdural hematoma following trauma: two case reports. J Med Case Rep. 2009;3:53.
58. Pothe H. Chronic subdural haematoma in prize fighters (In German). Beitr Neurochir. 1964;8:232–7.
59. Powell J, Barber-Foss K. Traumatic brain injury in high school athletes. JAMA. 1999;282:958–63.
60. Prabhu VC, Bailes JE. Chronic subdural hematoma complicating arachnoid cyst secondary to soccer-related head injury: case report. Neurosurgery. 2002;50:195–7.
61. Pretorius PM, McAuley DJ. Something old, something new? Br J Radiol. 2005;78:1063–4.
62. Raghupathi R, Mehr M, Heflaer M, Margulies S. Traumatic axonal injury is exacerbated following repetitive closed head injury in the neonatal pig. J Neurotrauma. 2004;21:307–16.
63. Rashid S, Watson C, Agarwal R. Episodic headache and arachnoid cyst related subdural hematoma. Headache. 2016;56:1354–5.
64. Robles LA, Hernandez V. Subdural and intracystic hematomas in an arachnoid cyst secondary to a boxing injury. Inj Extra. 2006;37:375–8.
65. Rogers MA, Klug GL, Siu KH. Middle fossa arachnoid cysts in association with subdural hematomas. A review and recommendations for management. Br J Neurosurg. 1990;4:497–502.
66. Roldan-Valadez E, Facha MT, Martinez-Lopez M, Herrera-Mora P. Subdural hematoma in a teenager related to roller-coaster ride. Eur J Paediatr Neurol. 2006;10:194–6.
67. Ross R, Oschner M. Acute intracranial boxing related injuries in US Marine Corps recruits: report of two cases. Mil Med. 1999;164:68–70.
68. Santarius T, Hutchinson P. Chronic subdural haematoma: time to rationalize treatment. Br J Neurosurg. 2004;18:328–32.
69. Seelig J, Becker D, Miller D, Greenberg R, Ward J, Choi S. Traumatic acute subdural hematoma: major mortality reduction in comatose patients treated within four hours. N Engl J Med. 1981;304:1511–8.
70. Senturk S, Guzel A, Bilici A, Takmaz I, Guzel E, Aluclu MU, et al. CT and MR imaging of chronic subdural hematomas: a comparative study. Swiss Med Wkly. 2010;140:335–40.
71. Shell D, Carico G, Patton R. Can subdural hematoma result from repeated minor head trauma? Phys Sportsmed. 1993;21:74–84.
72. Strahle J, Selzer B, Geh N. Sports participation with arachnoid cysts. J Neurosurg Pediatr. 2016;17:410–7.
73. Svien HJ, Gelety JE. On the surgical management of encapsulated subdural hematoma. A comparison of the results of membranectomy and simple evacuation. J Neurosurg. 1964;21:172–7.
74. Takizawa K, Sorimachi T, Honda Y, Ishizaka H, Baba T, Osada T. Chronic subdural hematomas associated with arachnoid cysts: significance in young patients with chronic subdural hematomas. Neurol Med Chir (Tokyo). 2015;55:727–34.
75. Torg JS, Vegso JJ, Sennelt B. The national football head and neck injury registry: 14-year report on cervical quadriplegia, 1971 through 1984. JAMA. 1985;254:3439–43.
76. Tsitsopoulos PP, Pantazis GC, Syrmou EC, Tsitsopoulos PD. Intracranial arachnoid cyst associated with traumatic intracystic hemorrhage and subdural haematoma. Hippokratia. 2008;12:53–5.
77. Tsuzuki N, Katoh H, Ohtani N. Chronic subdural hematoma complicating arachnoid cyst secondary to soccer-related head injury: case report. Neurosurgery. 2003;53:242–3.
78. Türkoğlu E, Serbes G, Sanli M, Sari O, Sekerci Z. Chronic subdural hematoma in capoeira sport. Turk Neurosurg. 2008;18:39–41.
79. Tyson G, Strachan WE, Newman P, Winn HR, Butler A, Jane J. The role of craniectomy in the treatment of chronic subdural hematomas. J Neurosurg. 1980;52:776–81.

80. Ulmer S, Engellandt K, Stiller U, Nabavi A, Jansen O, Mehdorn MH. Chronic subdural hemorrhage into a giant arachnoidal cyst (Galassi classification type III). J Comput Assist Tomogr. 2002;26:647–53.
81. Varma TRK, Sedzimir CB, Miles JB. Post-traumatic complications of arachnoid cysts and temporal lobe agenesis. J Neurol Neurosurg Psychiatry. 1981;44:29–34.
82. Wakai S, Hashimoto K, Watanabe N, Lnoh S, Ochiai C, Nagai M. Efficacy of closed-system drainage in treating chronic subdural hematoma: a prospective comparative study. Neurosurgery. 1990;26:7713.
83. Weinberg PE, Flom RA. Intracranial subarachnoid cysts. Radiology. 1973;106:329–33.
84. Wetjen N, Pichelmann M, Atkinson J. Second impact syndrome: concussion and second injury brain complications. J Am Coll Surg. 2010;211:553–7.
85. Yaldiz C, Kacira T, Ceylan D, Asil K. Chronic subdural hemorrhage associated with an arachnoid cyst after sports injury in childhood. Neurosurg Q. 2016;26:361–4.
86. Yokoyama K, Tonami N, Kimura M. Scintigraphic demonstration of intracranial communication between arachnoid cyst and associated subdural hematoma. Clin Nucl Med. 1989;14:350–3.
87. Zeng T, Shi S, Lin Y. Chronic subdural hematoma associated with sylvian arachnoid cyst in juvenile athletes: report of two cases and literature review. Chin J Traumatol. 2011;14:174–7.
88. Zhang H, Zhang JM, Chen G. Chronic subdural hematoma associated with arachnoid cyst: report of two cases. Chin Med J (Engl). 2007;120:2339–40.
89. Zhao KJ, Zhang RY, Sun QF, Wang XQ, Gu XY, Qiang Q, et al. Comparisons of 2/3Sh estimation technique to computer-assisted planimetric analysis in epidural, subdural and intracerebral hematomas. Neurol Res. 2010;32:910–7.
90. Zheng S-P, Li G, You C. Chronic subdural hematoma associated with arachnoid cysts in young people. Neurosurg Q. 2013;23:258–61.

第 26 章 慢性硬膜下血肿的神经影像学鉴别诊断（影像学层面）

Ali Akhaddar

译者：朱炳城

26.1 引言

慢性硬膜下血肿（chronic subdural hematoma，CSDH）通常可由计算机断层成像（CT）诊断。CSDH 典型的血肿表现为沿着颅骨凸面呈新月形的陈旧性积血。大多数情况下，血肿的密度较低；但是，也可以看到等密度、混合或不均匀密度的病变（图 26.1 a～d）。CSDH 通常是单侧的，有明显的占位效应。但也有部分 CSDH 可发生于双侧，大脑半球间以及颅后窝。在罕见病例中，可以观察到血肿发生机化、钙化甚至是骨化（图 26.1 e，f）[44, 55]。因为该病的神经影像学表现很可能与其他疾病相似，使得 CSDH 的诊断更具有挑战性。

除了病史资料外，临床信息和生物学数据对放射科医生的疾病确诊和鉴别诊断也发挥着重要作用。

在颅脑 CT 和（或）磁共振成像（MRI）结果中，创伤性、感染性、炎症性、肿瘤病变甚至正常成像结果都可能与 CSDH 相似。此外，一些硬膜下血肿的表现在 CT 上很难诊断（表 26.1）。另外，CSDH 与其他疾病同时存在的情况以前也有文献报道，因此，在处理任何形状的硬膜下血肿时都要考虑到与其他相关疾病的鉴别诊断[11, 20, 25, 28-29, 50, 59]。提及所有这些诊断难点并不在本章范围。根据病变的起源和发病机制，总结了慢性硬膜下血肿最常见的影像学鉴别诊断。

26.2 硬膜下脓肿

颅内硬膜下脓肿是发生在硬脑膜和软脑膜之间的脓性物质聚集。鼻窦炎、中耳炎或牙源性感染是硬膜下脓肿的主要感染源，其他常见病因包括脑膜

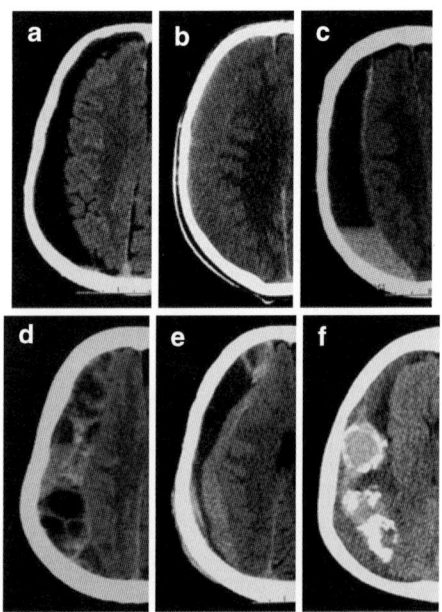

图 26.1 慢性硬膜下血肿的几种不同类型：（a）低密度，（b）等密度，（c）慢性硬膜下血肿的急性出血期，（d）混合型，（e）机化的慢性硬膜下血肿，（f）钙化的慢性硬膜下血肿

表 26.1 慢性硬膜下血肿的主要鉴别诊断

- 硬膜下脓肿
- 硬膜外脓肿
- 急性 / 亚急性硬膜下血肿
- 蛛网膜下腔出血
- 脑卒中
- 肿瘤 / 转移瘤
- 硬膜下积液
- 蛛网膜囊肿
- 儿童的特殊情况 慢性硬膜下积液 脑萎缩 脑积水 蛛网膜下腔增大 颅脑比例失调
- 肥厚性硬脑膜炎
- 软脑膜病变（Rosai-Dorfman 病）
- 正常颅内解剖变异
- CT 扫描未被明确诊断的 CSDH
- 伪影

炎、颅骨骨髓炎、开颅手术后并发症、外伤后感染和血流播散性感染[3, 12, 14]。

硬膜下脓肿 CT 扫描结果一般表现为等密度或低密度的新月形，有时可不显示病灶。脓肿的颅内转移常见原因是水肿（脑炎），而非脓肿本身播散。注射造影剂后可更好地分清脓肿边界，特别是脓肿脓腔的内侧（皮质缘）（图 26.2）。在 MRI 上，脓腔弥散加权成像（DWI）的弥散效应受限，表观弥散系数（ADC）图像为低信号，光谱检查乳酸浓度升高[3]。增强后，增厚的硬脑膜出现明显的强化。严重时可出现广泛的脑水肿、脑炎、血栓性静脉炎和静脉梗死（图 26.3）。

许多细菌性病原体、寄生虫可能是导致硬膜下脓肿的原因。有文献报道了两例硬膜下神经囊尾蚴病（寄生虫感染），在硬膜下出现了游离性的囊尾蚴，其影像学表现类似于慢性硬膜下出血[13, 21]。

26.3 急性/亚急性硬膜下血肿

急性和亚急性硬膜下血肿通常是继发于头部外伤后的常见损伤，有如下常见的原因：

1. 脑实质受伤出血导致血液积聚。
2. 头部受到剧烈撞击，脑皮质和（或）桥静脉因惯性力量（加速/减速）而破裂。

此外，一些急性/亚急性硬膜下血肿可能发生于没有外伤史但患有出血性疾病（接受抗凝治疗或患有凝血疾病）的患者身上，或其他罕见继发性病因如肿瘤或血管畸形患者。此外，也有少数病例发生于颅骨或脊柱手术后。详情请见本书第 2 章。

急性/亚急性血肿 CT 扫描结果主要表现为一个高密度（急性血肿）（图 26.4 和图 26.5）或等密度（亚急性血肿）（图 26.6）的新月形病灶，通常

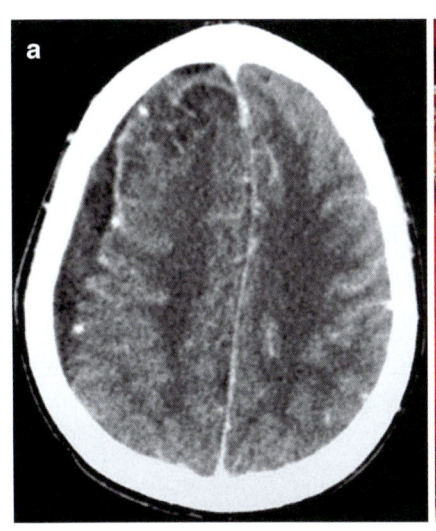
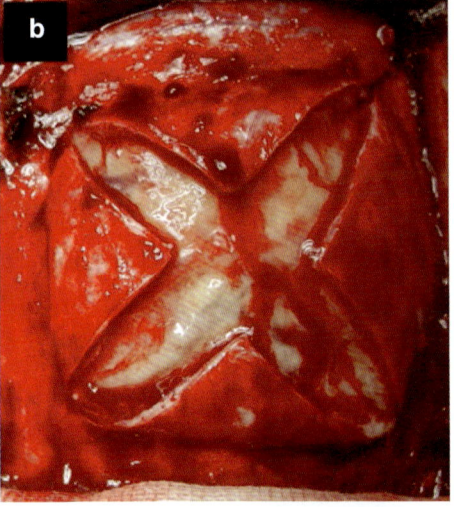

图 26.2 （a）CT 扫描显示右侧额部硬膜下脓肿。（b）硬膜开放后的额部硬膜下脓肿的手术视图

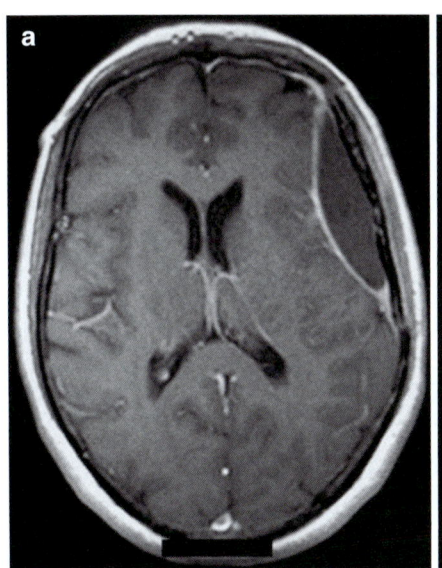
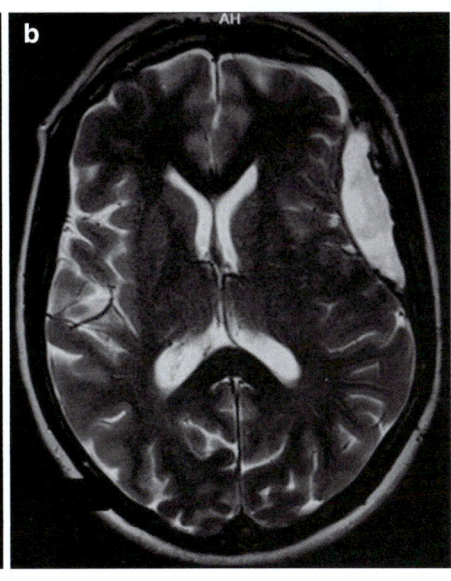

图 26.3 增强 MRI 的 T1 加权像（a）和 T2 加权像（b）显示左侧额部硬膜外脓肿

图 26.4 CT 显示右侧的创伤性急性硬膜下血肿

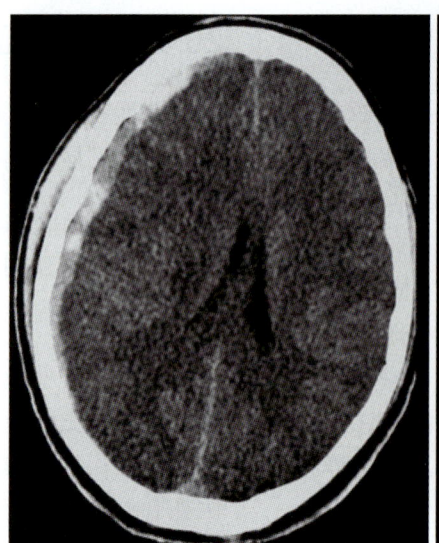
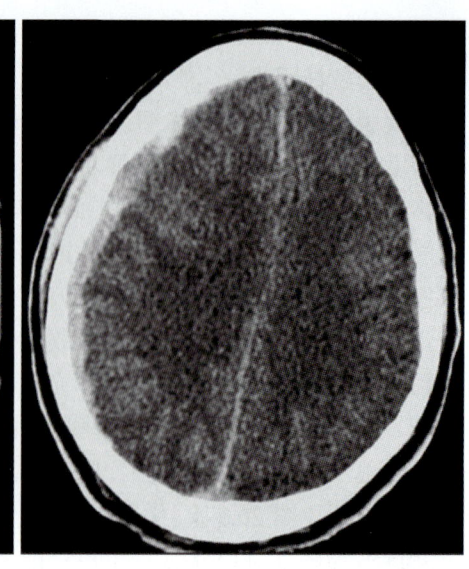

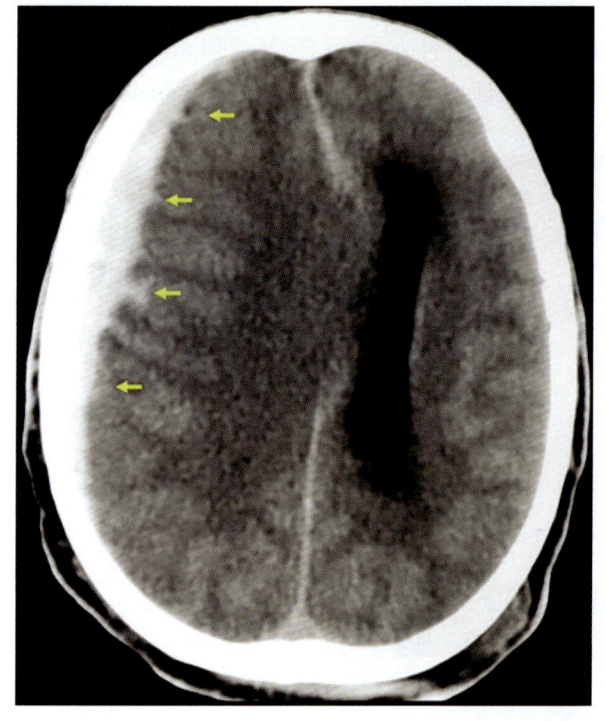

图 26.5 在一名接受抗凝治疗的患者 CT 成像中，观察到自发性的急性硬膜下血肿和蛛网膜下腔出血（黄色箭头所示）

伴有脑水肿、占位效应和中线移位。严重的硬膜下血肿表现伴有脑挫伤、脑实质内血肿、基底池消失和对侧颞角扩张。急性/亚急性血肿有时可能与 CSDH 混淆，特别是慢性低密度血肿中混有急性/亚急性出血血块（图 26.1c～e）。

26.4 蛛网膜下腔出血

日本的一些研究指出，迟发性的蛛网膜下腔出血可能被误诊为 CSDH[42, 51, 54]。在 CT 图像上，基底节或蛛网膜下腔空间内的等密度或高密度积血并不一定代表蛛网膜下腔出血（图 26.5）。Ohno 等学者研究证明，MRI 鉴别 CSDH 与蛛网膜下腔出血是有效的，特别是在 FLAIR 序列中[42]。

26.5 硬膜外血肿

硬膜外血肿（EDH）的特点是在颅骨和硬膜之间出现血液积聚。最常见的病因是颞骨骨折导致硬膜外腔的脑膜中动脉出血。在 CT 扫描中，EDH 通常表现为高密度的双凸形（图 26.7）。此外，EDH 通常不会跨越中线，除非有颅骨骨折或其他病变存在[1-2]。1987—2017 年间的文献报道了 15 例不典型外观的硬膜外血肿[45]。在这 15 名患者中，有 7 名 CSDH 患者的血肿边缘呈双凸形。CSDH 血肿表现为双凸形的原因尚不清楚，但可能是由于颅腔内组织粘连所造成的。值得注意的是，上述病例均接受了开颅血肿清除术[45]。

在既往的研究中，有些颅内血肿被描述为"硬膜间"的血肿。这种罕见的情况可能是由于出血将骨膜硬脑膜与脑膜硬脑膜分离所造成的。诊断这种罕见的病例并不容易，需要通过手术和（或）组织病理学结果才能做出判断[9, 46]。

26.6 脑卒中

尽管某些 CSDH 可能表现为缺血性发作，但根据 CT 成像结果区分缺血性卒中和硬膜下血肿并不困难。在一例特殊病例中，经头颅 CT 扫描高度

第 26 章 慢性硬膜下血肿的神经影像学鉴别诊断（影像学层面） 187

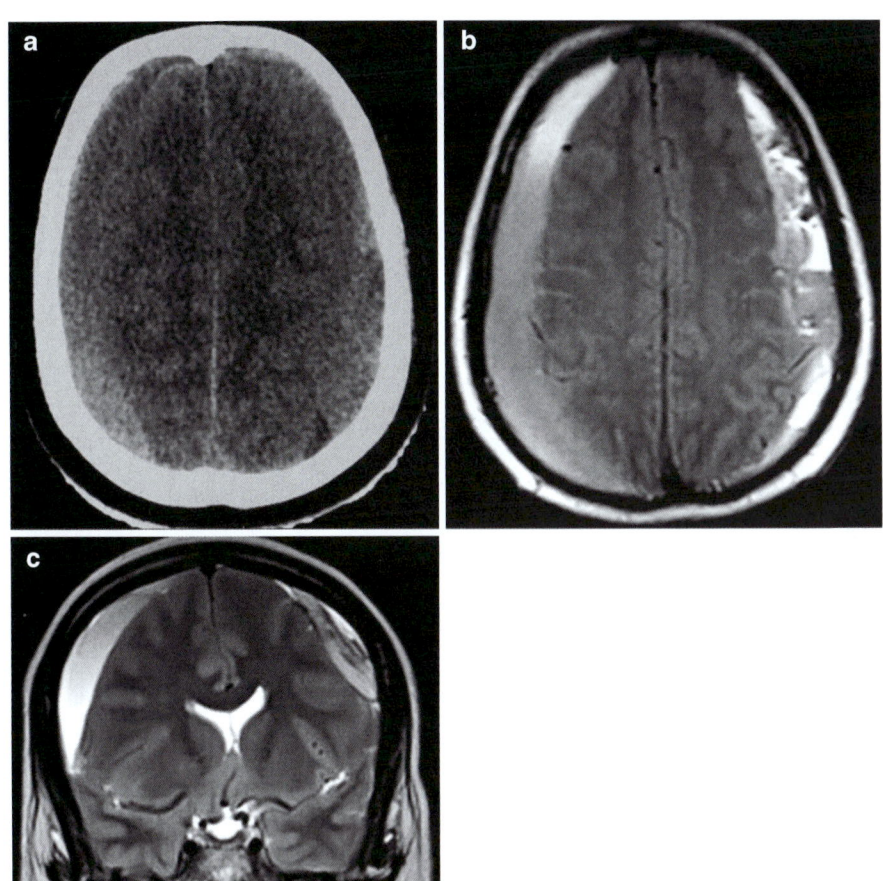

图 26.6 （a）双侧硬膜下血肿的 CT 图像，（b）双侧硬膜下血肿的轴状位 T2 加权像，（c）双侧硬膜下血肿的冠状位 T2 加权像

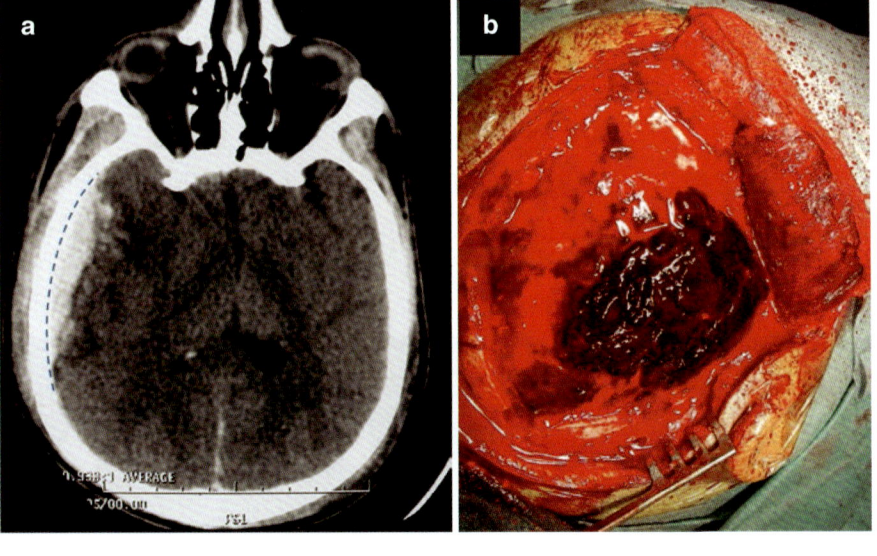

图 26.7 轴位 CT 扫描：右颞创伤后急性硬膜外血肿（a）。去除骨瓣手术后视图：硬膜外可见急性血肿（血凝块）（b）

怀疑是右颞枕部慢性异质性硬膜下血肿，但在 MRI 中得到了"脑卒中"的正确诊断（图 26.8）。根据 MRI 结果回顾 CT 图像，发现患者脑实质水肿，灰白分化消失，脑组织无受压。当 CSDH 与脑卒中无法区分时，MRI 可以有效地进行鉴别。Shimizu 等学者报道，非典型的脑梗死 CT 图像可表现为低密度区域与脑动脉分布区域不完全重合，与周围脑组织界限清楚[49]。临床接诊有脑血管疾病病史的老年人时应考虑不典型影像学特征的可能，最终诊断需依据 MRI 结果。

26.7 创伤性硬膜下积液

CSDH 和硬膜下积液通常都由轻微的脑部创伤

图 26.8 （a）CT 扫描怀疑右侧有慢性异质性硬膜下血肿，（b）轴向 MRI 的 FLAIR 序列显示脑部缺血区。注意脑实质水肿、灰白分化消失、无脑移位等特点

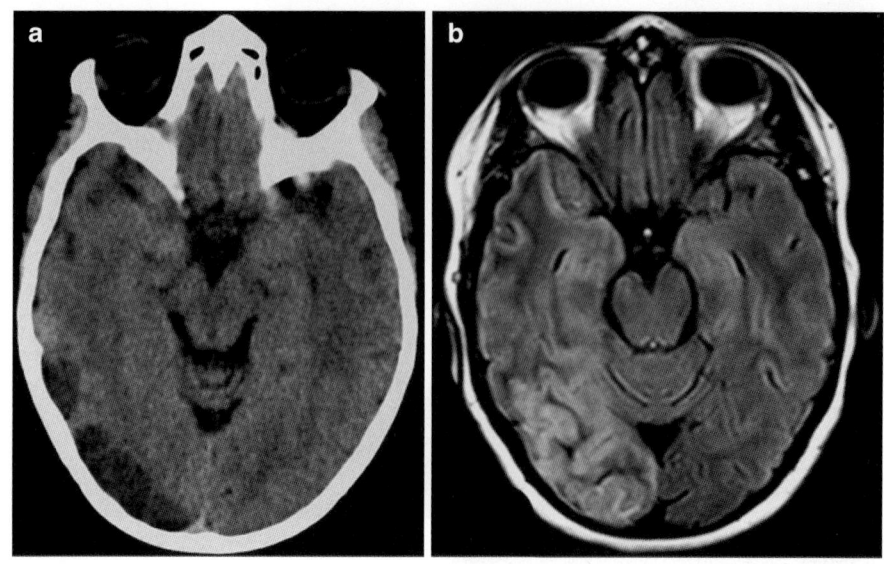

所引起。然而，CSDH 与硬膜下积液在许多方面都不同，如神经影像学外观和临床表现等[34]。因为硬膜下积液的内容物通常是血液和脑脊液的混合物，因此在某些情况下区分这两个疾病并不容易[30]。此外，硬膜下积液变成 CSDH 的情况也并不少见（见第 16 章颅脑创伤性硬膜下积液后的慢性硬膜下血肿）。

硬膜下积液一般被认为是外伤后硬膜/蛛网膜分离的结果，主要表现为硬膜下少量液体聚集。一般认为，脑膜（蛛网膜）撕裂是主要的致病机制[22]。此外，足够大的潜在硬膜下空间（尤其是老年人出现脑萎缩后）是硬膜下积液扩张的关键条件[22, 30]。大部分硬膜下积液发生于大脑侧裂和额叶凸起处。

在 CT 和 MRI 上，单纯硬膜下积液的密度和信号与脑脊液相似（图 26.9）。然而，也有文献指出当硬膜下积液中混杂着出血后，其 CT 图像上密度可能会增高，MRI 图像因混杂血液出现不均匀信号[30]。需要注意的是，皮质静脉不会穿过硬膜下积液区[36]。

26.8 肿瘤

多种硬脑膜和硬脑膜下肿瘤，包括淋巴瘤、转移瘤、肉瘤、胶质母细胞瘤、脑膜瘤和单发纤维瘤，在神经影像学上都可能与 CSDH 相混淆[8, 10, 18-20, 23, 31-32, 37, 39, 41, 48, 53]。此外，这些病变也可能是 CSDH 的病因[11, 29, 38]。临床病史中如果没有头部外伤史，但是硬膜下肿块出现结节状表现，以及随访时发现病变扩大，则应怀疑肿瘤的可能（图 26.9）。2016 年，一项关于硬膜下血肿的系统回顾研究发现，与 CSDH 最相似的病变是淋巴瘤

图 26.9 轴位头颅 CT 扫描显示左侧的硬膜下积液伴脑实质受压

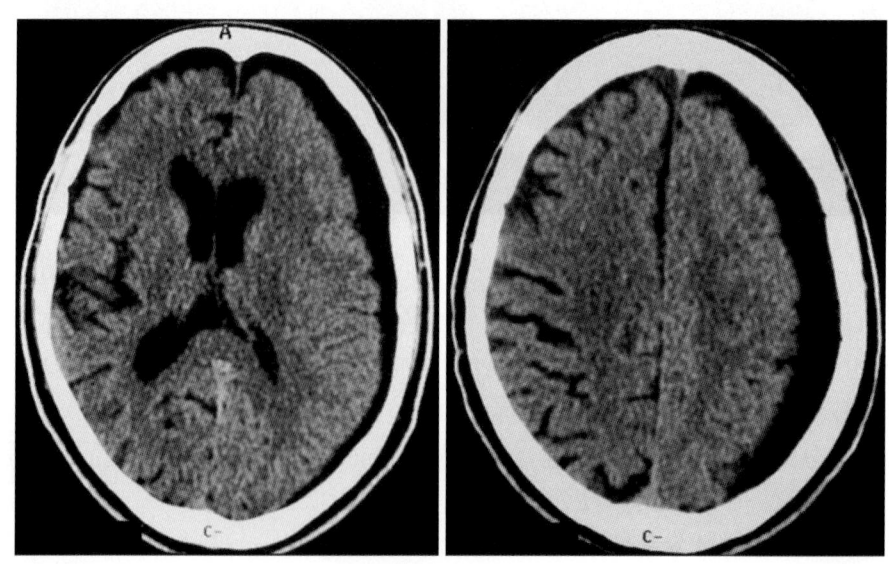

(29%)，其次是转移瘤（21%）和肉瘤（15%）[8]。平扫 CT 通常不足以区分肿瘤病变和 CSDH，只有通过手术才能明确区分[20, 41, 53]。然而，一些 CT 表现可以帮助鉴别 CSDH，包括骨质改变（脑膜瘤的骨质增生和硬脑膜转移的骨质侵蚀）、结节状和分叶状边界、多灶性病变以及不同时期出血的不均匀表象[11, 57]。出现脑水肿或脑皮质的扩展也提示肿瘤的可能（图 26.10a）。增强 CT 有助于鉴别肿瘤，但钆增强 MRI 可以提供更好的图像分辨率（图 26.10b）[32]。不同于 CSDH，钆增强 MRI 中肿瘤表现呈均匀强化[23]，硬脑膜转移瘤表现为增厚的均匀强化[18]。MRI 对检测小脑实质转移瘤也具有一定价值[29]。

26.9 儿童颅外积液

颅外积液是一个广泛用于儿童的颅外脑脊液积聚的术语。文献中对相同或类似的情况有不同的名称，如良性硬膜下积水、有症状的慢性颅外积水、外脑积水、硬膜下积水、假性脑积水、良性沟通性脑积水和脑室外梗阻性脑积水[17, 26, 33, 40, 59]。这种情况有时会与 CSDH 相混淆[30]。随着现代 MRI 技术的发展，鉴别诊断婴儿期的脑外积水已经变得容易[17]。在 CT 扫描结果中，主要表现为在额叶上出现低密度影，同时出现脑沟的扩张，而脑室通常呈正常或轻微膨胀[19, 30]。围产期外伤、颅内感染（如脑膜炎）、分流术后、窒息后以及凝血功能障碍均被怀疑是造成这种病变的原因[27, 33]。

26.10 肥厚性脑膜炎

已知某些形式的慢性硬膜下血肿在增强磁共振下包膜可能强化，这与纤维-胶原改变有关，而非是由于并存疾病（如感染或恶性肿瘤）所引起。肥厚性硬脑膜炎（hypertrophic pachymeningitis，HP）是一种以脑和（或）脊髓硬膜局限性或弥漫性纤维性增厚为特征的中枢神经系统罕见疾病。按发病部位可分为肥厚性硬脑膜炎和肥厚性硬脊膜炎（图 26.11）。肥厚性脑膜炎的病因主要包括炎症、自身免疫性疾病、感染和肿瘤[4, 6, 16, 43, 47]。然而某些病例的确切病因仍不清楚，这种情况下发生的肥厚性脑膜炎被称为"特发性"。在 CT 扫描结果中，增厚的硬脑膜可能会与慢性硬膜下血肿难以鉴别。在增强 MRI 结果中，肥厚性脑膜炎可能会存在脑膜瘤的特征——"硬膜尾征"[43]。此外，脑膜的增强可能与邻近的脑水肿有关（图 26.11）。

其他自身免疫性疾病如多血管炎肉芽肿病（以前称为韦格纳病），同样会出现与 CSDH 类似的病变特点[27, 32, 52, 58]。

26.11 正常解剖组织

各种正常的大脑和静脉结构在 CT 和 MRI 上的表现都可能与 CSDH 相混淆。其中，突出的静脉窦和皮质静脉可能被误诊为硬膜下血肿。增强 CT 扫描会显示正常组织中央均匀强化[24, 32]。

此外，一些脑叶实质结构（如延伸到颅中窝和

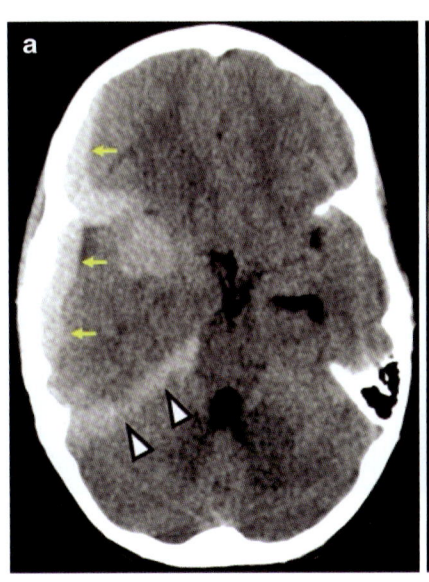
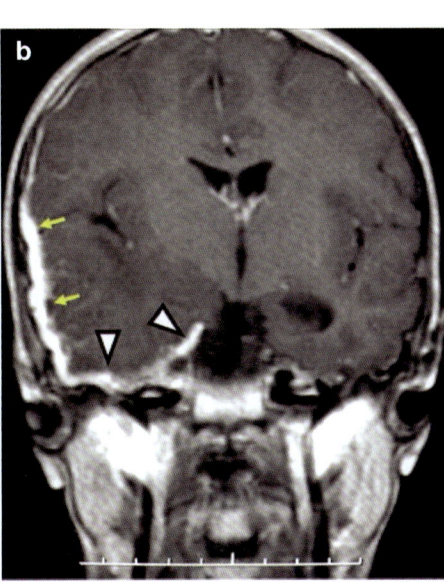

图 26.10　轴位颅脑平扫 CT 图像（a）及冠状位增强 MRI T1 加权图像（b）提示右额颞部的淋巴瘤（黄色箭头），并延伸至小脑幕和颅底（白色箭头）

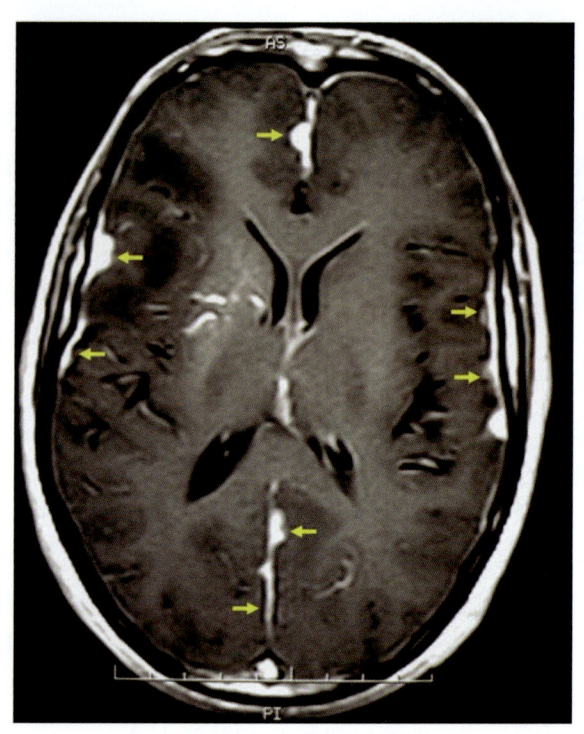

图 26.11　增强 MRI 扫描下的肥厚性脑膜炎。注意脑膜增厚等影像学特点（黄色箭头）

颅后窝的额叶和小脑球囊）也可能被误诊为 CSDH。因此，仔细观察相邻层面的扫描平片可以确定连续性的正常生理组织，有助于明确疾病判断[32]。

26.12　未被明确诊断的慢性硬膜下血肿

有时双侧或单侧等密度的 CSDH 可能会对 CT 中的结果诊断造成很大的困难（图 26.12）[1, 7, 15]，这是由于：①血肿呈等密度，很难与邻近的正常脑实质区分开来。②双侧大脑半球和侧脑室对称受压，使得占位效应不明显，没有中线移位的出现。"兔耳征"经常被认为是诊断 CSDH 的依据。"兔耳征"是指两个脑室的内侧受压，形成一个狭窄的、狭长的脑室（前额角尖锐，相互靠近）[35]。在难以区分的情况下，MRI 可以帮助对这种不典型的 CSDH 做出正确诊断（图 26.6）[7, 56]。

26.13　CT 图像上的伪影

一些伪影会降低 CT 扫描图像的质量[5]。沿着额部颅顶深面的线状伪影可能会与硬膜下血肿相似[32]。此外，患者的误动可导致重建的 CT 图像出现阴影、模糊或条纹。放射科医生必须优化图像质量，防止伪影的出现。

26.14　结论

CSDH 在临床中存在很多诊断误区与相似病变。在诊断有疑问或影像结果特征不典型的情况下，应尽可能要求患者接受增强 CT，甚至 MRI 检查。进一步的影像学检查可以明确病变形态和内部构造，确定病变的边缘，并明确与邻近组织的解剖结构关系，这些对后续治疗至关重要。

图 26.12　轴位 CT 平扫：（a）双侧硬膜下血肿（黄色箭头）很难与脑实质相鉴别。（b）单侧等密度的硬膜下血肿与邻近脑实质难以区分（黄色虚线所示）

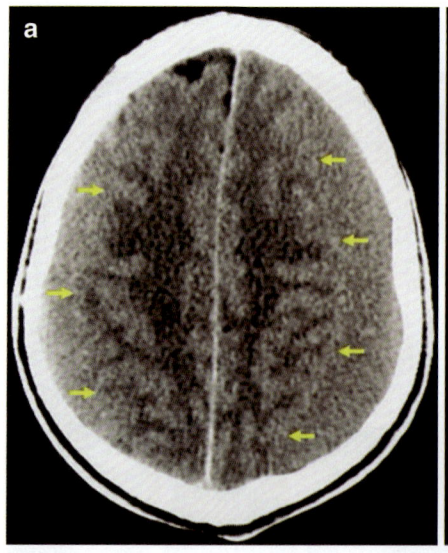
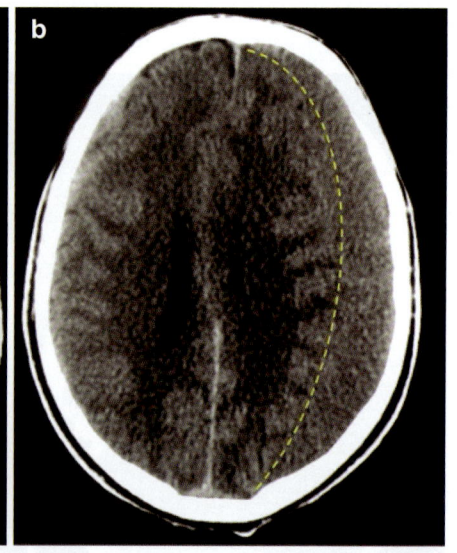

参考文献

1. Agrawal A. Bilateral biconvex frontal chronic subdural hematoma mimicking extradural hematoma. J Surg Tech Case Rep. 2010;2:90–1. https://doi.org/10.4103/2006-8808.73625.
2. Akhaddar A. The yin-yang shaped image following head injury. Pan Afr Med J. 2013;16:133. https://doi.org/10.11604/pamj.2013.16.133.3555.
3. Akhaddar A. Cranial subdural empyemas. In: Akhaddar A, editor. Atlas of infections in neurosurgery and spinal surgery. Cham: Springer International Publishing; 2017. p. 51–64.
4. Akhaddar A, Rharrassi I. Hypertrophic cranial pachymeningitis coinfection with tuberculosis and actinomycosis. Surg Neurol Int. 2020;11:201. https://doi.org/10.25259/SNI_383_2020.
5. Barrett JF, Keat N. Artifacts in CT: recognition and avoidance. Radiographics. 2004;24:1679–91. https://doi.org/10.1148/rg.246045065.
6. Blitshteyn S, Mechtler LL, Bakshi R. Diffuse dural gadolinium MRI enhancement associated with bilateral chronic subdural hematomas. Clin Imaging. 2004;28:90–2. https://doi.org/10.1016/S0899-7071(03)00205-5.
7. Boviatsis EJ, Kouyialis AT, Sakas DE. Misdiagnosis of bilateral isodense chronic subdural haematomas. Hosp Med. 2003;64:374–5. https://doi.org/10.12968/hosp.2003.64.6.374.
8. Catana D, Koziarz A, Cenic A, Nath S, Singh S, Almenawer SA, et al. Subdural hematoma mimickers: a systematic review. World Neurosurg. 2016;93:73–80. https://doi.org/10.1016/j.wneu.2016.05.084.
9. Chen KT, Huang HC, Lin YJ, Chen MH, Hsieh TC. The relationship between hematoma and pachymeninges in an interdural hematoma: diagnosis and surgical strategy. World Neurosurg. 2018;110:492–8.e3. https://doi.org/10.1016/j.wneu.2017.11.040.
10. Cheng YK, Wang TC, Yang JT, Lee MH, Su CH. Dural metastasis from prostatic adenocarcinoma mimicking chronic subdural hematoma. J Clin Neurosci. 2009;16:1084–6. https://doi.org/10.1016/j.jocn.2008.08.008.
11. Cherif El Asri A, El Mostarchid B, Akhaddar A, Boucetta M. Chronic subdural hematoma revealing skull metastasis. Intern Med. 2011;50:791. https://doi.org/10.2169/internalmedicine.50.4654.
12. Doan N, Patel M, Nguyen HS, Mountoure A, Shabani S, Gelsomino M, et al. Intracranial subdural empyema mimicking a recurrent chronic subdural hematoma. J Surg Case Rep. 2016;2016(9):rjw158. https://doi.org/10.1093/jscr/rjw158.
13. Feinberg WM, Valdivia FR. Cysticercosis presenting as a subdural hematoma. Neurology. 1984;34:1112–3. https://doi.org/10.1212/wnl.34.8.1112.
14. French H, Schaefer N, Keijzers G, Barison D, Olson S. Intracranial subdural empyema: a 10-year case series. Ochsner J. 2014;14:188–94.
15. Guénot M. Chronic subdural hematoma: diagnostic imaging studies. Neurochirurgie. 2001;47:473–8.
16. He Z, Ding F, Rong J, Gan Y. A case of idiopathic hypertrophic cranial pachymeningitis presenting as chronic subdural hematoma. Zhejiang Da Xue Xue Bao Yi Xue Ban. 2016;45:540–3.
17. Hellbusch LC. Benign extracerebral fluid collections in infancy: clinical presentation and long-term follow-up. J Neurosurg. 2007;107(2 Suppl):119–25. https://doi.org/10.3171/PED-07/08/119.
18. Houssem A, Helene C, Francois P, Salvatore C. "The subdural collection" a great simulator: case report and literature review. Asian J Neurosurg. 2018;13:851–3. https://doi.org/10.4103/ajns.AJNS_325_16.
19. Hussain ZB, Hussain AB, Mitchell P. Extra-axial cerebrospinal fluid spaces in children with benign external hydrocephalus: a case-control study. Neuroradiol J. 2017;30:410–7. https://doi.org/10.1177/1971400917719298.
20. Ichinose T, Ueno M, Watanabe T, Murakami KI, Minato H, Hayashi Y. A rare case of chronic subdural hematoma coexisting with metastatic tumor. World Neurosurg. 2020;139:196–9. https://doi.org/10.1016/j.wneu.2020.04.029.
21. Im SH, Park SH, Oh DH, Kang BS, Kwon OK, Oh CW. Subdural cysticercosis mimicking a chronic subdural hematoma. Case illustration. J Neurosurg. 2005;102:389. https://doi.org/10.3171/jns.2005.102.2.0389.
22. Kamezaki T, Yanaka K, Fujita K, Nakamura K, Nagatomo Y, Nose T. Traumatic acute subdural hygroma mimicking acute subdural hematoma. J Clin Neurosci. 2004;11:311–3. https://doi.org/10.1016/j.jocn.2003.10.013.

23. Kanazawa T, Miwa T, Akiyama T, Ohara K, Kosugi K, Nishimoto M, et al. A case of aggressive recurrent intracranial subdural hematoma associated with angiosarcoma originating from the skull. World Neurosurg. 2019;126:120–3. https://doi.org/10.1016/j.wneu.2019.02.168.
24. Kiliç T, Akakin A. Anatomy of cerebral veins and sinuses. Front Neurol Neurosci. 2008;23:4–15. https://doi.org/10.1159/000111256.
25. Komiyama M, Yasui T, Tamura K, Nagata Y, Fu Y, Yagura H. Chronic subdural hematoma associated with middle meningeal arteriovenous fistula treated by a combination of embolization and burr hole drainage. Surg Neurol. 1994;42:316–9. https://doi.org/10.1016/0090-3019(94)90400-6.
26. Kozubek D. Widening of the pericerebral space in infants—consultative problems. Arch Med Sadowej Kryminol. 2019;69:70–81. https://doi.org/10.5114/amsik.2019.89237.
27. Kumar KK, Menon G, Nair S, Radhakrishnan VV. Rosai-Dorfman disease mimicking chronic subdural hematoma. J Clin Neurosci. 2008;15:1293–5. https://doi.org/10.1016/j.jocn.2007.09.010.
28. Kwak YS, Hwang SK, Park SH, Park JY. Chronic subdural hematoma associated with the middle fossa arachnoid cyst: pathogenesis and review of its management. Childs Nerv Syst. 2013;29:77–82. https://doi.org/10.1007/s00381-012-1896-4.
29. Lecouvet FE, Annet L, Duprez TP, Cosnard G, Scordidis V, Malghem J. Uncommon magnetic resonance imaging observation of lumbar subdural hematoma with cranial origin. J Comput Assist Tomogr. 2003;27:530–3. https://doi.org/10.1097/00004728-200307000-00013.
30. Lee HC, Chong S, Lee JY, Cheon JE, Phi JH, Kim SK, et al. Benign extracerebral fluid collection complicated by subdural hematoma and fluid collection: clinical characteristics and management. Childs Nerv Syst. 2018;34:235–45. https://doi.org/10.1007/s00381-017-3583-y.
31. Lee J, Kim MS, Kim YZ. Extensive pachymeningeal dissemination of glioblastoma mimicking chronic subdural hematoma: a case report. Brain Tumor Res Treat. 2019;7:39–43. https://doi.org/10.14791/btrt.2019.7.e24.
32. Lim M, Kheok SW, Lim KC, Venkatanarasimha N, Small JE, Chen RC. Subdural haematoma mimics. Clin Radiol. 2019;74:663–75. https://doi.org/10.1016/j.crad.2019.04.013.
33. Litofsky NS, Raffel C, McComb JG. Management of symptomatic chronic extra-axial fluid collections in pediatric patients. Neurosurgery. 1992;31:445–50. https://doi.org/10.1227/00006123-199209000-00009.
34. Liu Y, Gong J, Li F, Wang H, Zhu S, Wu C. Traumatic subdural hydroma: clinical characteristics and classification. Injury. 2009;40:968–72. https://doi.org/10.1016/j.injury.2009.01.006.
35. Marcu H, Becker H. Computed-tomography of bilateral isodense chronic subdural hematomas. Neuroradiology. 1977;14:81–3. https://doi.org/10.1007/BF00339964.
36. McCluney KW, Yeakley JW, Fenstermacher MJ, Baird SH, Bonmati CM. Subdural hygroma versus atrophy on MR brain scans: "the cortical vein sign". AJNR Am J Neuroradiol. 1992;13:1335–9.
37. Miki K, Kai Y, Hiraki Y, Kamano H, Oka K, Natori Y. Malignant meningioma mimicking chronic subdural hematoma. World Neurosurg. 2019:S1878-8750(18)32952-8. https://doi.org/10.1016/j.wneu.2018.12.129.
38. Mirsadeghi SM, Habibi Z, Meybodi KT, Nejat F, Tabatabai SA. Malignant subdural effusion associated with disseminated adenocarcinoma: a case report. Cases J. 2008;1:328. https://doi.org/10.1186/1757-1626-1-328.
39. Neeley OJ, Al-Hreish KM, Aoun SG, El Ahmadieh TY, Plitt A, Vance AZ, et al. Tumoral mimics of subdural hematomas: case report and review of diagnostic and management strategies in primary B-cell lymphoma of the subdural space. World Neurosurg. 2020;133:49–54. https://doi.org/10.1016/j.wneu.2019.09.091.
40. Nguyen VN, Wallace D, Ajmera S, Akinduro O, Smith LJ, Giles K, et al. Management of subdural hematohygromas in abusive head trauma. Neurosurgery. 2020;86:281–7. https://doi.org/10.1093/neuros/nyz076.
41. O'Brien CE, Saratsis AM, Voyadzis JM. Granulocytic sarcoma in a patient with blast crisis mimicking a chronic subdural hematoma. J Clin Oncol. 2011;29:e569–71. https://doi.org/10.1200/JCO.2010.33.1272.
42. Ohno S, Ikeda Y, Onitsuka T, Nakajima S, Haraoka J. Bilateral chronic subdural hematoma in a young adult mimicking subarachnoid hemorrhage. No To Shinkei. 2004;56:701–4.
43. Park IS, Kim H, Chung EY, Cho KW. Idiopathic hypertrophic cranial pachymeningitis misdiagnosed as acute subtentorial hematoma. J Korean Neurosurg Soc. 2010;48:181–4. https://doi.org/10.3340/jkns.2010.48.2.181.
44. Per H, Gümüş H, Tucer B, Akgün H, Kurtsoy A, Kumandaş S. Calcified chronic subdural

hematoma mimicking calvarial mass: a case report. Brain Dev. 2006;28:607–9. https://doi.org/10.1016/j.braindev.2006.03.012.
45. Prasad GL, Menon GR. Lentiform subdural hematoma-a rare mimicker of extradural hematoma. World Neurosurg. 2017;97:738–41. https://doi.org/10.1016/j.wneu.2016.08.109.
46. Prieto R, Pascual JM, Subhi-Issa I, Yus M. Acute epidural-like appearance of an encapsulated solid non-organized chronic subdural hematoma. Neurol Med Chir (Tokyo). 2010;50:990–4. https://doi.org/10.2176/nmc.50.990.
47. Rossi S, Giannini F, Cerase A, Bartalini S, Tripodi S, Volpi N, et al. Uncommon findings in idiopathic hypertrophic cranial pachymeningitis. J Neurol. 2004;251:548–55. https://doi.org/10.1007/s00415-004-0362-y.
48. Semonche A, Gomez P, Kolcun JPG, Perez-Roman RJ, Starke RM. Primary central nervous system lymphoma presenting as chronic subdural hematoma: case report and review of the literature. Cureus. 2020;12:e7043. https://doi.org/10.7759/cureus.7043.
49. Shimizu S, Ozawa T, Irikura K, Sagiuchi T, Kan S, Fujii K. Huge chronic subdural hematoma mimicking cerebral infarction on computed tomography—case report. Neurol Med Chir (Tokyo). 2002;42:380–2. https://doi.org/10.2176/nmc.42.380.
50. Shrestha R, You C. Spontaneous chronic subdural hematoma associated with arachnoid cyst in children and young adults. Asian J Neurosurg. 2014;9:168–72. https://doi.org/10.4103/1793-5482.142739.
51. Son D, Kim Y, Kim C, Lee S. Pseudo-subarachnoid hemorrhage; chronic subdural hematoma with an unruptured aneurysm mistaken for subarachnoid hemorrhage. Korean J Neurotrauma. 2019;15:28–33. https://doi.org/10.13004/kjnt.2019.15.e11.
52. Song JS, Lim MK, Park BH, Park W. Acute pachymeningitis mimicking subdural hematoma in a patient with polyarteritis nodosa. Rheumatol Int. 2005;25:637–40. https://doi.org/10.1007/s00296-005-0615-9.
53. Tan LQ, Loh DD, Qiu L, Ng YP, Hwang PYK. When hoofbeats mean zebras not horses: tumour mimics of subdural haematoma—case series and literature review. J Clin Neurosci. 2019;67:244–8. https://doi.org/10.1016/j.jocn.2019.06.035.
54. Tokuno T, Sato S, Kawakami Y, Yamamoto T. Bilateral chronic subdural hematomas presented with subarachnoid hemorrhage: report of two cases. No Shinkei Geka. 1996;24:573–6.
55. Turgut M, Akhaddar A, Turgut AT. Calcified or ossified chronic subdural hematoma: a systematic review of 114 cases reported during last century with a demonstrative case report. World Neurosurg. 2020;134:240–63. https://doi.org/10.1016/j.wneu.2019.10.153.
56. Williams VL, Hogg JP. Magnetic resonance imaging of chronic subdural hematoma. Neurosurg Clin N Am. 2000;11:491–8.
57. Wu C, Liu J, Yang C. Meningioma mimics chronic subdural hematoma: a case report and discussion of differential diagnosis. Neurol India. 2012;60:549–50. https://doi.org/10.4103/0028-3886.103222.
58. Yagita K, Shinde A, Suenaga T. Rheumatoid meningitis can present MRI findings that mimic chronic subdural haematoma. BMJ Case Rep. 2019;12:e229642. https://doi.org/10.1136/bcr-2019-229642.
59. Zahl SM, Wester K, Gabaeff S. Examining perinatal subdural haematoma as an aetiology of extra-axial hygroma and chronic subdural haematoma. Acta Paediatr. 2020;109:659–66. https://doi.org/10.1111/apa.15072.

第 27 章 慢性硬膜下血肿的非手术治疗

Abad Cherif El Asri，Ali Akhaddar 和 Miloudi Gazzaz

译者：朱炳城

27.1 引言

随着人口老龄化的加剧，慢性硬膜下血肿（chronic subdural hematoma，CSDH）预计会越来越常见。现如今，CSDH 平均发病率约为每 10 万人中 13.1 人，在 70 岁或以上的人中达到每 10 万人中 58 人[7, 36]。虽然手术能够有效地清除血肿，减轻相关神经功能症状，但同样存在多种手术禁忌，并且复发风险高。因此，基于病理生理机制、动物实验和临床研究，我们发现 CSDH 的保守治疗方案同样值得研究，并在患者中表现出良好的效果[10, 15-16]。

27.1.1 保守治疗的合理性：为什么要讨论是否需手术治疗？

CSDH 患者的最佳治疗方法虽然尚未达成共识，但一般有两种治疗方式：对无症状的患者进行观察，对有症状的患者进行血肿引流。有一些研究报道过未经治疗的 CSDH 自行消失的案例。根据一篇 meta 分析报道，2.4%～18.0% 的 CSDH 病例在没有手术或医疗干预的情况可以自行消失[13, 16, 26]。除此之外，手术治疗一直被认为是 CSDH 的一线治疗方法[10]。虽然手术能有效清除血肿或减少血肿体积，但 27%～33% 的患者会出现血肿复发。经手术治疗的 CSDH 患者中总体死亡率高达 24%～32%[35, 38]。手术还与感染、出血和癫痫发作有关。此外，严重心肺疾病（心力衰竭和近期心肌梗死）、遗传性出血性疾病和颅内或全身感染也是手术禁忌证。由于这些手术禁忌证的存在，基于抑制毛细血管出血、抗炎等途径的非手术治疗可能有助于治疗 CSDH，并促进神经系统的恢复[3, 7, 35]。

27.1.2 探讨 CSDH 治疗中的合理用药

27.1.2.1 病理生理学支持：图 27.1

27.1.2.2 皮质类固醇：地塞米松（DXM）

近期，使用类固醇治疗 CSDH 已成为一种受欢迎的替代疗法[40]。既往研究显示，VEGF 和血管紧张素转换酶（ACE）等炎症介质和血管生成介质在 CSDH 的发生发展中起着关键作用[49]。因此，有人推测皮质类固醇通过抑制这些炎症和血管生成因子，抑制 CSDH 中炎症引起的血管生成反应[38, 42]。鉴于这一推测，多项观察性研究评估了类固醇作为单一疗法或作为手术引流的辅助疗法的疗效[4, 7, 36, 44-45, 52]。大多数研究认为，对于不适合手术治疗的 CSDH 患者来说，皮质类固醇可能是一种有效的治疗选择。在一项对 112 名患者的前瞻性队列研究中，比较了使用皮质类固醇（DXM 4 mg，每天 4 次，共 21 天）治疗的患者、使用钻孔引流和术后皮质类固醇治疗的患者、仅使用手术引流的患者以及既不接受手术也不使用皮质类固醇的患者的结果，研究者观察到所有组的住院时间、结果和死亡率都相当，并且没有明显的类固醇相关并发症出现[13]。另外，一项回顾性研究比较了使用皮质类固醇的保守治疗和手术治疗，发现皮质类固醇组有 2/3 的病例避免了手术，96% 的病例预后良好，而手术组只获得 93% 的良好预后。因此对出现轻度或中度神经系统症状的 CSDH 患者来说，使用皮质类固醇保守治疗是一种安全可行的治疗方法[8]。

一项回顾性研究认为，钻孔引流术后使用 DXM 作为手术辅助手段，可有效降低疾病复发风险[4, 36]。同样，近期 Yao 等学者进行的一项共涉及 523 名患者的 meta 分析表明，单独使用或作为辅助治疗的类固醇药物可降低 CSDH 的复发率，但不同研究结果存在很大的差异性[52]。

此外，Thotakura 和 Marabathina 确定了几个

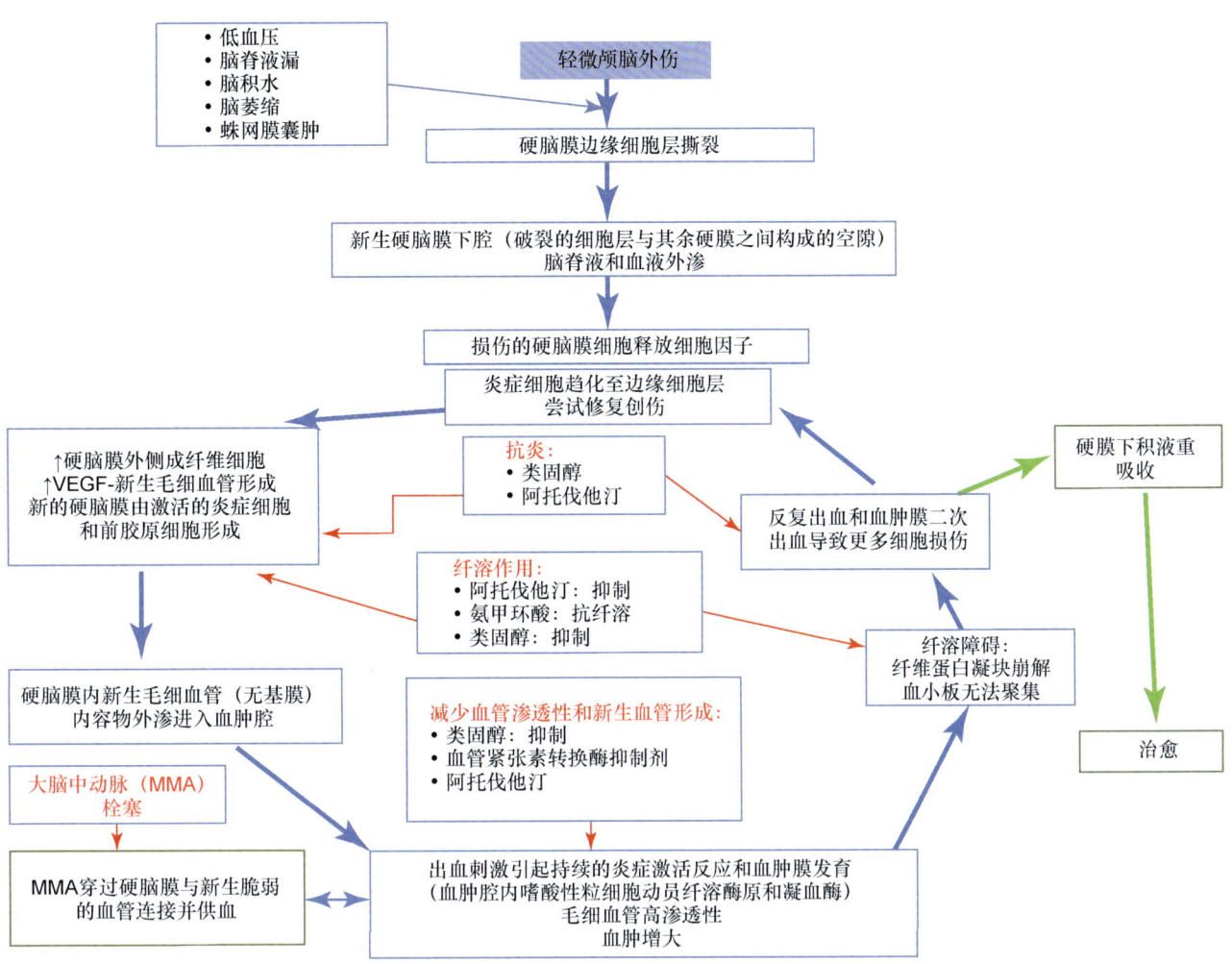

图 27.1　CSDH 保守治疗的病理生理学路径示意图

与 DXM 保守治疗后的良好临床结局有关的因素（女性、较小的中线移位距离和血肿厚度、较低的 CT 密度值）[44-45]。该项研究同样提出了一个影像学分级表（表 27.1），可以用于帮助预测用皮质类固醇成功治疗 CSDH 的概率。他们认为，相对于高等级（4 和 5）的患者，应用皮质类固醇治疗低等级（0～2）的患者可能更容易起效。

另外，Berghauser 等的研究表明，钻孔引流术前使用 DXM 可以有效降低 CSDH 复发率[4]。近期 Miah 等进行了一项研究，比较 DXM 单药治疗与手术治疗 CSDH 患者的临床结局[26]，结果发现这两项治疗方式的效果没有差别。

Almenawer 等最近在其系统回顾和 meta 分析中也报道了类似的研究结果。他们发现，皮质类固醇作为手术治疗后的辅助治疗在复发和治愈率方面并不能使患者获益更多，仍需要更多的证据来进一步证明类固醇能否作为轻度 CSDH 的治疗方法[1]。

使用 DXM 治疗的缺点是其具有较多的并发症，如糖尿病、感染以及精神异常，这也导致住院时间比钻孔引流手术长。在使用 DXM 治疗 CSDH 的研究中，使用 DXM 治疗的患者死亡率为 0.8%～4%[7, 16, 26]。

表 27.1　Amit-Rao 慢性硬膜下血肿的放射学分级 a

中线移位程度	
Ⅰ度（无中线移位）	0
Ⅱ度（中线移位小于 5 mm）	1
Ⅲ度（中线移位 5～10 mm）	2
Ⅳ度（中线移位大于 10 mm）	3
若为双侧血肿，则需加上下列评分	
血肿的 HU 值	
小于 30	0
31～40	1
大于 40	2

a 此表由 Thotakura 和 Marabathina 提出[44]。

鉴于这些不同的结果，一些评估类固醇在 CSDH 治疗中应用疗效的试验正在进行中，如 SUCRE、DESCA 和 Dex-CSDH 试验[11, 19, 25]。

综上所述，尽管 DXM 治疗存在副作用，但这一药物在 CSDH 的保守治疗中发挥了积极作用。此外，标准的治疗剂量、治疗时间以及适用患者群体仍有待确定。尽管现有的几项研究验证了初步结果，但使用 DXM 作为标准医疗手段的合理性仍然处于理论阶段，需要通过大型前瞻性随机研究来证明[53]。

27.1.2.3 阿托伐他汀

阿托伐他汀除了通过抑制 3-羟基-3-甲基戊二酰辅酶 A 还原酶来降低低密度脂蛋白水平外，其作为一种他汀类药物还可用于抑制局部炎症和血管生成[10, 12, 15]。

硬膜下血肿小鼠模型中低剂量的阿托伐他汀[3 mg/（kg·d）]可以提高外周血内皮祖细胞和血管生成因子的水平，促进血管生成和功能性血管的形成；更大剂量的阿托伐他汀[8 mg/（kg·d）]可导致血管内皮生长因子以及基质金属蛋白酶-9（MMP-9）水平的增加[2, 5, 22]。

作为一种保守治疗方法，阿托伐他汀也有望抑制血肿部位的炎症反应。炎症反应会破坏内皮细胞屏障，导致"渗漏性血管"的形成。阿托伐他汀可以通过减少炎症反应引起的血管渗漏和血管形成，防止血肿的形成并加速血肿的吸收，从而改善 CSDH 患者的神经功能[43, 48]。

通过这些机制，阿托伐他汀在治疗 CSDH 患者和减少手术需要方面可能存在一定的价值[33]。事实上，最近的一些研究表明阿托伐他汀在减少血肿体积和降低 CSDH 术后复发率方面有着明显的效果。

Wang 等进行的一项包含了 23 名使用阿托伐他汀（口服剂量为 20 mg，每天一次，为期 1～6 个月）保守治疗 CSDH 患者的前瞻性研究表明[49]，有 22 名患者在治疗的第一个月内血肿体积明显减小，在 36 个月的随访中没有出现复发或明显的不良事件，只有一名患者在保守治疗 4 周后因神经系统症状恶化而接受了手术[49]。

同样，Jiang 等进行的一项双盲、随机、安慰剂对照的临床试验也评估了阿托伐他汀在 CSDH 非手术治疗中的安全性和有效性，结果显示阿托伐他汀组的血肿体积缩小率和临床症状改善率更高，患者生活质量更好，8 周后需要手术的 CSDH 患者明显减少，且无明显不良事件。阿托伐他汀对年龄较大、血肿相对较大的患者似乎更有效。由于该试验中 11.2% 的患者对阿托伐他汀治疗无效，同一作者进行了一项 II 期随机试验，证明联合地塞米松和阿托伐他汀比单独使用阿托伐他汀在减小血肿体积和改善神经功能方面更有优势[15, 49]。一些研究甚至表明，阿托伐他汀对轻度 CSDH 患者的效果与手术治疗效果一样[39, 41]。

因此，无论 CSDH 患者是否需要进行手术治疗，使用阿托伐他汀是对已有治疗方案的有效补充[21]。在一项包含 756 名 CSDH 患者的 6 项研究的 meta 分析中，He 等发现阿托伐他汀在 CSDH 患者的保守治疗和手术治疗中都很有效，可以降低手术后的复发率，促进神经功能恢复[10]。目前正在进行的前瞻性研究显示，在使用阿托伐他汀治疗的 6 名轻度 CSDH 患者中，5 名患者的症状已经得到了明显改善（图 27.2）。

综上所述，阿托伐他汀似乎是无症状或轻度症状 CSDH 患者保守治疗的一个安全有效的选择[27, 47]。为了确定他汀类药物在 CSDH 保守治疗中的真正价值，需要进一步的前瞻性研究和更大的人群队列研究[41]。

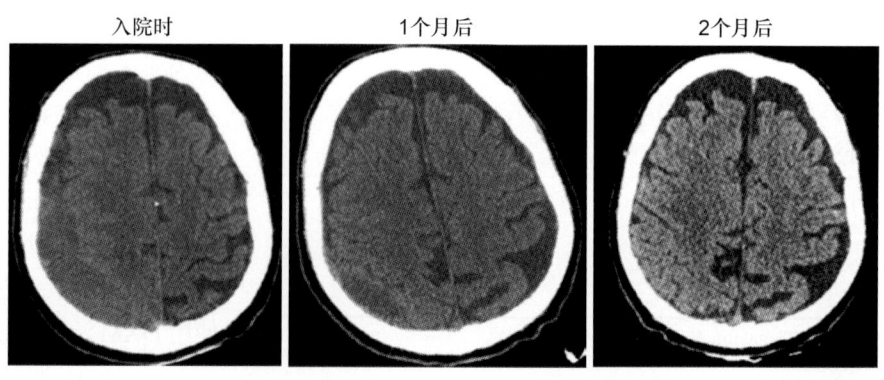

图 27.2 连续 3 次 CT 扫描结果显示一名 73 岁的男性的 CSDH 正在进行性吸收。在头部轻微创伤 3 周后患者出现偏瘫、头痛和记忆力障碍等症状。在使用阿托伐他汀治疗 8 周后，患者的血肿正逐渐被吸收

27.1.2.4　氨甲环酸

氨甲环酸（Txa）是一种已被广泛用于减少各类手术中出血的药物，其有效性已得到证实。最近氨甲环酸在 CSDH 保守治疗中的作用正被逐渐重视[7]。既往研究发现，纤维蛋白溶解和凝血功能亢进在 CSDH 的发生和进展中发挥着作用[27]。Txa 通过可逆性地与血浆蛋白原上的赖氨酸位点结合而降低血浆蛋白的活性，从而同时减少纤维蛋白溶解和炎症。理论上，Txa 打破了血肿包膜形成、血管再出血、炎症反应和毛细血管通透性升高的病理循环，从而使血肿体积不再扩大，并逐步在包膜内被重吸收[36]。基于这些假设，Kageyama 等进行的一项回顾性研究分析了 Txa 对 21 例保守治疗的 CSDH 患者的影响。研究结果显示，18 名接受 Txa 治疗的患者其血肿均完全吸收，且无不良反应[16]。另一项包括 232 名 CSDH 患者的研究比较了 Txa 和中药治疗对钻孔手术后的血肿复发率和残余血肿体积的影响。该研究发现，虽然两种药物在血肿复发率上无明显差异，但 Txa 组的残留血肿体积要小得多[51]。最近 Kutty 等进行了一项关于用 Txa（750 mg/d，分次服用）治疗 CSDH 的前瞻性观察研究。在这项研究中，所有患者的血肿都得到了很好的吸收，在保守治疗期间没有一例患者出现血肿进展，同时也没有并发症出现。因此该研究认为，在没有危及生命的症状时，用 Txa 对 CSDH 进行保守治疗是一种既安全又有效的选择[20]。

尽管这些观察性研究取得了可喜的结果，但 Txa 在治疗 CSDH 中的真正作用仍不确定，特别是它对存在血栓栓塞风险的 CSDH 患者的血肿吸收率和不良事件发生率的影响仍未明确。目前并没有任何研究发现与 Txa 有关的静脉血栓栓塞的不良反应。两个大型随机试验 CRASH225 和 CRASH 分别使用 Txa 治疗颅外和颅内的头部损伤，结果也没有发现 Txa 和安慰剂之间的血栓栓塞事件有任何明显差异[6, 37]。Txa 可能是一种可应用于 CSDH 保守治疗的药物，但由于其具有引起血栓栓塞或缺血性梗死的风险，应用 Txa 的安全性仍需进一步的评估，因此并不推荐作为日常治疗手段[45, 51]。

27.1.2.5　血管紧张素转换酶抑制剂（ACE 抑制剂）

根据 CSDH 的血管生成假说，人们认为 ACE 抑制剂可能会降低 CSDH 的发病率和复发率[34, 41]。ACE 抑制剂减少了血管内皮生长因子的产生，进而导致新生毛细血管的减少，抑制血液的外渗从而降低 CSDH 复发率。目前将 ACE 抑制剂应用于 CSDH 患者的研究并不多。Weigel 等的研究显示，ACE 抑制剂可降低 CSDH 的术后复发率，甚至可能通过其抗血管生成机制降低 CSDH 的发病风险[50]。然而，也有相反的研究结果。因为 ACE 抑制剂会增加缓激肽的水平，而缓激肽是一种血管活性肽，诱导血管扩张和通透性增加，从而导致血肿扩大[30]。Poulsen 等在一项使用培哚普利来控制术后残余血肿体积的实验中发现，培哚普利不能减少钻孔手术后 6 周残余血肿的大小，同样也不能减少 CSDH 复发率[34, 45]。

到目前为止，还没有进一步的权威研究证实 ACE 抑制剂在治疗 CSDH 中发挥的作用。基于现有研究结果，ACE 抑制剂作为辅助治疗手段对 CSDH 的术后治疗效果并不明确。ACE 抑制剂似乎不能有效降低 CSDH 的复发率，因此这类药物并不推荐用于临床[40]。

27.1.2.6　传统中药治疗

在日本，一些临床试验研究了五苓散在 CSDH 患者中的应用，五苓散是一种能够抑制水分子蛋白表达的中草药。Okamura 等在对 125 名患者的回顾性研究中指出，术前使用五苓散对预防 CSDH 术后复发有潜在作用[31]。最近，Katayama 等开展的随机多中心研究发现，术后使用五苓散治疗可以大幅度减少 CSDH 患者的复发率[17]。

27.1.3　保守治疗的适用人群

CSDH 的治疗方式可根据患者的症状、合并症和影像学特征以及患者和神经外科医生的偏好来决定。一些研究认为，症状较轻、血肿体积小的患者，其血肿自行消退的机会更大[41]，存在中度或重度神经系统症状并且血肿体积大的患者通常会被建议进行手术治疗。此外，有一些因素可能会影响慢性硬膜下血肿的药物治疗结果，如年龄、性别、神经系统状况、血肿厚度等。

27.1.3.1　年龄

众所周知，CSDH 的发病率随年龄增长而增加。老年人脑萎缩较为严重，硬膜下间隙增大从而导致血肿的占位效应不明显，因此症状较为轻微。一些研究者提出，年龄超过 70 岁伴有精神状况恶化、脑萎缩但是不存在颅内压增高导致的临床和影像学症状的患者，可以选择保守治疗[18, 33]。即使在外科手术治疗中，年龄也被报告为一个风险因素，大于 90 岁的手术患者中只有 24% 的患者取得了令人满意的结果[4, 8]。因此，对于处于早期 CSDH 的老年患者，保守治疗是一个值得考虑的选择。

27.1.3.2 神经系统状况

患者的神经系统状况是决定是否可以尝试保守治疗的最重要临床因素。一些研究已经表明，药物治疗一般在 3 天至 1 周内出现初步效果，CSDH 的消除或体积减少则需要 8～12 周的时间[7, 16, 31, 45]。对于昏迷或神经系统功能分级差的患者，则不应进行药物治疗。对于尝试不同的非手术治疗的患者，研究者纳入的均为神经功能状态较好的患者[2, 7, 41]。据报道，CSDH 自愈患者的临床症状主要是轻微的头痛和认知水平的轻微下降。尽管一些研究认为，患者出现偏瘫就需要手术的介入，但也有相关研究报道了两名出现偏瘫的患者在接受阿托伐他汀治疗 2～3 个月后，其偏瘫症状得到了治愈（图 27.2）[7, 13, 16]。因此，对 CSDH 患者的神经功能状况进行分级是很重要的。根据 Markwalder 的观点，CSDH 患者可根据其神经系统状况分为五个等级（0～4 级）[24]。一些作者通过格拉斯哥昏迷评分对 Markwalder 神经功能分级进行改良[23-24, 28, 45]。目前大多数研究认为，只有神经功能较好的患者（0～2）可以进行药物治疗。

27.1.3.3 性别

与男性相比，女性 CSDH 的发病率要低得多[16, 36, 45]。虽然这种现象还没有明确的解释，但目前存在着一些假说包括创伤原因、颅骨形态学原因和激素因素。Thotakura 和 Marabathina 指出，与男性患者相比，女性患者使用类固醇治疗的疾病结局更满意。6 名女性患者中有 5 人（83.3%）治疗成功，而 20 名男性患者中只有 6 人（30%）使用类固醇治疗成功[26]。Giuffrè 等在对血肿外膜的研究中发现，发生 CSDH 的男性患者体内雌激素受体和孕激素受体的含量高于女性[9]。据研究者称，男性由于其机体组织通常不适应雌激素的作用，可能导致组织型纤溶酶原激活剂的合成增加，从而维持局部纤溶亢进[35-36, 44-45, 47]。雌激素可以帮助女性减少发生 CSDH 的风险，也可能帮助她们通过类固醇治疗获得良好的效果[44]。

27.1.3.4 血肿大小

CSDH 血肿的大小同样也是影响患者临床症状的一个重要因素。根据中线移位的多少，CSDH 的大小可分为小、中、大和巨大血肿。对于双侧慢性硬膜下血肿，占位效应会更加明显，但是中线移位的发生率较低[46]。有研究将中线位移的可能分为 6 级，0 级为最小可能，5 级为最大可能。中线位移可能性低等级为 0～2 级，高等级为 4～5 级，剩下的 3 级为中等级[44]。一些研究认为，小体积的 CSDH 对药物治疗的反应更好。Horikoshi 等指出，无症状的额部硬膜下血肿有自行吸收的可能性[13]。Delgado-Lopez 等在他们的研究中指出，大或巨大的血肿会引起更严重的占位效应，该类患者大多临床分级较差需手术治疗[7]。

另外，中线移位也可以提示更多颅内病变信息，因为它代表了颅内压力的大小，而且在影像学上更容易测量。中线移位与患者的神经系统状况相关，因此在选择 CSDH 治疗方案时必须考虑中线移位的程度。

27.1.3.5 血肿密度

根据计算机断层成像（CT）上所显示密度，CSDH 被分为高密度型、混合密度型、等密度型和低密度型[32]。2001 年 Nakaguchi 等提出了血肿内部结构的影像学分类，即均质型、层状型、分离型和小梁型，这些不同的分类对应 CSDH 发展过程中的不同阶段[29]。Ito 等证明，血红蛋白的数量与硬膜下血肿的密度（HU）相关联。高密度的血肿含有更多的血红蛋白，需要手术介入的概率更大。密度较低的血肿则更容易被吸收，类固醇类药物的治疗效果更好[14]。Thotakura 和 Marabathina 在其进一步的工作中也得出了类似的结论[44]。Nakamura 等指出，正在吸收的血肿在 CT 扫描中表现多为低密度[18]。

27.2 结论

手术治疗依然是 CSDH 的主要治疗手段，但手术对高龄、并发症较多的患者存在较大的风险。因此在某些情况下，保守治疗是一种可靠的选择。可以在入院时根据临床症状和影像学特点对患者进行分类，并根据不同的分类给予合适的治疗方案。一旦选择了保守治疗，那么还要衡量选择药物的剂量、使用方法、治疗时间等。

目前的研究证实了阿托伐他汀与其他非手术治疗方案相比，其疗效更确切，副作用更少。为了确定每种药物在 CSDH 保守治疗中的真正价值，我们需要对更大的人群队列进行进一步的前瞻性研究。

参考文献

1. Almenawer SA, Farrokhyar F, Hong C, Alhazzani W, Manoranjan B, Yarascavitch B, et al. Chronic subdural hematoma management: a systematic review and meta-analysis of 34,829 patients. Ann Surg. 2014;259(3):449–57.
2. Araujo FA, Rocha MA, Mendes JB, Andrade SP. Atorvastatin inhibits inflammatory angiogenesis in mice through down regulation of VEGF, TNF-alpha and TGF-beta1. Biomed Pharmacother. 2010;64:29–34.
3. Bender MB, Christoff N. Nonsurgical treatment of subdural hematomas. Arch Neurol. 1974;31:73–9.
4. Berghauser Pont LM, Dirven CM, Dippel DW, Verweij BH, Dammers R. The role of corticosteroids in the management of chronic subdural hematoma: a systematic review. Eur J Neurol. 2012;19(11):1397–403.
5. Chan DYC, Chan DTM, Sun TFD, et al. The use of atorvastatin for chronic subdural haematoma: a retrospective cohort comparison study. Br J Neurosurg. 2017;31(1):72–7.
6. Collaborators Crash-3. Effects of tranexamic acid on death, disability, vascular occlusive events and other morbidities in patients with acute traumatic brain injury (CRASH-3): a randomised, placebo-controlled trial. Lancet. 2019;394:1713–23.
7. Delgado-Lopez PD, Martin-Velasco V, Castilla-Diez JM, Rodriguez-Salazar A, Galacho-Harriero AM, Fernandez-Arconada O. Dexamethasone treatment in chronic subdural haematoma. Neurocirugia (Astur). 2009;20(4):346–59.
8. Dran G, Berthier F, Fontaine D, Rasenrarijao D, Paquis P. Effectiveness of adjuvant corticosteroid therapy for chronic subdural hematoma: a retrospective study of 198 cases. Neurochirurgie. 2007;53:477–82.
9. Giuffrè R, Palma E, Liccardo G, Sciarra F, Pastore FS, Concolino G. Sex steroid hormones in the pathogenesis of chronic subdural haematoma. Neurochirurgia (Stuttg). 1992;35:103–7.
10. He C, Xia P, Xu J, Chen L, Zhang Q. Evaluation of the efficacy of atorvastatin in the treatment for chronic subdural hematoma: a meta-analysis. Neurosurg Rev. 2021;44(1):479–84. https://doi.org/10.1007/s10143-019-01218-w.
11. Henaux P-L, Le Reste P-J, Laviolle B, Morandi X. Steroids in chronic subdural hematomas (SUCRE trial): study protocol for a randomized controlled trial. Trials. 2017;18(1):252.
12. Holl DC, Volovici V, Dirven CMF, Peul WC, Jellema K, van der Gaag NA, et al. Pathophysiology and targets for non-surgical therapy of chronic subdural haematoma: evolution from past to present to future. World Neurosurg. 2018;116:402–11.
13. Horikoshi T, Naganuma H, Fukasawa I, Uchida M, Nukui H. Computed tomography characteristics suggestive of spontaneous resolution of chronic subdural hematoma. Neurol Med Chir (Tokyo). 1998;38:527–33.
14. Ito H, Maeda M, Uehara T, Yamamoto S, Tamura M, Takashima T. Attenuation values of chronic subdural hematoma and subdural effusion in CT scans. Acta Neurochir. 1984;72:211–7.
15. Jiang R, Zhao S, Wang R, Feng H, Zhang J, et al. Safety and efficacy of atorvastatin for chronic subdural hematoma in chinese patients: a randomized ClinicalTrial. JAMA Neurol. 2018;75(11):1338–46.
16. Kageyama H, Toyooka T, Tsuzuki N, Oka K. Nonsurgical treatment of chronic subdural hematoma with tranexamic acid. J Neurosurg. 2013;119(2):332–7.
17. Katayama K, Matsuda N, Kakuta K, Naraoka M, Takemura A, Hasegawa S, Akasaka K, Shimamura N, Itoh K, Asano K, Konno H, Ohkuma H. The effect of Goreisan on the prevention of chronic subdural hematoma recurrence: multi-center randomized controlled study. J

Neurotrauma. 2018;35(13):1537–42.
18. Kim HC, Ko JH, Yoo DS, Lee SK. Spontaneous resolution of chronic subdural hematoma: close observation as a treatment strategy. J Korean Neurosurg Soc. 2016;59(6):628–36.
19. Kolias AG, Edlmann E, Thelin EP, et al. Dexamethasone for adult patients with a symptomatic chronic subdural haematoma (Dex-CSDH) trial: study protocol for a randomised controlled trial. Trials. 2018;19(1):670.
20. Kutty RK, Leela SK, Sreemathyamma SB, Sivanandapanicker JL, Asher P, Peethambaran A, Prabhakar RB. The outcome of medical management of chronic subdural hematoma with tranexamic acid—a prospective observational study. J Stroke Cerebrovasc Dis. 2020;29(11):105273.
21. Laldjisinga ERA, Cornelissenb FMG, Gadjradj PS. Practice variation in the conservative and surgical treatment of chronic subdural hematoma. Clin Neurol Neurosurg. 2020;195:105899.
22. Li T, Wang D, Tian Y, Yu H, Wang Y, Quan W, et al. Effects of atorvastatin on the inflammation regulation and elimination of subdural hematoma in rats. J Neurol Sci. 2014;341:88–96.
23. Marcikic M, Hreckovski B, Samardzic J, Martinovic M, Rotim K. Spontaneous resolution of post-traumatic chronic subdural hematoma: case report. Acta Clin Croat. 2010;49:331–4.
24. Markwalder TM. Chronic subdural hematomas: a review. J Neurosurg. 1981;54:637–45.
25. Miah IP, Holl DC, Peul WC, et al. Dexamethasone therapy versus surgery for chronic subdural haematoma (DECSA trial): study protocol for a randomised controlled trial. Trials. 2018;19(1):575.
26. Miah IP, Herklots M, Roks G, Peul WC, Walchenbach R, Dammers R, Lingsma HF, den Hertog HM, Jellema K, Van der Gaag NA. Dexamethasone therapy in symptomatic chronic subdural hematoma (DECSA-R): a retrospective evaluation of initial corticosteroid therapy versus primary surgery. J Neurotrauma. 2020;37:366–72.
27. Min X, Pin C, Xun Z, Cun-Zu W, Xue-Qiang S, Bo Y. Effects of atorvastatin on conservative and surgical treatments of chronic subdural hematoma in patients. World Neurosurg. 2016;91:23–8.
28. Naganuma H, Fukamachi A, Kawakami M, Misumi S, Nakajima H, Wakao T. Spontaneous resolution of chronic subdural hematomas. Neurosurgery. 1986;19:794–8.
29. Nakaguchi H, Tanishima T, Yoshimasu N. Factors in the natural history of chronic subdural hematomas that influence their postoperative recurrence. J Neurosurg. 2001;95:256–62.
30. Neidert MC, Schmidt T, Mitova T, Fierstra J, Bellut D, Regli L, et al. Preoperative angiotensin converting enzyme inhibitor usage in patients with chronic subdural hematoma: associations with initial presentation and clinical outcome. J Clin Neurosci. 2016;28:82–6.
31. Okamura A, Kawamoto Y, Sakoda E, Murakami T, Hara T. Evaluation of recurrence factors and Gorei-san administration for chronic subdural hematoma after percutaneous subdural tapping. Hiroshima J Med Sci. 2013;62:77–82.
32. Park HR, Lee KS, Shim JJ, Yoon SM, Bae HG, Doh JW. Multiple densities of the chronic subdural hematoma in CT scans. J Korean Neurosurg Soc. 2013;54:38–41.
33. Parlato C, Guarracino A, Moraci A. Spontaneous resolution of chronic subdural hematoma. Surg Neurol. 2000;53(4):312–5; discussion 315–7.
34. Poulsen FR, Munthe S, Søe M, Halle B. Perindopril and residual chronic subdural hematoma volumes six weeks after burr hole surgery: a randomized trial. Clin Neurol Neurosurg. 2014;123:4–8.
35. Prud'homme M, Mathieu F, Marcotte N, Cottin S. A pilot placebo controlled randomized trial of dexamethasone for chronic subdural hematoma. Can J Neurol Sci. 2016;43:284–90.
36. Qian Z, Yang D, Sun F, Sun Z. Risk factors for recurrence of chronic subdural hematoma after burr hole surgery: potential protective role of dexamethasone. Br J Neurosurg. 2017;31:84–8.
37. Roberts I, Shakur H, Coats T, Hunt B, Balogun E, Barnetson L, et al. The CRASH-2 trial: a randomised controlled trial and economic evaluation of the effects of tranexamic acid on death, vascular occlusive events and transfusion requirement in bleeding trauma patients. Health Technol Assess. 2013;17:1–79.
38. Santarius T, Lawton R, Kirkpatrick PJ, Hutchinson PJ. The management of primary chronic subdural haematoma: a questionnaire survey of practice in the United Kingdom and the Republic of Ireland. Br J Neurosurg. 2008;22:529–34.
39. Shofty B, Grossman R. Treatment options for chronic subdural hematoma. World Neurosurg. 2016;87:529–30.
40. Soleman J, Taussky P, Fandino J, Muroi C. Chapter 12: Evidence-based treatment of chronic subdural hematoma. Traumatic brain injury. In: Sadaka F. IntechOpen; 2014. https://doi.org/10.5772/57336.

41. Soleman J, Nocera F, Mariani L. The conservative and pharmacological management of chronic subdural haematoma. Swiss Med Wkly. 2017;147:w14398.
42. Sun TF, Boet R, Poon WS. Non-surgical primary treatment of chronic subdural haematoma: preliminary results of using dexamethasone. Br J Neurosurg. 2005;19(4):327–33.
43. Tang R, Shi J, Li X, et al. Effects of atorvastatin on surgical treatments of chronic subdural hematoma. World Neurosurg. 2018;117:e425–9.
44. Thotakura AK, Marabathina NR. Nonsurgical treatment of chronic subdural hematoma with steroids. World Neurosurg. 2015;84:1968–72.
45. Thotakura AK, Marabathina NR. The role of medical treatment in chronic subdural hematoma. Asian J Neurosurg. 2018;13(4):976–83.
46. Tsai TH, Lieu AS, Hwang SL, Huang TY, Hwang YFA. Comparative study of the patients with bilateral or unilateral chronic subdural hematoma: precipitating factors and postoperative outcomes. J Trauma. 2010;68:571–5.
47. Wang D, Li T, Tian Y, Wang S, Jin C, Wei H, et al. Effects of atorvastatin on chronic subdural hematoma: a preliminary report from three medical centers. J Neurol Sci. 2014;336(1–2):237–42.
48. Wang D, Li T, Wei H, et al. Atorvastatin enhances angiogenesis to reduce subdural hematoma in a rat model. J Neurol Sci. 2016;362:91–9.
49. Wang D, Gao C, Xu X, et al. Treatment of chronic subdural hematoma with atorvastatin combined with low-dose dexamethasone: phase II randomized proof-of-concept clinical trial. J Neurosurg. 2020:1–9.
50. Weigel R, Hohenstein A, Schlickum L, Weiss C, Schilling L. Angio-tensin converting enzyme inhibition for arterial hypertension reduces the risk of recurrence in patients with chronic subdural hematoma possibly by an antiangiogenic mechanism. Neurosurgery. 2007;61(4):788–92; discussion 792–3.
51. Yamada T, Natori Y. Prospective study on the efficacy of orally administered tranexamic acid and Goreisan for the prevention of recurrence after chronic subdural hematoma burr hole surgery. World Neurosurg. 2020;134:e549–53.
52. Yao Z, Hu X, Ma L, You C. Dexamethasone for chronic subdural haematoma: a 449 systematic review and meta-analysis. Acta Neurochir (Wien). 2017;159(11):2037–44.
53. Zarkou S, Aguilar MI, Patel NP, Wellik KE, Wingerchuk DM, Demaerschalk BM. The role of corticosteroids in the management of chronic subdural hematomas: a critically appraised topic. Neurologist. 2009;15(5):299–302.

第 28 章 慢性硬膜下血肿的麻醉治疗

Kathryn Rosenblatt，Ji Yoon Baek，Fenghua Li 和 Reza Gorji

译者：李姝

28.1 慢性硬膜下血肿的麻醉治疗

28.1.1 慢性硬膜下血肿对脑生理的影响

慢性硬膜下血肿（chronic subdural hematoma，CSDH）是最常见的神经外科疾病之一，尤其是在老年患者中。CSDH 是大脑表面蛛网膜和硬脑膜之间由液体、血液和血液降解产物聚积而成的积液腔。CSDH 的发病率约为每年 17 人/10 万人，且随着年龄的增长而增加[99]。CSDH 患者可能会出现精神状态改变、局灶性神经功能障碍、头痛、跌倒、癫痫发作和一过性神经功能障碍。CSDH 的危险因素包括高龄、使用抗凝药、男性、酗酒以及直接或间接头部创伤病史[1]。虽然体积小和无症状的 CSDH 可以保守治疗，但手术治疗仍然是 CSDH 治疗的首选[65]。手术方式根据患者的特点和外科医生的经验而有所不同，但钻孔开颅手术是最首选的手术方式[17, 65]。在外科手术中，局部麻醉和全身麻醉均会被使用。许多研究表明局部麻醉比全身麻醉更有优势[13, 63, 78]，但一项大型回顾研究中发现不同麻醉方法患者预后结局没有差别[44]。而在最近的一项前瞻性研究中，93% 的钻孔开颅手术是在全身麻醉下进行的[17]。麻醉类型必须根据患者的情况与神经外科医生共同制订。

CSDH 对脑生理的影响主要取决于硬膜下血肿的大小及其对脑组织的压迫。CSDH 患者的颅内压（ICP）升高，全脑血流量（CBF）减少[57]。由于 CSDH 的缓慢扩张，ICP 值的显著增加并不常见，但未经治疗的 CSDH 最终可导致 ICP 升高和脑疝。CSDH 患者的局部和远端脑的 CBF 减少，但丘脑和壳核的 CBF 减少比脑皮质更严重[111]。据推测，慢性硬膜下血肿主要通过导致中央脑区的机械性变形引发神经功能障碍[67, 111]。因此，CSDH 对颅内压和脑血流的影响不是发生神经功能障碍的主要原因，远端脑结构的变形比局部脑结构的受压在导致局部脑血流下降方面起着更显著的作用[59, 67, 111]。

大脑半球 CBF 的减少也可能与功能失调大脑的代谢减少有关[122]。研究表明，通过增加局部氧摄取分数（rOEF），脑氧代谢在皮质区域得以维持，但丘脑、纹状体和扣带回的氧代谢降低[67]。尽管脑血流量发生变化，但 CSDH 患者的大脑自主调节功能（在动脉血压和颅内压波动下维持恒定微血管血流的能力）通常得以保留[106, 113]。麻醉的目标是避免颅内压进一步升高，通过保持脑灌流压在 60～80 mmHg 维持脑灌注，并防止继发性脑损伤。麻醉药物的选择应根据患者的个体需求量身定制，以优化大脑生理功能。

28.1.2 慢性硬膜下血肿术前评估

麻醉术前评估是围手术期管理的基石，其基本目的是全面了解患者的相关病史，并对术中风险进行评估和必要的围手术期优化。术前患者教育以及与患者和患者家属或代理人的沟通可以减少患者和家属对麻醉过程和围手术期神经外科治疗的焦虑和恐惧[64, 108]。全面而周到的术前评估，以及神经外科医生与患者和患者家属讨论计划中的操作，可以减少手术并发症，改善患者的预后。

虽然有一些患者是在手术当天才由麻醉师进行首次评估，但越来越多的患者在手术日之前就在术前项目或诊所进行评估并为手术做好准备。考虑到 CSDH 患者的年龄通常较大，同时伴随的医疗风险和合并症也随之增加，因此建议在对这些患者进行神经外科干预之前进行术前评估。非急诊神经外科手术的术前评估涉及患者神经系统状态、患者总体健康状况和手术计划。

28.1.3 术前评估会影响术中麻醉的神经功能状态

硬膜下血肿的发展速度会对神经功能状态和围手术期的治疗方式产生影响。明确硬膜下出血的病史和相关神经症状的时间线将有助于指导麻醉处理。CSDH 可能会出现轻微但通常持续时间较长的症状，这通常表明患者具备足够的颅内代偿。然而，新发症状或症状的恶化提示颅内顺应性和自我调节能力降低，颅内稳态接近极限，任何额外可导致颅内压-容量曲线变化的因素都可能导致稳态到达极限。神经病学上，颅内压升高的迹象包括新发头痛或头痛加剧、恶心、呕吐、视物模糊、嗜睡增加或意识水平下降。

与 CSDH 相关或无关的既往神经系统疾病和损伤史都是有意义的信息，既往检查和治疗记录也很重要。卒中病史或脑血管功能不全症状（如短暂性神经功能缺损）是围手术期卒中的有力预测因素[69]。缺血性卒中的病因和治疗通常与 CSDH 密切相关，为治疗 CSDH 和准备手术而停用抗血栓药物会增加围手术期因心房颤动、机械性心脏瓣膜、颈动脉疾病或左心房或左心室血栓而发生卒中的概率。目前，关于卒中后多久麻醉和手术是安全的还缺乏高质量的数据。如果在急性缺血性卒中后不久需要进行 CSDH 手术，则需要严格监测和控制血压，以防止再灌注损伤并维持侧支循环。

癫痫发作可能是 CSDH 的后遗症和危险因素。如果存在原有或新发的癫痫发作，应在术前评估时确定癫痫发作的类型、频率和症状，并记录抗癫痫药物的服用时间和剂量（以及患者对药物的依从性）。控制癫痫发作的药物有多种副作用，包括白细胞减少、血小板减少、低钠血症、巨幼红细胞性贫血、PR 间期延长和骨髓抑制。术前检查应根据病史和体格检查结果，针对可疑的异常情况进行。通常需要进行心电图、全血细胞计数、血小板计数和电解质水平检查。除非对抗癫痫药物的毒性有疑虑，否则不需要常规检测抗癫痫药物（AED）的血药浓度，因为患者充分控制癫痫发作的药物浓度可能超出治疗范围。由于诱导（苯妥英、苯巴比妥、卡马西平）或抑制（丙戊酸）细胞色素 P450 同工酶活性，或竞争蛋白质结合位点（苯妥英、苯二氮䓬、丙戊酸），许多 AED 与麻醉剂和其他 AED 存在广泛的药物相互作用，从而影响肝脏代谢和多种麻醉剂的游离药物水平。

28.1.4 术前麻醉评估中神经系统检查的重要性

基本的术前体格检查应包括重点神经评估，记录精神状态、语言、脑神经、运动和感觉功能以及步态方面的缺陷（或无缺陷）。尽管将评估重点只放在之前的记录或可预测的异常进行评估十分简便，但每次检查都应该以统一的方式进行，并从高到低进行整合，以免遗漏新的发现。神经系统检查涉及外周和中枢神经系统功能的评估，大部分检查可在询问病史时完成。其他器官系统的体格检查，如心脏和肺部检查，可在神经系统检查之前或之后进行。然而，为了将 CSDH 相关的神经系统症状与其他器官或肌肉骨骼功能障碍的表现适当区分开来，有必要将全身体格检查结果与神经系统异常表现结合起来。采用格拉斯哥昏迷量表评估意识水平具有快速、简便、可重复的特点，且兼具诊断、治疗指导及预后判断价值。较低的格拉斯哥昏迷量表（GCS）评分向麻醉医生提示，催眠/镇静剂可能会在麻醉诱导过程中产生过大或更快的效果，从而导致气道保护功能的过早丧失。在一些中心，使用小型精神状态检查（Mini-Mental State Exam，MMSE）对老年患者进行基线神经认知功能测试是术前麻醉评估的常规组成部分。与没有认知障碍的患者相比，围手术期 MMSE 确定有认知障碍的患者术后谵妄、院内死亡率和 1 年内死亡率更高[20]。而通过充分练习，可以简明扼要地对所有 12 条脑神经进行详细检测。嗅觉障碍最近因其与 SARS-CoV-2 感染有关而受到关注。然而，嗅觉神经功能障碍也提示颅内压增高、额叶或垂体病变、脑膜炎、脑积水、临床前神经变性疾病（如阿尔茨海默病和帕金森病）或颅前窝颅骨骨折。嗅觉神经可通过让患者辨别一些常见气味来评估。ICP 增高的其他体格检查体征包括警觉性下降、乳头水肿、单侧瞳孔放大、外展神经（脑神经Ⅵ）或动眼神经（脑神经Ⅲ）麻痹和颈部僵硬。评估乳头水肿需要使用眼底镜进行眼底检查，通常由眼科医生进行。评估瞳孔大小、反应能力和反应时间对确定相对颅内压同样重要，在强光下可以看到明显的结果，如异视和反应能力减弱。瞳孔测定仪可用于测定神经瞳孔指数（NPi）和检测细微的眼球运动神经变化[21]。NPi 结合了瞳孔大小、潜伏期、收缩速度和扩张速度等变量，提供了一个基于正常瞳孔计数值模型的比例值[105]。眼球运动神经功能障碍使患者无法向下、向上或向内侧看。双眼水平复视可能表明 ICP 增高继发了脑神经瘫痪，检查将发现受累眼不能侧视。

应评估肌肉力量、张力和大小是否不对称，以及肌肉被动拉伸阻力是否增加。反射测试和外周感觉系统评估对于检测和记录基线病变也很重要。CSDH 被称为"伟大的神经模仿者"，因为它可以模仿痴呆、缺血性卒中、帕金森病或脊髓损伤。这是因为其最常出现的症状和体征是偏瘫和头痛，其次是精神状态改变、意识减退、乳头水肿、癫痫发作和表达性失语。大多数接受 CSDH 手术的患者症状都会得到缓解。然而，神经系统检查结果的基线记录可用于比较术后出现的新缺陷。

28.1.5　检测影响总体健康状况的原有合并症

心血管、呼吸、肾脏、内分泌和胃肠道系统与神经麻醉相互影响，需要进行彻底的术前评估。确定器官或系统疾病的严重程度、当前或近期的病情加重情况和稳定性以及之前的治疗或计划中的干预措施对于确定疾病的存在同样重要。疾病的控制程度、范围以及因疾病导致的任何活动限制也同样重要。应注意处方药和非处方药（包括补充剂和草药）的剂量和频率，以及最近停药的情况。有必要询问过敏反应以及接触乳胶或放射染色剂等药物和物质的具体反应，并记录使用烟草、酒精或违禁药物的情况。在系统检查中应特别强调气道异常、与麻醉相关的不良事件的个人或家族病史、打鼾和白天嗜睡（如果尚未诊断出睡眠呼吸暂停）以及与反流相关的严重烧心病史。术前应查明个人或家族是否有恶性高热或假性胆碱酯酶缺乏症病史，以便在术前做出适当安排。以前的麻醉记录总是有用的，可以澄清病史中不确定的因素。

28.1.5.1　心血管健康术前评估

心血管风险分层是术前评估、共享手术决策和优化管理的重要组成部分。需要有重点的病史采集和体格检查，以确定缺血性心脏病、严重瓣膜疾病、严重高血压、肺动脉高压、心律失常和心力衰竭的体征和症状。应该询问患者是否可以执行 4 个或更多代谢当量（MET）的工作量，例如爬上两层或更多层楼梯或步行上山而没有症状限制。40 多年前开发了 Goldman 心脏风险指数量表，随后由 Lee 等提出并由美国心脏病学会和美国心脏协会特别工作组修订的心脏风险指数使用六点量表来确定手术后 30 天内发生围手术期主要不良心血管事件（MACE）的低风险（< 1%）和高风险（≥ 1%）的个体[42, 50, 70]。然而，由 21 个组成部分组成的美国外科医师学会国家外科质量改进计划（ACS NSQIP）通用手术风险计算和新的心血管风险指数可能提供更好的预测性区分[4, 11, 28, 52, 116-117]（表 28.1）。虽然心血管检查如运动心电负荷试验、运动负荷（运动或药物）影像学检查如超声心动图、核灌注或心脏磁共振成像等很少适用于 MACE 的低风险患者，但如果测试结果会改变围手术期的医疗、麻醉或手术处理，则可考虑在风险较高的患者（由 < 4 METs 确定）[107]中进行负荷试验（图 28.1）。脑灌注和氧合取决于心血管健康状况，反之，CSDH 常见的血管源性水肿和颅内高压等颅内病理可能会改变心血管功能。

28.1.5.2　术前肺健康评估

慢性阻塞性肺疾病（如支气管炎和肺气肿、哮喘、肺部和肺外限制性肺疾病）患者术前的病史、症状和体格检查有助于进行进一步的定向评估和诊断性检查（如有）。在采集病史时，应重点询问气短、胸闷、咳嗽、痰量变化、痰液颜色、近期病情加重情况、治疗或吸氧情况、住院情况、插管情况、既往麻醉后病情加重情况以及最佳运动量。应通过简单的听诊评估呼吸音的质量、喘息程度和空气流动量。用脉搏血氧仪测定血氧饱和度有助于确定基线状况，除非是确定初步诊断或评估急性或进行性恶化、感染或气胸[41]，否则无须进行动脉血气分析、胸片和肺功能检查（PFT）。肺部并发症的风险因素包括吸烟超过 40 包 / 年，美国麻醉医师协会身体状况评分超过 2 分，年龄超过 70 岁，慢性阻塞性肺疾病，神经系统、主动脉、上腹部、胸部或颈部手术，预计手术时间超过 2 h，低白蛋白血症，体重指数超过 30 kg/m^2 和低于 4 METs[7]。虽然多达 1/4 的术后 1 周内死亡病例与肺部并发症有关，但研究表明，术前动脉血气分析、PFT 和胸片检查结果并不能预测非胸部和非心脏手术后的并发症风险[7, 85, 121]。但 PFT 和胸部扫描可能有助于区分肺部疾病引起的呼吸困难和心力衰竭，或评估是否需要使用抗生素、支气管扩张剂或类固醇。吸烟会增加许多围手术期并发症的风险，但戒烟的最大益处只有在戒烟数月

表 28.1 风险评分和计算

			国家手术质量改进计划		
			风险计算		
	戈德曼心脏风险指数[21]，1977	修订后心脏风险指数[78]，1999	围手术期心肌梗死和心搏骤停[105]，2011年	通用外科手术[50]，2013年	老年敏感围手术期心脏风险指数[70]，2017年	心血管风险指数[42]，2019
标准	• 年龄大于70岁（5分）	• 缺血性心脏病（1分）	• 年龄	• 年龄	• 年龄	• 年龄≥75岁（1分）
	• 6月内有过一次MI（10分）	• 脑血管疾病（1分）	• ASA分级	• 性别	• 性别	• 心脏病史（1分）
	• 颈静脉扩张或听诊出现第三心音（11分）	• 充血性心力衰竭病史（1分）	• 术前功能	• ASA分级	• ASA分级	• 心绞痛或呼吸困难症状
	• ≥5 PVCs/min（7分）	• 胰岛素治疗糖尿病（1分）	• 肌酐水平	• 功能状态	• 高风险手术	• 血红蛋白水平＜12 mg/dl（1分）
	• 术前ECG显示无窦性心律或PAC（7分）	• 血清肌酐水平≥2.0 mg/dl（1分）	• 手术类型：肛门直肠，主动脉，减肥，脑，乳腺，心脏，耳鼻喉，肝胆胰，胆囊，阑尾，肾上腺，脾肠，颈部，产科或妇科，整形外科，其他腹部，外周血管，皮肤，脊柱，胸部，泌尿或静脉	• 急诊手术	• 心力衰竭病史	• 血管外科
	• 主动脉瓣狭窄（3分）	• 计划中的高风险手术（腹腔内、胸腔内或血管手术）（1分）		• 使用类固醇治疗慢性病	• 脑卒中	• 急诊手术（1分）
	• 腹腔内、胸腔内或主动脉手术（3分）			• 术前30天内出现腹水	• 胰岛素治疗	
	• 紧急手术（4分）			• 术前48小时内出现系统性败血症	• 糖尿病	
				• 需要呼吸机支持	• 透析治疗	
				• 扩散性癌症	• 治疗高血压的药物	
				• 糖尿病	• 目前吸烟情况	
				• 需要药物治疗的高血压	• COPD病史	
				• 曾发生心脏事件	• 功能状态（部分依赖与完全依赖）	
				• 术前30天内出现充血性心力衰竭	• 肌酐水平	

（续表）

	国家手术质量改进计划风险计算				
	戈德曼心脏风险指数[21]，1977	修订后心脏风险指数[78]，1999	围手术期心肌梗死和心搏骤停[105]，2011年	通用外科手术[50]，2013年	老年敏感围手术期心脏风险指数[70]，2017年	心血管风险指数[42]，2019
得分范围	• Ⅰ级：0~5分（风险最低） • Ⅱ级：6~12分 • Ⅲ级：13~25分 • Ⅳ级：≥26分（最高风险）	• Ⅰ级：0分（风险最低） • Ⅱ级：1分 • Ⅱ级：2分 • Ⅱ级：≥3分（最高风险）	0~100%（0，最低风险；100%，最高风险）	0~100%（0，最低风险；100%，最高风险）	0~100%（0，最低风险；100%，最高风险）	• 0分（风险最低） • 1分 • 2分 • 3分
表示风险升高的阈值	≥Ⅱ级（≥6分）	>1分	>1%	>1%	>1%	≥2分 ≥3分（最高风险）
临床结局	术中或术后MI，肺水肿，VT，心源性死亡	MI，肺水肿，心室颤动，完全性心脏传导阻滞，心源性死亡	术中或术后30天内发生MI或心搏骤停	心搏骤停，MI，30天全因死亡	心搏骤停，MI，30天因死亡	30天死亡，心肌梗死或脑卒中
	Goldman index of cardiac risk[21]，1977	Revised cardiac risk index[78]，1999	Perioperative MI and cardiac arrest[105]，2011	Universal surgical[50]，2013	Geriatric-sensitive perioperative cardiac risk index[70]，2017	Cardiovascular risk index[42]，2019
推导人群	1001	1422	11 414 006	584 931	3284	
ROC						
推导	0.61	0.76	0.88	0.90（心搏骤停或MI）；0.94（死亡率）	0.9	
验证	0.7	0.81；0	0	0.88（心搏骤停或MI）；0.94（死亡率）	0.83（≥65岁成年人为0.76）	0

缩写：ASA 美国麻醉医师协会，BMI 体重指数，BUN 血（血清）尿素氮，COPD 慢性阻塞性肺疾病，CPT 通用过程术语学，EDG 心电图，MI 心肌梗死，PAC 房性早搏，PVC 室性早搏，ROC 接受者操作特征曲线，VT 室。

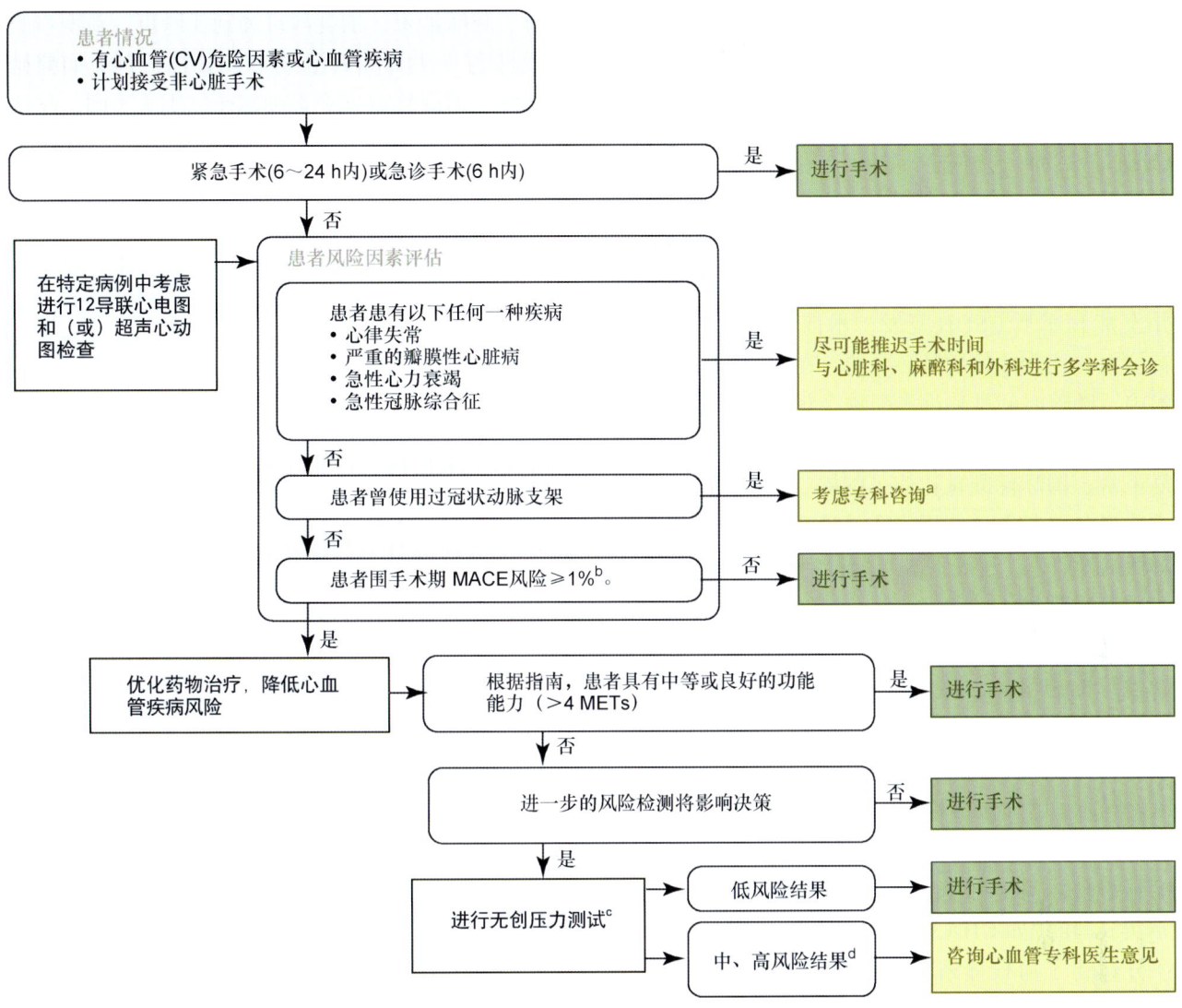

图 28.1 一项围手术期心血管风险评估流程。该流程尚未经过验证。MACE 表示主要心血管不良事件；METs 表示代谢当量（Reproduced with permission from JAMA. 2020；324（3）：279-290. Copyright©2020 American Medical Association. All rights reserved）。[a] 会诊围手术期注意事项（见来源文章 doi：https://doi.org/10.1001/jama.2020.7840）。[b] 临床风险计算器确定围手术期 MACE 风险。[c] 测试选项包括：①无心肌成像的运动心电图压力测试；或②合并如超声心动图、单光子发射计算机断层扫描核灌注成像、正电子发射断层成像或心脏磁共振等成像的压力测试（运动或药物）。[d] 压力测试发现的中高危结果可能包括中重度心肌缺血、低负荷诱发出的缺血、运动后低血压反应、短暂性缺血扩张和压力测试期间出现室性心律失常。

后才能显现。

28.1.5.3 内分泌功能障碍与糖尿病的术前评估

糖尿病患者面临多器官功能障碍的风险，包括肾功能不全、周围神经病变、卒中、自主神经功能障碍、心血管疾病、胃瘫和视网膜病变，糖尿病被认为是与心绞痛或既往心肌梗死类似的围手术期心脏并发症的中介风险因素。评估器官损伤和优化围手术期血糖控制应是术前麻醉评估的重点。脑缺血前或脑缺血期间的高血糖将导致神经预后恶化，这一点已得到公认。缺血前血糖水平升高为无氧糖酵解提供额外的底物，从而加速乳酸酸中毒的有害影响。相反，强化血糖控制会带来低血糖的风险，进而导致葡萄糖沿着浓度梯度净移出大脑。根据美国临床内分泌医师协会和美国糖尿病协会的建议及现有证据，在更多前瞻性研究针对特定神经损伤或神经外科手术的血糖管理目标得到结论前，将围手术期血糖水平维持在 140～180 mg/L（7.8～10.0 mmol/L）是一个合理的目标[49, 88]。

28.1.5.4 围手术期凝血障碍评估

任何程度或类型的凝血障碍（包括遗传性或获得性疾病）患者都可能会自发或因轻微外伤而发生 CSDH。然而，抗血栓药物可能用于针对 CSDH 的择期手术治疗中，尤其是在 CSDH 稳定的病例中，抗血栓治疗的益处大于出血风险。然而，考虑到手术期间血肿扩大的可能性，以及为了防止围手术期并发症和术后 CSDH 复发，术前停止和（或）逆转抗血栓药物的作用是必要的。在非急诊的择期手术中，随着时间推移许多药物在肾脏和肝脏中被逐渐清除。术前活化的凝血酶原时间（APTT）应恢复正常，国际标准化比值（INR）应小于 1.4。服用维生素 K 拮抗剂（使用华法林患者通常 > 5 天）将降低抗凝效果。建议手术当日早上复查 INR 水平确认逆转情况。

对于有明显高凝状态或已有血栓负担需要抗凝治疗的患者中，围手术期采用普通肝素或低分子量肝素等短效药物进行"桥接"治疗的风险与获益尚不明确，因此需审慎权衡血栓栓塞与出血风险[110]。增加血栓栓子出现风险的主要因素是房颤、人工心脏瓣膜和前 3 个月的静脉或动脉血栓栓塞事件。具有这些危险因素的患者形成了不同分类人群，如 CHA3DS2-VASc 和 HAS-BLED 等评分包含了血栓栓塞和出血风险分层的其他重要临床变量[95]。然而，在围手术期使用风险评分尚未经过前瞻性验证，也没有任何评分系统可以替代临床判断。对于血栓栓塞症风险极高的患者，如 3 个月内发生过缺血性脑卒中，或术前 1 个月抗凝不足的非瓣膜性房颤患者，应尽可能推迟择期手术，直到风险恢复到基线水平。如果无法推迟手术，或者血栓风险长期升高且正在接受华法林治疗的患者，应尽可能在临近手术时停止抗凝治疗，并对这些使用华法林的患者采用过渡药物。肝素过渡治疗通常在计划手术前 3 天（即停用华法林 2 天后）开始使用，此时 INR 已开始降至治疗范围以下。低分子量肝素的消除半衰期为 3～5 h，因此可在计划手术前 24 h 停用低分子量肝素；而普通肝素消除半衰期约为 45 min，因此治疗性普通肝素的输注可持续到手术前 4～6 h。

越来越多的血栓栓塞风险的患者使用直接口服抗凝药（DOAC）和肠外直接作用抗凝药，如达比加群、阿哌沙班、依度沙班和利伐沙班。新型口服抗凝药与华法林和其他维生素 K 拮抗剂（如醋硝香豆醇、苯丙羟基香豆素和氟茚二酮）不同，华法林和其他维生素 K 拮抗剂通过阻断肝脏中维生素 K 环氧化物还原酶复合体的功能，导致还原形式的维生素 K 耗尽，从而间接发挥作用，还原形式的维生素 K 是维生素 K 依赖的凝血因子 Ⅱ、Ⅶ、Ⅸ 和 Ⅹ 的 γ-羧化的辅助因子，而这些直接凝血酶（因子 Ⅱ）和直接凝血因子 Xa 抑制物阻止了与纤维蛋白凝块生成有关的主要促凝血活性[6]。直接的凝血酶抑制剂，如比伐芦定、阿加曲班、地西芦定和达比加群，可阻止凝血酶将纤维蛋白原裂解成纤维蛋白并直接与凝血酶结合，而不是像肝素那样增强抗凝血酶的活性。包括利伐沙班、阿哌沙班、依度沙班和贝曲沙班在内的直接 Xa 因子抑制剂可阻止 Xa 因子将凝血酶原裂解为凝血酶，并直接与 Xa 因子结合。鉴于 CSDH 手术治疗的出血风险较高，建议无论肾功能如何，在手术前 2 天内不使用直接 Xa 因子抑制剂，肾功能正常的患者在手术前 2 天内不使用直接凝血酶抑制剂，因为 DOACs 的消除半衰期为 9～14 h。对于肌酐清除率为 30～50 ml/min 的达比加群患者，基于药代动力学方法建议在 CSDH 干预前 4 天开始停药，其依据是肾功能受损患者的消除半衰期为 18～24 h[48]。与血栓栓塞风险高的患者停用维生素 K 拮抗剂不同，直接作用抗凝药不需要过渡治疗。

患有 CSDH 并在发病前 12 个月内有经皮冠状动脉介入治疗（PCI）史的患者可能正在服用如阿司匹林和血小板 P2Y12 受体阻滞剂等抗血小板药物，以预防冠状动脉支架血栓形成。根据大型 POISE-2 试验的结果，建议接受阿司匹林单抗治疗以一级或二级预防心血管疾病的患者在术前 5～7 天内暂停此类治疗[33]。对于在使用支架的 PCI 术后服用双抗血小板疗法（DAPT）的患者，在建议的双抗治疗周期（裸金属支架或药物洗脱支架术后至少 6 个月，使用球囊血管成形术的 PCI 术后 14 天）之前停止双抗治疗与心肌梗死、支架血栓形成和死亡等不良心血管事件的风险增加相关[74]。建议在使用支架进行 PCI 后将择期非心脏手术推迟 6 个月，以防止 DAPT 中断，但对于无法等待 6 个月的手术，尽可能将 DAPT 的最短持续时间维持为支架PCI术后4～6周，在球囊血管成形术后48 h[38, 56, 114]。CSDH患者可能需要更及时的干预。此外，对CSDH进行神经外科治疗的DAPT导致出血的风险可能比停药后发生不良心血管事件的风险更大，因此这些治疗应该在围手术期进行。对于服用氯吡格雷、替卡格雷和普拉格雷的患者，根据每种药物制造商的包装说明书，建议分别在术前5天、3～5天和7天暂停使用。

28.1.6　术前麻醉评估中的体格检查

28.1.6.1　气道检查

气道检查是术前查体中最重要的一项内容。虽然它占用的术前时间最少，但要进行充分的气道评估，就必须在气道评估和管理方面接受专门培训并积累经验。气道评估的主要目的是检查患者的特定身体和生理特征，这些特征可预测患者在需要进行气道管理的手术时可能遇到的困难。气道检查的内容包括Mallampati分级、牙齿检查、颈部活动范围、颈围、甲状腺距离、体型、相关畸形和胸部听诊。研究人员和专家根据对困难气道管理的有效研究，将这些身体物理属性变量纳入了记忆法。美国外科医生学会高级创伤生命支持（ATLS）课程采用的LEMON评估和ROMAN记忆法就是这样两种经过验证的工具，它们分别用于评估喉镜插管困难和面罩通气困难[5, 68, 103]。当发现有气道插管困难时，则需要让患者做好准备，以便在适当情况下进行清醒纤支镜插管，并提前计划以确保有必要的设备和熟练的人员可用。

28.1.6.2　一般体格检查

听诊心脏，包括第三或第四心音、杂音、心律紊乱和啰音，检查脉搏、外周静脉和中央静脉，以及四肢是否出现水肿，有助于制订围手术期计划。体格检查应重点关注容量超负荷、颈静脉扩张、腹水和肝肿大的体征，以及听诊颈部是否有淤血。听诊是否有喘息、哮鸣音或呼吸音异常、减弱或其他异常也有助于制订术前计划。还应注意患者是否有呼吸费力、发绀、杵状指和辅助呼吸肌的使用。颈围过大、高血压和肥胖会增加阻塞性睡眠呼吸暂停（OSA）的发病率。有数据表明，疑似OSA患者的术后并发症和死亡发生率增加，而且已知未经治疗的OSA患者插管困难、入住重症监护室、术后并发症和住院时间延长的发生率更高[15]。目前已开发出使用STOP-Bang问卷、柏林问卷和ASA（美国麻醉医师协会）检查表等工具检测OSA，以识别有OSA风险的患者[24-26]。如果患者通过术前门诊筛查而及早接受OSA治疗，可能会减少与OSA相关的围手术期不良事件，并为患者带来长期健康益处。虽然夜间多导睡眠图是诊断OSA的标准方法，但其费用昂贵且不方便，而且在CSDH手术治疗的术前时间安排中，睡眠医学会诊的时间通常很少。相反，采取围手术期预防措施，如使用短效麻醉剂、为可能出现的困难面罩通气和困难插管做好准备、充分的神经肌肉阻滞剂逆转、术后使用CPAP和术后持续脉搏血氧监测，可能有助于预防被STOP-Bang问卷调查归类为OSA高风险的患者出现不良后果[97]。

28.1.7　评估麻醉风险

虽然多个医学专业发布的循证指南已经为患者准备了麻醉和手术的评估方案，但麻醉医生是唯一能够真正评估与麻醉相关的风险、与患者和手术团队讨论这些风险并在术中管理这些风险的术前医生。关于评估风险-收益比和告知患者麻醉相关风险，麻醉医生在术前的作用是独一无二的。麻醉给患者带来了风险却没有直接的益处，麻醉的益处是帮助主刀医生顺利完成对患者的手术。由于CSDH的神经外科手术已经随着微创、内窥镜和血管内技术的创新而发展，需要强效药物的全身麻醉、气道器械、机械通气以及相关的生理紊乱可能会给某些患者群体带来比手术本身更大的重大风险。美国麻醉医师协会（ASA）的身体状况分级系统是在80年前开发的，至今仍在使用[84]。ASA分级系统的目的是主观地评估和确定患者麻醉前的医疗合并症，而不考虑麻醉类型或手术程序。一些研究表明，ASA分级与不良的心肺结局、更长的住院时间和意外的重症监护病房入院之间存在相关性。虽然ASA分级系统本身并不量化风险，但该系统同时纳入了美国国家卫生研究院NSQI和RCRI。像这样的患者病情和手术风险组合的工具为围手术期临床医生和患者提供了全面的风险评估，允许对并发症发生的可能性进行一定程度的估计，并帮助决定是否应该推迟手术，直到干预措施改善风险，如控制不佳的高血压或不稳定的缺血性心脏病。

28.2 慢性硬膜下血肿术中处理

28.2.1 麻醉方法的选择

麻醉选择取决于患者和外科医生的倾向，并考虑到手术患者的相关临床和心理因素。

28.2.1.1 局部麻醉

小骨瓣开颅治疗慢性硬膜下血肿复发率较低。Mahmood 及其同事发现，在局部麻醉的情况下，CSDH 的小骨瓣开颅手术与全身麻醉同样有效[79]。在一项比较右美托咪定镇静和全身麻醉治疗慢性硬膜下血肿的前瞻性随机研究中，右美托咪定联合局部麻醉被发现在通过钻孔清除慢性硬膜下血肿时有效。该技术具有手术时间短、血流动力学改变少、术后并发症少等优点。另一个好处是住院时间更短[109]。与咪达唑仑-芬太尼联合应用相比，右美托咪定用于麻醉监测管理（MAC）与术中患者活动更少、恢复时间更快以及更好的外科医生和患者满意度评分相关[12]。进一步的研究比较了右美托咪定和氯胺酮（DK）和右美托咪啶-咪达唑仑-芬太尼（DMF）药物"鸡尾酒"组合，发现两组在恢复时间、起效时间、心肺变量和止痛方面具有相似的疗效。然而，DMF 组表现出更好的镇静质量和满意度评分，尽管右美托咪定剂量较低，脑电双频指数 < 60 的发生率高于 DK 组[23]。

28.2.1.2 局部麻醉与全身麻醉

一项包含 1029 名患者的大型研究发现，接受全身麻醉的患者术后并发症的发生率远高于接受局部麻醉的患者。多变量分析显示，接受全身麻醉的患者出现术后问题的概率是接受局部麻醉患者的 1.8 倍（aOR 1.8, 95% CI: 1.0～3.3）。值得注意的是，在根据手术医院进行调整后，这种关联性降低了。同一研究还发现局部麻醉病例的住院时间更短[13]。

由于文献资料有限，很难真正区分一种手术方式对 CSDH 的益处。在回顾文献时也可以发现，不严谨的研究设计也会对实验结果产生影响。此外，全身麻醉有时被认为与术后认知问题有关，但事实上这可能与麻醉无关，而是与炎症反应、细胞因子增加和手术压力等其他因素有关[14, 102]。其他因素，如患者因不适而移动，也会增加手术不适[62]。

28.2.2 术中全身麻醉管理

当液化的 CSDH 无法自发吸收时，钻孔并引流血肿是一种有效的治疗方法[83]。引流能有效防止血肿复发，还能降低与手术相关的发病率和死亡率[101]。通过开颅手术排出血凝块和血凝块周围的相关组织膜，对预防 CSDH 的再发生有效[71, 90, 118]。

在大多数情况下，CSDH 患者的 ICP 会增高。因此，需要为脑部降压做好准备。这包括使用利尿剂、渗透疗法和糖皮质激素，以及控制二氧化碳分压（$PaCO_2$）、麻醉药物和脑脊液（CSF）引流。

28.2.2.1 监护

在清除小型 CSDH 的过程中，可以使用美国麻醉医师协会（ASA）要求的监护仪来完成监测。监护项目包括心电图、血压、脉搏血氧饱和度、体温、氧气分析仪和呼气末二氧化碳（$ETCO_2$）。在进行小骨瓣开颅手术时，可以使用一套类似的监护仪。但在大多数情况下，需要进行创伤性的监测。

在需要开颅手术的情况下，建议使用动脉内导管持续监测动脉血压（ABP）。连续 ABP 监测有助于优化脑灌注压（CPP）、评估血容量状态，并允许采血进行术中电解质和葡萄糖测量。

如果手术部位高于心脏水平，则需要考虑到空气栓塞的可能性。在坐位开颅手术中，空气栓塞是一种常见且严重的并发症[80]。然而，空气栓塞也可能在沿静脉窦开颅时发生，也可能发生在上头架时头钉固定头骨的地方[51]。所有接受全身麻醉的患者都必须进行 $ETCO_2$ 监测。在检测静脉空气栓塞方面，$ETCO_2$ 非常敏感，可检测到低至 0.25 mg/kg 的水平[39]。

患者在进入手术室之前可能有脑室外引流管（EVD）。EVD 可用于 CSF 引流或 ICP 监测，引流 CSF 可进一步降低 ICP。

在硬脑膜被打开之前，EVD 监测结果最有意义，当硬脑膜被剪开后，此时的 ICP 等同于环境压力。

有些 CSDH 病例可能还需要神经电生理监测。脑电图（EEG）和诱发电位的使用将决定麻醉的选择。例如，运动诱发电位（经颅）监测通常伴随着全静脉麻醉的使用。

28.2.2.2 必须建立静脉通路

CSDH 的清除需要建立足够的静脉通道。本章作者们常规都建立两个外周静脉通路（除非有中心通路）。如有中心静脉通路，一个外周静脉通路就足够了。

CSDH 患者可能需要中心静脉通路，使用血管活性药物和容量复苏是放置中心静脉导管的主要原因。如果放置了中心静脉导管，则应进行胸部 X 线检查以排除气胸。如果可能发生静脉空气栓塞（VAE）且术前没有放置静脉通路，则需要放置一条多孔单腔中心静脉导管。在上腔静脉下方 2 cm、右心房稍上方放置的中心静脉导管可通过荧光透视确认位置，并能显示导管的空气抽吸状况良好[18]。

28.2.2.3 全麻诱导

全身麻醉诱导的目的是降低脑代谢率（CMR）、脑血流量和颅内压（或不改变后者）。可以使用的方法有很多，通常使用多种药物的组合来诱导麻醉。

异丙酚会降低 CMR、脑血流量和颅内压[96, 115]，维持自身调节和对二氧化碳（CO_2）的反应[43]。

由于巴比妥类药物在美国难以获取，因此该类药物在美国很少用于诱导麻醉。由于和异丙酚相似，硫喷妥钠和美索比妥以前也用于诱导麻醉，它们在维持脑血流自主调节能力和二氧化碳反应性的同时，降低 CMR、CBF 和颅内压。

依托咪酯可用于 CSDH 患者的麻醉诱导，然而存在严重的术后恶心[19]和呕吐以及肾上腺皮质类固醇抑制[32]的问题。依托咪酯可维持 CPP 并降低 ICP 和 CBF[27]。依托咪酯也可保留患者对二氧化碳的反应性[27]。

氯胺酮在神经麻醉中的使用，特别是在开颅手术中的使用是有争议的。氯胺酮对 CBF、CMR 和颅内压的影响是有争议的，一些研究表明这些参数升高，而另一些研究则表明其没有变化[3, 29, 58]。我们认为在慢性硬膜下血肿患者中应慎用氯胺酮。没有文献明确在 CSDH 患者中使用或不使用氯胺酮的立场。

阿片类药物不仅被用来诱导麻醉，也被用来维持麻醉。有多种药物可供选择，如芬太尼、舒芬太尼和瑞芬太尼。这些药物对 CBF、ICP 和 CMR 的影响很小[72]。

28.2.2.4 全麻的维持

麻醉诱导完成后，麻醉师将着手建立额外的静脉通路和一条动脉导管。

在安装 Mayfield 头架后，由于要处理其他手术问题（导航设置、皮肤准备），在切皮前可能会有一段或长或短的时间。在此期间，通常有必要减少麻醉量以获得最佳的血流动力学变量（避免低血压）。

在上 Mayfield 头架的过程中，通常会有一段短暂的疼痛刺激，这可能会导致高血压和心动过速。可以使用各种药物来减弱这些反应。芬太尼（50 ~ 150 μg IV）、瑞芬太尼（25 ~ 50 μg IV）、异丙酚（20 ~ 50 mg IV）、利多卡因（1 mg/kg IV）、艾司洛尔（1030 ~ 30 mg IV）可滴定至起效。局部麻醉也可能有助于减弱头钉固定的反应[47, 104]。

CSDH 患者可能有颅内压升高，但与急性 SDH 不同的是，CSDH 存在代偿机制。麻醉药物的使用要考虑到颅内病变的程度以及其他并发症。此外，神经生理监测将对所使用的麻醉类型产生影响。

对于可能有明显的颅内压升高的患者，麻醉方式可以选择挥发性麻醉药和静脉麻醉剂（输液或单次注入）。一氧化二氮（N_2O）在开颅手术中的使用是有争议的。麻醉医生对最佳麻醉类型［全凭静脉麻醉（TIVA）和吸入麻醉］没有明确的一致意见。在一项观察各种麻醉方式的大型研究中，基于异丙酚的麻醉方式（TIVA）和使用挥发性麻醉药物的颅内压评分相似。在异丙酚维持麻醉中，ICP 值和 CPP 值得到了较好的控制，但对神经系统的发病率和死亡率尚不能得出明确的结论[22]。

所有挥发性药物（七氟醚、异氟烷、地氟烷和氟烷）都是脑血管扩张剂[76, 112]。具体来讲，七氟醚导致大血管扩张，但小动脉水平的血管收缩可能是由于 CMR 降低引起的[89]。CMR 降低，自主调节降低，从而导致 CBF 和代谢的解耦（过度灌注）[31]。这种效应具有剂量依赖性，解耦反应通常发生在 1 MAC 以上[77]。

全凭静脉麻醉（TIVA）可作为慢性硬膜下血肿患者的唯一麻醉剂。这可能是因为丙泊酚输注可以降低 CMR、CBF、CBV 和 ICP，同时保持 CO_2 反应性。阿片类药物在开颅手术中很常见，它们对 CBF 和 ICP 的影响最小，有时可作为 TIVA 的一部分，右美托咪定也可以用作辅助用药。右美托咪定是一种具有镇静和镇痛特性的 α2 受体激动剂，可降低 CBF 和 CMR[35]，右美托咪定会引起脑血管收缩，但没有证据表明脑血管受损的患者应用右美托咪定会出现脑缺血[119]。

CSDH 术中的血流动力学管理必须考虑患者的因素以及 CSDH 的大小和影响。麻醉的目标是维持 CPP，避免脑缺血、脑卒中、更多的脑损伤和高血压。这种处理方式类似于因颅内占位病变而行开颅手术的患者。

一些机构在术中使用抗癫痫药物。在许多情况下，患者术中继续使用术前抗癫痫药物。CSDH 患者即使无癫痫史也可能发生癫痫，尽管发病率很低（5.3%）[120]。在急性硬膜下血肿患者中，创伤后癫痫是一种常见病。我们认为预防性使用抗癫痫药物是合理的，以避免这种严重的并发症。

在 CSDH 的清除过程中，应给予近等渗晶体溶液。低渗盐水可引起间质水肿。在血脑屏障受损的情况下，高渗盐水溶液会导致脑组织体积增加[73]。胶体溶液在开颅手术中的使用是有争议的，但如果患者血容量低，可以使用白蛋白。

通常采用过度通气松弛脑组织。其目的是通过将 $PaCO_2$ 控制在 25～30 mmHg[45] 来改善手术条件。动脉血气监测有助于指导临床医生如何调整 $PaCO_2$。过度通气常用于颅内出血患者，以降低颅内压，放松紧绷的大脑。但该方法是否改善患者预后尚未在文献中得到证实[123]。

28.3 一般术后护理

开颅手术清除硬膜下血肿后，患者可在 PACU（术后护理病房）康复，或直接被送往重症监护室。不管在哪里，都应对患者进行密切监测，其目的是及早发现严重的术后并发症，并便于干预[100]。控制血压，治疗疼痛，预防和治疗谵妄和术后恶心呕吐，是优化康复的关键。同时应慎重考虑何时是为这些患者重新使用抗凝药的最佳时机。

28.3.1 术后神经学评估

必须在术后即刻进行神经学评估，以便及时发现任何术后脑部并发症[40]。一般采用格拉斯哥（Glasgow）昏迷评分、脑神经检查、感觉、运动、语言和小脑功能检查。当出现新的神经功能缺陷时，应立即进行脑部 CT 扫描，以排除神经外科并发症[40]。

28.3.2 术后恶心和呕吐

术后恶心和呕吐是全身麻醉最常见的副作用之一。恶心和呕吐会升高患者的血压，增加腹内和胸腔内压力，这可能会导致颅内压升高，并导致术后颅内出血[37]。此外，患者在开颅手术后可能出现吞咽反射受损，因此在呕吐后误吸的风险可能会增加[37]。

因此，建议采取多模式结合的方法来治疗开颅术后患者的恶心。最常用的药物包括静脉注射甲氧氯普胺和昂丹司琼[37]。

28.3.3 疼痛管理

尽管普遍认为开颅术后患者的疼痛程度比其他外科患者要低，但约 60% 的患者报告术后有中度至重度疼痛[30]。未有效控制的疼痛可能会导致交感神经刺激，从而导致高血压，并有可能导致继发性颅内出血[9]。然而，过量的止痛药可能会导致镇静，这也可能会掩盖新发神经缺陷。此外，过量使用阿片类止痛药产生的呼吸抑制效应可能会导致高碳酸血症，从而导致颅内压升高。因此，最重要的是维持适当的神经状态，同时为这些患者提供足够的镇痛。

为了达到这种微妙的平衡，可以对开颅术后患者实施多模式镇痛[9]。常用的术后镇痛一线药物是阿片类药物和静脉注射对乙酰氨基酚。芬太尼单次给药由于其高效力而被广泛使用，尽管其作用时间短。静脉注射吗啡是芬太尼的替代品，其作用时间更长。缓慢滴定并密切监测患者，可以避免严重的副作用，如过度镇静和呼吸抑制[36]。一旦患者清醒，拔管，并能够开始经口进食，他们可以过渡到口服药物，包括曲马多、羟考酮和口服对乙酰氨基酚。

28.3.4 血压控制

血压高于 160/90 mmHg 的患者极易发生开颅

术后颅内血肿[9]。当血压超过脑自主调节能力上限时，会导致脑血流量增加，进而破坏血脑屏障，继而可能发生血管内液体渗出和出血。颅内血肿可导致颅内压升高，加重脑水肿，并导致局部和全脑缺血，继而可能导致危及生命的脑疝[61]。

血管扩张剂（硝普钠、硝酸甘油和肼屈嗪）、钙通道阻滞剂（尼卡地平）和 β 受体阻滞剂（拉贝洛尔和艾司洛尔）已用于治疗开颅术后患者的高血压。

在这些药物中，静脉注射尼卡地平和拉贝洛尔是最常用的。拉贝洛尔被认为是开颅术后患者理想的降压药物，因为它不影响脑部血流或脑血流自主调节[94, 98]。在滴定长效拉贝洛尔的同时，可以安全地使用艾司洛尔（半衰期约为 9 min），以达到安全的血压范围，而不会导致低血压。然而，对于那些对这些药物反应不佳的患者，或者那些患有肺部疾病（即哮喘和慢性阻塞性肺疾病）而禁止使用 β 受体阻滞剂的患者，可以替代使用静脉注射钙通道阻滞剂（即尼卡地平）。但需注意有报道尼卡地平静脉推注引起心动过缓、心动过速和低血压。此外，还存在尼卡地平剂量依赖性脑血管扩张和脑自动调节受到抑制的问题[66]，这些效应会导致局部脑血流量减少[2]。然而，许多研究表明，当持续输注时，尼卡地平在快速降低血压方面有很好的疗效，副作用发生最少[93]。

术后应避免低血压（平均血压较标准下降 30% 以上），因为它可能导致脑低灌注，从而导致术后脑缺血[10]。

去甲肾上腺素和去氧肾上腺素是低血压患者术后常用的升压药物。然而，需要注意的是，去甲肾上腺素增加动脉压，但不会增加脑灌注压，而且如果剂量较高，它会对脑氧合产生负面影响[16, 91]。研究发现，去氧肾上腺素也可能通过减少心输出量来降低脑氧饱和度[86]，维持正常的血液碳酸含量可以避免去氧肾上腺素的这种作用[87]。

28.3.5　谵妄预防

谵妄是一种常见而重要的术后并发症，其特征是难以识别、预防和治疗。谵妄的危险因素包括睡眠障碍、感觉障碍、疼痛、脱离社会、光照性抑郁、感染、戒断综合征、脱水、贫血、输血、电解质异常、酸碱异常、低氧血症、体温紊乱、癫痫发作和内分泌功能障碍[46, 81-82]。预防和治疗谵妄的方法是及早解除肢体束缚、导尿管、侵入性导管、气管插管和外科引流，因为这些可能会给患者带来不必要的不适和不安[60]。抗精神病药物经常被用于治疗谵妄患者的躁动，但其对预后的影响仍不清楚[53-54, 75]。术后疼痛管理是治疗谵妄的另一个因素，疼痛可以导致精神错乱，但阿片类止痛药也可以导致谵妄，因此术后对疼痛的管理需要医生谨慎权衡。易发生谵妄的患者应考虑使用非镇静镇痛药，在有严重术后疼痛的患者中，阿片类止痛药已被证明可以缓解疼痛和谵妄[34]。

如上文所述，及早认识到谵妄，并采取非药理学和药理学干预措施是降低术后谵妄发生率的关键。

28.3.6　重新进行抗凝治疗

CSDH 通常与长期使用抗凝药治疗血栓栓塞和心血管疾病有关。此外，受伤前使用抗凝药与血肿清除后 CSDH 复发风险增加有关[92]。

血肿复发的风险必须与出现血栓栓塞事件的风险相权衡。

房颤患者在抗凝治疗中断的 90 天内发生早期血栓栓子事件的风险很高[8]。事实上，7 天内发生卒中的风险为 2.5%～5%[55]。早期恢复抗凝治疗可以降低这一风险，但也可能增加 CSDH 复发的风险[92]。很少有研究对 CSDH 患者进行抗凝治疗的最佳时机进行研究，而且这些研究受到样本量小和方法学欠佳的限制。

因此，对于 CSDH 清除后早期或晚期重新使用抗凝药治疗这一问题，相关的研究数据结果存在很大的差异。目前较为广泛使用的术后恢复抗凝方案有两种：手术后约 1 周开始早期抗凝治疗，或手术后约 4 周开始晚期抗凝治疗[92]。

此外，在决定何时重新进行抗凝治疗之前，需要考虑患者的个体情况。例如，在患者进行抗凝治疗时，通过 CHADS 评分评估卒中的基线风险可能会影响未来对患者卒中风险的预测[92]。相反，高风险出血特征（如凝血功能障碍）可能会促使临床医生尽早恢复使用抗凝药[92]。

参考文献

1. Adhiyaman V, Asghar M, Ganeshram Bhowmick KNBK. Chronic subdural haematoma in the elderly. Postgrad Med J. 2002;78:71–5. https://doi.org/10.1136/pmj.78.916.71.
2. Akopov S, et al. Regional cerebral blood flow in patients with internal carotid artery stenosis: effects of nifedipine and nimodipine. Int J Angiol. 2011;2(01):16–21. https://doi.org/10.1007/bf02651556.
3. Albanèse J, Arnaud S, Rey M, et al. Ketamine decreases intracranial pressure and electroencephalographic activity in traumatic brain injury patients during propofol sedation. Anesthesiology. 1997;87:1328.
4. Alrezk R, Jackson N, Al Rezk M, et al. Derivation and validation of a geriatric-sensitive perioperative cardiac risk index. J Am Heart Assoc. 2017;6(11):e006648. https://doi.org/10.1161/JAHA.117.006648.
5. American College of Surgeons, Committee on Trauma. Advanced trauma life support: student course manual. American College of Surgeons; 2018.
6. Ansell J, Hirsh J, Hylek E, Jacobson A, Crowther M, Palareti G. Pharmacology and management of the vitamin K antagonists: American College of Chest Physicians evidence-based clinical practice guidelines (8th edition). Chest. 2008;133(6 Suppl):160S–98S. https://doi.org/10.1378/chest.08-0670.
7. Arozullah AM, Daley J, Henderson WG, Khuri SF. Multifactorial risk index for predicting postoperative respiratory failure in men after major noncardiac surgery. The National Veterans Administration Surgical Quality Improvement Program. Ann Surg. 2000;232(2):242–53. https://doi.org/10.1097/00000658-200008000-00015.
8. Baechli H, et al. Demographics and prevalent risk factors of chronic subdural haematoma: results of a large single-center cohort study. Neurosurg Rev. 2004;27(4):263–6. https://doi.org/10.1007/s10143-004-0337-6.
9. Basali A, et al. Relation between perioperative hypertension and intracranial hemorrhage after craniotomy. Anesthesiology. 2000;93(1):48–54. https://doi.org/10.1097/00000542-200007000-00012.
10. Bijker JB, Gelb AW. Review article: the role of hypotension in perioperative stroke. Can J Anaesth. 2012;60(2):159–67. https://doi.org/10.1007/s12630-012-9857-7.
11. Bilimoria KY, Liu Y, Paruch JL, Zhou L, Kmiecik TE, Ko CY. Development and evaluation of the universal ACS NSQIP surgical risk calculator: a decision aid and informed consent tool for patients and surgeons. J Am Coll Surg. 2013;217(5):833-42.e1–3.
12. Bishnoi V, Kumar B, Bhagat H, Salunke P, Bishnoi S. Comparison of dexmedetomidine versus midazolam-fentanyl combination for monitored anesthesia care during Burr-hole surgery for chronic subdural hematoma. J Neurosurg Anesthesiol. 2016;28(2):141–6. https://doi.org/10.1097/ANA.0000000000000194. PMID: 26018670.
13. Blaauw J, Jacobs B, den Hertog HM, van der Gaag NA, Jellema K, Dammers R, Lingsma HF, van der Naalt J, Kho KH, Groen RJM. Neurosurgical and perioperative management of chronic subdural hematoma. Front Neurol. 2020;11:550. https://doi.org/10.3389/fneur.2020.00550. eCollection 2020. PMID: 32636797; PMCID: PMC7317017.
14. Bodenham AR, Howell SJ. General anaesthesia vs local anaesthesia: an ongoing story. Br J Anaesth. 2009;103:785–9. https://doi.org/10.1093/bja/aep310.
15. Bolden N, Posner KL, Domino KB, et al. Postoperative critical events associated with obstructive sleep apnea: results from the Society of Anesthesia and Sleep Medicine Obstructive Sleep Apnea Registry. Anesth Analg. 2020;131(4):1032–41. https://doi.org/10.1213/ANE.0000000000005005.
16. Brassard P, et al. Is cerebral oxygenation negatively affected by infusion of norepinephrine in healthy subjects? Br J Anaesth. 2009;102(6):800–5. https://doi.org/10.1093/bja/aep065.
17. Brennan PM, Kolias AG, Joannides AJ, Shapey J, Marcus HJ, Gregson BA, et al. The management and outcome for patients with chronic subdural hematoma: a prospective, multicenter, observational cohort study in the United Kingdom. J Neurosurg. 2017;127:732–9. https://doi.org/10.3171/2016.8.JNS16134.
18. Bunegin L, Albin MS, Helsel PE, Hoffman A, Hung TK. Positioning the right atrial catheter: a model for reappraisal. Anesthesiology. 1981;55(4):343–8. https://doi.org/10.1097/00000542-198110000-00003. PMID: 7294368.
19. Camu F, Lauwers MH, Verbessem D. Incidence and aetiology of postoperative nausea and vomiting. Eur J Anaesthesiol Suppl. 1992;6:25.

20. Cao S, Chen D, Yang L, Zhu T. Effects of an abnormal mini-mental state examination score on postoperative outcomes in geriatric surgical patients: a meta-analysis. BMC Anesthesiol. 2019;19(1):74. https://doi.org/10.1186/s12871-019-0735-5.
21. Chen JW, Gombart ZJ, Rogers S, Gardiner SK, Cecil S, Bullock RM. Pupillary reactivity as an early indicator of increased intracranial pressure: the introduction of the Neurological Pupil index. Surg Neurol Int. 2011;2:82. https://doi.org/10.4103/2152-7806.82248.
22. Chui J, Mariappan R, Mehta J, Manninen P, Venkatraghavan L. Comparison of propofol and volatile agents for maintenance of anesthesia during elective craniotomy procedures: systematic review and meta-analysis. Can J Anaesth. 2014;61(4):347–56. https://doi.org/10.1007/s12630-014-0118-9. Epub 2014 Jan 31. PMID: 24482247.
23. Chun EH, Han MJ, Baik HJ, Park HS, Chung RK, Han JI, Lee HJ, Kim JH. Dexmedetomidine-ketamine versus dexmedetomidine-midazolam-fentanyl for monitored anesthesia care during chemoport insertion: a prospective randomized study. BMC Anesthesiol. 2016;16(1):49. https://doi.org/10.1186/s12871-016-0211-4. PMID: 27484227; PMCID: PMC4970235.
24. Chung F, Yegneswaran B, Liao P, et al. STOP questionnaire: a tool to screen patients for obstructive sleep apnea. Anesthesiology. 2008;108(5):812–21. https://doi.org/10.1097/ALN.0b013e31816d83e4.
25. Chung F, Yegneswaran B, Liao P, et al. Validation of the Berlin questionnaire and American Society of Anesthesiologists checklist as screening tools for obstructive sleep apnea in surgical patients. Anesthesiology. 2008;108(5):822–30. https://doi.org/10.1097/ALN.0b013e31816d91b5.
26. Chung F, Subramanyam R, Liao P, Sasaki E, Shapiro C, Sun Y. High STOP-Bang score indicates a high probability of obstructive sleep apnoea. Br J Anaesth. 2012;108(5):768–75. https://doi.org/10.1093/bja/aes022.
27. Cold GE, Eskesen V, Eriksen H, et al. CBF and CMRO2 during continuous etomidate infusion supplemented with N2O and fentanyl in patients with supratentorial cerebral tumour. A dose-response study. Acta Anaesthesiol Scand. 1985;29:490.
28. Dakik HA, Chehab O, Eldirani M, et al. A new index for pre-operative cardiovascular evaluation. J Am Coll Cardiol. 2019;73(24):3067–78. https://doi.org/10.1016/j.jacc.2019.04.023.
29. Dawson B, Michenfelder JD, Theye RA. Effects of ketamine on canine cerebral blood flow and metabolism: modification by prior administration of thiopental. Anesth Analg. 1971;50:443.
30. De Benedittis G, et al. Postoperative pain in neurosurgery: a pilot study in brain surgery. Neurosurgery. 1996;38(3):466–70. https://doi.org/10.1097/00006123-199603000-00008.
31. De Deyne C, Joly LM, Ravussin P. Les nouveaux agents volatils halogénés en neuro-anesthésie: quelle place pour le sévoflurane ou le desflurane? [Newer inhalation anaesthetics and neuro-anaesthesia: what is the place for sevoflurane or desflurane?]. Ann Fr Anesth Reanim. 2004;23(4):367–74. https://doi.org/10.1016/j.annfar.2004.01.012. French. PMID: 15120783.
32. de Jong FH, Mallios C, Jansen C, et al. Etomidate suppresses adrenocortical function by inhibition of 11 beta-hydroxylation. J Clin Endocrinol Metab. 1984;59:1143.
33. Devereaux PJ, Mrkobrada M, Sessler DI, et al. Aspirin in patients undergoing noncardiac surgery. https://doi.org/10.1056/NEJMoa1401105.
34. Dhallu MS, et al. Perioperative management of neurological conditions. Health Serv Insights. 2017;10:117863291771194. https://doi.org/10.1177/1178632917711942.
35. Drummond JC, Dao AV, Roth DM, et al. Effect of dexmedetomidine on cerebral blood flow velocity, cerebral metabolic rate, and carbon dioxide response in normal humans. Anesthesiology. 2008;108:225.
36. Durieux ME, Himmelseher S. Pain control after craniotomy: off balance on the tightrope? J Neurosurg. 2007;106(2):207–8. https://doi.org/10.3171/jns.2007.106.2.207.
37. Eberhart LHJ, et al. Prevention and control of postoperative nausea and vomiting in post-craniotomy patients. Best Pract Res Clin Anaesthesiol. 2007;21(4):575–93. https://doi.org/10.1016/j.bpa.2007.06.007.
38. Egholm G, Kristensen SD, Thim T, et al. Risk associated with surgery within 12 months after coronary drug-eluting stent implantation. J Am Coll Cardiol. 2016;68(24):2622–32. https://doi.org/10.1016/j.jacc.2016.09.967.
39. English JB, Westenskow D, Hodges MR, Stanley TH. Comparison of venous air embolism monitoring methods in supine dogs. Anesthesiology. 1978;48(6):425–9. https://doi.org/10.1097/00000542-197806000-00009. PMID: 666025.
40. Fàbregas N, Bruder N. Recovery and neurological evaluation. Best Pract Res Clin

Anaesthesiol. 2007;21(4):431–47. https://doi.org/10.1016/j.bpa.2007.06.006.
41. Feely MA, Collins CS, Daniels PR, Kebede EB, Jatoi A, Mauck KF. Preoperative testing before noncardiac surgery: guidelines and recommendations. Am Fam Physician. 2013;87(6):414–8.
42. Fleisher LA, Fleischmann KE, Auerbach AD, et al. 2014 ACC/AHA guideline on perioperative cardiovascular evaluation and management of patients undergoing noncardiac surgery: executive summary: a report of the American College of Cardiology/American Heart Association Task Force on Practice Guidelines. Circulation. 2014;130(24):2215–45. https://doi.org/10.1161/CIR.0000000000000105.
43. Fox J, Gelb AW, Enns J, et al. The responsiveness of cerebral blood flow to changes in arterial carbon dioxide is maintained during propofol-nitrous oxide anesthesia in humans. Anesthesiology. 1992;77:453.
44. Gelabert-González M, Iglesias-Pais M, García-Allut Martínez-Rumbo AR. Chronic subdural haematoma: surgical treatment and outcome in 1000 cases. Clin Neurol Neurosurg. 2005;107:223–9. https://doi.org/10.1016/j.clineuro.2004.09.015.
45. Gelb AW, Craen RA, Rao GS, et al. Does hyperventilation improve operating condition during supratentorial craniotomy? A multicenter randomized crossover trial. Anesth Analg. 2008;106:585.
46. George J, et al. Causes and prognosis of delirium in elderly patients admitted to a district general hospital. Age Ageing. 1997;26(6):423–7. https://doi.org/10.1093/ageing/26.6.423.
47. Geze S, Yilmaz AA, Tuzuner F. The effect of scalp block and local infiltration on the haemodynamic and stress response to skull-pin placement for craniotomy. Eur J Anaesthesiol. 2009;26(4):298–303. https://doi.org/10.1097/EJA.0b013e32831aedb2. PMID: 19262392.
48. Godier A, Dincq A-S, Martin A-C, et al. Predictors of pre-procedural concentrations of direct oral anticoagulants: a prospective multicentre study. Eur Heart J. 2017;38(31):2431–9. https://doi.org/10.1093/eurheartj/ehx403.
49. Godoy DA, Di Napoli M, Biestro A, Lenhardt R. Perioperative glucose control in neurosurgical patients. Anesthesiol Res Pract. 2012;2012:690362. https://doi.org/10.1155/2012/690362.
50. Goldman L, Caldera DL, Nussbaum SR, et al. Multifactorial index of cardiac risk in non-cardiac surgical procedures. N Engl J Med. 1977;297(16):845–50. https://doi.org/10.1056/NEJM197710202971601.
51. Grinberg F, Slaughter TF, McGrath BJ. Probable venous air embolism associated with removal of the Mayfield skull clamp. Anesth Analg. 1995;80(5):1049–50. https://doi.org/10.1097/00000539-199505000-00036. PMID: 7726406.
52. Gupta PK, Gupta H, Sundaram A, et al. Development and validation of a risk calculator for prediction of cardiac risk after surgery. Circulation. 2011;124(4):381–7. https://doi.org/10.1161/CIRCULATIONAHA.110.015701.
53. Hatta K, et al. Antipsychotics for delirium in the general hospital setting in consecutive 2453 inpatients: a prospective observational study. Int J Geriatr Psychiatry. 2013;29(3):253–62. https://doi.org/10.1002/gps.3999.
54. Hawkins SB, et al. Quetiapine for the treatment of delirium. J Hosp Med. 2013;8(4):215–20. https://doi.org/10.1002/jhm.2019.
55. Hohnloser SH, Eikelboom JW. The hazards of interrupting anticoagulation therapy in atrial fibrillation. Eur Heart J. 2012;33(15):1864–6. https://doi.org/10.1093/eurheartj/ehs032.
56. Holcomb CN, Graham LA, Richman JS, Itani KMF, Maddox TM, Hawn MT. The incremental risk of coronary stents on postoperative adverse events: a matched cohort study. Ann Surg. 2016;263(5):924–30. https://doi.org/10.1097/SLA.0000000000001246.
57. Horinaka N, Yasumoto Y, Kumami K, Matsumura K. Evaluation of regional cerebral blood flow in chronic subdural hamatoma. Keio J Med. 2000;49(Suppl 1):A156–8.
58. Hougaard K, Hansen A, Brodersen P. The effect of ketamine on regional cerebral blood flow in man. Anesthesiology. 1974;41:562.
59. Inao S, Kawai T, Kabeya R, Sugimoto T, Yamamoto M, Hata N, Isobe T, Yoshida J. Relation between brain displacement and local cerebral blood flow in patients with chronic subdural hematoma. J Neurol Neurosurg Psychiatry. 2001;71:741–6.
60. Inouye SK. Precipitating factors for delirium in hospitalized elderly persons. JAMA. 1996;275(11):852. https://doi.org/10.1001/jama.1996.03530350034031.
61. Jian M, et al. Flurbiprofen and hypertension but not hydroxyethyl starch are associated with post-craniotomy intracranial haematoma requiring surgery. Br J Anaesth. 2014;113(5):832–9. https://doi.org/10.1093/bja/aeu185.
62. Kim SE, Kim E. Local anesthesia with monitored anesthesia care for patients undergoing

thyroidectomy—a case series. Korean J Anesthesiol. 2016;69:635–9. https://doi.org/10.4097/kjae.2016.69.6.635.
63. Kim SO, Jung Il S, Won YS, Choi Yang CSJY. A comparative study of local versus general anesthesia for chronic subdural hematoma in elderly patients over 60 years. Korean J Neurotrauma. 2013;9:47–51. https://doi.org/10.13004/kjnt.2013.9.2.47.
64. Klopfenstein CE, Forster A, Van Gessel E. Anesthetic assessment in an outpatient consultation clinic reduces preoperative anxiety. Can J Anesth. 2000;47(6):511. https://doi.org/10.1007/BF030189.
65. Kolias AG, Chari A, Santarius Hutchinson TPJ. Chronic subdural haematoma: modern management and emerging therapies. Nat Rev Neurol. 2014;10:570–8. https://doi.org/10.1038/nrneurol.2014.163.
66. Kross RA, et al. A comparative study between a calcium channel blocker (nicardipine) and a combined α-β-blocker (labetalol) for the control of emergence hypertension during craniotomy for tumor surgery. Anesth Analg. 2000;91(4):904–9. https://doi.org/10.1097/00000539-200010000-00024.
67. Kuwabara H. Regional cerebral blood flow and metabolism in chronic subdural hematoma. Neurosurg Clin N Am. 2000;11:499–502.
68. Langeron O, Masso E, Huraux C, et al. Prediction of difficult mask ventilation. Anesthesiology. 2000;92(5):1229–36.
69. Leary MC, Varade P. Perioperative stroke. Curr Neurol Neurosci Rep. 2020;20(5):12. https://doi.org/10.1007/s11910-020-01033-7.
70. Lee TH, Marcantonio ER, Mangione CM, et al. Derivation and prospective validation of a simple index for prediction of cardiac risk of major noncardiac surgery. Circulation. 1999;100(10):1043–9. https://doi.org/10.1161/01.cir.100.10.1043.
71. Lee JY, Ebel H, Ernestus RI, Klug N. Various surgical treatments of chronic subdural hematoma and outcome in 172 patients: is membranectomy necessary? Surg Neurol. 2004;61(6):523–7; discussion 527–8. https://doi.org/10.1016/j.surneu.2003.10.026. PMID: 15165784.
72. Leone M, Albanèse J, Viviand X, et al. The effects of remifentanil on endotracheal suctioning-induced increases in intracranial pressure in head-injured patients. Anesth Analg. 2004;99:1193.
73. Lescot T, Degos V, Zouaoui A, et al. Opposed effects of hypertonic saline on contusions and noncontused brain tissue in patients with severe traumatic brain injury. Crit Care Med. 2006;34:3029.
74. Levine GN, Bates ER, Bittl JA, et al. 2016 ACC/AHA guideline focused update on duration of dual antiplatelet therapy in patients with coronary artery disease: a report of the American College of Cardiology/American Heart Association task force on clinical practice guidelines. J Am Coll Cardiol. 2016;68(10):1082–115. https://doi.org/10.1016/j.jacc.2016.03.513.
75. Liu C-Y, et al. Efficacy of risperidone in treating the hyperactive symptoms of delirium. Int Clin Psychopharmacol. 2004;19(3):165–8. https://doi.org/10.1097/00004850-200405000-00008.
76. Lutz LJ, Milde JH, Milde LN. The cerebral functional, metabolic, and hemodynamic effects of desflurane in dogs. Anesthesiology. 1990;73:125.
77. Madsen JB, Cold GE, Hansen ES, Bardrum B. The effect of isoflurane on cerebral blood flow and metabolism in humans during craniotomy for small supratentorial cerebral tumors. Anesthesiology. 1987;66:332.
78. Mahmood SD, Waqas M, Baig Darbar MZA. Mini-craniotomy under local anesthesia for chronic subdural hematoma: an effective choice for elderly patients and for patients in a resource-strained environment. World Neurosurg. 2017;106:676–9. https://doi.org/10.1016/j.wneu.2017.07.057.
79. Mahmood SD, Waqas M, Baig MZ, Darbar A. Mini-craniotomy under local anesthesia for chronic subdural hematoma: an effective choice for elderly patients and for patients in a resource-strained environment. World Neurosurg. 2017;106:676–9. https://doi.org/10.1016/j.wneu.2017.07.057. Epub 2017 Jul 19. PMID: 28735131.
80. Mammoto T, Hayashi Y, Ohnishi Y, Kuro M. Incidence of venous and paradoxical air embolism in neurosurgical patients in the sitting position: detection by transesophageal echocardiography. Acta Anaesthesiol Scand. 1998;42(6):643–7. https://doi.org/10.1111/j.1399-6576.1998.tb05295.x. PMID: 9689268.
81. Marcantonio ER. A clinical prediction rule for delirium after elective noncardiac surgery. JAMA. 1994;271(2):134–9. https://doi.org/10.1001/jama.271.2.134.
82. Marcantonio ER, et al. The association of intraoperative factors with the development of postoperative delirium. Am J Med. 1998;105(5):380–4. https://doi.org/10.1016/

s0002-9343(98)00292-7.
83. Mayer S, Rowland L. Head injury. In: Rowland L, editor. Merritt's neurology. Philadelphia: Lippincott Williams & Wilkins; 2000. p. 401.
84. Mayhew D, Mendonca V, Murthy BVS. A review of ASA physical status—historical perspectives and modern developments. Anaesthesia. 2019;74(3):373–9. https://doi.org/10.1111/anae.14569.
85. McAlister FA, Bertsch K, Man J, Bradley J, Jacka M. Incidence of and risk factors for pulmonary complications after nonthoracic surgery. Am J Respir Crit Care Med. 2005;171(5):514–7. https://doi.org/10.1164/rccm.200408-1069OC.
86. Meng L, et al. Effect of phenylephrine and ephedrine bolus treatment on cerebral oxygenation in anaesthetized patients. Br J Anaesth. 2011;107(2):209–17. https://doi.org/10.1093/bja/aer150.
87. Meng L, et al. Impact of phenylephrine administration on cerebral tissue oxygen saturation and blood volume is modulated by carbon dioxide in anaesthetized patients †. Br J Anaesth. 2012;108(5):815–22. https://doi.org/10.1093/bja/aes023.
88. Moghissi ES, Korytkowski MT, DiNardo M, et al. American Association of Clinical Endocrinologists and American Diabetes Association Consensus Statement on inpatient glycemic control. Diabetes Care. 2009;32(6):1119–31. https://doi.org/10.2337/dc09-9029.
89. Molnár C, Settakis G, Sárkány P, Kálmán S, Szabó S, Fülesdi B. Effect of sevoflurane on cerebral blood flow and cerebrovascular resistance at surgical level of anaesthesia: a transcranial Doppler study. Eur J Anaesthesiol. 2007;24(2):179–84. https://doi.org/10.1017/S0265021506001335. Epub 2006 Sep 14. PMID: 16970835.
90. Moon HG, Shin HS, Kim TH, Hwang YS, Park SK. Ossified chronic subdural hematoma. Yonsei Med J. 2003;44(5):915–8. https://doi.org/10.3349/ymj.2003.44.5.915. PMID: 14584111.
91. Moppett IK. Sympathetic activity and cerebral oxygenation. Br J Anaesth. 2009;103(5):769–70. https://doi.org/10.1093/bja/aep281.
92. Nassiri F, et al. Reinitiation of anticoagulation after surgical evacuation of subdural hematomas. World Neurosurg. 2020;135:e616–22. https://doi.org/10.1016/j.wneu.2019.12.080.
93. Neutel JM, et al. A comparison of intravenous nicardipine and sodium nitroprusside in the immediate treatment of severe hypertension. Am J Hypertens. 1994;7(7 Pt 1):623–8. https://doi.org/10.1093/ajh/7.7.623.
94. Olsen KS, et al. Effect of labetalol on cerebral blood flow, oxygen metabolism and autoregulation in healthy humans. Br J Anaesth. 1995;75(1):51–4. https://doi.org/10.1093/bja/75.1.51.
95. Omran H, Bauersachs R, Rübenacker S, Goss F, Hammerstingl C. The HAS-BLED score predicts bleedings during bridging of chronic oral anticoagulation. Thromb Haemost. 2012;108(07):65–73. https://doi.org/10.1160/TH11-12-0827.
96. Petersen KD, Landsfeldt U, Cold GE, et al. Intracranial pressure and cerebral hemodynamic in patients with cerebral tumors: a randomized prospective study of patients subjected to craniotomy in propofol-fentanyl, isoflurane-fentanyl, or sevoflurane-fentanyl anesthesia. Anesthesiology. 2003;98:329.
97. Practice guidelines for the perioperative management of patients with obstructive sleep apnea: a report by the American Society of Anesthesiologists Task Force on perioperative management of patients with obstructive sleep apnea. Anesthesiology. 2006;104(5):1081–93. https://doi.org/10.1097/00000542-200605000-00026.
98. Qureshi AI, et al. Pharmacologic reduction of mean arterial pressure does not adversely affect regional cerebral blood flow and intracranial pressure in experimental intracerebral hemorrhage. Crit Care Med. 1999;27(5):965–71. https://doi.org/10.1097/00003246-199905000-00036.
99. Rauhala M, Luoto TM, Huhtala H, Iverson GL, Niskakangas T, Öhman J, et al. The incidence of chronic subdural hematomas from 1990 to 2015 in a defined Finnish population. J Neurosurg. 2019;22:1–11. https://doi.org/10.3171/2018.12.JNS183035.
100. Rhondali O, et al. Do patients still require admission to an intensive care unit after elective craniotomy for brain surgery? J Neurosurg Anesthesiol. 2011;23(2):118–23. https://doi.org/10.1097/ana.0b013e318206d5f8.
101. Santarius T, Kirkpatrick PJ, Ganesan D, Chia HL, Jalloh I, Smielewski P, Richards HK, Marcus H, Parker RA, Price SJ, Kirollos RW, Pickard JD, Hutchinson PJ. Use of drains versus no drains after burr-hole evacuation of chronic subdural haematoma: a randomised controlled trial. Lancet. 2009;374(9695):1067–73. https://doi.org/10.1016/S0140-6736(09)61115-6. PMID: 19782872.

102. Shapira-Lichter I, Beilin B, Ofek K, Bessler H, Gruberger M, Shavit Y, et al. Cytokines and cholinergic signals co-modulate surgical stress-induced changes in mood and memory. Brain Behav Immun. 2008;22:388–98. https://doi.org/10.1016/j.bbi.2007.09.006.
103. Sharrock MF, Rosenblatt K. Acute airway management and ventilation in the neurocritical care unit. In: Nelson SE, Nyquist PA, editors. Neurointensive care unit: clinical practice and organization. Cham: Springer International Publishing; 2020. p. 31–47. https://doi.org/10.1007/978-3-030-36548-6_3.
104. Shiau JM, Chen TY, Tseng CC, Chang PJ, Tsai YC, Chang CL, Lee CG. Combination of bupivacaine scalp circuit infiltration with general anesthesia to control the hemodynamic response in craniotomy patients. Acta Anaesthesiol Sin. 1998;36(4):215–20. PMID: 10399517.
105. Shoyombo I, Aiyagari V, Stutzman SE, et al. Understanding the relationship between the neurologic pupil index and constriction velocity values. Sci Rep. 2018;8(1):6992. https://doi.org/10.1038/s41598-018-25477-7.
106. Slotty PJ, Kamp MA, Steiger HJS, Cornelius JF, Macht S, Stumer W, Turowski B. Cerebral perfusion changes in chronic subdural hematoma. J Neurotrauma. 2013;30:347–51.
107. Smilowitz NR, Berger JS. Perioperative cardiovascular risk assessment and management for noncardiac surgery: a review. JAMA. 2020;324(3):279. https://doi.org/10.1001/jama.2020.7840.
108. Stamenkovic DM, Rancic NK, Latas MB, et al. Preoperative anxiety and implications on postoperative recovery: what can we do to change our history. Minerva Anestesiol. 2018;84(11):1307–17. https://doi.org/10.23736/S0375-9393.18.12520-X.
109. Surve RM, Bansal S, Reddy M, Philip M. Use of dexmedetomidine along with local infiltration versus general anesthesia for Burr hole and evacuation of chronic subdural hematoma (CSDH). J Neurosurg Anesthesiol. 2017;29(3):274–80. https://doi.org/10.1097/ANA.0000000000000305. PMID: 27100913.
110. Tafur A, Douketis J. Perioperative management of anticoagulant and antiplatelet therapy. Heart. 2018;104(17):1461–7. https://doi.org/10.1136/heartjnl-2016-310581.
111. Tanaka A, Nakayama Y, Yoshinaga S. Cerebral blood flow and intracranial pressure in chronic subdural hematoma. Surg Neurol. 1997;47:346–52.
112. Todd MM, Drummond JC. A comparison of the cerebrovascular and metabolic effects of halothane and isoflurane in the cat. Anesthesiology. 1984;60:276.
113. Trofimova AO, Kalentiev G, Voennov O, Yuriev M, Agarkova D, Trofimov S, Bragin DE. Comparison of two algorithms for analysis of perfusion computed tomography (PCT) data for evaluation of cerebral microcirculation in chronic subdural hematoma. Adv Exp Med Biol. 2016;923:407–12.
114. Valgimigli M, Bueno H, Byrne RA, et al. 2017 ESC focused update on dual antiplatelet therapy in coronary artery disease developed in collaboration with EACTS: the Task Force for dual antiplatelet therapy in coronary artery disease of the European Society of Cardiology (ESC) and of the European Association for Cardio-Thoracic Surgery (EACTS). Eur Heart J. 2018;39(3):213–60. https://doi.org/10.1093/eurheartj/ehx419.
115. Vandesteene A, Trempont V, Engelman E, et al. Effect of propofol on cerebral blood flow and metabolism in man. Anaesthesia. 1988;43(Suppl):42–3.
116. Vaziri S, Wilson J, Abbatematteo J, et al. Predictive performance of the American College of Surgeons universal risk calculator in neurosurgical patients. J Neurosurg. 2018;128(3):942–7. https://doi.org/10.3171/2016.11.JNS161377.
117. Vaziri S, Abbatematteo JM, Fleisher MS, et al. Correlation of perioperative risk scores with hospital costs in neurosurgical patients. J Neurosurg. 2019;132(3):818–24. https://doi.org/10.3171/2018.10.JNS182041.
118. Victor M, Ropper A. Craniocerebral trauma. In: Victor M, Ropper A, editors. Adams and Victor's principles of neurology. 7th ed. New York: McGraw-Hill; 2001. p. 925.
119. Wang X, Ji J, Fen L, Wang A. Effects of dexmedetomidine on cerebral blood flow in critically ill patients with or without traumatic brain injury: a prospective controlled trial. Brain Inj. 2013;27(13–14):1617–22. https://doi.org/10.3109/02699052.2013.831130. Epub 2013 Oct 8. PMID: 24102571.
120. Won SY, Konczalla J, Dubinski D, Cattani A, Cuca C, Seifert V, Rosenow F, Strzelczyk A, Freiman TM. A systematic review of epileptic seizures in adults with subdural haematomas. Seizure. 2017;45:28–35. https://doi.org/10.1016/j.seizure.2016.11.017. Epub 2016 Nov 25. PMID: 27914224.
121. Wong DH, Weber EC, Schell MJ, Wong AB, Anderson CT, Barker SJ. Factors asso-

ciated with postoperative pulmonary complications in patients with severe chronic obstructive pulmonary disease. Anesth Analg. 1995;80(2):276–84. https://doi.org/10.1097/00000539-199502000-00013.

122. Yoshida K, Furuse M, Izawa A, Lizima N, Hirano T, Kuchiwaki H, Inao S, Sugita K. Dynamics of cerebral metabolism in patients with chronic subdural hematoma evaluated with phosphorus 31MR spectroscopy before and after surgery. AJNR Am J Neuroradiol. 1994;15:1681–6.

123. Zhang Z, Guo Q, Wang E. Hyperventilation in neurological patients: from physiology to outcome evidence. Curr Opin Anaesthesiol. 2019;32(5):568–73. https://doi.org/10.1097/ACO.0000000000000764. PMID: 31211719; PMCID: PMC6735527.

第29章 慢性硬膜下血肿的外科治疗

Kemal Ertilav，Ümit Kocaman 和 Arif Önder

译者：吴量

29.1 引言

硬膜下血肿（SDH）通常是由于皮质桥静脉破裂，血液进入蛛网膜和硬脑膜之间的潜在间隙而引起的。硬脑膜窦、蛛网膜下腔肉芽肿或小皮质动脉损伤也可引起硬膜下血肿[1]。由于硬膜下腔的阻力较低，出血可在该腔内的半球表面呈新月形扩散。此外，由于出血可沿大脑镰和小脑幕扩散，该空间内的出血可能比实际看起来更薄[6]。出血通常是由于创伤时的加速-减速机制，导致桥静脉的撕裂[28]。血肿常见于出血晚期和老年，因为随着大脑萎缩，脑组织的顺应性降低。出血分为4天内的急性出血、4～21天的亚急性出血和21天后的慢性出血[28]。慢性硬膜下血肿最可能以急性硬膜下血肿开始，存在的血凝块会引发炎症反应。然后，成纤维细胞进入血凝块并在最初的24 h内覆盖硬脑膜的内表面，成纤维细胞导致血肿膜的形成并逐渐完全包围血凝块。7天形成壁层血肿膜，21天形成脏层血肿膜，血肿膜形成之后是新生血管的形成。现有血凝块的溶解产生了纤维蛋白降解产物，从而阻碍了止血。慢性硬膜下血肿包膜内形成的新生血管窦状结构较脆弱，容易出血，反复出血使硬膜下血肿内的压力降低至静脉压和毛细血管压以下，使血液进入新生血管然后进入包膜。由于止血功能受损，源自新生血管的出血不能完全停止。此外，脆弱的新生血管导致的出血及其溶解后形成的纤维蛋白降解产物也会形成恶性循环，破坏止血。因此，由于新形成的出血灶以及低压的作用，慢性硬膜下血肿不断吸收血液并逐渐扩张[1, 4, 6, 28]。

29.2 手术原则

直到20世纪70年代，最常用的治疗硬膜下血肿的方法是开颅手术；20世纪80年代以后，钻孔引流术成为最常用的方法；床旁颅骨钻孔术于1977年问世；闭式引流仍是开颅术后最常用的引流方法。手术引流可迅速改善症状[16]。在208例患者中，67.8%的患者出现神经功能缺损[20]，手术消除了脑疝发生的风险。急诊神经外科手术治疗适用于有症状的慢性硬膜下血肿。手术治疗是治疗有症状的慢性硬膜下血肿的基础方法[8, 22]，在手术与非手术治疗难以抉择时，做出联合治疗决策更为合适[16]。

治疗的主要原则是降低颅内压，保持再出血和液体吸收的平衡。这两个独立存在的情况分别需要手术治疗和保守治疗。因为在厚度为1 cm或以上的慢性硬膜下血肿中，再出血和液体吸收之间的平衡被破坏，因此经常出现进行性的出血。在这种情况下，即使患者无症状，也需要手术治疗[8]。当颅内压升高时，症状就会出现。患者可能表现出广泛的症状，如头痛、定向障碍、癫痫发作、局灶缺陷、嗜睡、精神错乱或昏迷[8, 28]。对于小于1 cm的慢性硬膜下血肿，如果出现局灶缺陷、精神状态改变或癫痫发作而没有其他原因，也需要手术治疗[8]。对于厚度小于1 cm且无其他体征或症状的慢性硬膜下血肿，可采取保守方法，并缩短随访时间。对于厚度小于1 cm的慢性硬膜下血肿，并且在随访中尺寸未增大且无症状或体征表现，无手术指征[8]。

29.3 双孔钻孔术

在颞上线冠状缝合线前方1 cm处开一个额部骨孔和一个后顶骨骨孔[15, 21]。我们建议钻孔直径为12 mm，这一长度为硬膜下引流管提供了合适的推进角度。打开硬脑膜，用双极电凝将硬脑膜电凝在颅骨内平板上。然后使用温盐水和尖端柔软钝化的引流管通过额部和顶端的骨孔对血肿腔进行4个方向的冲洗，使用生理盐水不断冲洗，直至液体变清[8, 15, 21]。最后使用一根柔软钝头的硬脑膜下引流管，小心地通过前额和顶骨的钻孔插入，用于血肿的持续引流。关颅时首先关闭顶骨骨孔，以防止气颅发生；硬膜下区域通过额部骨孔充满生理盐水，使空气随生理盐水排出[15]，也可根据术者的喜好进行 Valsalva 手法。然后关闭正面骨孔，并使用双封闭自由排水系统。术后平均 48 h 后拔除引流管。

29.4 单孔钻孔术

在颞上线上钻开一个直径 20～25 mm 的颞顶钻孔[8, 15]。在双极电凝的帮助下，打开硬脑膜并将其黏附到骨板上。如果观察到壁膜应首先电凝，然后切开血肿膜，排出膜下血肿。使用温盐水和尖端柔软钝化的引流管通过额部和顶端的骨孔对血肿进行 4 个方向的冲洗，生理盐水持续冲洗直到液体变清[8, 15]。最后在背侧向前基底方向放置柔软钝头的硬膜下引流管，并在其上填塞相同大小的明胶海绵后关闭骨孔。硬膜下区域填满生理盐水，并置于封闭的自由引流管中，术后 48 h 后拔除引流管。

29.5 床旁颅骨钻孔术

床旁颅骨钻孔引流术适用于无分隔的慢性硬膜下血肿的高危手术患者。该手术的优点和主要特点是可以在局部麻醉下于床边进行。在冠状缝前方 10 mm 处，于颞上线上标记入路[8, 17, 34]。使用这种方法的重要前提是硬膜下血肿的厚度至少是 CT 扫描上骨厚度的 2 倍。如果满足上述条件，在用酒精和聚维酮碘溶液消毒头皮后，给予 2% 利多卡因溶液麻醉。使用 15 号手术刀在记号切口处做一个约 5 mm 长的切口，颅骨与硬膜用麻花钻垂直钻孔[8, 17]。垂直钻孔可防止钻头滑动，安全地将硬脑膜与血肿膜分离，然后用麻花钻以 45°角刨削颅腔内壁，以防止导管穿透损伤皮质[8, 17]。使用标准脑室造瘘引流管，向后下方向朝向耳朵前推约 50 mm。术中不进行冲洗和抽吸，术后采用封闭排水系统，48 h 后拔出导管[8, 17]。

29.6 扩大开颅术

开颅手术适用于存在多分隔、含有其他组织、钙化或骨化的慢性硬膜下血肿，该手术也适用于具有较厚血肿膜的慢性硬膜下血肿。通过开颅术，可以获得更广阔的骨化膜的视野[32]。根据慢性硬膜下血肿的位置进行开颅手术，传统的方法是通过额-颞-顶-枕开颅术治疗扩散到整个半球表面的硬膜下血肿。打开硬脑膜后，通过顶膜切开术排出硬膜下血肿[21]（图 29.1 和图 29.2）。这种膜切开术的目的不是切除膜，而是在膜结构上做一个开口，类似于硬脑膜开口，膜切开术也可以通过以包膜或皮瓣的形式切开来进行。在切开之前，对任何脆弱的、易因新生血管形成而出血的血肿膜进行电凝。如前所述[8, 21]，应再次使用温盐水向血肿四周进行冲洗。在血肿膜切开之前，必须将脏膜与蛛网膜区分开。脏膜比壁膜薄，通常呈淡黄色，在厚度和外观上与蛛网膜相似（图 29.3），这层组织可以被剥离和切除。应在一个没有血管形成的区域切开血肿膜，切开脏膜时应避免用力动作[8, 21]。通过增加大

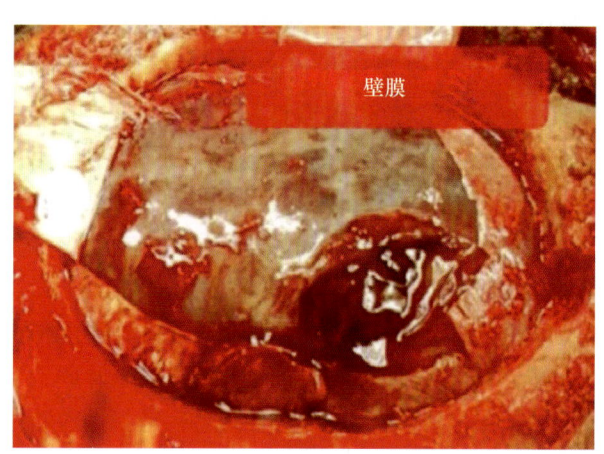

图 29.1　77 岁女性患者行大骨瓣开颅手术后，从硬脑膜上方看到血肿周围的壁膜

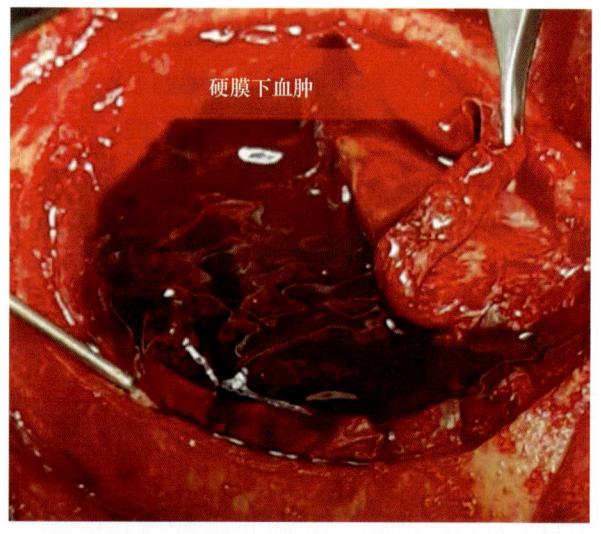

图 29.2　77 岁女性患者，经壁膜切除术后出现慢性硬膜下血肿块

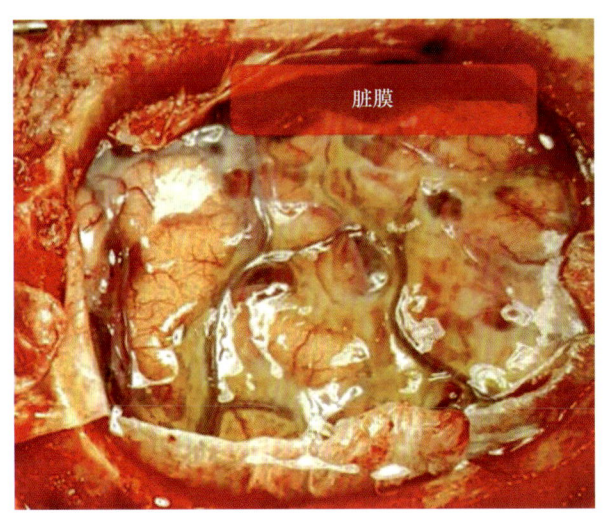

图 29.3　77 岁女性硬膜下血块切除后黄色脏膜部分黏附蛛网膜和大脑皮质

脑扩张度确保硬膜下间隙消失，从而防止复发[13]。控制出血后，在硬膜下空间放置引流管，闭合硬脑膜，将骨瓣固定回原位，48 h 后拔除引流管。

29.7　内镜技术

内镜手术适用于有组织和多分隔的慢性硬膜下血肿在直视下去除血凝块。内镜治疗可以提供清晰的术中视野，使手术更安全，该技术可以识别和去除血肿膜[34]。内镜下引流慢性硬膜下血肿时，根据血肿的位置，在头盖骨最弯曲的顶骨区做 40 mm 的皮肤切口，最好行 30 mm 的小开颅手术。使用内窥镜在血肿膜上钻孔，以提供血肿的直线视图[2, 9, 35]。硬脑膜以信封的形式打开并保留。分离壁膜并行血肿膜切开术后，将内窥镜向前穿过壁膜和脏膜以提供血肿内部视野。在吸引器的帮助下吸除血肿，然后在内窥镜的帮助下打开分隔，在不同的隔室中进行血肿引流。用温盐水向血肿四周冲洗，并用引流管引流。在远端硬脑膜下隙放置引流管，关闭硬脑膜，向腔内注入生理盐水，骨瓣重新固定，48 h 后拔出引流管[31, 34]。

29.8　硬脑膜中动脉栓塞

脑膜中动脉（MMA）栓塞术可定义为"硬膜下血管断流术"。该手术有助于打破持续渗出和血液降解产物不断积累的恶性循环，将血肿出血与重吸收重新平衡。脑膜中动脉是上颌动脉的一个分支，起源于颈动脉，它通过颅骨底部的棘孔进入颅骨，然后其额支和顶支进入硬脑膜。MMA 通过脑膜前动脉和脑膜后动脉供应脑膜，换言之 MMA 为位于大脑前凸和后凸的慢性硬膜下血肿提供营养支持。MMA 远端分支通过脑膜中动脉与眼动脉吻合，MMA 也与耳后动脉吻合。栓塞颗粒意外进入这些血管的吻合口可引起眼神经和面神经损伤。13% 的受试者眼动脉起源于 MMA，这种情况是 MMA 栓塞治疗慢性硬膜下血肿的禁忌[5]。MMA 栓塞治疗可以通过三种方式进行：①作为单一治疗；②作为术前附加治疗；③作为术后附加治疗[26]。用于栓塞的经典方案是聚乙烯醇（PVA）颗粒栓塞，另一种方法是使用液体栓塞剂。PVA 栓塞的优点是其具有更强的远端穿透性，是一种用于阻断供应血肿血管的很好材料。缺点是聚乙烯醇是一种透明的物质，微导管中的视野只能提供有限的 PVA 颗粒分散效果，因此很难确定栓塞效果。可以分布大量的液体栓塞剂则可以清晰显示[5]。

29.9　小开颅和基底（内）膜切开术

小开颅和基底（内）膜切开术是扩大开颅术和单孔钻孔术的改进，钻孔直径一般为 40 mm[13]，以马蹄形打开硬脑膜。打开壁膜后，将膜间硬膜下血肿排出。打开分隔，排出密闭区域的血肿。脏膜结构外观为脏黄色，厚度类似于洋葱膜，这层结构与蛛网膜的不同之处在于它的颜色和厚度。小心地打开脏膜[13, 21]，通过内膜和蛛网膜之间的裂隙，向四个方向伸入软引流管，用温盐水进行冲洗。脏膜切开术的最大优点是通过促进大脑扩张来封闭硬膜下间隙，这可以显著减少复发。最后，在硬脑膜下放置引流管，关闭硬脑膜，骨瓣复位，术后 48 h 终止引流[13]。

29.10　针对复发性硬膜下血肿，手术方式选择，引流问题，青少年和儿童患者及其他问题的讨论

慢性硬膜下血肿的复发并不罕见，手术引流失败率为 9.4%～30%，钻孔引流术术后复发率为 18% 左右[20]。一旦首次手术治疗不成功，重复手术治疗的复发率可高达 46%。Oslo 复发检测和分级系

统可以指导外科医生[27]，判断慢性硬膜下血肿钻孔引流后需要再次手术的复发概率（表29.1）。根据该预测系统，所有总分为0分的患者均未发生需要重复手术的慢性硬膜下血肿。需要再次手术的CSDH在1分或2分患者中占6%，在3分或4分患者中占30%，在5分患者中占63%。

对291例患者进行的一项研究认为，钻孔开颅术后第7天脑容量下降是决定复发的最重要因素。临界脑组织体积值为51.6 cm³，敏感性和特异性分别为79.3%和67.9%[11]。

一项包括461例患者的研究确定，增加复发风险的因素是中线移位超过10 mm、严重脑萎缩、术后严重的气颅和血肿引流超过100 ml[24]。

需要手术的对侧SDH可能在SDH引流手术后发生。一些研究指出，第一次手术后对侧血肿体积是这些患者的危险因素。血肿临界体积值有报道为37.84 cm³[23]。

硬膜下-腹膜分流术或放置Ommaya囊重复穿刺是多次复发的慢性硬膜下血肿的手术治疗选择。

从这些研究中得出的一个普遍结论是，术后任何不扩张的脑组织都为慢性硬膜下血肿复发的发展提供了条件。

决定合适的手术方式需要综合评估多种因素，患者的年龄、Karnofsky评分、其他潜在疾病、抗血小板或抗凝治疗的使用以及血肿的影像学特征将是决定手术方式选择的重要因素。在"Oslo复发检测和分级系统"中，慢性硬膜下血肿钻孔引流术后需要手术的复发评分为5分的患者，应优先选择可以打开分隔和血肿膜的手术方法。我们推荐的治疗方法是"单孔钻孔技术""小开颅和基底膜切开术""开颅术"和"内窥镜法"。外科医生通过考虑上述所有因素来决定使用哪种方法。例如，如果患者年事已高且合并其他潜在疾病，则可能优先选择需要较短手术时间和较少麻醉并产生较低手术创伤的方法。另一个重要的问题是抗凝药的使用，在一些研究系列中，大约50%的患者使用了抗凝药。使用抗凝药的患者可能不适合进行大手术，应首选微创手术技术[14, 20]。"双钻孔技术"是一种传统的微创方法，对于评分低于5分的患者可能是首选。单孔术式也可能是一种潜在的选择。一项meta分析显示，单钻孔和双钻孔在复发率、并发症发生率、发病率和死亡率方面没有显著差异[32]。床旁颅骨钻孔术，也是一种创伤较小的手术方法，可以作为一种治疗替代方法。在另一项研究中，比较了局麻下床旁颅骨钻孔术与全麻下钻孔引流术的应用。在此比较中，血肿排出、复发率和住院时间没有明显差异，局部麻醉对帕金森病、阿尔茨海默病等既往存在的神经系统疾病的患者影响较小[3]。

我们已经研究了"复发"和"手术技术"的细微差别，对手术细节的评估也是必要的。治疗CSDH最常用的两种方法是钻孔引流和开颅术。外科医生的倾向是决定使用哪种方法的最重要因素。一项研究发现开颅手术的复发率为15.7%，而其他方法的复发率为7.5%。两组患者的高龄和低GCS评分均与预后不良相关。研究还发现阿司匹林的使用增加了开颅患者的30天死亡率，华法林的使用也增加了钻孔引流患者的30天死亡率[19]。将钻孔引流术与小开颅术进行比较的研究强调，两种技术在死亡率和复发率方面没有显著差异，而其他研究报道，小开颅术促进脑扩张可显著降低复发率[10, 13]。我们也倾向于第二种选择，即小开颅术既可以切开内膜，又可以避免大开颅手术的并发症。

内窥镜手术的平均手术时间为45 min，经验丰富的外科医生进行内窥镜手术时对患者造成的创伤很小。内窥镜手术也能有效预防复发，因为它们允许进行分隔造口术和血肿膜切开术[2, 9, 35]。内镜入路可以减少老年患者的复发，特别是那些超过85岁的患者，因为内窥镜可以对血肿分隔进行造口。因此，患者可以避免手术复发的风险[19]。

MMA栓塞可以作为手术引流前后的联合治疗，也可以在不能进行手术的情况下作为单独的治

表29.1 针对CSDH钻孔引流术后需要手术的复发的Oslo复发检测和分级系统ᵃ

– 基于CT密度	
等密度/高密度亚型和层状/分隔型	2
低密度/渐变亚型和小梁型	0
– 术前体积	
大于130 ml	1
小于130 ml	0
– 术后残留腔的体积	
大于200 ml	2
80～200 ml	1
小于80 ml	0
– 总分	0～5

ᵃ 这个表格取自Stanišic和Pripp[27]。

疗方法。虽然有研究发现该技术治疗慢性硬膜下血肿的复发率明显较低，但其并发症发生率无明显差异[26]。从神经外科的角度来看，伴有外科指征的慢性硬膜下血肿属于神经外科急症，应立刻行急诊手术减压。在这种情况下，特别是在复发风险高的慢性硬膜下血肿中，将 MMA 栓塞考虑作为一种额外的治疗是合适的。

目前常规方式是将引流管放置在硬膜下间隙，对血肿进行引流。硬脑膜下引流管要柔软，尖端要钝，我们建议将引流管向前推进伸入至距脑表面约 3～4 cm。如果用双孔进行钻孔引流，两孔均应留置硬膜下引流。尖锐的硬质引流管有移位的危险，将引流管伸入超过 4 cm 也可能造成穿透大脑皮质的风险。此外，有证据表明，随着引流管深度的增加，复发率可能显著增加[33]。在同一项研究中，硬膜下引流管的深度小于 4.3 cm 时血肿复发率最小[33]。在伸入引流管时避免皮质损伤的另一个要点是至少要有 12 mm 直径的钻孔，以确保适当的引流管伸入角度。在一项研究中，290 例患者行钻孔引流术，并使用硬膜下引流，其中 73 例（15.8%）患者出现引流管移位，5 例（6.9%）患者出现医源性出血，9 例（12.3%）患者出现神经系统症状[12]。在一些研究中，使用骨膜下引流术可以避免硬膜下引流管移位的风险。在复发率、感染率和医源性引流损伤方面，骨膜下引流优于硬膜下引流[25]。一项多中心的引流位置（额孔/顶孔）、持续时间和引流管定位（骨膜下/硬膜下）的研究也产生了值得注意的结果。本研究比较了这三个因素的复发率，得出引流位置、持续时间和引流管定位对慢性硬膜下血肿的复发没有影响[7]。

虽然慢性硬膜下血肿常见于老年，但在 40 岁以下也可以看到。需要强调的是，头部创伤是年轻脑室–腹膜分流或蛛网膜囊肿患者发生慢性硬膜下血肿的危险因素。这些患者大多表现为头痛和头晕。然而，在没有分流术或蛛网膜囊肿的年轻患者中，头部创伤并不是慢性硬膜下血肿发生的危险因素[18]。

手术伤口愈合后的皮肤凹陷也会引起患者显著的不满，但大多数神经外科医生至今仍未使用钻孔保护套。我们相信钻孔保护套将在未来被常规使用[30]。

钙化的 SDH 是非常罕见的 SDH 亚型，占所有慢性硬膜下血肿的 0.3%～2.7%。这个过程是缓慢的，可能多年无症状。手术是有症状病例的主要治疗方法。一项数据库综述显示 72.8% 钙化的硬膜下血肿需要手术治疗，建议开颅切除钙化肿块，同时仔细解剖内膜和外膜是很重要的[29]。

硬膜下–腹膜分流术可用于儿童硬膜下血肿的治疗，分流泵应选择低压阀门。硬膜下穿刺是另一种选择。对于三次穿刺后仍存在的血肿，应采用分流术治疗[28]。

29.11 结论

尽管目前已有多种手术方法被报道或在临床中使用，但最终还是将由医生来选择使用何种方法。患者的年龄、表现评分、基础疾病、使用的药物、其他风险因素和外科医生的经验均会影响手术决策。需要注意的问题是血肿清除和复发之间的关系。避免再次手术应是最重要的目标，尤其是对存在基础疾病的老年人群。我们认为，如果最终让患者接受了多次手术治疗，那么最初使用微创手术的决定是不合适的。医生应综合考虑所有因素，为患者做出正确的手术决定。在选择手术或保守治疗以及在选择最佳手术方法有困难的情况下，应与本科室的其他神经外科医生共同决定。

参考文献

1. Akpınar E, Cila A. Radiology in a head injury patient (in Turkish). In: Ozgen T, Ziyal I, editors. Emergency neurosurgery. Ankara; 2009. p. 64–6.
2. Ca Q, Guo Q, Zhang F, Sun D, Zhang W, Ji B, Chen Z, Mao S. Evacuation of chronic and subacute subdural hematoma via transcranial neuroendoscopic approach. Neuropsychiatr Dis Treat. 2019;15:385–90.
3. Certo F, Maione M, Altieri R, Garozzo M, Toccaceli G, Peschillo S, Barbagallo GMV. Pros and cons of a minimally invasive percutaneous subdural drainage system for evacuation of chronic subdural hematoma under local anesthesia. Clin Neurol Neurosurg. 2019;187:105559.
4. Feghali J, Yang W, Huang J. Updates in chronic subdural hematoma: epidemiology, etiology, pathogenesis, treatment and outcome. World Neurosurg. 2020;141:339–45.

5. Fiorella D, Arthur AS. Middle meningeal artery embolization for the management of chronic subdural hematoma. J Neurointerv Surg. 2019;11(9):912–5.
6. Gentry LR. Imaging of closed head Injury. Radiology. 1994;191(1):1–17.
7. Glancz LJ, Poon MTC, Coulter JC, Hutchinson PJ, Kolias AG, Brennan PM, British Neurosurgical Trainnee Research Collaborative (BNTRC). Does drain position and duration influence outcomes in patients undergoing burr-hole evacuation of chronic subdural hematoma? Lessons from a UK multicenter prospective cohort study. Neurosurgery. 2019;85(4):486–93.
8. Greenberg Mark S. In: Hakan OH, editor. Handbook of neurosurgery (Turkish translation). Ankara; 2013. p. 674–6.
9. Guan F, Peng WC, Huang H, Dai B, Zhu GT, Mao BB, Xiao ZY, Lin ZY, Hu ZQ. Efficacy analysis of soft neuroendoscopic techniques in the treatment of chronic subdural hematoma. Zhonghua Yi Xue Za Zhi. 2019;99(9):695–9.
10. Haron S, Bogduk N, Hansen M. A retrospective analysis of chronic subdural haematoma recurrence rates following burr hole trephination versus minicraniotomy. J Clin Neurosci. 2019;59:47–50.
11. Jang KM, Choi HH, Mun HY, Nam TK, Park YS, Kwon JT. Critical depressed brain volume influences the recurrence of chronic subdural hematoma after surgical evacuation. Sci Rep. 2020;10(1):1–8.
12. Kamenova M, Wanderer S, Lipps P, Marbacher S, Mariani L, Soleman J. When the drain hits the brain. World Neurosurg. 2020;138:e426–36.
13. Kocaman U, Yilmaz H. Description of a modified technique (mini craniotomy-basal membranotomy) for chronic subdural hematoma surgery and evaluation of the contribution of basal membranotomy performed as part of this technique to cerebral expansion. World Neurosurg. 2019;122:e1002–6.
14. Kotwica Z, Saracen A, Dziuba I. Chronic subdural hematoma (CSH) is still an important clinical problem. Analysis of 700 consecutive patients. Tranl Neurosci. 2019;10:260–3.
15. Kutty SA, Jony M. Chronic subdural hematoma: a comparison of recurrence rates following burr-hole craniostomy with and without Drains. Turk Neurosurg. 2014;24:494–7.
16. Lee KS. How to treat chronic subdural hematoma? Past and now. J Korean Neurosurg Soc. 2019;62(2):144–52.
17. Lee SJ, Hwang SC, Im SB. Twist-drill or burr hole craniostomy for draining chronic subdural hematomas: how to choose it for chronic subdural hematoma drainage. Korean J Neurotrauma. 2016;12(2):107–11.
18. Ou Y, Dong J, Wu L, Xu L, Wang L, Liu B, Li J, Liu W. The clinical characteristics, treatment, and outcomes of chronic subdural hematoma in young patients. World Neurosurg. 2019;125:e1241–6.
19. Raghavan A, Smith G, Onyewadume L, Peck MR, Herring E, Pace J, Rogers M, Momotaz H, Hoffer SA, Hu Y, Liu H, Tatsuoka C, Sajatovic M, Sioan AE. Morbidity and mortality after burr hole craniostomy versus craniotomy for chronic subdural hematoma evacuation: a single-center experience. World Neurosurg. 2020;134:e196–203.
20. Ridwan S, Bohrer AM, Grote A, Simon M. Surgical treatment of chronic subdural hematoma: predicting recurrence and cure. World Neurosurg. 2019;128:e1010–23.
21. Salcman M, Heros RC, Laws ER Jr, Volker K, Sonntag H. Subdural hematoma. Chapter 15: Kempe's Operative Neurosurgery. Springer-Verlag New York, Inc. 2004. p. 155–8.
22. Scerrati A, Visani J, Ricciardi L, Dones F, Rustemi O, Cavallo MA, Bonis PD. To drill or not to drill, that is the question: nonsurgical treatment of chronic subdural hematoma in the elderly. A systematic review. Neurosurg Focus. 2020;49(4):E7.
23. Shen J, Shao X, Gao Y, Li Q, Ge R, Wang Q, Zhou W, Jiang X. Risk factors for contralateral hematoma progression after unilateral evacuation of bilateral chronic subdural hematomas. World Neurosurg. 2019;126:e773–8.
24. Shen J, Yuan L, Ge R, Wang Q, Zhou W, Jiang XC, Shao X. Clinical and radiological factors predicting recurrence of chronic subdural hematoma: a retrospective cohort study. Injury. 2019;50(10):1634–40.
25. Soleman J, Lutz K, Schaedelin S, Kamenova M, Guzman R, Mariani L, Fanding J. Subperiosteal vs subdural drain after burr-hole drainage of chronic subdural hematoma: a randomized clinical trial (cSDH-Drain-Trial). Neurosurgery. 2019;85(5):E825–34.
26. Srivatsan A, Mohanty A, Nascimento FA, Hafeez MU, Srinivasan VM, Thomas A, Chen SR, Johnson JN, Kan P. Middle meningeal artery embolization for chronic subdural hematoma: meta-analysis and systematic review. World Neurosurg. 2019;122:613–9.
27. Stanišic M, Pripp AH. A reliable grading system for prediction of chronic subdural hema-

toma recurrence requiring reoperation after initial burr-hole surgery. Neurosurgery. 2017;81(5):752–60.
28. Tahta K. Traumatic intracranial hematomas (in Turkish). In: Aksoy K, editor. Basic neurosurgery. Ankara; 2005. p. 328–30.
29. Turgut M, Akhaddar A, Turgut AT. Calcified or ossified chronic subdural hematoma: a systematic reviewof 114 cases reported during last century with a demonstrative case report. World Neurosurg. 2020;134:240–63.
30. Velz J, Vasella F, Akeret K, Dias S, Jehli E, Bosinov O, Regli L, Germans MR, Stienen MN. Patterns of care: Burr-hole cover application for chronic subdural hematoma trepanation. Neurosurg Focus. 2019;47(5):E14.
31. Wakuta N, Abe H, Fukuda K, Nonaka M, Morishita T, Arima H, Inoue T. Feasibility and safety of endoscopic procedure in burr-hole surgery for chronic subdural hematoma in patients of very advanced age. World Neurosurg. 2020;134:e1037–46.
32. Wan Y, Xie D, Xue Z, Xie J, Song Z, Wang Y, Yang S. Single versus double burr hole craniostomy in surgical treatment of chronic subdural hematoma: a meta-analysis. World Neurosurg. 2019;131:e149–54.
33. Weng W, Li H, Zhao X, Yang C, Wang S, Hui J, Mao Q, Gao G, Feng J. The depth of catheter in chronic subdural haematoma: does it matter? Brain Inj. 2019;33(6):717–22.
34. Yadav YR, Parihar V, Namdev H, Bejaj J. Chronic subdural hematoma. Asian J Neurosurg. 2020;11(4):330–42.
35. Yadav YR, Ratre S, Parihar V, Bajaj J, Sinha M, Kumar A. Endoscopic management of chronic subdural hematoma. J Neurol A Cent Eur Neurosurg. 2020;81(4):330–41.

第30章 神经内镜在慢性硬膜下血肿手术治疗中的作用

Ali Hazama，Said Shukri，Fakhri Awawdeh 和 Walter A. Hall

译者：郭旭飞

30.1 慢性硬膜下血肿的发病率

慢性硬膜下血肿（chronic subdural hematoma，CSDH）的年发病率约为（1～5.3）/10万人[10]。高龄、男性和使用抗凝药是增加CSDH发生率的危险因素[17]。芬兰的一项研究记录了1990—2015年间CSDH的发病率，发现CSDH的发病率从1990年的8.2/10万人显著增加到2015年的17.6/10万人[9]。这一变化是由于抗凝药使用的增加以及世界人口老龄化的趋势[9]。在该研究中，CSDH患者的中位年龄在73～79岁，80岁以上的人群中则更为普遍。

30.2 慢性硬膜下血肿的危险因素

CSDH最常见的危险因素是老年、男性和头部损伤[15]。其他已知的硬膜下血肿的危险因素包括癫痫、过量饮酒、凝血功能障碍、抗凝药、蛛网膜囊肿、糖尿病、血小板减少症和心血管疾病等[11]。然而，慢性肾脏疾病和心脏病等对发生CSDH具有保护作用，这可能是因为它们限制了患者的活动能力，降低了患者遭受头部损伤的可能性[15]。

30.3 内镜在慢性硬膜下血肿治疗中的作用

内镜技术是指通过头皮小切口将一个细长的器械插入硬膜下腔，其尖端带有一个摄像装置。该种技术允许外科医生对血肿内部及其组织结构的细节进行直接可视化评估，同时使手术医生能够在对正常结构破坏最小的情况下进行手术，切除纤维组织和引流血肿液。内镜手术对CSDH的治疗是有益的。通常，CSDH的治疗包括开颅、小骨瓣开颅、钻孔开颅术、麻花钻开颅伴硬膜下引流。最近，神经内镜治疗CSDH也被证明其有效性[4]，已被成功用于清除硬膜下血肿[15]。在Yadav等的研究中，CSDH在神经内镜技术下于35～80 min内清除[15]，而开颅手术则可能至少需要3～5 h[16]。

关于神经内镜技术的相关研究认为血管生成是导致CSDH复发的主要原因之一[2]。传统的手术操作通常很难完全清除这些新生血管，而通过神经内镜则可以直接观察和切除这些异常血管，进一步降低CSDH复发的风险。评估内镜作为慢性硬膜下血肿治疗方法的研究尚未发现与内镜技术相关的显著不良影响[2, 15]。在Yadav的研究中，68例接受内镜下CSDH引流术的患者没有出现硬膜下复发、急性出血、脑损伤或颅内感染的报道[15]。尽管如此，内镜手术的风险仍包括神经外科手术相关的常见风险，如感染和再出血等。

Guan等证实了内镜下CSDH引流术的安全性和有效性，该研究证实内镜手术能显著降低患者血肿复发率和并发症发生率，因此应该被认为是一种更安全的CSDH治疗方法[1]。他们的研究得出结论：内镜手术治疗CSDH是一种高效、安全的方法。众所周知，小骨瓣开颅和钻孔开颅对整个CSDH腔的可视性非常有限，这种局限的视野限制了对整个硬膜下腔的评估，并增加了硬膜下血肿不完全排出的风险。此外，内镜辅助手术的平均手术时间为37.4 min，明显短于非内镜手术的43.1 min[5]。除了能更完整地清除硬膜下血肿外，内镜可以提供更佳手术区视野，为术中保护大脑表面和桥静脉创造了有利的条件[5]。

30.4　内镜技术

CSDH 的开颅手术通常在全身麻醉下进行。然而，使用小切口和单一钻孔的内镜手术可以在局部麻醉下对部分患者进行血肿清除[3]。随着患者年龄的增长和合并症的增加，侵入性治疗策略的风险更高[8]。这部分患者可能会受益于侵入性较小的内镜技术，并避免了与气管插管和全身麻醉相关的风险。内镜操作如下：头皮切开一个 4 cm 的切口，在颅骨上钻孔，然后打开硬脑膜，此时通常会有血肿液流出。然后将一个柔性内镜插入硬膜下腔并排出血肿，进一步的血肿清除和血肿膜去除可以在内镜的直视下进行。通过内镜检查硬膜下腔，识别任何可能的出血点并在直视下电凝。在止血完全并彻底清除 CSDH 后，可以在硬膜下间隙放置引流管，然后关闭切口[13]。术后进行 CT 检查并确认大脑扩张是否充分[3]。

30.5　内镜检查费用

进行内镜手术的费用在各国之间差别很大。在美国，全国平均费用约为 2750 美元[7]，全国范围内在 1250 美元到 4800 美元之间[2]。在世界其他地区，如印度，内镜手术相对便宜。在印度，这种手术的费用可能在 15 美元到 100 美元之间，具体取决于患者接受治疗的机构。在美国各种因素会影响内镜手术的费用，包括医疗设施、保险类型以及不同的州等。就医疗设施而言，与门诊中心相比，住院条件下执行手术的成本更高。与清除 CSDH 的其他治疗方案相比，内镜手术的成本明显较低。在美国，开颅手术的费用在 20 936 美元到 50 090 美元之间[14]。钻孔手术的成本虽然低于开颅手术，但仍是内镜手术的 2 倍，费用约为 7588 美元[6]。与全身麻醉相比，镇静和局麻下清除 CSDH 不仅更安全，而且更具成本效益。

30.6　手术干预的生存结局

根据 Lee 等完成的一项研究，接受 CSDH 手术干预的患者存活率在统计学上具有显著意义。随访时，92.9% 和 81.4% 的手术组患者分别存活至少 30 天和 6 个月。在相同的时间内，保守组的存活率分别为 58.1% 和 41.9%[12]。此外，与钻孔开颅手术相比，内镜辅助手术治疗 CSDH 的复发率和并发症发生率明显降低，但两组死亡率无显著差异[1]。当比较内镜和开颅手术作为脑出血的治疗选择时，Sun 等报道在他们的研究中，内镜组表现出更少的平均失血量、输血量和更短的手术时间。此外，内镜组的平均血肿清除率和术后日常生活活动评分均有所增加[18]。与标准钻孔开颅术相比，内镜辅助钻孔开颅术患者的总住院时间也更短[18]。根据血肿造成的脑损伤的大小，患者可以在内镜手术干预后的 2 周到几个月的时间内完全恢复[15]。

30.7　结论

神经内镜手术是治疗 CSDH 的有效手段。该技术提供了更好的手术视野，帮助手术医生更好地评估硬膜下腔。内镜手术的血肿清除率更高，新生血管的切除更完整，从而降低了 CSDH 复发的可能性。在特定情况下，由于不需要全身麻醉和气管插管，因此避免这些治疗可能的并发症。因此，神经内镜技术应该作为 CSDH 可用的手术治疗方案之一。

参考文献

1. Guan F, Peng W, Huang H, Dai B, Zhu G, Xiao Z, Hu Z. Efficacy analysis of flexible neuroendoscopy combined with dry-field techniques in the treatment of chronic subdural hematoma. Chin Med J. 2019;132(11):1359–62.
2. Guo S, Gao W, Cheng W, Liang C, Wu A. Endoscope-assisted surgery vs. burr-hole craniostomy for the treatment of chronic subdural hematoma: a systematic review and meta-analysis. Front Neurol. 2020;11(3):1–6.
3. Kawasaki T, Kurosaki Y, Fukuda H, et al. Flexible endoscopically assisted evacuation of acute and subacute subdural hematoma through a small craniotomy: preliminary results. Acta Neurochir. 2018;160:241–8.

4. Kim D-J, et al. Continuous monitoring of the Monro-Kellie doctrine: is it possible? J Neurotrauma. 2012;29(7):1354–63.
5. Kon H, et al. Endoscopic surgery for traumatic acute subdural hematoma. Case Rep Neurol. 2014;5(3):208–13.
6. Lee L, et al. Outcomes of chronic subdural hematoma drainage in nonagenarians and centenarians: a multicenter study. J Neurosurg. 2016;124(2):546–51.
7. Leuthardt EC, Voigt J, Kim AH, Sylvester P. A single-center cost analysis of treating primary and metastatic brain cancers with either brain laser interstitial thermal therapy (LITT) or craniotomy. Pharmacoecon Open. 2017;1(1):53–63.
8. Maryua J. Endoscopic hematoma evacuation following emergent Burr hole surgery for acute subdural hematoma in critical conditions: technical note. Interdiscip Neurosurg. 2018;12:48–51.
9. Rauhala M, Luoto TM, Huhtala H, Iverson GL, Niskakangas T, Ohman J, Helen P. The incidence of chronic subdural hematomas from 1990 to 2015 in a defined Finnish population. J Neurosurg. 2019;22(3):1–11.
10. Sahyouni R, Goshtasbi K, Mahmoodi A, Tran D, Chen J. Chronic subdural hematoma: a historical and clinical perspective. World Neurosurg. 2017;108:948–53.
11. Sim Y, Min K, Lee M, Kim Y, Kim D. Recent changes in risk factors of chronic subdural hematoma. J Korean Neurosurg Soc. 2012;52(3):234–9.
12. Sun G, et al. Comparison of keyhole endoscopy and craniotomy for the treatment of patients with hypertensive cerebral hemorrhage. Medicine. 2019;98(2):e14123.
13. Vanvuren C. What is the cost of an endoscopy? New Choice Health; 2020. https://www.newchoicehealth.com/endoscopy/cost#:~:text=The%20average%20cost%20of%20an,or%20an%20outpatient%20surgery%20center. Accessed 15 Dec 2020.
14. Wick JY. The true cost of chronic subdural hematoma. HCPLive; 2015. www.hcplive.com/view/the-true-cost-of-chronic-subdural-hematoma. Accessed 20 Dec 2020.
15. Yadav YR, Ratre S, Parihar V, Bajaj J, Sinha M, Kumar A. Endoscopic management of chronic subdural hematoma. J Neurol Surg. 2020;81(4):330–41.
16. Yan K, Gao H, Wang Q, Xu X, Wu W, Zhou X. Endoscopic surgery to chronic subdural hematoma with neovessel septation: technical notes and literature review. Neurol Res. 2016;38(5):467–76.
17. Yang W, Huang J. Chronic subdural hematoma: epidemiology and natural history. Neurosurg Clin N Am. 2017;28(2):205–10.
18. Zhang J, et al. The use of endoscopic-assisted burr-hole craniostomy for septated chronic subdural haematoma: a retrospective cohort comparison study. Brain Res. 2018;1678:245–53.

第31章 脑膜中动脉栓塞治疗慢性硬膜下血肿

Stephanie Zyck 和 Harish Babu

译者：马永杰

31.1 血管内治疗的理论和生理学基础

慢性硬膜下血肿（chronic subdural hematoma，CSDH）的经典治疗方式为开颅引流或钻孔引流灌洗。然而，经典方式治疗后 CSDH 的复发率出奇的高。文献报道的复发率差异很大，平均范围在 10%～30%[3]。高龄、合并多种疾病以及抗血栓药物的使用在 CSDH 患者中常见，这使得血肿复发时治疗的决策进一步复杂化。

理解 CSDH 复发背后的病理生理机制对于采取相应治疗方式有着重要的意义。在最初的某些因素引起硬膜下腔出血后（例如头部的微创伤引起桥静脉破裂），一系列促炎症级联反应被触发。这一事件导致炎症细胞和成纤维细胞从硬膜上迁移，导致硬膜下间隙内的液体被一层膜包裹。这层膜引起随后的血管再生和新生血管化膜的形成[13]。研究已经表明这些外层的新生血管化膜包含着脆弱的窦状通道和缺乏基底膜或内皮细胞连接的毛细血管。这些新的血管没有平滑肌细胞或周细胞，导致血浆和红细胞持续渗漏至硬膜下腔[13-14, 20]。这导致了进一步炎症反应的发生，引起恶性循环。

脑膜中动脉（middle meningeal artery，MMA），是起源于颈外动脉的颅内动脉，通过其额叶和顶叶的分支向硬脑膜供血。组织学和影像学已经提供证据表明，MMA 为 CSDH 的外层膜供血[17-18]。还有一项研究表明，CSDH 同侧的 MMA 直径明显大于对侧[16]。MMA 栓塞已经被作为一种治疗 CSDH 的方法，其原理为阻断 MMA 对 CSDH 的血供和阻止未成熟血管的微出血。

31.2 目前的证据

Komiyama 于 1994 年第一次报道了使用 MMA 栓塞治疗复发 CSDH[11]。从那时起，多个单中心和多中心研究报道了他们将 MMA 栓塞作为主要或补救措施治疗大脑凸面 CSDH 的经验。常见的应用指征包括与血肿相关的临床症状，中线移位大于 5 mm 或既往手术干预后复发。对于那些不适合手术治疗的患者，如高龄、潜在的凝血功能障碍或患有其他严重疾病的患者，MMA 栓塞是一种更优的治疗方式。MMA 栓塞治疗既可以单独进行，也可以作为手术血肿清除、钻孔引流、床旁放置硬膜下引流系统的辅助手段[7, 9]。MMA 栓塞的作用是防止血肿持续出血，血肿会随着时间的推移被逐渐吸收，因此 MMA 栓塞的治疗效果不是即刻产生的。当出现血肿肿块占位效应引起肢体对侧无力等临床症状时，我们更倾向于 MMA 栓塞辅助开颅或床边放置硬膜下引流系统治疗来缓解占位引起的症状。

存在潜在肿瘤、严重肾衰竭和非大脑凸面 SDH（MMA 血管区域不向血肿膜供血）的患者，通常不考虑进行血管内治疗。术前头颈部 CTA 对于规划介入方式和技术考虑有帮助，也有助于排除栓塞的解剖学禁忌证。其中一个重要的例子就是眼动脉起源于 MMA，栓塞治疗可能会引起术后的视力下降。尽管血管畸形如硬脑膜动静脉瘘涉及 MMA 供血的可能会与 SDH 有关联，并且在某些情况下适合进行栓塞治疗，但这些情况通常应被视为一种独立的疾病，而不是归入 CSDH。

31.3 血管内治疗技术

MMA 栓塞是患者入院以后在神经介入治疗组进行的。MMA 栓塞可以在适度镇静或全麻下进行，这取决于患者对镇静状态下手术的耐受能力和整体健康状态。经桡或经股动脉置入 5 F 或 6 F 鞘是常规安全的方式，然后使用一根引导导管进入颈外动脉的近端，进行选择性造影以确定MMA确实来源于颌内动脉，然后在透视路图引导下将微导管引入MMA，后进行超选择血管造影来识别危险吻合，大约10%的病例中可以观察到岩支或泪腺支[9]。这些吻合血管在栓塞时必须小心保护以防止发生术后神经功能缺损。

栓塞治疗既可以在MMA主干处进行，也可以选择性地在近端额叶或枕叶分支处进行。血肿的位置，MMA分支的关系以及重要侧支从主干的起源点，可能决定选择用于栓塞的血管。当发现眼支和岩支时，微导管应在这些侧支的远端进行靶向栓塞，以免引起失明或面神经瘫。栓塞材料可以包括液体栓塞剂如Onyx或NBCA、弹簧圈或颗粒（例如PVA或栓塞微颗粒球）。在临床上，发现这些危险血管时更倾向于使用弹簧圈而不是栓塞剂。栓塞在透视路图下持续进行直至观察到目标血管血流停滞。血肿患者在进行造影时常可见血管"脸红"样的染色（"vascular blush"），在治疗结束后会消失（图31.1）。

31.4 临床和放射学结果

已经有多项Meta分析评估MMA栓塞治疗CSDH的安全性和有效性。Srivatsan及其同事的一项meta分析汇集三项双臂研究从血肿复发率、并发症和mRS评分（modifed Rankin Scale score）来比较MMA栓塞组（伴或不伴传统手术）和传统手术治疗组[15]。其中有两项研究将钻孔引流作为MMA栓塞队列治疗方案的一部分，而第三项研究仅对血管内介入治疗队列中有症状的患者使用钻孔引流联合MMA栓塞治疗[1, 10, 12]。在该Meta分析中，相比传统手术治疗组，栓塞组的血肿复发率更低（2.1%和27.7%）。在汇集了三项双臂研究后，发现并发症和mRS评分无显著的统计学差异[15]。另一项由Jumah及其同事的Meta分析纳入11项研究，包括单臂研究和小数量的病例系列汇报；栓塞组在血肿复发率、需要手术干预的比例以及并发症发生率方面均比传统治疗组低[8]。这一数据表明，无论伴或不伴钻孔引流，MMA栓塞相比单独钻孔引流均可以提高对CSDH的疗效，且没有显著提高并发症发生率。

第三项Meta分析由Haldrup及其同事进行，其纳入18项研究共计191例接受MMA栓塞作为首选或复发补救治疗的患者。其中119例CSDH患者接受MMA栓塞作为最初治疗方式，72例复发硬膜下血肿患者接受MMA栓塞治疗。在上述两组中，复发率无显著统计学差异，说明MMA栓塞对于治疗CSDH可以是一种首要或补救的治疗措施[6]。在纳入Meta分析的研究中，没有报道与血管内介入治疗直接相关的并发症。

然而，已知的介入治疗风险包括血管通路相关的并发症、造影剂引起的肾损伤以及卒中。还需要考虑栓塞剂反流入眼支和岩支引起的失明以及面神经瘫痪的风险，必须极力避免并发症的出现。在154例因CSDH接受MMA栓塞治疗的患者中，有1例出现术中症状性MMA破裂，1例出现术后癫痫，1例出现面瘫[9]。其他文献中报道的并发症与介入治疗无关或与开放手术治疗相关，如伤口相关或术后血肿相关并发症。在同一系列研究中，90.3%的患者血肿厚度明显减小，70.8%的患者在随访时达到了血肿厚度减少50%或减少的更多[10]。在不同的随访时间下，mRS评分以及美国国立卫生研

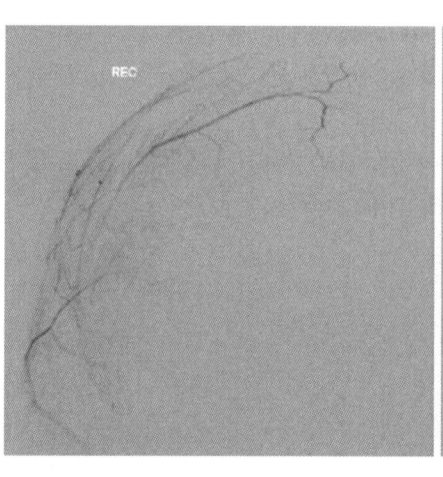 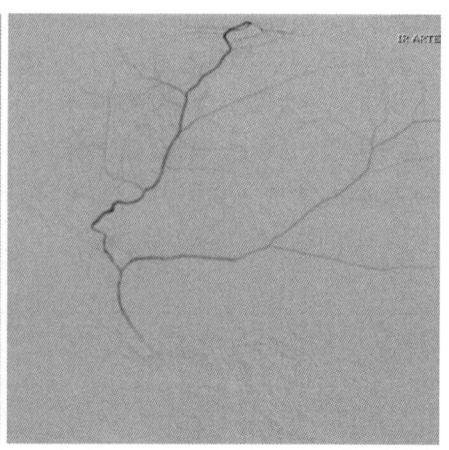

图31.1 右侧脑膜中动脉超选造影的前后位（左侧）和侧位（右侧）观，显示MMA血管轻轻"泛红"，与潜在的慢性硬膜下血肿相关（CSDH）

究院卒中量表（National Institutes of Health Stroke Scale，NIHSS）的改善分别为 44% 和 30%[9]。当采取同样的方法衡量患者临床结果时，分别有 79% 和 46% 的病例无显著性统计学差异[9]。

总之，目前的证据表明，无论使用或不使用手术引流，MMA 治疗 CSDH 作为首发或复发后补救的治疗方式是安全和有效的。

31.5 典型病例

一名 80 岁男性，几周前出现头晕和频繁的跌倒，既往有高血压、糖尿病及近期左侧卒中病史，并持续服用阿司匹林和氯吡格雷。患者此前卒中引起的右侧肢体无力已经缓解，但自从最近摔倒后无力症状逐渐加重。头颅 CT 显示左侧凸面混合密度的硬膜下血肿，血肿成分主要为亚急性和慢性。血肿的最大直径为 24 mm，中线移位 7 mm。因为患者有抗血小板药物服用史，因此被转诊进行神经外科评估。在神经系统评估中，较前相比，右侧旋前肌偏移及腿部移动缓慢。由于高龄和患有其他疾病，决定放置左侧硬膜下引流系统（subdural evacuating port system）进行治疗。他接受了这个疗法并且耐受性很好。该患者的术后 CT 提示有残存的血液，但血肿大小和中线移位程度都有显著的减小。他的旋前肌偏移及腿部移动缓慢也得到改善，只残留右上肢无力。

该患者出院后到一家康复中心 2 周后，出现多次跌倒和右侧肢体无力加重。他的头部 CT 扫描发现左侧硬膜下血肿再次聚积。由于血肿的占位效应，患者同意接受重复的硬膜下引流系统治疗。每次进行硬膜下引流治疗术前术后的 CT 见图 31.2。

由于 SDH 容易复发，MMA 栓塞也被采取用于治疗这类复发患者。该患者既往 CTA 提示无介入治疗禁忌证，如眼动脉起源于 MMA。因此该患者进行了血管内介入治疗，行左侧颈外动脉造影，通过微导管进入脑膜中动脉（图 31.3）。由

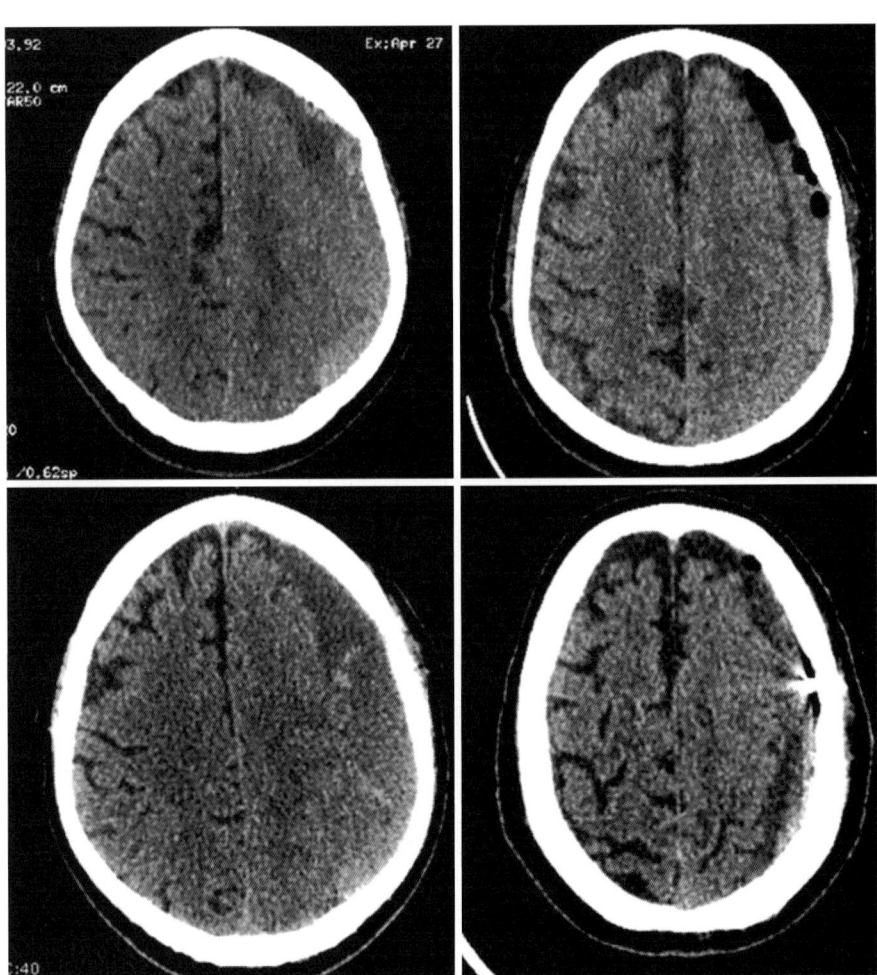

图 31.2 最初头颅 CT 显示混合亚急性和慢性左侧凸面慢性硬膜下血肿（左上）。硬膜下钻孔引流后血肿体积减小（右上）。2 周后出现血肿复发（左下），经再次钻孔引流后血肿体积再次缩小（右下）

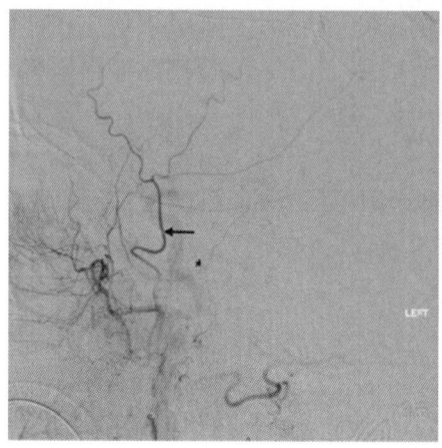
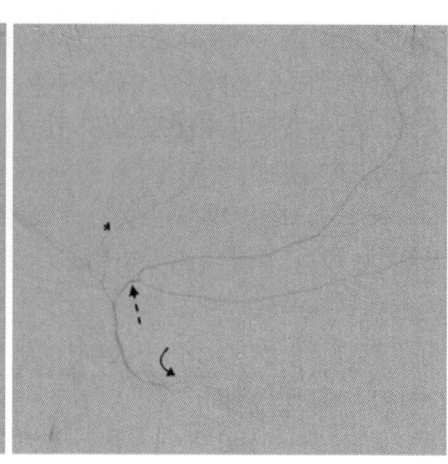

图 31.3 左侧颈外动脉造影（左）显示颈外动脉显影正常，可见 MMA（星号）和颞浅动脉（箭头）。右图显示了 MMA 的超选造影，可见额支（星号）和顶支（虚线箭头）。隐约可见岩支（弯曲的箭头）

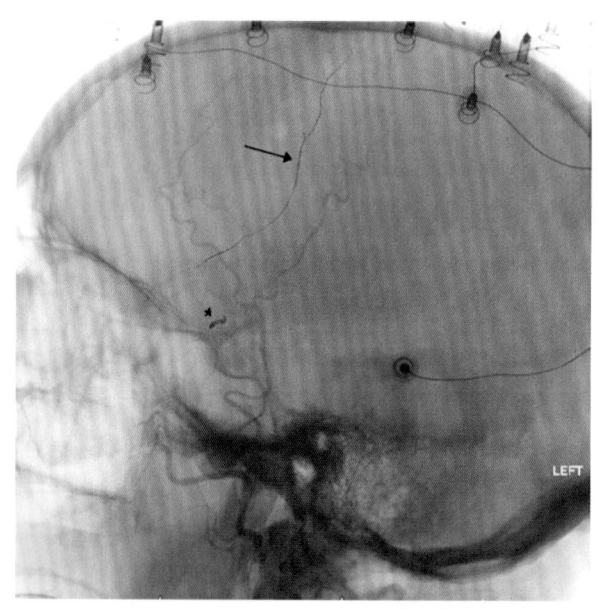

于造影显示岩支靠近顶支，故选择弹簧圈栓塞顶支来防止液体栓塞剂意外反流入岩支。之后，又通过 Onyx 精确栓塞额支。术后没有发生任何并发症（图 31.4）。

患者术后表现良好，术后 1 个月随访时，血肿体积缩小。术后 2 个月随访 CT 显示 SDH 几乎消失（图 31.5）。

31.6　未来方向

目前有多项随机对照研究正在进行，以比较 MMA 栓塞和手术引流之间的临床结果[2, 4-5, 19]。未来的研究还应针对首发和复发 SDH 单独 MMA 栓塞和不同手术方法治疗的对比，以及哪些栓塞剂能够达到最好的临床结果。

图 31.4　最终颈外血管造影显示 MMA 完全栓塞，无造影剂显影。额支可见 Onyx 铸型（箭头）。顶支采用弹簧圈栓塞（星号）。可见紧邻栓塞后的 MMA 的颞浅动脉造影剂显影

图 31.5　MMA 栓塞后 1 个月（左）和 2 个月（右）的 CT 显示，随着时间推移，血肿逐渐消退

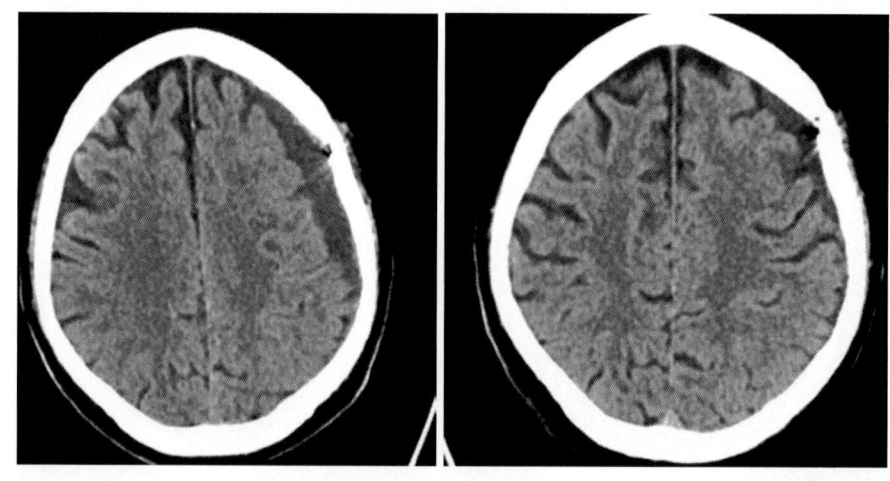

参考文献

1. Ban SP, et al. Middle meningeal artery embolization for chronic subdural hematoma. Radiology. 2018;286(3):992–9.
2. Dartmouth Middle Meningeal Embolization Trial (DaMMET). ClinicalTrials.gov Identifier: NCT04270955.
3. Ducruet AF, et al. The surgical management of chronic subdural hematoma. Neurosurg Rev. 2012;35(2):155–69.
4. Embolization of the Middle Meningeal Artery for the Prevention of Chronic Subdural Hematoma Recurrence in High Risk Patients (EMPROTECT). ClinicalTrials.gov Identifier: NCT04372147.
5. Embolization of the Middle Meningeal Artery With ONYX™ Liquid Embolic System for Subacute and Chronic Subdural Hematoma. ClinicalTrials.gov Identifier: NCT04402632.
6. Haldrup M, et al. Embolization of the middle meningeal artery in patients with chronic subdural hematoma-a systematic review and meta-analysis. Acta Neurochir (Wien). 2020;162(4):777–84.
7. Joyce E, et al. Middle meningeal artery embolization treatment of nonacute subdural hematomas in the elderly: a multiinstitutional experience of 151 cases. Neurosurg Focus. 2020;49(4):E5.
8. Jumah F, et al. Efficacy and safety of middle meningeal artery embolization in the management of refractory or chronic subdural hematomas: a systematic review and meta-analysis. Acta Neurochir (Wien). 2020;162(3):499–507.
9. Kan P, et al. Middle meningeal artery embolization for chronic subdural hematoma: a multicenter experience of 154 consecutive embolizations. Neurosurgery. 2021;88(2):268–77.
10. Kim E. Embolization therapy for refractory hemorrhage in patients with chronic subdural hematomas. World Neurosurg. 2017;101:520–7.
11. Komiyama M, et al. Chronic subdural hematoma associated with middle meningeal arteriovenous fistula treated by a combination of embolization and burr hole drainage. Surg Neurol. 1994;42(4):316–9.
12. Matsumoto H, et al. Which surgical procedure is effective for refractory chronic subdural hematoma? Analysis of our surgical procedures and literature review. J Clin Neurosci. 2018;49:40–7.
13. Moshayedi P, Liebeskind DS. Middle meningeal artery embolization in chronic subdural hematoma: implications of pathophysiology in trial design. Front Neurol. 2020;11:923.
14. Sato S, Suzuki J. Ultrastructural observations of the capsule of chronic subdural hematoma in various clinical stages. J Neurosurg. 1975;43(5):569–78.
15. Srivatsan A, et al. Middle meningeal artery embolization for chronic subdural hematoma: meta-analysis and systematic review. World Neurosurg. 2019;122:613–9.
16. Takizawa K, et al. Enlargement of the middle meningeal artery on MR angiography in chronic subdural hematoma. J Neurosurg. 2016;124(6):1679–83.
17. Tanaka T, et al. [Superselective angiographic findings of ipsilateral middle meningeal artery of chronic subdural hematoma in adults]. No Shinkei Geka. 1998;26(4):339–47.
18. Tanaka T, Kaimori M. [Histological study of vascular structure between the dura mater and the outer membrane in chronic subdural hematoma in an adult]. No Shinkei Geka. 1999;27(5):431–6.
19. The SQUID Trial for the Embolization of the Middle Meningeal Artery for Treatment of Chronic Subdural Hematoma (STEM). ClinicalTrials.gov Identifier: NCT04410146.
20. Weigel R, Hohenstein A, Schilling L. Vascular endothelial growth factor concentration in chronic subdural hematoma fluid is related to computed tomography appearance and exudation rate. J Neurotrauma. 2014;31(7):670–3.

第 32 章 慢性硬膜下血肿围手术期管理

Mohammed Benzagmout，Tokpo Armel Junior 和 Said Boujraf

译者：马永杰

32.1 引言

慢性硬膜下血肿（chronic subdural hematoma，CSDH）是指在硬脑膜下腔病理性的血液积聚，且病情发生发展过程隐匿[15]。CSDH 的发病率随着年龄的增长而增加，主要见于老年人。CSDH 可以通过药物治疗，然而在某些情况下手术引流治疗是必要的。手术适用于有症状的患者，特别是最初的保守治疗失败后或在 CT 上显示血肿最大厚度大于 10 mm 时[65]。

CSDH 很常见，其相关手术方法存在多种。出现多种不同的治疗方法是因为缺乏一级证据制定治疗指南来规范这一危重疾病的围手术期管理[65]。

在本章中，我们将主要说明在手术治疗 CSDH 之前，术中和术后使用的医疗策略，并讨论它们的局限性和有效性。

32.2 术前医疗管理

32.2.1 凝血功能障碍的纠正

凝血功能障碍是导致 CSDH 发展和复发的主要危险因素之一。因此，为避免任何可能立即危及生命的情况发生，在手术清除血肿前控制凝血功能障碍是至关重要的。CSDH 主要见于有多种并发症的老年人，因此老年 CSDH 多存在医源性凝血功能障碍。

32.2.1.1 医源性的凝血功能障碍

抗凝治疗的患者管理需要多学科的介入，包括神经外科医生、心脏相关学科医生、血液科医生和麻醉医师。主要目标是在一定时间内停止抗凝治疗，保证手术安全进行且不会发生血栓事件。实际上，所使用的医疗策略取决于患者的相应情况和受益-风险比。

关于维生素拮抗剂（VKA）的使用，在择期手术的情况下，要口服维生素 K 来纠正国际标准化比值（INR）。新鲜冰冻血浆（FFP）、凝血酶原复合物（PCC）或重组活化因子Ⅶ（rfⅦa）可在危急情况下使用。此外，FFP 可能不能用于肾功能不全的患者，PCC 可成为另外一种选择[65]。

2017 年，法国团队修改了一项有关直接口服抗凝药物的指南，他们主要研究术前止血问题。考虑到 CSDH 手术清除是涉及颅内的手术，他们提议在术前停止服用沙班类药物至少 3 天。达比加群的使用取决于肌酐清除率；因此，如果肌酐清除率在 30～50 ml/min，至少需要停止 5 天；如果清除率大于 50 ml/min，则停止 4 天即可。在紧急情况下，使用 PPC 或 FFP 仍然有效[1,73]。此外，Andexanet alfa 是一种特异性拮抗沙班类药物的拮抗剂，建议可在紧急情况下谨慎使用[14]并在使用前监测凝血功能[73]。

此外，另外一种策略也可以采用：使用肝素如低分子量肝素（LWMH）或普通肝素（UFH）。这一策略虽然存在争议但在临床中普及率较高。已经有人指出，它可以降低非瓣膜性房颤或机械瓣膜置换患者在围手术期发生血栓栓塞事件的风险。

欧洲心脏病学会（ESC）和美国心脏病学会（ACC）分别在 2016 年和 2017 年提出了一些值得注意的指导方针[72]。

关于机械瓣膜假体，ESC 建议在 INR 降到治疗范围后使用 UFH。术前 4～6 h 停止使用 UFH。另外，ACC 针对非瓣膜房颤患者提出了详细的抗凝管理准则。采用 CHA_2DS_2-VASc 评分来评估血栓事件风险，采用 HAS-BLED 评分评估出血风险[19,81]。表 32.1 和表 32.2 展示了 2 项详细评分。这两项是迄今为止推荐的最可靠和最实用的评分系统。ACC 的建议汇总于图 32.1。

32.2.1.2 病理性凝血功能障碍

文献中已经报道了 CSDH 合并先天性出血疾

表 32.1 CHA$_2$DS$_2$-VASc 评分。低风险（总分＝0）；中度风险（总分＝1）；高风险（总分＞1）[19]

CHA$_2$DS$_2$-VASc 首字母缩略词	得分
C	充血性心力衰竭/左心室功能障碍（射血分数小于35%）	1
H	高血压	1
A$_2$	年龄≥75岁	2
D	糖尿病	1
S$_2$	卒中/短暂性脑缺血发作（TIA）/体循环动脉血栓栓塞	2
V	血管相关疾病	1
A	年龄为65～74岁	1
Sc	性别（女性）	1

表 32.2 HAS-BLED 评分 [HAS-BLED：Hypertension 高血压，Abnormal Renal/Liver Function 肾/肝功能异常，Stroke 卒中，Bleeding History or Predisposition 出血史或出血倾向，Labile INR INR不稳定，Elderly 老人，Drugs/Alcohol Concomitantly 药物/酒精同时摄入]。低风险（最高评分＝0）；中等风险（最高评分＝1～2）；高风险（最高评分≥3）[81]。（缩写：AST，谷草转氨酶；ALT，谷丙转氨酶；Cr，肌酐；INR，国际标准化比值；NSAIDs，非甾体抗炎药）

HAS-BLED 首字母缩略词	得分
高血压	1
肾脏病（透析，移植，Cr＞2.26 mg/dl 或 200 μmol/L）	1
肝脏病（肝硬化或胆红素＞2×正常值，AST/ALT＞3×正常值）	1
卒中病史	1
出血病史（既往有大出血或有出血倾向）	1
INR 值不稳定（不稳定/高 INR）	1
年龄＞65岁	1
药物使用相关易出血倾向 阿司匹林、氯吡格雷、NSAIDs	1
酒精滥用	1
满分	9分

病的案例。通常来说，这些情况需要协调神经外科医生、麻醉医生和血液科医生，通过特殊和（或）一般的措施来解决主要的问题。

在2017年，有一项研究报道了16名患有自发性CSDH的年轻男性（27～59岁）。凝血因子完全筛选结果显示，1例患者表现为血管性血友病，而另外6名患者表现为凝血因子Ⅶ的改变。CSDH复发与4例患者具有未知凝血因子Ⅶ缺陷相关[12]。此前，圣卡罗医院的神经外科团队（波坦察，意大利）报道了3例年轻"O"型血血管性血友病患者患有CSDH[39-40]。因此，他们建议，在对不明原因患CSDH的年轻人进行手术前，先对凝血因子进行系统的检查。

在2019年，有研究报道一名患者与凝血因子Ⅴ严重缺乏相关。该病例通过FFP得到了很好的治疗[43]。在另一个病例中，CSDH的发生与凝血因子ⅩⅢ低活性相关[66]。

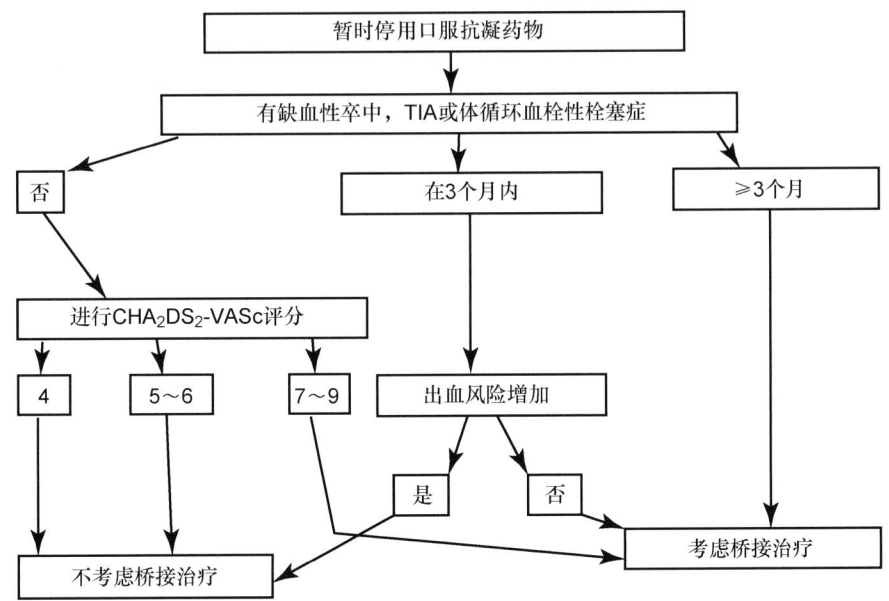

图 32.1 根据美国心脏病学会，非瓣膜性房颤患者手术前的衔接治疗[6]

32.2.2 血栓性疾病的纠正

32.2.2.1 医源性血栓性疾病

众所周知，围手术期抗血小板药物的使用与出血风险增加相关，虽然这种说法存在争议[14]。另外，停止抗血小板治疗会导致患者面临心肌梗死、支架内血栓形成甚至引起死亡的风险增加。因此，围手术期抗血小板治疗应该由多学科商议决定。治疗时要同时考虑出血和出现血栓的风险，特别是当抗血小板药物已经用于心血管事件的一级或二级预防时。目前，多种不同治疗策略已经被提出。此外，其他因素也应考虑在内，如患者是否正在服用单一或双重抗血栓药物，患者是否迫切需要手术或可以推迟 CSDH 手术。

事实上，进行 CSDH 血肿清除前，作为一级或二级预防的阿司匹林停用 7～10 天被认为是安全的[52, 64]。术前通常建议改用氯吡格雷[52]。

相比之下，双重抗血小板治疗（DAPT）的管理更加复杂。事实上，阿司匹林和腺苷二磷酸受体拮抗剂（氯吡格雷、普拉格雷、替格瑞洛等）的组合通常应用于高凝状态[52]。支架置入术后，在支架完全内皮化之前过早中断 DAPT 可能会造成严重的后果。事实上，血栓形成的风险在术后第一个月最高，在 2～6 个月、6～12 个月和 1 年以上时逐渐减低[30, 64]。对于这些高风险的情况，强烈建议在危险性最小时进行手术。如果不存在高风险情况，虽然桥接治疗相关的证据很少，也建议应在停用 2 种药物和桥接治疗后 5 天进行治疗[30, 52]。此外，使用肝素药物在桥接治疗无效时，通常会采用静脉注射短效糖蛋白 Ⅱb/Ⅲa 抑制剂，例如坎格雷洛、依替巴肽和替罗非班[33, 38, 56, 62]。替罗非班和依替巴肽均可使用，分别在术前 3～6 h 和 4～12 h 停止。

在紧急情况下，当患者已经使用一种或两种抗血小板药物后，建议在最后一次使用阿司匹林 2 h 后和氯吡格雷 12～24 h 后输注血小板[30, 52]。然而需要注意的是，输注血小板会增加支架内血栓形成的风险。

32.2.2.2 病理性血栓相关疾病

遗传性血小板功能障碍（IPFD）是一种罕见疾病[2, 28]，我们尚未发现任何与 CSDH 相关的病例。在这种情况下进行止血需要与血液科医生密切合作，特别是在术前阶段。围手术期管理方案取决于是否需要紧急手术[2]。根据疾病的类型，可以相应输注血小板、使用重组活化凝血因子Ⅶ、去氨加压素或抗纤溶药物。

32.2.3 辅助治疗

32.2.3.1 抗癫痫类药物

由于血肿对大脑皮质的刺激和（或）引起颅内压升高，部分神经外科医生更喜欢提前预防癫痫的发生。然而，由于缺乏随机对照研究，这种做法并没有得到 1 级证据的支持。一篇 2013 年开展的文献回顾没有发现关于这一问题的随机对照研究[42]。此外，已经发布的相关资料相当不统一。一些学者推荐术前使用抗癫痫药物（AED），因为它们可以降低术后癫痫发作的风险[21]，并且对患者的出院没有影响。然而其他学者没有发现预防性使用 AED 有任何好处[37, 59]，考虑到 AED 对于老年人神经认知功能方面的负面影响，他们反对预防性使用 AED[16]。

最近，一项病例报道报告了癫痫病灶与 MRI Flair 上脑沟高密度有着明确的关联[53]。随后，作者暗示对于脑沟 Flair 序列高信号的 CSDH 患者需要进行癫痫的预防；也同时假设了其他相关的风险因素，如术前的中线移位、颅脑内的积气、开颅手术和 CSDH 膜切除术都被认为是术后发生癫痫的危险因素[20]。此外，酗酒、左侧和混合型 CSDH 也被认为与术后癫痫发生相关[11, 63]。

相反，一项针对 2010—2017 年诊断为 CSDH 的系统回顾并没有发现血肿体积、中线移位、手术策略和术后气颅是急性癫痫发作/癫痫持续状态的重要预测因素。然而，卒中、格拉斯哥昏迷评分为 13 分或更低以及 14 天内血肿的复发是癫痫发作的危险因素[78]。也有文献报道，左乙拉西坦是上述情况最适宜的 AED[78]。

根据这些相互矛盾的文献报道，我们认为术前和术后使用脑电图是决定是否开始 AED 的最好检查方法[78]。

32.2.3.2 激素治疗

由于炎症反应是 CSDH 形成的潜在原因，类固醇类药物被推荐为临床保守治疗的一部分或手术清除的辅助治疗。

1962年，类固醇被首次成功应用于治疗3名CSDH患者[3]。自那时起，各种类固醇类药物被应用于临床，但却没有明确的指南指导。事实上，治疗的适应证、剂量以及使用时间随不同医疗团队而不尽相同[5]。

类固醇已经在临床中被广泛应用但没有任何高水平的证据证明[15]。据报道，地塞米松作为主要治疗方式，对CSDH有较好的疗效[7, 70]。此外，多项研究已经报道类固醇有促进CSDH血肿吸收以及防治复发的作用[6, 8, 47, 60]。上述对于防治复发的积极效果，让类固醇成为手术清除血肿的辅助治疗方式，但仍没有标准化的相关使用方案。

最近，两项双盲、随机对照研究探讨了糖皮质激素治疗的适应证、剂量和使用时长问题。首先是SUCRE研究探究甲泼尼龙对没有严重临床症状或影像学表现的CSDH的疗效[22]。第二项研究是dex-CSDH研究，针对地塞米松对于有症状CSDH成人疗效的探究[35]。第二项研究的结果表明，地塞米松组相比安慰剂组，在使用6个月后其良好的临床结果较少而不良事件发生较多。然而，地塞米松组CSDH患者的再手术率低[24]。

32.2.3.3 其他药物

基于CSDH膜内新生血管形成和血管高通透性，一些药物被用于在手术清除后加快血肿吸收和减少复发。血管紧张素转换酶抑制剂（ACEI）已经在不同研究中得到了探究，疗效存在争议[4, 49, 77]。从理论上讲，ACEI可以减少血管内皮生长因子产生，抑制血肿膜内新生血管生成和发育，进而降低血管的通透性[77]。ACEI也参与控制动脉高压；因此，它可能通过减少脆性血管破裂导致的微出血从而促进血肿的吸收[4, 65]。

他汀类药物是用于治疗冠心病和高胆固醇的药物。最常使用的是阿托伐他汀钙片，众所周知它对老年人有显著的效果。他汀类药物具有抗炎和促进血管修复的功能[51]。阿托伐他汀无论是单独使用还是联合手术使用，均能减少CSDH体积和改善预后[10, 74, 79]。所报道的研究结果已被一项双盲随机安慰剂对照临床试验所证实[27]。目前，另外两项评估阿托伐他汀钙片安全性和有效性的随机对照试验正在进行中，包括REACH和ATOCH[15]。等到试验结果被公布，关于适应证、剂量和治疗时间的临床数据可能在临床实践中更进一步改善CSDH预后。

另一种值得关注的药物是氨甲环酸，这是一种抗纤溶药物，它是一种激肽释放酶-激肽系统抑制剂，可促进血肿消退。小数量患者样本的回顾性研究报道了良好的临床结果。第一例是在未经手术治疗的患者中达到血肿的完全消退[29]。第二例显示术后空腔内残余血肿缩小[69]。在2020年，Raja等对27例患者进行了前瞻性观察研究，发现氨甲环酸是一种安全有效的替代治疗方式[36]。目前，有5项正在进行的临床研究来确定该项药物的受益和风险，以进一步优化其在临床实践中的使用[15]。

32.3 围手术期管理

32.3.1 麻醉的选择

基于手术过程和患者既往病史，麻醉选择一直是老年人群中普遍存在的问题。术前应在外科医生、麻醉医生和患者家属讨论后决定麻醉方式，同时考虑患者的健康状况。

目前，关于麻醉和手术相关结果的研究有限，并且这些研究存在方法和解释上的偏差，包括样本量和研究组间的异质性[65]。即使全身麻醉（GA）和监测麻醉管理（MAC）相结合，在全身麻醉后老年患者心脏相关并发症的发生率仍然很高[31]。

2017年一项研究报道了两组患者，分别采用GA或局部麻醉对CSDH患者进行微创开颅手术，局部麻醉组的并发症风险更少[41]。此外，与GA组相比，局部麻醉组术后不需要重症监护，有着较短的手术时间和住院时间。这种麻醉模式更适宜资源有限的医疗机构在治疗老年CSDH患者时选择[41]。

2020年Blaauw等对923例进行手术治疗的CSDH患者进行了研究。他们报道了更多的GA后并发症，这些患者在3个月内的死亡率没有显著差异[9]。本回顾性研究包括3个中心，每个中心都有自己的麻醉模式选择标准。最后，在本中心局部麻醉实验中发现，右美托咪定（1 μg/kg）在MAC中比舒芬太尼更安全，并且在术中患者表现出更好的舒适度，更少的抢救发生率，术后住院时间更短并且外科医生满意度更高[75]。因此，当全身麻醉不适用时，局部麻醉可以很好地替代全身麻醉。

32.3.2 氧疗

麻醉前病情评估可以充分了解患者的病史，并评估其呼吸和心血管功能。在 CSDH 手术中，维持良好的氧合是必需的。因为低氧血症对脑组织的损害很大，是术后出现并发症的主要原因。因此，特别是当在局部麻醉下进行手术时，在手术中应系统性地予以患者鼻导管或面罩高浓度氧气吸氧。

低氧血症是由于麻醉和术后膈肌功能障碍的联合作用引起的，导致肺萎缩和肺内分流[4]。此外，阻塞性呼吸暂停的发作可能是由于残留的麻醉药物效应或睡眠障碍，特别是在老年人当中[4]。因此，患者在术中和术后不久均应采用脉搏血氧仪系统性监测血氧。

32.3.3 镇痛治疗

颅脑手术后，完善的疼痛管理对于确保患者的舒适和促进快速恢复至关重要[4]。目前的镇痛策略优化了疼痛的控制并且限制了潜在的不良反应。疼痛管理应从围手术期开始且在术后继续进行。适当的术前风险评估，对患者手术信息和术前老年人的用药情况的了解有利于进行术后疼痛管理[50]。

众所周知，CSDH 术中对头皮切口进行局部麻醉剂浸润，可以减少头皮切口炎症和疼痛信号，以此来减轻术后的疼痛[46]。

根据患者的疼痛程度，患者的基础疾病以及可能出现的副作用和并发症来使用不同药物。扑热息痛通常单独或联合用于治疗轻至中度疼痛，而中至重度疼痛最常使用阿片类药物[50, 55]。

32.4 术后医疗护理

32.4.1 补液

静脉输液（IVFA）被认为可以促进脑组织的扩张，已被广泛应用于 CSDH 术后预防复发。CSDH 患者的临床表现多为脱水，并且已经有证据表明脱水可以引起脑容量减低[25-26]。

Janowski 等之前研究过 IVFA 对 CSDH 患者术后的作用[26]。在这项研究中，他们发现术后 3 天每静脉输入 2000 ml 的晶体与较低的血肿复发和更好的临床结果相关。该研究还强调了这种做法的两项好处，包括在给药期间患者需要卧床休息能够促进脑组织扩张，在液体输完后患者还能够通过走动来预防体位相关的并发症[26]。

在 2017 年，Montano 等已经证明术后充足的输液可以增加脑容量并显著减少术后 SDH 的残余，这确保了术后患者良好的临床预后和影像学结果[45]。输液治疗方案包括术后静脉注射生理盐水和口服补水，这是一种安全有效的治疗残余 SDH 的辅助方法。补液治疗的优点主要是没有副作用，然而对有心脏病史和体质差的老年人应用时应特别注意。

32.4.2 血栓栓塞的预防

静脉血栓栓塞的预防是 CSDH 术后护理的一部分，特别是对于有多种基础疾病的老年人。另外，血栓的预防也可能导致术后再出血和血肿复发等相关问题。

使用下肢气囊持续加压装置对患者是有价值的。此外，术后 24~72 h 内给予肝素通常认为是安全的[34]。自 2003 年以来，LWMH 一直被推荐在术前和术后 12 h 使用[18, 32]。然而，一些学者报道了使用肝素会增加血肿的复发率[48, 68]，与之矛盾的是其他学者已经注意到早期给予预防性剂量的 LWMH 可以降低再手术的风险[57]。

在 2017 年，Fornebo 等学者观察到无论是否正在接受抗血栓治疗，患者 CSDH 确诊率均相同[17]。作者还表明，在 CSDH 手术后 30 天内早期给予抗血栓治疗与较低的血栓栓塞事件发生率相关。在 2020 年，一项前瞻性法国多中心研究显示，不使用抗血栓药物与血栓栓塞的显著高风险相关[71]。相反，术后第一个月抗血栓药物的使用增加了血肿复发的风险[71]。因此，他们建议术后延迟 1 个月使用抗血栓药物。

由于缺乏共识，血栓栓塞预防的问题应在精准医疗的基础上考虑患者的疾病情况和影像学特点。

32.4.3 抗凝血和抗血小板药物的使用

2016 年一项 meta 研究显示，抗凝血药和抗血小板药物已被确定为血肿复发的危险因素，但恢复药物使用又可以减少血栓栓塞事件的发生[76]。在2018年，一项系统回顾和meta分析已经回答了CSDH术后恢复抗血栓药物使用的问题[55]。作者指出，尽早开始抗血栓治疗不会有任何额外的出血性或血栓栓塞风险。尽管如此，他们认为这个过程是高度个性化的并且依赖于患者的情况。

随后，Zanaty等报道了一个前瞻性收集596例患者的研究。他们进行了回顾性多变量分析，并确定重新开始口服抗凝的最佳时间范围在术后2～21天。他们得出的结论是，这一时间范围内血肿复发和卒中的发生风险都很低[80]。

颅内手术后恢复抗血栓药物的使用通常是由多学科共同决定的。在CSDH清除术后，抗凝治疗的开始时间缺乏明确相关的指南[71]。然而，HAS-BLED和CHA_2DS_2-VASc风险评分可能有助于确定抗凝治疗的理想时间和策略。

关于之前讨论过的VKA，是否重新开始抗凝治疗取决于出血的风险，并且VKA可以在术后第一天使用，因为VKA只在术后4～7天后才会生效。在此期间，建议进行血栓栓塞预防或替代治疗[73]。替代治疗应在手术后尽快重新开始，特别是对于那些有心脏机械瓣膜换瓣手术史的患者[72]。

口服抗凝药物可在术后48～72 h内使用，如果需要静脉血栓预防，应该使用肝素[73]。术后第一次口服抗凝药物治疗应在最后一次使用肝素至少12 h后使用[1]。

对于抗血小板药物，没有关于术后恢复使用最佳时间的指南，需要进一步临床试验[65]。迄今为止，老年人的抗血小板药物使用与再出血风险之间还没有明确的联系[48]。

32.4.4　抗癫痫治疗

为了预防癫痫发作，一项随机对照研究评估了术后使用AED的情况[59]。研究结果于2019年公布，结果表明AED的使用与否对癫痫发作的发生无明显影响。此外，8%的患者出现了AED的不良反应[59]。

尽管多项研究已经证实了相关预测危险因素[3, 11, 63, 78]，这些危险因素与癫痫发作的发生之间没有很强的关系。然而，这类研究所报道的结果也是相当的矛盾。

CSDH钻孔引流后，术后癫痫发作的发生率低，约为2.3%。因此，考虑到副作用会带来更大的风险，不应系统地预防性使用AED[16]。最后，我们发现在开始任何AED治疗之前进行脑电图评估是非常有意义的[3, 20]。

32.4.5　皮质激素治疗

正如上文所述，已知类固醇激素可诱导CSDH的自发性消退并降低手术血肿清除后的复发率[6, 47]。然而，这些药物在某种程度上仍在被盲目使用，未来的研究可能会更好地阐明治疗的适应证、剂量和效果，期待未来的相关共识的产生。

实际上，CSDH无论在术前还是术后均推荐使用皮质类固醇。Berghauser等报道在CSDH术前使用较长一段时间的地塞米松与CSDH较低的复发率相关[6]。此外，Drapkin推荐对有持续或复发性症状的患者进行常规的术后皮质激素治疗[63]。

32.4.6　其他治疗

有几种药物被建议作为CSDH术后阶段的辅助治疗来防止复发。血管紧张素转换酶抑制剂、氨甲环酸和阿托伐他汀均有相关文献报道[61, 67, 77, 79]。口服氨甲环酸[69]和依替唑仑[23]与随访时SDH体积的显著减小相关。然而，口服培哚普利[58]和链激酶-链道酶[54]与残留的SDH无显著相关性。

32.5　结论

CSDH是一种良性疾病，最常见于老年人。虽然CSDH是神经外科中最常见的疾病，但其在临床治疗中的几个方面仍然存在争议。

合并多种基础疾病的CSDH围手术期医疗管理可能是棘手的，特别是抗血栓药物的停用和恢复使用。关于这一方面的文献较少且缺乏指南和一般建议。

此外，各种治疗方法包括皮质醇、他汀类药物或氨甲环酸等，被用来防止手术血肿清除后的复发，但是仍然缺乏高级别的证据。目前，许多前瞻性随机对照研究正在进行，来评估常见的经验性药物使用疗效，如皮质醇疗法和像阿托伐他汀、氨甲环酸这类有应用前景的药物。

参考文献

1. Albaladejo P, Bonhomme F, Blais N, et al. Management of direct oral anticoagulants in patients undergoing elective surgeries and invasive procedures: updated guidelines from the French Working Group on Perioperative Hemostasis (GIHP)—September 2015. Anaesth Crit Care Pain Med. 2017;36(1):73–6.
2. Al-Huniti A, Kahr WH. Inherited platelet disorders: diagnosis and management. Transfus Med Rev. 2020;34(4):277–85.
3. Ambrosetto C. Post-traumatic subdural hematoma. Further observations on nonsurgical treatment. Arch Neurol. 1962;6:287–92.
4. Baillard C. Oxygen supplementation in the postoperative period: when and how? Le Praticien en Anesthésie Réanimation. 2011;15(5):310–4.
5. Bartek J Jr, Sjåvik K, Schaible S, et al. The role of angiotensin-converting enzyme inhibitors in patients with chronic subdural hematoma: a Scandinavian population-based multicenter study. World Neurosurg. 2018;113:e555–60.
6. Baschera D, Tosic L, Westermann L, Oberle J, Alfieri A. Treatment standards for chronic subdural hematoma: results from a survey in Austrian, German, and Swiss neurosurgical units. World Neurosurg. 2018;116:e983–95.
7. Berghauser Pont LM, Dammers R, Schouten JW, Lingsma HF, Dirven CM. Clinical factors associated with outcome in chronic subdural hematoma: a retrospective cohort study of patients on pre-operative corticosteroid therapy. Neurosurgery. 2012;70(4):873–80.
8. Berghauser Pont LM, Dirven CM, Dippel DW, Verweij BH, Dammers R. The role of corticosteroids in the management of chronic subdural hematoma: a systematic review. Eur J Neurol. 2012;19(11):1397–403.
9. Blaauw J, Jacobs B, den Hertog HM, et al. Neurosurgical and perioperative management of chronic subdural hematoma. Front Neurol. 2020;11:550.
10. Chan DY, Chan DT, Sun TF, et al. The use of atorvastatin for chronic subdural hematoma: a retrospective cohort comparison study. Br J Neurosurg. 2016;31(1):72–7.
11. Chen CW, Kuo JR, Lin HJ, et al. Early post-operative seizures after burr-hole drainage for chronic subdural hematoma: correlation with brain CT findings. J Clin Neurosci. 2004;11:706–9.
12. Dobran M, Iacoangeli M, Scortichini AR, et al. Spontaneous chronic subdural hematoma in young adult: the role of missing coagulation factors. G Chir. 2017;38(2):66–70.
13. Drapkin AJ. Chronic subdural hematoma: pathophysiological basis for treatment. Br J Neurosurg. 1991;5:467–73.
14. Enriquez A, Lip GY, Baranchuk A. Anticoagulation reversal in the era of the non-vitamin K oral anticoagulants. Europace. 2016;18(7):955–64.
15. Feghali J, Yang W, Huang J. Updates in chronic subdural hematoma: epidemiology, etiology, pathogenesis, treatment, and outcome. World Neurosurg. 2020;141:339–45.
16. Flores G, Vicenty JC, Pastrana EA. Post-operative seizures after burr hole evacuation of chronic subdural hematomas: is prophylactic anti-epileptic medication needed? Acta Neurochir (Wien). 2017;159:2033–6.
17. Fornebo I, Sjåvik K, Alibeck M, et al. Role of antithrombotic therapy in the risk of hematoma recurrence and thromboembolism after chronic subdural hematoma evacuation: a population-based consecutive cohort study. Acta Neurochir (Wien). 2017;159(11):2045–52.
18. Gerlach R, Scheuer T, Beck J, Woszczyk A, Seifert V, Raabe A. Risk of postoperative hemorrhage after intracranial surgery after early nadroparin administration: results of a prospective study. Neurosurgery. 2003;53:1028–34.
19. Giralt-Steinhauer E, Cuadrado-Godia E, Ois A, et al. Comparison between $CHADS_2$ and CHA_2DS_2-VASc score in a stroke cohort with atrial fibrillation. Eur J Neurol. 2013;20(4):623–8.
20. Goertz L, Speier J, Schulte AP, et al. Independent risk factors for postoperative seizures in chronic subdural hematoma identified by multiple logistic regression analysis. World Neurosurg. 2019;132:e716–21.
21. Grobelny BT, Ducruet AF, Zacharia BE, et al. Preoperative antiepileptic drug administration and the incidence of postoperative seizures following bur hole-treated chronic subdural hematoma. J Neurosurg. 2009;111(6):1257–62.
22. Henaux PL, Le Reste PJ, Laviolle B, Morandi X. Steroids in chronic subdural hematomas (SUCRE trial): study protocol for a randomized controlled trial. Trials. 2017;18(1):252.

23. Hirashima Y, Kuwayama N, Hamada H, Hayashi N, Endo S. Etizolam, an antianxiety agent, attenuates recurrence of chronic subdural hematoma. Evaluation by computed tomography. Neurol Med Chir (Tokyo). 2002;42:53–5.
24. Hutchinson PJ, Edlmann E, Bulters D, et al. Trial of dexamethasone for chronic subdural hematoma. N Engl J Med. 2020;383(27):2616–27.
25. Jack A, O'Kelly C, McDougall C, Findlay JM. Predicting recurrence after chronic subdural haematoma drainage. Can J Neurol Sci. 2015;42:34–9.
26. Janowski M, Kunert P. Intravenous fluid administration may improve post-operative course of patients with chronic subdural hematoma: a retrospective study. PLoS One. 2012;7(4):e35634.
27. Jiang R, Zhao S, Wang R, et al. Safety and efficacy of atorvastatin for chronic subdural hematoma in Chinese patients: a randomized clinical trial. JAMA Neurol. 2018;75(11):1338–46.
28. Jung N, Shim YJ. Current knowledge on inherited platelet function disorders. Clin Pediatr Hematol Oncol. 2020;27(1):1–13.
29. Kageyama H, Toyooka T, Tsuzuki N, et al. Nonsurgical treatment of chronic subdural hematoma with tranexamic acid. J Neurosurg. 2013;119:332–7.
30. Keeling D, Tait RC, Watson H, British Committee of Standards for Haematology. Peri-operative management of anticoagulation and antiplatelet therapy. Br J Haematol. 2016;175(4):602–13.
31. Kim SO, Jung SI, Won YS, Choi CSYJ. A comparative study of local versus general anesthesia for chronic subdural hematoma in elderly patients over 60 years. Korean J Neurotrauma. 2013;9(2):47–51.
32. Kleindienst A, Harvey HB, Mater E, et al. Early antithrombotic prophylaxis with low molecular weight heparin in neurosurgery. Acta Neurochir (Wien). 2003;145:1085–90.
33. Koenig-Oberhuber V, Filipovic M. New antiplatelet drugs and new oral anticoagulants. Br J Anaesth. 2016;117(S2):ii74–84.
34. Kolias AG, Chari A, Santarius T, Hutchinson PJ. Chronic subdural haematoma: modern management and emerging therapies. Nat Rev Neurol. 2014;10:570–8.
35. Kolias AG, Edlmann E, Thelin EP, et al. Dexamethasone for adult patients with a symptomatic chronic subdural haematoma (Dex-CSDH) trial: study protocol for a randomised controlled trial. Trials. 2018;19(1):670.
36. Kutty RK, Leela SK, Sreemathyamma SB, et al. The outcome of medical management of chronic subdural hematoma with tranexamic acid—a prospective observational study. J Stroke Cerebrovasc Dis. 2020;29(11):10527372.
37. Lavergne P, Labidi M, Brunet MC, et al. Efficacy of anti-seizure prophylaxis in chronic subdural hematoma: a cohort study on routinely collected health data. J Neurosurg. 2019;1:1–5.
38. Lizza BD, Kauflin MJ. Extended-infusion eptifibatide to prevent stent thrombosis in a patient undergoing orthopedic surgery. Ann Pharmacother. 2011;45(5):e28.
39. Luongo M, Pizzuti M, Godano U. Bilateral chronic subdural non-traumatic hematoma associated with von Willebrand's type I disease: a case report. Acta Neurochir (Wien). 2012;154(6):1087–8.
40. Luongo M, Pizzuti M, Godano U. Chronic subdural non traumatic hematoma associated with von Willebrand's disease: a real clinical association or just a mere coincidence? Clin Neurol Neurosurg. 2013;115(8):1569–70.
41. Mahmood SD, Waqas M, Baig MZ, Darbar A. Mini-craniotomy under local anesthesia for chronic subdural hematoma: an effective choice for elderly patients and for patients in a resource-strained environment. World Neurosurg. 2017;106:676–9.
42. Mehta V, Harward SC, Sankey EW, Nayar G, Codd PJ. Evidence based diagnosis and management of chronic subdural hematoma: a review of the literature. J Clin Neurosci. 2018;50:7–15.
43. Meidert AS, Kinzinger J, Möhnle P, et al. Perioperative management of a patient with severe factor V deficiency presenting with chronic subdural hematoma: a clinical report. World Neurosurg. 2019;127:409–13.
44. Merrill SA, Khan D, Richards AE, Kalani MA, Patel NP, Neal MT. Functional recovery following surgery for chronic subdural hematoma. Surg Neurol Int. 2020;11:450.
45. Montano N, Stifano V, Skrap B, Mazzucchi E. Management of residual subdural hematoma after burr-hole evacuation. The role of fluid therapy and review of the literature. J Clin Neurosci. 2017;46:26–9.
46. Mulligan P, Raore B, Liu S, Olson JJ. Neurological and functional outcomes of subdural hematoma evacuation in patients over 70 years of age. J Neurosci Rural Pract. 2013;4(3):250–6.
47. Nagatani K, Wada K, Takeuchi S, Nawashiro H. Corticosteroid suppression of vascular endothelial growth factor and recurrence of chronic subdural hematoma. Neurosurgery. 2012;70(5):E1334.

48. Nathan S, Goodarzi Z, Jette N, Gallagher C, Holroyd-Leduc J. Anticoagulant and antiplatelet use in seniors with chronic subdural hematoma: systematic review. Neurology. 2017;88(20):1889–93.
49. Neidert MC, Schmidt T, Mitova T, et al. Preoperative angiotensin converting enzyme inhibitor usage in patients with chronic subdural hematoma: associations with initial presentation and clinical outcome. J Clin Neurosci. 2016;28:82–6.
50. Oh HJ, Lee KS, Shim JJ, Yoon SM, Yun IG, Bae HG. Postoperative course and recurrence of chronic subdural hematoma. J Korean Neurosurg Soc. 2010;48(6):518–23.
51. Oikonomou E, Siasos G, Zaromitidou M, et al. Atorvastatin treatment improves endothelial function through endothelial progenitor cells mobilization in ischemic heart failure patients. Atherosclerosis. 2015;238:159–64.
52. Oprea AD, Popescu WM. Perioperative management of antiplatelet therapy. Br J Anaesth. 2013;111(Suppl 1):i3–i17.
53. Oshida S, Akamatsu Y, Matsumoto Y, et al. A case of chronic subdural hematoma demonstrating the epileptic focus at the area with sulcal hyperintensity on fluid-attenuated inversion recovery image. Radiol Case Rep. 2019;14(9):1109–12.
54. Park M, Kim JM, Kim HJ. Effects of oral streptokinase-streptodornase on remnant chronic subdural hematomas. Korean J Neurotrauma. 2015;11:131–4.
55. Phan K, Abi-Hanna D, Kerferd J, et al. Resumption of antithrombotic agents in chronic subdural hematoma: a systematic review and meta-analysis. World Neurosurg. 2018;109:e792–9.
56. Pickett AM, Taylor DA, Ackman ML. Prolonged infusion of eptifibatide as bridge therapy between bare-metal stent insertion and cardiovascular surgery: case report and review of the literature. Pharmacotherapy. 2010;30(4):127e–33e.
57. Pinggera D, Unterhofer C, Görtz P, Thomé C, Ortler M. Postoperative thromboembolic prophylaxis with low-molecular-weight heparin and risk of rebleeding in patients with chronic subdural hematomas: a comparative retrospective cohort study. World Neurosurg. 2017;104:284–90.
58. Poulsen FR, Munthe S, Soe M, Halle B. Perindopril and residual chronic subdural hematoma volumes six weeks after burr hole surgery: a randomized trial. Clin Neurol Neurosurg. 2014;123:4–8.
59. Pradhanang AB, Sedain G, Shilpakar SK, Sharma MR. Prophylactic use of antiepileptic drug (Phenytoin) in preventing early postoperative seizure in patients with chronic subdural hematoma: a randomized control trial. Indian J Neurosurg. 2019;08(03):168–78.
60. Prud'homme M, Mathieu F, Marcotte N, Cottin S. A pilot placebo controlled randomized controlled trial of Dexamethasone for Chronic Subdural Haematoma. Can J Neurol Sci. 2016;43(2):284–90.
61. Qiu S, Zhuo W, Sun C, Su Z, Yan A, Shen L. Effects of atorvastatin on chronic subdural hematoma: a systematic review. Medicine (Baltimore). 2017;96(26):e7290.
62. Rassi AN, Blackstone E, Militello MA, et al. Safety of "bridging" with eptifibatide for patients with coronary stents before cardiac and non-cardiac surgery. Am J Cardiol. 2012;110(4):485–90.
63. Samokhvalov AV, Irving H, Mohapatra S, Rehm J. Alcohol consumption, unprovoked seizures, and epilepsy: a systematic review and meta-analysis. Epilepsia. 2010;51:1177–84.
64. Savonitto S, Caracciolo M, Cattaneo M, DE Servi S. Management of patients with recently implanted coronary stents on dual antiplatelet therapy who need to undergo major surgery. J Thromb Haemost. 2011;9(11):2133–42.
65. Shapey J, Glancz LJ, Brennan PM. Chronic subdural haematoma in the elderly: is it time for a new paradigm in management? Curr Geriatr Rep. 2016;5:71–7.
66. Shimogawa T, Morioka T, Sayama T, et al. Impact of low coagulation factor XIII activity in patients with chronic subdural hematoma associated with cerebrospinal fluid hypovolemia: a retrospective study. Surg Neurol Int. 2017;8:192.
67. Son S, Yoo CJ, Lee SG, Kim EY, Park CW, Kim WK. Natural course of initially non-operated cases of acute subdural hematoma: the risk factors of hematoma progression. J Korean Neurosurg Soc. 2013;54:211–9.
68. Tahsim-Oglou Y, Beseoglu K, Hänggi D, Stummer W, Steiger H-J. Factors predicting recurrence of chronic subdural hematoma: the influence of intraoperative irrigation and low-molecular-weight heparin thromboprophylaxis. Acta Neurochir. 2012;154(6):1063–8.
69. Tanweer O, Frisoli FA, Bravate C, et al. Tranexamic acid for treatment of residual subdural hematoma after bedside twist-drill evacuation. World Neurosurg. 2016;91:29–33.
70. Thotakura AK, Marabathina NR. Non-surgical treatment of chronic subdural hematoma with steroids. World Neurosurg. 2015;84:1968–72.

71. Todeschi J, Ferracci FX, Metayer T, et al. Impact of discontinuation of antithrombotic therapy after surgery for chronic subdural hematoma. Neurochirurgie. 2020;66(4):195–202.
72. Volovár Š, Tancošová R, Rokyta R. Bridging anticoagulation therapy. Cor Vasa. 2018;60(4):e400–6.
73. Wagner J, Lock JF, Kastner C, et al. Perioperative management of anticoagulant therapy. Innov Surg Sci. 2019;4(4):144–51.
74. Wang D, Li T, Tian Y, et al. Effects of atorvastatin on chronic subdural hematoma: a preliminary report from three medical centers. J Neurol Sci. 2013;336:237–42.
75. Wang W, Feng L, Bai F, Zhang Z, Zhao Y, Ren C. The safety and efficacy of dexmedetomidine vs. sufentanil in monitored anesthesia care during burr-hole surgery for chronic subdural hematoma: a retrospective clinical trial. Front Pharmacol. 2016;7:410.
76. Wang Y, Zhou J, Fan C, et al. Influence of antithrombotic agents on the recurrence of chronic subdural hematomas and the quest about the recommencement of antithrombotic agents: a meta-analysis. J Clin Neurosci. 2017;38:79–83.
77. Weigel R, Hohenstein A, Schlickum L, Weiss C, Schilling L. Angiotensin converting enzyme inhibition for arterial hypertension reduces the risk of recurrence in patients with chronic subdural hematoma possibly by an antiangiogenic mechanism. Neurosurgery. 2007;61:788–92.
78. Won SY, Dubinski D, Sautter L, et al. Seizure and status epilepticus in chronic subdural hematoma. Acta Neurol Scand. 2019;140(3):194–203.
79. Xu M, Chen P, Zhu X, Wang C, Shi X, Yu B. Effects of atorvastatin on conservative and surgical treatments of chronic subdural hematoma in patients. World Neurosurg. 2016;91:23–8.
80. Zanaty M, Park BJ, Seaman SC. Predicting chronic subdural hematoma recurrence and stroke outcomes while withholding antiplatelet and anticoagulant agents. Front Neurol. 2020;10:1401.
81. Zeng J, Yu P, Cui W, Wang X, Ma J, Zeng C. Comparison of HAS-BLED with other risk models for predicting the bleeding risk in anticoagulated patients with atrial fibrillation: a PRISMA-compliant article. Medicine (Baltimore). 2020;99(25):e20782.

第 33 章　颅内慢性硬膜下血肿术后并发症

Ali Akhaddar

译者：李云飞

33.1　引言

尽管大都认为清除颅内硬膜下血肿的手术是一种相对简单、安全、并发症发生率低的手术，但术后并发症发生率在 5% 至 38% 之间 [5-6, 10, 14, 17, 32, 34, 41, 48-49, 57]。并发症包括与手术及与手术技术直接相关并发症，也包括非手术（常见内科）并发症。所有并发症都会对疾病预后和死亡率产生不利影响，并大大增加治疗和住院费用 [6, 55]。经验不足的外科医生更容易出现术后并发症 [3]。不过，并发症的发生率也取决于患者的自身因素（如高龄、全身及神经系统状况和其他相关疾病）以及血肿类型、潜在病因和手术方法 [10, 37]。

本章全面概述了手术清除颅内慢性硬膜下血肿后可能出现的主要问题（表 33.1），目的是帮助医疗团队避免并发症的发生。

33.2　复发/硬膜下积液

硬膜下间隙残留的血肿不被认为是复发血肿，因为这是手术引流后 CT 扫描的常见表现，除非神经系统症状与此相关，否则大多数患者可以保守治疗（图 33.1）。术后 3 个月有复发症状的病例占 4.9%～28% [1, 17, 21, 35-36, 39, 41-42, 48, 53, 55, 60]。然而，在某些人群中，这种并发症的发生率可达 1/3 [58]。有症状的硬膜下积液（如复发）是一种棘手的临床情况，许多患者需要再次手术，这增加了并发症的发病率和患者的死亡率（图 33.2）。

许多因素似乎与并发症的发生相关。例如，在抗凝/抗血小板治疗 [42, 64]、患者合并症 [37, 39]、血肿类型 [11, 40, 44]、手术方式 [36-37] 等方面仍存在争议。术后复发症状的治疗通常采用手术治疗，但参考 CT 扫描结果若仅存在积液并不需要系统治疗，除非积液有增大或患者恶化或临床症状复发。简而言之，医生应该根据患者具体情况进行治疗调整。

表 33.1　手术清除慢性硬膜下血肿后主要并发症

- 复发及硬膜下积液
- 手术部位感染
  - 硬膜下脓肿
  - 切口感染
  - 脑膜炎
  - 脑脓肿
- 新发急性颅内出血
  - 硬膜外血肿
  - 硬膜下血肿
  - 蛛网膜下腔出血
  - 医源性出血/损伤
- 癫痫发作和癫痫持续状态
- 张力性气颅
- 其他罕见并发症
  - 脑组织疝入硬膜下腔
  - 脊髓硬膜下血肿
  - 高灌注综合征
  - 缺血性脑卒中
- 医疗（非手术）并发症
  - 肺部
  - 泌尿系统
  - 心血管
  - 血栓栓塞
  - 消化系统
  - 肾脏
  - 败血症
  - 弥散性血管内凝血
  - 神经心理

在 Nayil 和同事的研究中，1181 例患者中有 57 例（4.82%）出现一次症状复发，其中 43 例血肿复发在同侧（3.6%），14 例对侧出现血肿（1.2%）。57 例患者均再次行血肿引流手术。其中 9 例 2 次复发（0.76%），行开颅清除血肿、切除血肿包膜手术 [46]。年龄、性别、血肿厚度、中线移位、血肿位置等参数与复发无关。然而，Nayil 的团队发现血肿的内部结构和出血倾向影响复发率 [46]。

Rauhala 等手术治疗了 1048 例 CSDH 患者。278

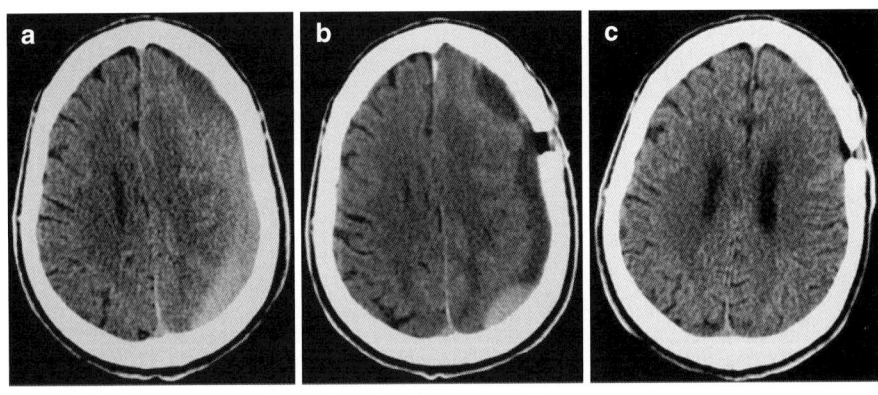

图 33.1 初始术前（a）、术后 1 周（b）和术后 3 个月（c）CT 显示，术后硬膜下腔残留积液（b）的无症状患者经过保守治疗后于术后 3 个月硬膜下血肿完全消失

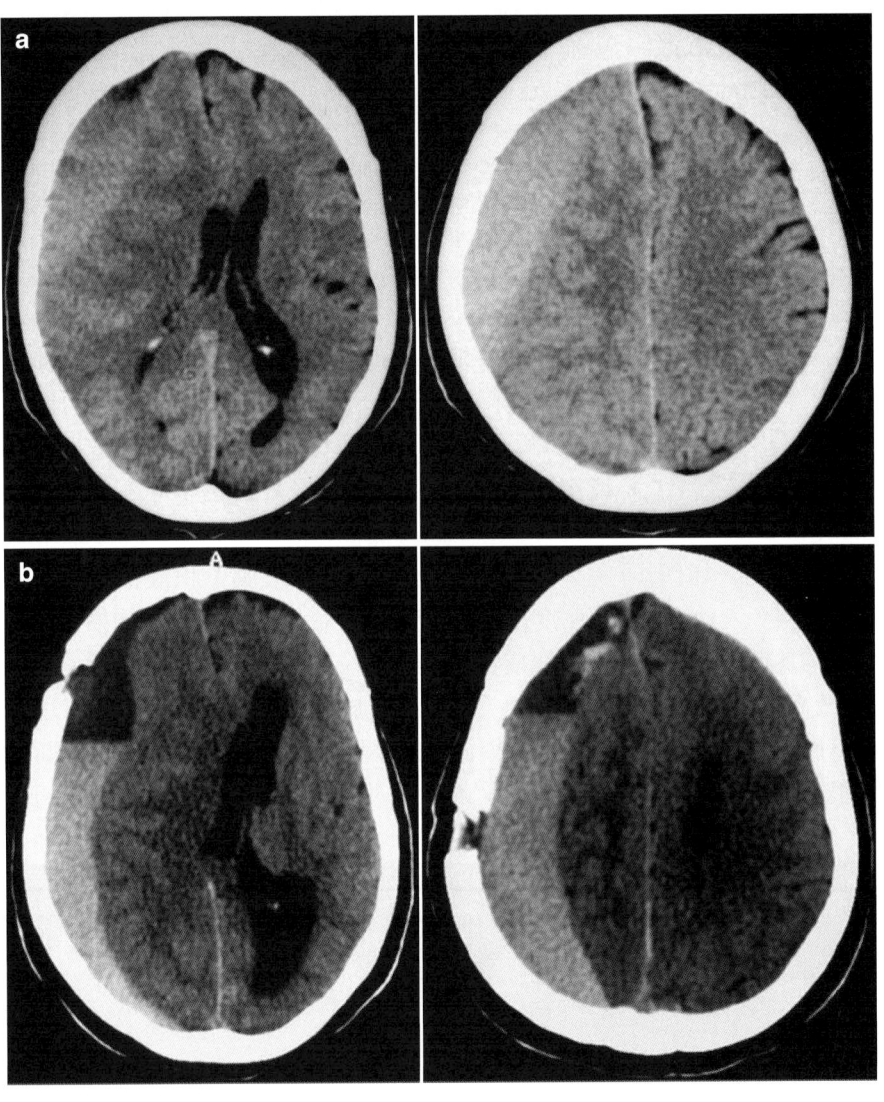

图 33.2 右侧慢性硬膜下血肿复发 6 周前通过两个钻孔引流（神经功能障碍复发）。初始（a）和术后 6 周后的对照 CT 扫描（b）

例（28%）因血肿复发再次手术。229 例复发血肿有临床症状，49 例因随访 CT 扫描发现大量 CSDH 而行手术治疗[55]。根据 Motoie 的研究，787 例患者中有 96 例（12.2%）出现 CSDH 复发。2 次以上手术 11 例，3 次手术 9 例，4 次手术 2 例[43]。

在 Shen 的研究中，中线移位大于 10 mm、严重脑萎缩、术后严重的气颅、引流量大于 100 ml 是复发的独立危险因素[60]。然而，Huang 等认为硬膜下血肿的体积与复发无关[21]。对于 CSDH 的类型，如层状或分层血肿、较厚硬膜下膜状结构、血肿高密度和混合密度以及多腔积血与复发率增加有关[11, 21, 40, 44, 46]。对于 Mori 等来说，第一次手术部位对侧存在薄层硬膜下血肿或积液会导致复发的风险增高[41]。

术后引流可降低复发率。然而，插入引流管的位置（硬膜下或骨膜下）似乎不影响复发[36]。利用重力可以帮助大脑复张。根据 Abouzari 的研究结果，CSDH 术后短时间内直立与复发率增加有关[1]。

尽管许多研究表明抗血小板/抗凝药物可能导致 CSDH 的复发[42, 64]，但 Motoie 在对 96 例因 CSDH 复发而再次手术的患者进行研究后发现，这些药物并不是 CSDH 复发的独立预测因素[43]。

在文献中，几乎所有的复发患者在第一次手术后 2 个月内可通过开颅和钻孔引流成功治疗[36, 41, 46, 55]。因此，CSDH 患者术后应至少随访 10 周，以检查是否复发。根据我们的个人经验，皮质类固醇可作为单一疗法或辅助手术治疗一些缺乏症状的患者。难治性 CSDH 可通过多种手术方式治疗，包括开颅术、硬膜下-腹膜分流术、脑膜中动脉介入栓塞或硬膜下引流管注射组织型纤溶酶原激活剂[25, 30]。

CSDH 手术引流后硬膜下积液再次出现的机制尚不完全清楚，仍需进一步研究[37]。

33.3 硬膜下脓肿

硬膜下脓肿是目前为止 CSDH 术后最严重的手术部位感染。其他感染性并发症不太常见，如伤口深部感染（图 33.3）、脑膜炎和脑脓肿[2, 57]。

硬膜下脓肿虽然罕见（少于所有手术并发症的 2.5%），但却是患者复发和死亡的重要原因[29, 35, 46, 55-56, 59, 66]。大多数硬膜下脓肿病例发生在术后 1～2 周，其临床症状差别很大。除了发热

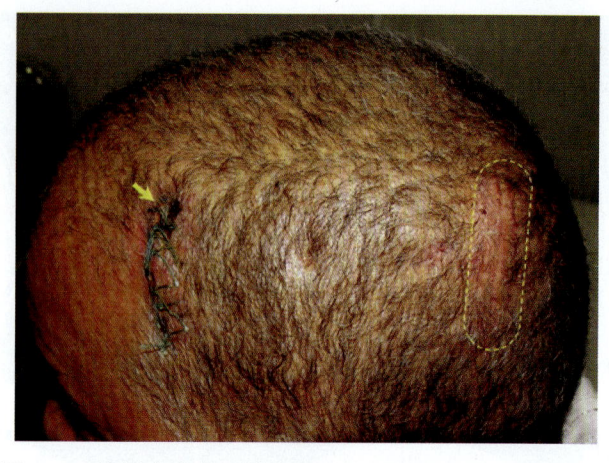

图 33.3　糖尿病患者 2 周前因慢性硬膜下血肿接受手术治疗后切口愈合良好（虚线）；然而，前部创面在切口附近出现局部炎症和感染征象，浅表创面裂开，愈合延迟（箭头）（Reproduced from Akhaddar A（editor）Atlas of Infections in Neurosurgery and Spinal surgery（2017）. Springer International Publishing；with permission）

和化脓性液体渗出外，大多数病例往往表现为出现新的局灶性神经缺损或原有神经缺损的恶化，体温正常或升高，意识水平逐渐受损。有些病例可能是隐匿的，很少或没有症状（例如，只有间歇性低热或全身不适）。因此，神经外科医生应考虑这些患者硬膜下感染的可能性，并制订适当的治疗策略。

CT 扫描显示，感染的硬膜下积液密度低或呈等密度，周围增强（图 33.4 和图 33.5）。如果无法行磁共振成像（MRI）检查，很难区分复发性 CSDH 和术后相关性硬膜下脓肿。这种情况下，进行增强后 T1 加权图像和弥散加权成像评估对疾病诊断可能是有意义的[45]（见第 26 章慢性硬膜下血肿的神

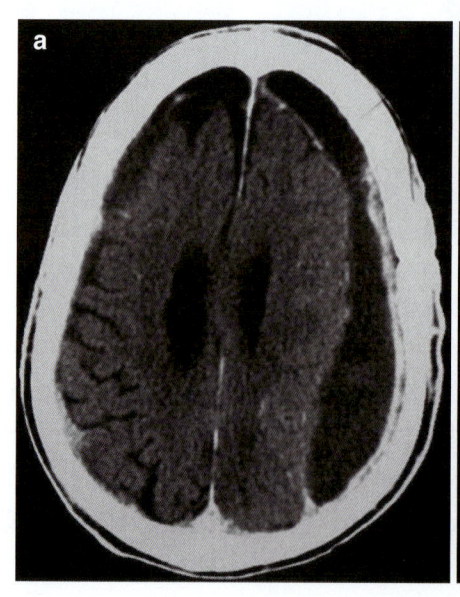
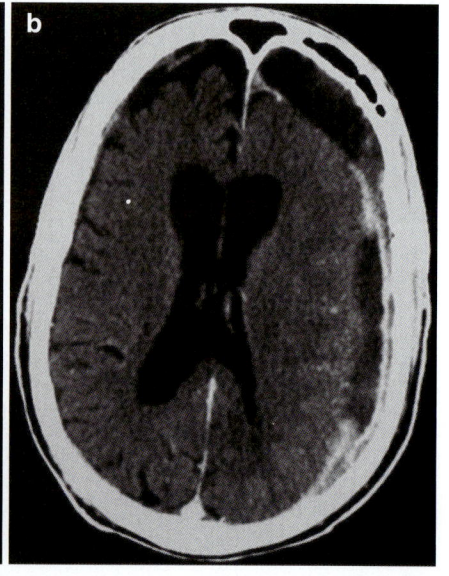

图 33.4　术后硬膜下脓肿，80 岁男性，4 周前因慢性硬膜下血肿行手术治疗。头颅 CT 扫描轴位与增强图像（a，b）（Reproduced from Akhaddar A（editor）Atlas of Infections in Neurosurgery and Spinal surgery（2017）. Springer International Publishing；with permission）

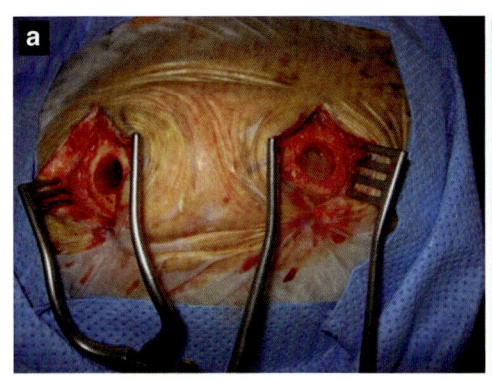
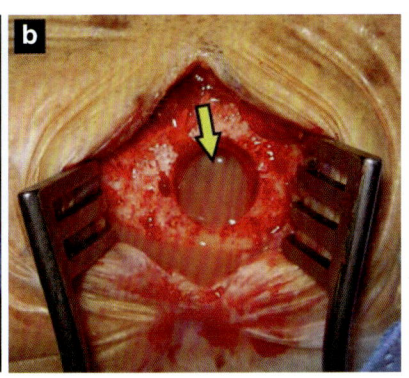

图 33.5 同一患者的手术视图显示颅内硬膜下化脓性内容物（箭头）（a，b）（Reproduced from Akhaddar A（editor）Atlas of Infections in Neurosurgery and Spinal surgery（2017）. Springer International Publishing；with permission）

经影像学鉴别诊断）。术后炎症生物标志物的表达变化很大。C 反应蛋白（CRP）和降钙素原水平的变化对鉴别诊断硬膜下脓肿是有意义的。医源性硬膜下脓肿的致病病原体报道并不多，主要是金黄色葡萄球菌、链球菌和革兰氏阴性菌[13, 35]。

硬膜下脓肿通常需要再次手术，清洗、排出化脓性积液、清创、引流和仔细地缝合伤口。治疗首先需应用广谱抗生素，然后根据药敏试验结果进行有针对性的治疗[2, 46]。

Nayil 和他的同事在 2012 年的研究中，报道了 1181 名接受手术治疗的患者中有 9 名出现硬膜下脓肿（0.76%）。该 9 名患者中有 6 例既往接受过一次慢性硬膜下血肿手术治疗，3 例既往接受过 2 次手术治疗。这 9 例患者存在偏瘫，2 例患者出现新发癫痫，4 例患者出现意识水平改变。对于大多数患者来说，感染性硬膜下积液会在最后一次手术后的 2 周或 3 周内被诊断出来。对于这 9 例患者，需再次进行外科手术治疗包括开颅、排空脓肿和切除血肿外膜。然而不幸的是，其中 2 例患者最终死亡[46]。

如果能够及时有效对症治疗，硬膜下脓肿可不遗留后遗症。然而可能发生许多神经系统并发症，甚至死亡。后遗症包括持续的癫痫发作、残留的局灶性神经功能缺损和精神状态的永久性改变[29]。

33.4 新发急性颅内出血

急性颅内出血虽然不常见（占不到所有并发症的 4%）[32, 41, 55, 57]，但却是 CSDH 手术后最严重的并发症之一，急性颅内出血的出现会增加 CSDH 的发病率和（或）死亡率，这种术后并发症可能发生在 CSDH 的开颅或钻孔手术之后。急性硬膜下血肿（图 33.6 和图 33.7）、硬膜外血肿（图 33.8）和蛛网膜下腔出血是手术部位发生最多的出血类型。然而，原发部位的远端脑出血可能出现在不同部位，如同侧（图 33.9）、对侧、脑室内或颅后窝[4, 22, 50, 62]。Patibandla 报道了一例 CSDH 手术引流后颅内多个部位（脑干、脑和小脑脚、右小脑半球、右丘脑和两个大脑半球）同时出现多处脑实质内出血的罕见病例[51]。

远端脑实质出血的确切发病机制尚不清楚，但这种出血被怀疑是多种复杂因素共同导致的结果，如高血压、低颅内压、颅内压改变、抽吸引流、脑脊液过度引流、先前未发现的挫伤区域出血和血小板减少[4, 12]。因此，许多学者建议缓慢渐进的脑部减压，以防止血流的快速变化。Kaneshiro 和同事考虑对所有疑似术后颅内出血的患者进行术后早期 CT 扫描[27]。面对这些不同形式的术后出血，手术治疗指征需要神经外科医生根据患者的具体情

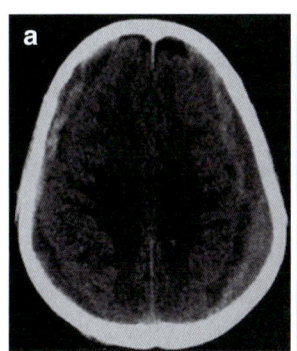
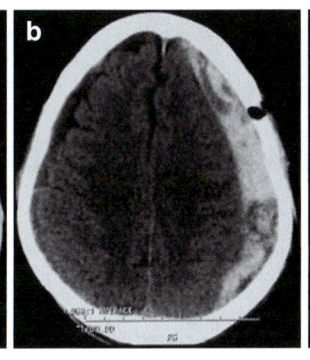
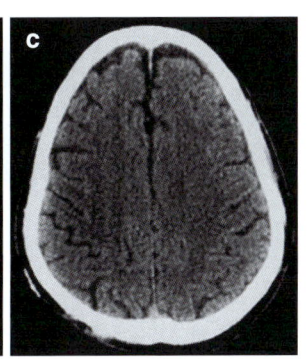

图 33.6 术后第三天急性硬膜下血肿。患者再次行开颅手术，预后良好。颅脑 CT 扫描初始轴位（a）、术后第三天（b）和 3 个月后（c）图像

图 33.7 慢性 SDH 钻孔引流术后立即出现硬膜下出血。术前（a）和术后紧急 CT 扫描（b）

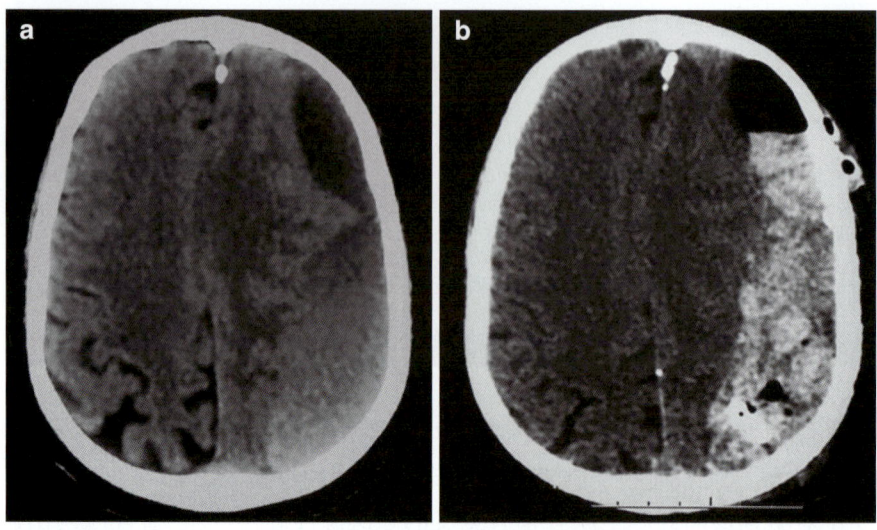

图 33.8 慢性硬膜下血肿钻孔引流术后出现急性硬膜外血肿（星号）。患者通过开颅手术获得了良好的预后。术后立即 CT 扫描（a）和第二次手术后 CT 扫描（b）

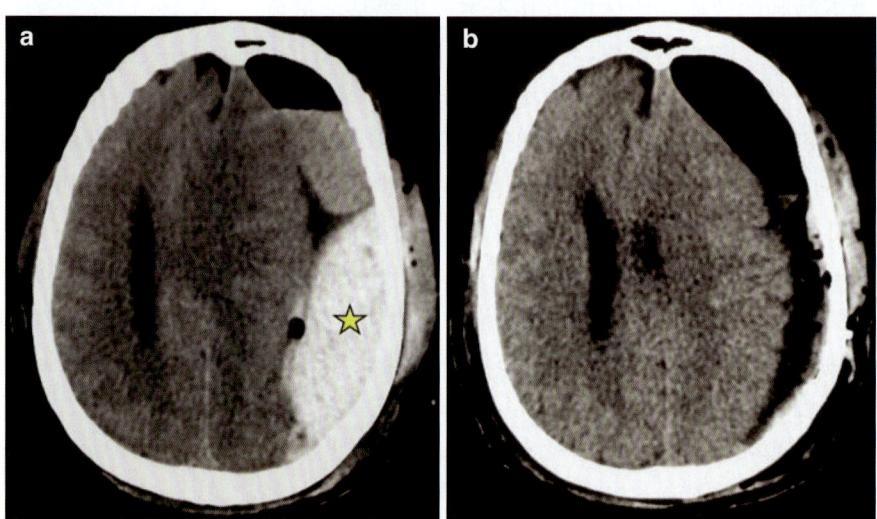

图 33.9 慢性硬膜下血肿术后右额叶远端脑血肿。初次头颅轴位 CT 扫描（a）和术后第三天（b）图像

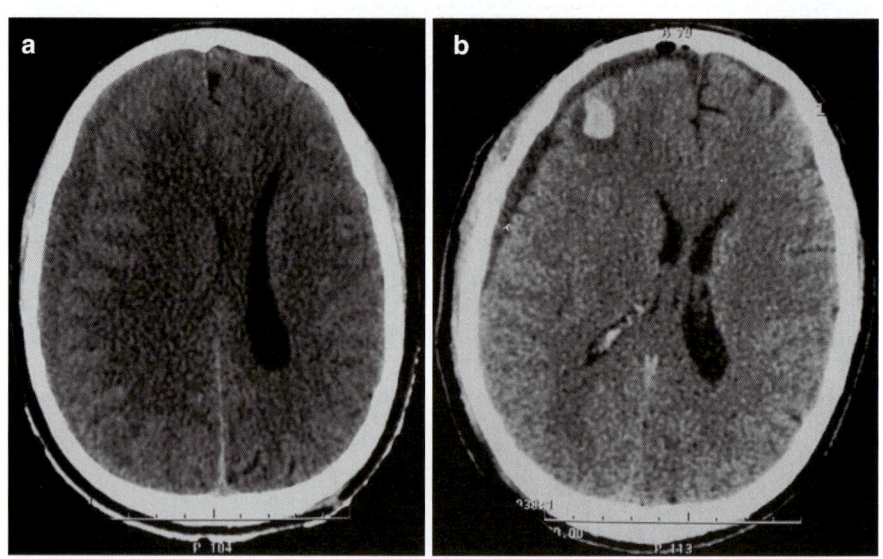

况决定。

根据 Lee 的经验，395 例患者中有 14 例（3.54%）在 CSDH 手术后发生了新的急性颅内出血。7 例患者为急性硬膜外血肿，其中 2 例需要开颅血肿清除术，术后效果良好。急性硬膜下血肿 6 例，其中 4 例患者行去骨瓣减压术及硬膜下血肿清除术。不幸

的是，其中 1 例未手术的患者死亡，另 1 例在钻孔附近可见小的脑实质内血肿[32]。Rohde 等在 376 例 CSDH 手术患者中，发现新发急性颅内出血 13 例（3.45%），其中脑出血 8 例（2.12%），急性硬膜外血肿 5 例（1.33%）[57]。

在 Nayil 等的另一项研究中，1181 例患者中有 5 例（0.42%）出现急性硬膜下血肿，但其中 2 例术前接受了抗凝治疗。5 例患者均行硬膜下血肿清除手术，2 例死亡。急性硬膜外血肿 1 例，术后恢复良好。1 例患者术后立即出现大面积丘脑血肿死亡[46]。

此外，慢性硬膜下血肿引流术后的医源性出血也不容忽视。颅骨穿孔器的错误使用（图 33.10）、引流管插入位置不当（图 33.11）、硬膜下的引流管放置位置错误（图 33.12）、脑损伤灌洗等，这些情况已出现少数病例报道[9, 26, 32, 46, 52, 65]。在我们的临床实践中，当我们需要引流硬膜下血肿时，我们只使用帽状腱膜下软引流（而不是硬膜下引流），这将减少脑损伤的机会。在任何情况下，在插入和拔除引流管时都必须采取适当的护理并警惕并发症出现。

33.5 癫痫发作和癫痫持续状态

据报道，CSDH 术后癫痫发作的全球发生率为 0.67%～23%[7, 20, 32, 35, 46, 48, 55, 57, 67]，癫痫发作对患者具有致死性[33]。术后癫痫发作发生率在开颅手术患者中尤其高[15]。Hirakawa 等发现，开颅清除血肿术后患者癫痫发作的发生率高于单纯钻孔引流术患者[19]。然而不仅是手术清除血肿，最初的头部损伤和压迫性血肿本身也可能是癫痫发作的原因。另外，有癫痫病史的患者术后癫痫发作风险更大[57]。Cameron 等建议术前开始使用预防性抗癫痫药，并于术后持续使用 6 个月[7]。然而，预防性抗癫痫药物在减少术后新发作发生方面的作用尚不清楚[7, 18]。

在 Lee 等报道的研究中，8 名患者（2%）在钻孔引流术后出现新的癫痫发作，其中 5 例患者因颅内新发病变加重癫痫发作。因此，对新发癫痫患者应及时进行 CT 扫描评估[32]。Nayil 等在术后急

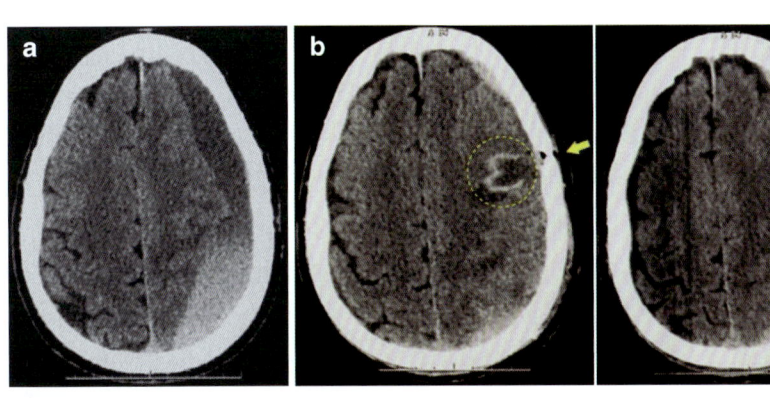

图 33.10 慢性硬膜下血肿（a，b）的钻孔清除（箭头）术后额叶皮质脑挫伤（虚线圈）。外科医生在手术过程中未报告任何特殊事件，但很可能是由于颅骨穿孔器的错误使用

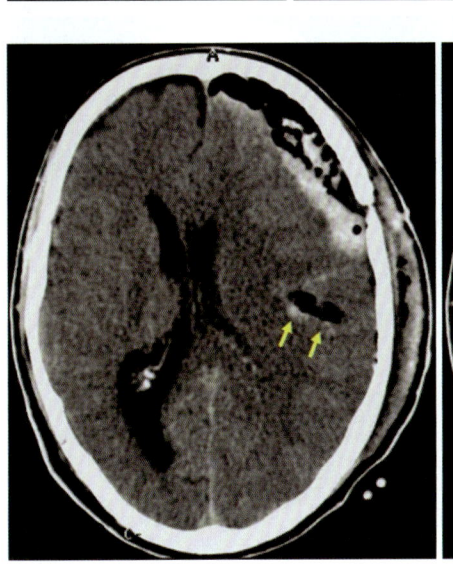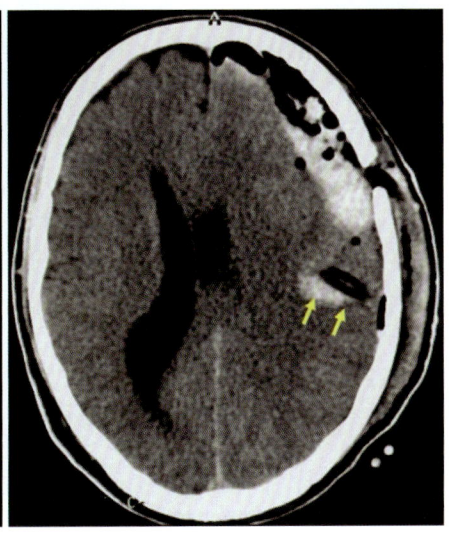

图 33.11 术后 CT 扫描轴位显示脑实质内深部脑挫伤（箭头），慢性硬膜下血肿引流管错误地插入

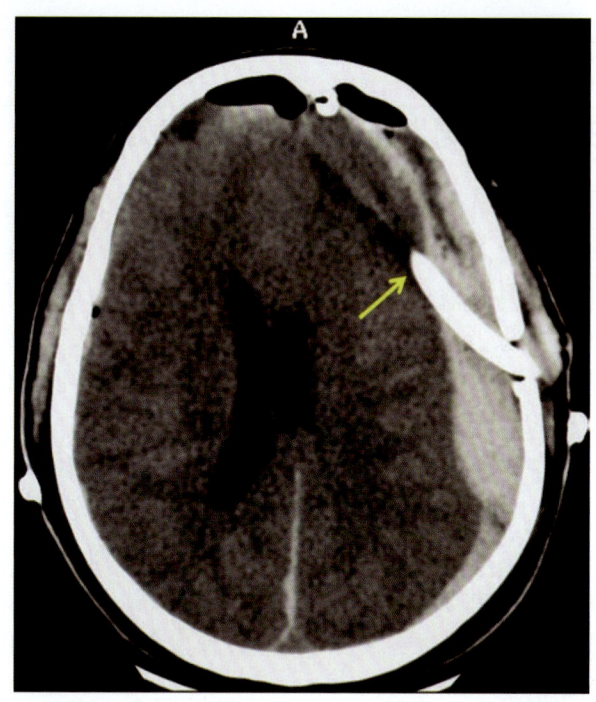

图 33.12 术后 CT 轴位扫描显示急性硬膜下出血和额皮质脑损伤，原因是钻孔后硬膜下引流管放置位置错位（箭头）

性期观察到 8 例（0.67%）患者出现新发癫痫发作，进行 CT 扫描均显示了单纯性张力性气颅，1 例出现急性硬膜下血肿[46]。然而，考虑到在 Nayil 和 Rohde 的研究中患者癫痫发作的发生率非常低，他们不建议慢性硬膜下血肿患者常规使用抗癫痫预防药物[46, 57]。此外，在 2013 年由 Ratial 等进行的基于 Cochrane register 的研究中，他们得出的结论是不推荐对于慢性硬膜下血肿手术患者使用预防性抗癫痫药物[54]。

需要补充的是，既往癫痫发作史是公认的慢性硬膜下血肿清除术后复发的危险因素[11, 68]。有关详细信息，请参阅本书第 10 章"慢性硬膜下血肿与癫痫"的相关论述。

33.6 张力性气颅

气颅症是指颅内存在空气，这是慢性硬膜下血肿手术后早期 CT 扫描常见的征象，近一半的患者可能会在术后出现气颅[23]。然而，大多数单纯性气颅没有症状，不需要治疗。相反，张力性气颅是罕见的（不到 10%），最严重的情况是空气聚集，于压力下压迫脑实质，导致神经症状恶化（图 33.13）[41, 53, 56-57]。由于最终会导致脑疝，既往报道存在张力性气颅导致患者死亡的病例[61]。

对于张力性气颅的发生发展，普遍接受的假设是球-阀机制。许多学者认为，手术中空气流入硬膜下间隙与血肿复发率高甚至硬膜下脓肿有关[41]。在 Ihab 的研究中，在 9 例 CSDH 复发患者中有 7 例发现气颅[23]。在 Shen 的研究中，CSDH 手术后脑萎缩与术后气颅之间无相关性[60]。

张力性气颅患者临床表现包括头痛、恶心/呕吐、癫痫发作、偏瘫、眩晕和进行性神经功能恶化。张力性气颅通常需要紧急处理[23, 41]。张力性气颅的诊断基于先前报道的单侧（图 33.13）或双侧 CT 扫描张力性气颅相关症状。"富士山征"是 CT 扫描中双侧额叶张力性气颅的一个特征性表现：硬膜下空气分离并压迫额叶，在额叶尖端之间形成一个宽的半球间隙，类似于日本富士山的阴影（图 33.14）。

图 33.13 慢性硬膜下血肿钻孔引流术后出现单侧张力性气颅。首次头颅轴位 CT 扫描（a）和术后第三天（b）图像

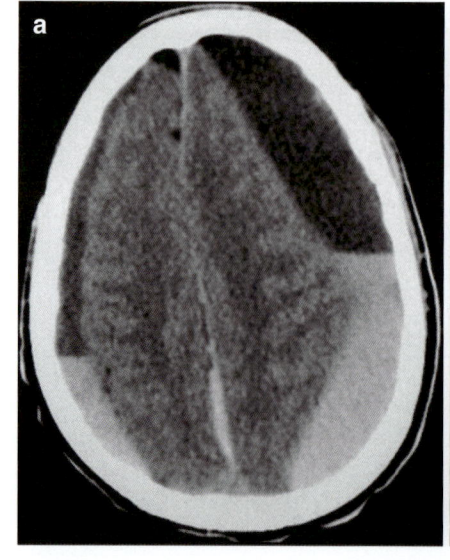
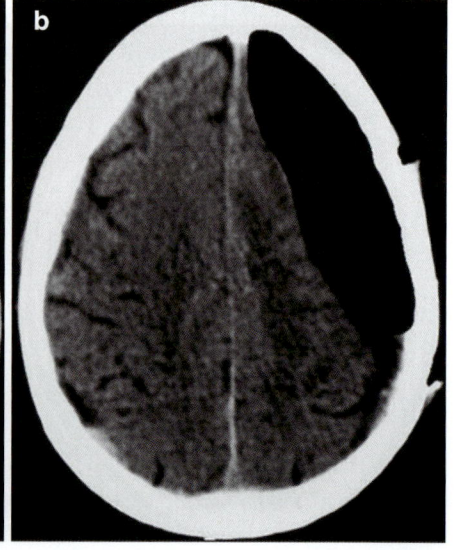

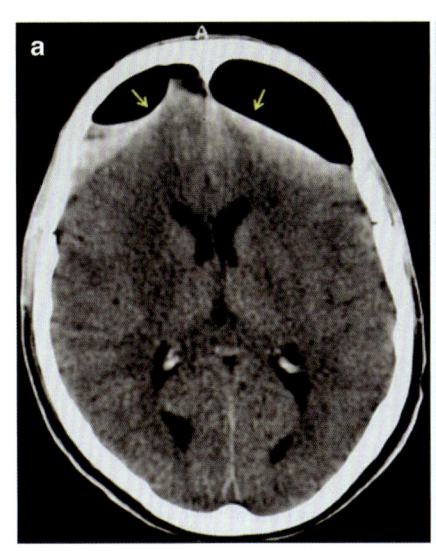 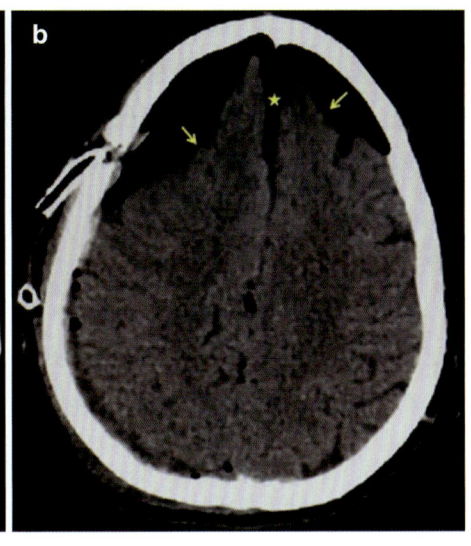

图 33.14 两例双侧慢性硬膜下血肿钻孔引流手术后双侧张力性气颅（箭头）患者（a，b）的术后头颅轴位 CT 扫描。注意额叶半球间性气颅（星号）和"富士山标志"

一些用于防止术后张力性气颅发展的方法已经被报道。最著名的方法包括术中腰椎鞘内注射等渗生理盐水、林格液或空气，对患者大量补液，采取 Trendelenburg 体位，术后加强卧床休息，Valsalva 手法，术中行生理盐水冲洗，用二氧化碳气体或氧气置换血肿，或将引流管插入硬膜下间隙并置入皮下储液器[8,23,31]。对于一些学者来说，硬膜下或皮下引流可以减少气颅的发生，并且有助于伤口愈合。其他一些操作简单的方法已被证明是有帮助的，如向积气腔充入 100% 的氧气和通过注射器抽吸积气对硬膜下进行减压[23,53]。Ramachandran 等用注射器抽吸减压有效地应用于 3 例张力性气颅患者，这些患者预后良好[53]。此外，Mori 及其同事报告的 4 例患者发现张力性气颅后，均立即通过重新打开头皮伤口以排出压迫性硬膜下空气。值得注意的是，Mori 的团队在手术结束时会例行进行颅脑 X 线检查，以确认是否存在潜在的颅内积气[41]。Kawabata、Shen 和 You 最近分别发表的研究表明，术后严重的气颅是慢性硬膜下血肿手术引流后复发的独立危险因素[28,60,69]。

33.7 其他罕见并发症

文献报道了其他一些罕见的并发症，如脑组织疝入硬膜下间隙、脊髓硬膜下血肿、术后高灌注综合征和缺血性卒中[16,24,38,47,70]。所有这些并发症临床医生都应保持警惕。

33.8 非手术（医疗）并发症

如同所有的神经外科手术一样，CSDH 的术后并发症也与各种非手术性的"医学"并发症有关。术后并发症的出现与患者的年龄、一般情况和基础疾病有关[46,53,55]，0.8%～22.3% 的患者会出现非手术并发症[32,41,46,57,63]。肺部（尤其是肺炎）和泌尿系统问题是最常见的医学并发症[32,57,63]。其他并发症不太常见，如胃肠道问题、血栓栓塞、心脏问题、肾脏问题、败血症、弥散性血管内凝血、神经心理并发症和认知障碍。

在 Lee HS 和其同事的研究中，39 例患者中有 2 例死亡与住院期间的非手术并发症有关，肺炎和心搏骤停是这两例患者的死亡原因。根据 Lee 的团队进行的多变量风险因素分析，肺部并发症和住院时间长、患者卧床有关。此外，老年是钻孔引流术后认知功能障碍的危险因素，麻醉类型与任何非手术并发症无关[32]。相反，Rauhala 等推测，通过减少手术血肿清除量和改变麻醉方式，可以减少医疗并发症的发生频率[55]。然而通过局部麻醉方式进行手术，患者的情绪应激可能使焦虑患者出现心脏并发症。

肺炎是在 Rohde 的研究中最常见的医学并发症（29 例，7.7%）。在 376 例手术患者中，有 24 例出现了致命的并发症。尽管进行了足量的抗生素治疗，仍有 10 名患者死于肺炎；9 例患者出现心律失常，其中 5 例死亡；7 例发生血栓栓塞性并发症；6 例发生其他脓毒性并发症[57]。在 Rauhala 等的研究中，CSDH 手术后近一半患者死亡是因出现了医学并发症[55]。

33.9 结论

慢性硬膜下血肿术后并发症的总体发生率被临床医生们低估。此外，由于数据收集方法和报告并发症的标准差异很大，不同研究之间的比较仍然很困难。术前应了解相关并发症并向患者或其家属清楚说明手术的主要风险和并发症。治疗这些并发症有多种方法，但没有公认的标准治疗方法。当考虑二次手术时，应根据收益-风险比选择对患者最佳的治疗方法。最后，围手术期和手术过程中必须非常谨慎，以减少术后并发症的发生率和死亡率。

参考文献

1. Abouzari M, Rashidi A, Rezaii J, Esfandiari K, Asadollahi M, Aleali H, et al. The role of postoperative patient posture in the recurrence of traumatic chronic subdural hematoma after burr-hole surgery. Neurosurgery. 2007;61:794–7. https://doi.org/10.1227/01.NEU.0000298908.94129.67.
2. Akhaddar A. Surgical site infections in cranial surgery. In: Akhaddar A, editor. Atlas of infections in neurosurgery and spinal surgery. Cham: Springer International Publishing; 2017. p. 191–215. https://doi.org/10.1007/978-3-319-60086-4_21.
3. Akhaddar A. Letter to the editor: talking about our own complications: is it still a taboo subject in neurosurgery? World Neurosurg. 2020;142:579. https://doi.org/10.1016/j.wneu.2020.07.191.
4. Akhaddar A, Ajja A, Boucetta M. Combined epidural and intracerebral hematomas after evacuation of bilateral chronic subdural hematoma. Neurochirurgie. 2008;54:728–30. https://doi.org/10.1016/j.neuchi.2008.09.001.
5. Borger V, Vatter H, Oszvald Á, Marquardt G, Seifert V, Güresir E. Chronic subdural haematoma in elderly patients: a retrospective analysis of 322 patients between the ages of 65-94 years. Acta Neurochir (Wien). 2012;154:1549–54. https://doi.org/10.1007/s00701-012-1434-x.
6. Bucher B, Maldaner N, Regli L, Sarnthein J, Serra C. Standardized assessment of outcome and complications in chronic subdural hematoma: results from a large case series. Acta Neurochir (Wien). 2019;161:1297–304. https://doi.org/10.1007/s00701-019-03884-7.
7. Cameron MM. Chronic subdural haematoma: a review of 114 cases. J Neurol Neurosurg Psychiatry. 1978;41:834–9. https://doi.org/10.1136/jnnp.41.9.834.
8. Caron JL, Worthington C, Bertrand G. Tension pneumocephalus after evacuation of chronic subdural hematoma and subsequent treatment with continuous lumbar subarachnoid infusion and craniostomy drainage. Neurosurgery. 1985;16:107–10. https://doi.org/10.1227/00006123-198501000-00025.
9. Chan KW, Datta NN. Iatrogenic acute subdural hematoma due to drainage catheter. Surg Neurol. 2000;54:444–6. https://doi.org/10.1016/s0090-3019(00)00323-2.
10. Chari A, Hocking KC, Edlmann E, Turner C, Santarius T, Hutchinson PJ, et al. Core outcomes and common data elements in chronic subdural hematoma: a systematic review of the literature focusing on baseline and peri-operative care data elements. J Neurotrauma. 2016;33:1569–75. https://doi.org/10.1089/neu.2015.4248.
11. Chon KH, Lee JM, Koh EJ, Choi HY. Independent predictors for recurrence of chronic subdural hematoma. Acta Neurochir (Wien). 2012;154:1541–8. https://doi.org/10.1007/s00701-012-1399-9.
12. Cohen-Gadol AA. Remote contralateral intraparenchymal hemorrhage after overdrainage of a chronic subdural hematoma. Int J Surg Case Rep. 2013;4:834–6. https://doi.org/10.1016/j.ijscr.2013.06.014.
13. Dabdoub CB, Adorno JO, Urbano J, Silveira EN, Orlandi BM. Review of the management of infected subdural hematoma. World Neurosurg. 2016;87:663.e1–8. https://doi.org/10.1016/j.wneu.2015.11.015.
14. Farhat Neto J, Araujo JL, Ferraz VR, Haddad L, Veiga JC. Chronic subdural hematoma: epidemiological and prognostic analysis of 176 cases. Rev Col Bras Cir. 2015;42:283–7. https://doi.org/10.1590/0100-69912015005003.
15. Fugate JE. Complications of neurosurgery. Continuum (Minneap Minn). 2015;21(5 Neurocritical Care):1425–44. https://doi.org/10.1212/CON.0000000000000227.
16. Fujita T, Iwamoto Y, Takeuchi H, Tsujino H, Hashimoto N. Lumbar subdural hematoma

detected after surgical treatment of chronic intracranial subdural hematoma. World Neurosurg. 2020;134:472–6. https://doi.org/10.1016/j.wneu.2019.11.053.

17. Gelabert-González M, Iglesias-Pais M, García-Allut A, Martínez-Rumbo R. Chronic subdural haematoma: surgical treatment and outcome in 1000 cases. Clin Neurol Neurosurg. 2005;107:223–9. https://doi.org/10.1016/j.clineuro.2004.09.015.
18. Goertz L, Speier J, Schulte AP, Stavrinou P, Krischek B, Goldbrunner R, et al. Independent risk factors for postoperative seizures in chronic subdural hematoma identified by multiple logistic regression analysis. World Neurosurg. 2019;132:e716–21. https://doi.org/10.1016/j.wneu.2019.08.032.
19. Hirakawa K, Hashizume K, Fuchinoue T, Takahashi H, Nomura K. Statistical analysis of chronic subdural hematoma in 309 adult cases. Neurol Med Chir (Tokyo). 1972;12:71–83. https://doi.org/10.2176/nmc.12.71.
20. Huang YH, Yang TM, Lin YJ, Tsai NW, Lin WC, Wang HC, et al. Risk factors and outcome of seizures after chronic subdural hematoma. Neurocrit Care. 2011;14:253–9. https://doi.org/10.1007/s12028-011-9509-8.
21. Huang YH, Lin WC, Lu CH, Chen WF. Volume of chronic subdural haematoma: is it one of the radiographic factors related to recurrence? Injury. 2014;45:1327–31. https://doi.org/10.1016/j.injury.2014.02.023.
22. Hyam JA, Turner J, Peterson D. Cerebellar haemorrhage after repeated burr hole evacuation for chronic subdural haematoma. J Clin Neurosci. 2007;14:83–6. https://doi.org/10.1016/j.jocn.2005.12.048.
23. Ihab Z. Pneumocephalus after surgical evacuation of chronic subdural hematoma: is it a serious complication? Asian J Neurosurg. 2012;7:66–74. https://doi.org/10.4103/1793-5482.98647.
24. Ito S, Miyazaki H, Iino N, Shiokawa Y, Saito I. Acute carotid arterial occlusion after burr hole surgery for chronic subdural haematoma in moyamoya disease. J Clin Neurosci. 2004;11(7):778–80. https://doi.org/10.1016/j.jocn.2003.10.028.
25. Joyce E, Bounajem MT, Scoville J, Thomas AJ, Ogilvy CS, Riina HA, et al. Middle meningeal artery embolization treatment of nonacute subdural hematomas in the elderly: a multiinstitutional experience of 151 cases. Neurosurg Focus. 2020;49:E5. https://doi.org/10.3171/2020.7.FOCUS20518.
26. Kamenova M, Wanderer S, Lipps P, Marbacher S, Mariani L, Soleman J. When the drain hits the brain. World Neurosurg. 2020;138:e426–36. https://doi.org/10.1016/j.wneu.2020.02.166.
27. Kaneshiro Y, Yamauchi S, Urano Y, Murata K. Remote hemorrhage after burr-hole surgery for chronic subdural hematoma: a report of two cases. Surg Neurol Int. 2019;10:18. https://doi.org/10.4103/sni.sni_108_18.
28. Kawabata S, Tani S, Imamura H, Adachi H, Sakai N. Postoperative subdural air collection is a risk factor for chronic subdural hematoma after surgical clipping of cerebral aneurysms. Neurol Med Chir (Tokyo). 2018;58:247–53. https://doi.org/10.2176/nmc.oa.2018-0019.
29. Kim YS, Joo SP, Song DJ, Kim SH, Kim TS. Delayed intracranial subdural empyema following burr hole drainage: case series and literature review. Medicine (Baltimore). 2018;97:e0664. https://doi.org/10.1097/MD.0000000000010664.
30. Lam J, Lee DJ, Oladunjoye A. Subdural catheter injection of tissue plasminogen activator for residual hematoma post drainage of acute-on-chronic subdural hematoma: novel case report of 2 patients. World Neurosurg. 2020;133:266–70. https://doi.org/10.1016/j.wneu.2019.10.007.
31. Lavano A, Benvenuti D, Volpentesta G, Donato G, Marotta R, Zappia M, et al. Symptomatic tension pneumocephalus after evacuation of chronic subdural haematoma: report of seven cases. Clin Neurol Neurosurg. 1990;92:35–41. https://doi.org/10.1016/0303-8467(90)90005-p.
32. Lee HS, Song SW, Chun YI, Choe WJ, Cho J, Moon CT, et al. Complications following burr hole craniostomy and closed-system drainage for subdural lesions. Korean J Neurotrauma. 2018;14:68–75. https://doi.org/10.13004/kjnt.2018.14.2.68.
33. Lee KJ, Eom KS, Park JT, Kim TY. Fatal post-operative epilepticus after burr-hole drainage for chronic subdural hematoma. Korean J Neurotrauma. 2015;11:144–6. https://doi.org/10.13004/kjnt.2015.11.2.144.
34. Lee L, Ker J, Ng HY, Munusamy T, King NK, Kumar D, et al. Outcomes of chronic subdural hematoma drainage in nonagenarians and centenarians: a multicenter study. J Neurosurg. 2016;124:546–51. https://doi.org/10.3171/2014.12.JNS142053.
35. Leung GK, Fan JK, Tam MC, Fan YW. Surgical complications of chronic subdural haematoma: a 5-year audit. Ann Coll Surg Hong Kong. 2001;5:99–103. https://doi.org/10.1046/j.1442-2034.2001.00111.x.
36. Lutz K, Kamenova M, Schaedelin S, Guzman R, Mariani L, Fandino J, et al. Time to and possible risk factors for recurrence after burr-hole drainage of chronic subdural hematoma: a sub-

analysis of the cSDH-drain randomized controlled trial. World Neurosurg. 2019;132:e283–9. https://doi.org/10.1016/j.wneu.2019.08.175.
37. Maher Hulou M, McLouth CJ, Hayden CS, Sheldrake AK, Parekh M, Dillen WL, et al. Predictors of re-operation in the setting of non-acute subdural hematomas: a 12-year single center retrospective study. J Clin Neurosci. 2020;81:334–9. https://doi.org/10.1016/j.jocn.2020.09.052.
38. Marini A, Spennato P, Aliberti F, Imperato A, Cascone D, Nastro A, et al. Brain herniation into the subdural space: rare iatrogenic complication of treatment of a giant calcified subdural hematoma. World Neurosurg. 2020;140:65–70. https://doi.org/10.1016/j.wneu.2020.05.057.
39. Martinez-Perez R, Tsimpas A, Rayo N, Cepeda S, Lagares A. Role of the patient comorbidity in the recurrence of chronic subdural hematomas. Neurosurg Rev. 2021;44(2):971–6. https://doi.org/10.1007/s10143-020-01274-7.
40. Miki K, Abe H, Morishita T, Hayashi S, Yagi K, Arima H, Inoue T. Double-crescent sign as a predictor of chronic subdural hematoma recurrence following burr-hole surgery. J Neurosurg. 2019;131:1905–11. https://doi.org/10.3171/2018.8.JNS18805.
41. Mori K, Maeda M. Surgical treatment of chronic subdural hematoma in 500 consecutive cases: clinical characteristics, surgical outcome, complications, and recurrence rate. Neurol Med Chir (Tokyo). 2001;41:371–81. https://doi.org/10.2176/nmc.41.371.
42. Motiei-Langroudi R, Stippler M, Shi S, Adeeb N, Gupta R, Griessenauer CJ, et al. Factors predicting reoperation of chronic subdural hematoma following primary surgical evacuation. J Neurosurg. 2018;129:1143–50. https://doi.org/10.3171/2017.6.JNS17130.
43. Motoie R, Karashima S, Otsuji R, Ren N, Nagaoka S, Maeda K, et al. Recurrence in 787 patients with chronic subdural hematoma: retrospective cohort investigation of associated factors including direct oral anticoagulant use. World Neurosurg. 2018;118:e87–91. https://doi.org/10.1016/j.wneu.2018.06.124.
44. Nagatani K, Takeuchi S, Sakakibara F, Otani N, Nawashiro H. Radiological factors related to recurrence of chronic subdural hematoma. Acta Neurochir (Wien). 2011;153:1713. https://doi.org/10.1007/s00701-011-0971-z.
45. Narita E, Maruya J, Nishimaki K, Heianna J, Miyauchi T, Nakahata J, et al. Case of infected subdural hematoma diagnosed by diffusion-weighted imaging. Brain Nerve. 2009;61:319–23.
46. Nayil K, Ramzan A, Sajad A, Zahoor S, Wani A, Nizami F, et al. Subdural hematomas: an analysis of 1181 Kashmiri patients. World Neurosurg. 2012;77:103–10. https://doi.org/10.1016/j.wneu.2011.06.012.
47. Ogasawara K, Ogawa A, Okuguchi T, Kobayashi M, Suzuki M, Yoshimoto T. Postoperative hyperperfusion syndrome in elderly patients with chronic subdural hematoma. Surg Neurol. 2000;54:155–9. https://doi.org/10.1016/s0090-3019(00)00281-0.
48. Ohno K, Maehara T, Ichimura K, Suzuki R, Hirakawa K, Monma S. Low incidence of seizures in patients with chronic subdural haematoma. J Neurol Neurosurg Psychiatry. 1993;56:1231–3. https://doi.org/10.1136/jnnp.56.11.1231.
49. Pang CH, Lee SE, Kim CH, Kim JE, Kang HS, Park CK, et al. Acute intracranial bleeding and recurrence after bur hole craniostomy for chronic subdural hematoma. J Neurosurg. 2015;123:65–74. https://doi.org/10.3171/2014.12.JNS141189.
50. Park KJ, Kang SH, Lee HK, Chung YG. Brain stem hemorrhage following burr hole drainage for chronic subdural hematoma-case report. Neurol Med Chir (Tokyo). 2009;49:594–7. https://doi.org/10.2176/nmc.49.594.
51. Patibandla MR, Thotakura AK, Shukla D, Purohit AK, Addagada GC, Nukavarapu M. Postoperative hematoma involving brainstem, peduncles, cerebellum, deep subcortical white matter, cerebral hemispheres following chronic subdural hematoma evacuation. Asian J Neurosurg. 2017;12:259–62. https://doi.org/10.4103/1793-5482.144163.
52. Pavlov V, Bernard G, Chibbaro S. Chronic subdural haematoma management: an iatrogenic complication. Case report and literature review. BMJ Case Rep. 2012;2012:bcr1220115397. https://doi.org/10.1136/bcr.12.2011.5397.
53. Ramachandran R, Hegde T. Chronic subdural hematomas—causes of morbidity and mortality. Surg Neurol. 2007;67:367–72. https://doi.org/10.1016/j.surneu.2006.07.022.
54. Ratilal BO, Pappamikail L, Costa J, Sampaio C. Anticonvulsants for preventing seizures in patients with chronic subdural haematoma. Cochrane Database Syst Rev. 2013;2013(6):CD004893. https://doi.org/10.1002/14651858.CD004893.pub3.
55. Rauhala M, Helén P, Huhtala H, Heikkilä P, Iverson GL, Niskakangas T, et al. Chronic subdural hematoma-incidence, complications, and financial impact. Acta Neurochir (Wien). 2020;162:2033–43. https://doi.org/10.1007/s00701-020-04398-3.

56. Reinges MH, Hasselberg I, Rohde V, Küker W, Gilsbach JM. Prospective analysis of bedside percutaneous subdural tapping for the treatment of chronic subdural haematoma in adults. J Neurol Neurosurg Psychiatry. 2000;69:40–7. https://doi.org/10.1136/jnnp.69.1.40.
57. Rohde V, Graf G, Hassler W. Complications of burr-hole craniostomy and closed-system drainage for chronic subdural hematomas: a retrospective analysis of 376 patients. Neurosurg Rev. 2002;25:89–94. https://doi.org/10.1007/s101430100182.
58. Schaumann A, Klene W, Rosenstengel C, Ringel F, Tüttenberg J, Vajkoczy P. COXIBRAIN: results of the prospective, randomised, phase II/III study for the selective COX-2 inhibition in chronic subdural haematoma patients. Acta Neurochir (Wien). 2016;158:2039–44. https://doi.org/10.1007/s00701-016-2949-3.
59. Schulz W, Saballus R, Flügel R, Harms L. Das chronische Subduralhämatom. Ein Vergleich zwischen Bohrlochtrepanation und Kraniotomie [Chronic subdural hematoma. A comparison of bore hole trepanation and craniotomy]. Zentralbl Neurochir. 1988;49:280–9.
60. Shen J, Yuan L, Ge R, Wang Q, Zhou W, Jiang XC, et al. Clinical and radiological factors predicting recurrence of chronic subdural hematoma: a retrospective cohort study. Injury. 2019;50:1634–40. https://doi.org/10.1016/j.injury.2019.08.019.
61. Shin HS, Lee SH, Ko HC, Koh JS. Extended pneumocephalus after drainage of chronic subdural hematoma associated with intracranial hypotension: case report with pathophysiologic consideration. J Korean Neurosurg Soc. 2016;59:69–74. https://doi.org/10.3340/jkns.2016.59.1.69.
62. Sun HL, Chang CJ, Hsieh CT. Contralateral acute subdural hematoma occurring after evacuation of subdural hematoma with coexistent contralateral subdural hygroma. Neurosciences (Riyadh). 2014;19:229–32.
63. Thomas PAW, Mitchell PS, Marshman LAG. Early postoperative morbidity after chronic subdural hematoma: predictive usefulness of the physiological and operative severity score for enumeration of mortality and morbidity, American College of Surgeons National Surgical Quality Improvement Program, and American Society of Anesthesiologists Grade in a Prospective Cohort. World Neurosurg. 2019;S1878-8750(18)32942–5. https://doi.org/10.1016/j.wneu.2018.12.119.
64. Torihashi K, Sadamasa N, Yoshida K, Narumi O, Chin M, Yamagata S. Independent predictors for recurrence of chronic subdural hematoma: a review of 343 consecutive surgical cases. Neurosurgery. 2008;63:1125–9. https://doi.org/10.1227/01.NEU.0000335782.60059.17.
65. Vogel TW, Dlouhy BJ, Howard MA 3rd. Don't take the plunge: avoiding adverse events with cranial perforators. J Neurosurg. 2011;115:570–5. https://doi.org/10.3171/2011.3.JNS101310.
66. Weir B. Oncotic pressure of subdural fluids. J Neurosurg. 1980;53:512–5. https://doi.org/10.3171/jns.1980.53.4.0512.
67. Won SY, Konczalla J, Dubinski D, Cattani A, Cuca C, Seifert V, et al. A systematic review of epileptic seizures in adults with subdural haematomas. Seizure. 2017;45:28–35. https://doi.org/10.1016/j.seizure.2016.11.017.
68. Yamamoto H, Hirashima Y, Hamada H, Hayashi N, Origasa H, Endo S. Independent predictors of recurrence of chronic subdural hematoma: results of multivariate analysis performed using a logistic regression model. J Neurosurg. 2003;98:1217–21. https://doi.org/10.3171/jns.2003.98.6.1217.
69. You CG, Zheng XS. Postoperative pneumocephalus increases the recurrence rate of chronic subdural hematoma. Clin Neurol Neurosurg. 2018;166:56–60. https://doi.org/10.1016/j.clineuro.2018.01.029.
70. Zavatto L, Marrone F, Allevi M, Ricci A, Taddei G. Bilateral oculomotor palsy after surgical evacuation of chronic subdural hematoma. World Neurosurg. 2019;127:241–4. https://doi.org/10.1016/j.wneu.2019.04.043.

第 34 章 慢性硬膜下血肿的术后处理及随访策略

Meryem Himmiche，Mohammed Benzagmout 和 Faycal Lakhdar

译者：吴量

34.1 引言

慢性硬膜下血肿（CSDH）是一种常见的神经外科疾病，常见于老年人。随着抗凝血和抗血小板药物的广泛使用以及老年人群预期寿命的延长，本病的发病率不断增加[58]。

慢性硬膜下血肿的治疗因患者病情而各异，最佳治疗策略仍存在争议[55]。事实上，对有症状的患者进行手术清除和引流血肿应该会带来更好的临床结果。然而，慢性硬膜下血肿的术后管理仍然是高度经验性的，导致我们目前对慢性硬膜下血肿的认识存在一些空白，这些认知上的空白导致了许多关于术后护理悬而未决的问题，例如辅助药物对改善预后的潜在价值。迄今为止，对于慢性硬膜下血肿的最佳管理和随访尚无统一的治疗方案[7]。

术后阶段需要制订标准的治疗方案，这是减少并发症、防止复发、促进康复和改善患者预后的基本要求[8]。有几个重要的因素需要考虑，如抗凝纠正的方法，预防性或治疗性抗凝/抗血小板治疗的开始/恢复，患者早期活动与卧床休息，引流时间，围手术期抗生素的应用，以及辅助药物的使用（如抗癫痫药或类固醇）。

在接下来的章节中，我们将总结对患有慢性硬膜下血肿的神经外科患者的术后处理以及临床和影像学随访策略。

34.2 术后管理

无论患者的临床情况如何及选择何种手术方式治疗，在慢性硬膜下血肿的术后处理中应考虑以下几个细节。这种术后管理从手术室就应开始，包括监测头部位置以及血流动力学和呼吸参数。主要目标是确保最佳的医疗治疗，以稳定患者的临床状态，防止早期并发症，避免任何潜在的神经功能缺损[7]。

34.2.1 患者护理和监护

血肿清除后的恢复过程需要时间，患者最好应能逐渐恢复到正常水平[7]。根据患者手术前的意识水平和围手术期患者的临床状况，患者预计术后在标准内科监护病房或神经外科重症监护病房住院 2～5 天[52, 56]。

在少数情况下，可能需要全身麻醉，患者拔出气管插管可以在手术结束后不久进行，也可以推迟[7, 50]。所有患者术后至少 6 h 内应进行仔细的神经系统监测[7]。

手术后，神经状况恶化的慢性硬膜下血肿患者需要在重症监护病房（ICU）行重症医疗护理[13]。应及时建立颅内压（ICP）监测，以控制患者的颅灌注压以防止颅内压升高和影像学提示脑疝的出现[12]。因此，必须管理几个关键要素[7]：

- 控制血压、心率和呼吸参数
- 麻醉复苏
- 警惕和发现早期手术并发症：癫痫发作、卒中、瞳孔不等大、神经功能缺损、脑脊液漏、感染
- 维持体温和正常血糖水平
- 引流监测

一般情况下，老年或易感患者术后需要重症监护 12～24 h，当患者恢复至术前神经水平时，可转至普通神经外科[23]。术后第二天早期活动有助于预防术后并发症而不增加血肿复发风险[3, 31]。

34.2.2 患者活动

手术治疗后，患者活动的时机仍然存在争议，在早期活动与长时间卧床休息方面，临床治疗模式差异很大[28, 65]。早期活动被认为可以减少术后与体位相关的并发症[31]。然而，卧床休息也可以促进脑复张，从而降低慢性硬膜下血肿排空后复发的风险[35]。

在这方面，外科医生的态度各不相同。一些人建议在最初24 h内早期活动，而另一些人则倾向于将活动时间推迟到引流管移除后，以促进脑复张和液体排出[48]。事实上，术后水平卧床有利于硬膜下积液的重力引流，降低复发率，促进脑复张，从而对临床进程产生积极影响[35, 65]。

此外，研究报道术后第一天早期活动与3天后甚至更晚的延迟活动在复发率方面没有差异。同时，该研究强调了患者术后早期活动的价值，以降低并发症（尿路感染、肺炎、深静脉血栓形成和褥疮形成）的风险[17, 28, 31, 35, 42]。

34.2.3 头部位置

术后头部的位置在慢性硬膜下血肿复发中的作用尚未得到充分研究[27]。术后，头部平卧与头部直立似乎并不会显著增加术后并发症的发生率[4]。

在慢性硬膜下血肿病例中，头部与水平位呈30°并不影响治疗结果，特别是对于症状复发、二次手术或医疗并发症的发生频率[27, 62]。然而，当床头水平升高超过30°～40°而未出现其他头部位置相关并发症时，患者的血肿复发率增加[2]。

在一些研究中，钻孔手术后不久便保持直立姿势与慢性硬膜下血肿复发率增加有关，但与其他姿势相关的术后并发症发生率没有显著变化[29]。根据这一结果，尤其不建议老年患者术后立即直立站立[2]。

目前的结论是，术后患者/头部的位置应根据患者的手术侧来确定。然而，特别是老年虚弱患者，应特别注意长期卧床休息所带来的并发症。

34.2.4 引流监测与拔除

通过封闭系统引流的钻孔引流术是治疗慢性硬膜下血肿最常用的手术方式[16, 53, 64, 74]。事实上，多项研究表明，使用血肿引流可显著降低慢性硬膜下血肿患者6个月的复发率和死亡率[20, 57]。

使用像Jackson-Pratt引流管（译者注：带负压球囊的引流管）这种可调节球囊压力的引流管必须得到适当的护理。球囊内的液体应及时清除。负压球囊产生的真空吸力，可逐渐将血肿液从硬膜下吸入球囊。在操作引流管时，观察周围皮肤以发现任何可能的伤口感染或颅脑脊液漏的迹象是很重要的。

长时间引流对慢性硬膜下血肿的功能结果和复发率的影响尚未得到充分研究[20]。然而，有研究推测，术后慢性硬膜下血肿外膜至少需要经过3天引流才能恢复凝血与纤溶的正常平衡[74]。

迄今为止，关于慢性硬膜下血肿手术后引流的必要时间没有达成共识。一些作者在术后48 h系统性地拔除引流[35, 63]。然而，其他人更喜欢保持引流管超过48 h[34, 40-41, 63, 74]。通常，治疗慢性硬膜下血肿的有效选择是在钻孔引流术后进行2～4天的封闭系统引流，但将引流时间延长至5～7天可以减少术后残留血肿厚度，从而在不增加其他并发症风险的情况下将复发风险降至最低，这样效果更好[29]。

34.2.5 药物治疗

34.2.5.1 辅助激素治疗

越来越多的证据表明炎症介质在慢性硬膜下血肿的发病机制中起重要作用。因此，类固醇经常被用作手术的辅助治疗[26, 54, 65]。甲泼尼龙和地塞米松是神经外科中广泛使用的两种药物，它们既改善了患者术后预后，又对患者存活率有益[37, 67]。

类固醇使用时长为21天至1个月，甲泼尼龙首日剂量为1 mg/(kg·d)，地塞米松首日剂量为4 mg/(h·d)，此后用量逐渐减少[36, 49]，平均总治疗时间约为2个月[65, 75]。并非所有慢性硬膜下血肿手术患者都推荐激素治疗[24]，辅助激素治疗适用于复发率高的患者，如老年人、中线明显移位或CT扫描显示有混合密度血肿患者[5]。为了减少皮质类固醇使用的不良反应，有必要进行临床和生物学随访[49]。

34.2.5.2 抗癫痫预防

尽管抗癫痫预防治疗在减少术后癫痫发作方面

的真正有效性仍存在争议，但许多学者建议在慢性硬膜下血肿患者中使用抗癫痫预防治疗，特别是当合并有其他脑损伤相关危险因素时，应预防性使用抗癫痫治疗。

总体而言，慢性硬膜下血肿患者术后癫痫发作的发生率较低，但由于气体对皮质的刺激，当术后患者存在大量颅内积气时，其癫痫发作的风险要高得多。此外，术后早期癫痫发作似乎在慢性酒精中毒者[10, 51]和术前CT扫描显示有混合密度血肿的患者中发生率很高[11]。

识别高风险患者和急性症状性癫痫发作/癫痫持续状态（ASZ/SE）的预测因素很重要，因为它们与出院时和随访时较差的功能结局有关[69]。远端卒中、入院时GCS ≤ 13和血肿复发都是ASZ/SE发生的预测因素，ASZ/SE的预测因素不同于引流术结局的预测因素[69]。

与Flores等一样，我们认为，如果存在上述任何癫痫发作危险因素，则需要常规预防性使用抗癫痫药物[18]。然而，在开始预防性抗癫痫治疗之前，强烈建议术前和术后进行CT扫描和脑电图监测。术后癫痫的最终预后一般是良好的。

34.2.5.3 抗生素治疗

根据标准临床治疗模式，大多数患者通常在术中或术后一天接受预防性抗生素的单次注射[65]。然而，虽然术后使用硬膜下引流被广泛接受，但没有科学数据支持长期预防性使用抗生素治疗。实际上没有外来物质与脑实质的直接接触会使术后脑脓肿的风险降到最低。

34.2.5.4 静脉血栓栓塞（VTE）预防

尽管接受神经外科手术治疗的患者发生静脉血栓栓塞的风险很高，但慢性硬膜下血肿患者的静脉血栓栓塞预防问题在文献中仍然存在争议。由于他们行动不便和有各种血管合并症，如冠状动脉疾病和心房颤动，因此手术血肿清除后往往需要预防血栓栓塞，临床医生面临的挑战是如何平衡此类治疗的风险和益处。

在许多医疗机构中，静脉血栓栓塞的药物预防通常在引流后开始[50]。也有人认为在病情稳定的患者手术干预后的24 h内早期使用静脉血栓栓塞预防药物是合理和安全的，对慢性硬膜下血肿复发没有影响[1, 50]。

另外，关于使用抗凝药物的争议因较高的CSDH复发率和VTE相关并发症而会持续[1, 50]。术后应用血栓栓塞预防治疗一直对外科医生的决策起着重要作用，这显然造成了选择偏差，需要更多的研究来比较术后早期静脉血栓栓塞药物预防的风险和益处，并确定何时是开始治疗的理想时间[1]。

34.2.5.5 抗凝/抗血小板药物的恢复使用

抗凝和抗血小板药物的围手术期管理是复杂的，其恢复使用时间仍有争议[60]。虽然有符合使用这些药物的适应证，但在慢性硬膜下血肿的手术治疗中往往需要暂时停用，但这可能使患者暴露于血栓栓塞或心血管并发症[19]。在血栓栓塞事件或冠状动脉疾病的病例中，抗血小板药物和抗凝治疗都被用作根治性治疗及一级和二级预防措施。这些药物与慢性硬膜下血肿的发生和复发都有关系[68]，术后管理使这些药物不增加出血或血栓栓塞事件的风险是很复杂的[47]。

在文献中，多个变量仍然不明确和有争议，包括抗凝和抗血栓治疗的适应证，术后恢复的最合适时间，恢复的药物选择，未来跌倒和头部创伤的风险，以及术后抗凝达到治疗水平的剂量和时间[10, 43]。

在接受慢性硬膜下血肿钻孔治疗的患者中，早期恢复低剂量ASA（乙酰水杨酸）治疗与出血的高风险无关[30]。然而，术前有抗栓治疗史的患者发生血栓栓塞并发症的风险较高；因此，术后第三天早期恢复抗栓治疗是合理的，术后出血风险低[22]。

对于维生素K拮抗剂，欧洲心脏病学会和欧洲卒中倡议建议在口服抗凝相关颅内出血后暂停所有口服抗凝治疗7～14天，即使是有机械心脏瓣膜的高危患者[43]。

迄今为止，对于如何在术后处理这些药物尚无共识[47]，因此这是一个高度个性化的问题，通常由神经外科团队和研究人员在充分考虑患者年龄、合并症以及各自的出血和血栓栓塞风险的情况下，平衡治疗的利弊，建立适当的方案[10, 43, 47]。

34.2.5.6 其他治疗

一些药物已被研究并被建议作为潜在的辅助治疗慢性硬膜下血肿的药物，包括血管紧张素转换酶（ACE）抑制剂、他汀类药物、氨甲环酸、塞来昔布和五苓散，但这些药物都没有足够的证据支持其常规使用[17]。

这些药物可能通过发挥不同的抗炎和抗血管生成作用来降低慢性硬膜下血肿复发的风险。事实上，ACE抑制剂的作用是减少血肿壁中未成熟血管的形成[17]，而他汀类药物具有抗炎作用，并通过募集内皮祖细胞促进血管修复[17]。

氨甲环酸已被用作儿科患者的抗纤溶药物控制出血，可通过抑制纤维蛋白溶解和激肽-激肽释放酶炎症系统有效解决慢性硬膜下血肿[17, 66]。塞来昔布是一种非甾体抗炎药，通过抑制环氧化酶-2起作用，环氧化酶-2在慢性硬膜下血肿液中明显较高；因此，认为它可以缩小血肿体积[17]。最近有报道称阿托伐他汀可有效预防慢性硬膜下血肿复发[32, 71]，有证据表明阿托伐他汀在减少血肿体积和改善患者神经功能方面安全有效[25]。

最后，日本传统中药Goreisan被广泛用于预防慢性硬膜下血肿术后复发的辅助治疗[72]。在缺血性脑卒中小鼠模型中，该药已被用作利尿剂，增加尿量，减少脑水肿，也可作为慢性硬膜下血肿术后患者治疗的辅助药物[17]。

34.2.6 患者出院

所有手术治疗的慢性硬膜下血肿患者在拔除引流管和恢复后很快出院。然而，一些患者出院回家，一些到养老院，还有一些需要医疗康复治疗，并被转移到适当的卫生保健机构[13, 39]。

无早期并发症的患者通过手术治疗，其住院时间中位数为3天；有些老年患者住院需要更长的时间。由于手术技术的进步，CSDH手术特别是局部麻醉下进行的钻孔开颅引流术，住院时间逐年缩短[6]。

34.3 随访

34.3.1 临床随访

患者术后和出院后的随访计划是必要的，可以减少并发症的发生，并可以早期发现需要再次手术的患者。

1个月、2~3个月和6个月的随访间隔似乎足以监测患者恢复的进展，而一些研究表明，患者会在术后60天内恢复[45, 55]。

事实上，慢性硬膜下血肿患者的临床资料表明，对于大多数无症状患者来说，钻孔手术后3个月的随访期可能足够了，因为患者术后复发的风险似乎很低[33]。

临床随访需要特别注意：

- 残留的神经系统问题，包括癫痫发作、伤口感染、脑脊液漏、发热、头痛、言语或运动障碍。
- 行为和认知障碍，主要使用包括改良Rankin量表在内的神经精神测试进行评估。
- 类固醇或抗血栓药物引起的任何潜在不良反应。

最后，慢性硬膜下血肿患者术后运动和认知方面的临床改善将导致并促进早日良好的恢复。

34.3.2 影像学随访

术后影像学的应用仍有争议，特别是在无症状患者中。在临床中，会使用多种影像学方法对患者进行随访。一些学者常规进行术后CT扫描作为对照[70]，而另一些作者则会在临床恶化的情况下进行CT扫描[59]。

术后常规CT扫描对最终结果的改变没有产生令人信服的影响[46]。然而，对于神经功能恶化或持续神经功能缺损的患者，应进行CT扫描[61]。

在临床症状与颅内压升高和（或）脑皮质受刺激相关的情况下，似乎有理由进行影像学CT扫描进行对比。此外，术后早期CT扫描可能有助于更好地了解可能影响脑复张的任何潜在的硬膜下残余积液，并发现任何其他复发危险因素[38]或癫痫发作的潜在预测因素，如中线移位和术后颅内空气潴留[69]。

硬膜下残余积液是CSDH引流后常见的特征[15]，必要时可进行药物治疗[66]。Ng等[44]发现可以通过术前血肿量预测术后残留血肿量。因为可以根据术前血肿体积计算的疑似残留体积来评估脑复张的程度，因此术后CT扫描可能不再需要[44]。

基于前面的讨论，我们认为应根据每个患者的具体情况来决定是否进行术后 CT 扫描作为对照，以减少患者辐射暴露的风险。

34.4 康复治疗计划

老年慢性硬膜下血肿患者可能表现出广泛的神经功能障碍，包括运动、言语、认知和行为障碍[21]。尽管手术成功，但手术后患者的活动和功能状态可能仍然受限[73]。因此，适当的康复计划可以帮助老年患者在完全康复之前早日出院[9]。物理治疗在改善步态平衡和运动无力方面起着重要作用，语言治疗可以帮助解决语言和沟通问题，而心理支持可以促进快速重新融入社会[14]。

34.5 结论

慢性硬膜下血肿是日常神经外科临床中最常见的疾病之一。然而，由于我们对其的认知存在一定误差，其治疗方案仍然是高度经验性的，因此产生了一些关于适当的手术技术和术后处理等相关悬而未决的问题。迄今为止，没有标准化的术后方案和常规随访计划来治疗这一常见的疾病。提高神经外科团队的专业水平，制订标准化的术后和随访方案，可以进一步改善患者临床结果。因此，更多的基础研究和建立慢性硬膜下血肿多学科治疗体系是非常必要的（图 34.1 至图 34.5）。

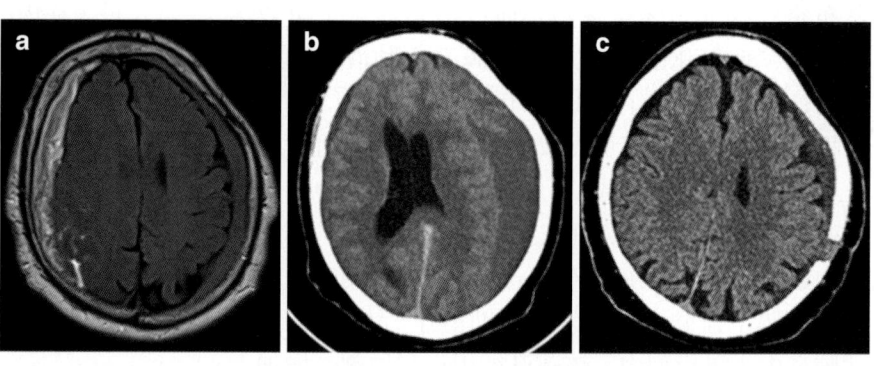

图 34.1 （a）术前脑部 MRI 显示双侧无症状额顶 CSDH 经保守治疗。（b）随访 1 个月 CT 扫描显示左侧 CSDH 体积明显增大，右侧 CSDH 体积明显减小。（c）术后 CT 扫描显示左侧硬膜下积液

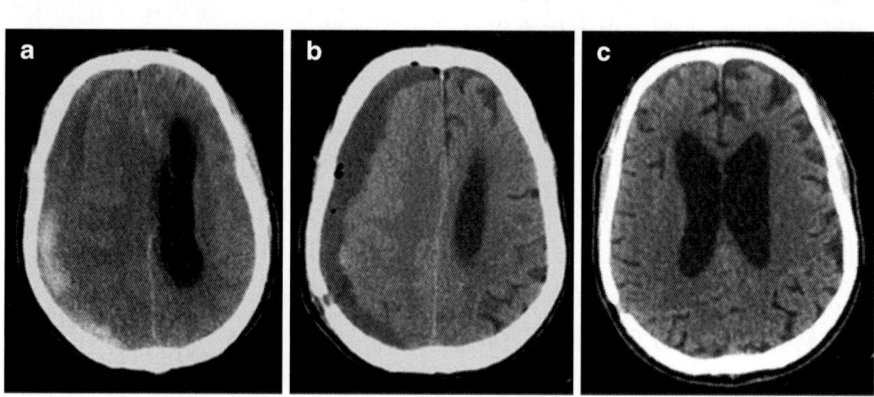

图 34.2 （a）初始 CT 扫描显示右侧额顶较大慢性硬膜下血肿。（b）随访 3 周的 CT 扫描显示慢性硬膜下血肿复发。（c）随访 4 个月的 CT 扫描显示右侧血肿完全消失

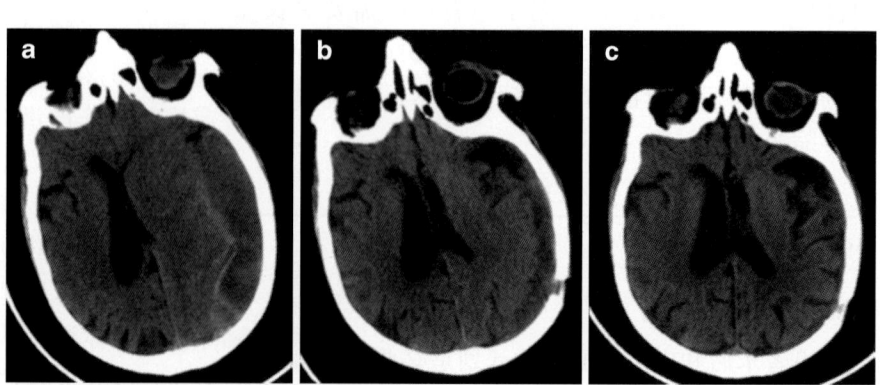

图 34.3 （a）老年患者左侧压缩性 CSDH 的初始脑 CT 扫描。（b）随访 1 个月的 CT 扫描显示慢性硬膜下血肿明显减少，中线结构的占位效应明显减弱。（c）随访 4 个月的 CT 扫描显示慢性硬膜下血肿完全消失

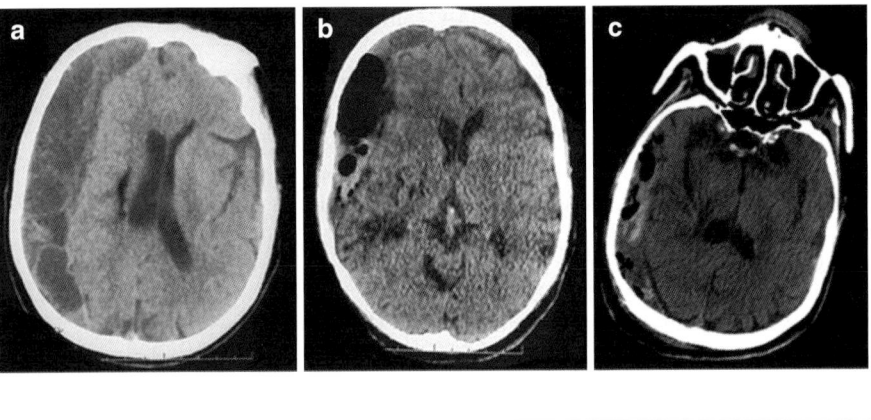

图 34.4 （a）初始脑部 CT 扫描显示右侧压迫性额顶慢性硬膜下血肿。（b、c）术后立即 CT 扫描显示血肿腔内术后积气

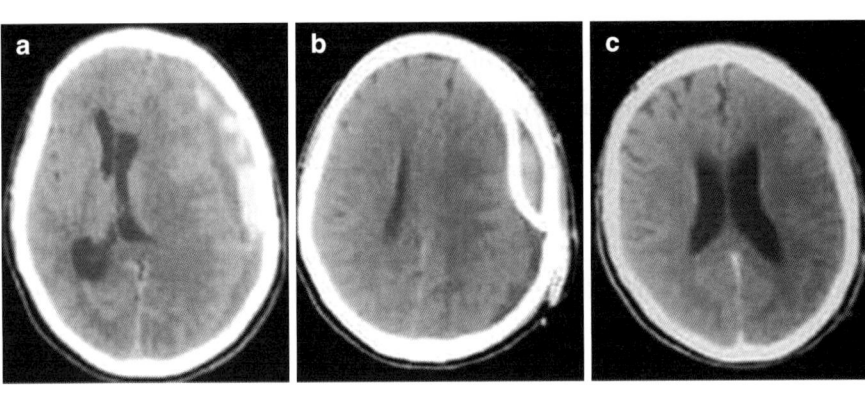

图 34.5 （a）初始脑部 CT 扫描显示左侧慢性硬膜下血肿伴急性再出血。（b）术后立即 CT 扫描显示引流管位置。（c）后期 CT 扫描显示慢性硬膜下血肿消除

参考文献

1. Abboud T, Dührsen L, Gibbert C, Westphal M, Martens T. Influence of antithrombotic agents on recurrence rate and clinical outcome in patients operated for chronic subdural hematoma. Neurocirugia (Astur). 2018;29(2):86–92.
2. Abouzari M, Rashidi A, Rezaii J, et al. The role of postoperative patient posture in the recurrence of traumatic chronic subdural hematoma after burr-hole surgery. Neurosurgery. 2007;61(4):794–7.
3. Adeolu AA, Rabiu TB, Adeleye AO. Post-operative day two versus day seven mobilization after burr-hole drainage of subacute and chronic subdural haematoma in Nigerians. Br J Neurosurg. 2012;26(5):743–6.
4. Alcalá-Cerra G, Moscote-Salazar LR, Paternina-Caicedo Á, Gutiérrez-Paternina JJ, Niño-Hernández LM, Sabogal-Barrios R. Postoperative bed header position after burr-hole drainage of chronic subdural haematoma: systematic review and meta-analysis of randomised controlled trials. Neurocirugia (Astur). 2014;25(3):99–107.
5. Altaf I, Shams S, Vohra AH. Radiological predictors of recurrence of chronic subdural hematoma. Pak J Med Sci. 2018;34(1):194–7.
6. Balser D, Rodgers SD, Johnson B, Shi C, Tabak E, Samadani U. Evolving management of symptomatic chronic subdural hematoma: experience of a single institution and review of the literature. Neurol Res. 2013;35(3):233–42.
7. Bose G, Luoma AMV. Postoperative care of neurosurgical patients: general principles. Anaesth Intensive Care Med. 2017;18(6):296–303.
8. Brennan PM, Kolias AG, Joannides AJ, et al. The management and outcome for patients with chronic subdural hematoma: a prospective, multicenter, observational cohort study in the United Kingdom. J Neurosurg. 2017;17:1–8.
9. Carlisi E, Feltroni L, Tinelli C, Verlotta M, Gaetani P, Dalla Toffola E. Postoperative rehabilitation for chronic subdural hematoma in the elderly. An observational study focusing on balance, ambulation and discharge destination. Eur J Phys Rehabil Med. 2017;53(1):91–7.
10. Chari A, Clemente Morgado T, Rigamonti D. Recommencement of anticoagulation in chronic subdural haematoma: a systematic review and meta-analysis. Br J Neurosurg. 2014;28(1):2–7.
11. Chen CW, Kuo JR, Lin HJ, et al. Early post-operative seizures after burr-hole drain-

age for chronic subdural hematoma: correlation with brain CT findings. J Clin Neurosci. 2004;11(7):706–9.
12. China Neurosurgical Critical Care Specialist Council (CNCCSC), Zhao JZ, Zhou DB, et al. The experts consensus for patient management of neurosurgical critical care unit in China. Chin Med J (Engl). 2015;128(9):1252–67.
13. Christopher E, Poon MTC, Glancz LJ, et al. Outcomes following surgery in subgroups of comatose and very elderly patients with chronic subdural hematoma. Neurosurg Rev. 2019;42(2):427–31.
14. Dang B, Chen W, He W, Chen G. Rehabilitation treatment and progress of Traumatic Brain Injury Dysfunction. Neural Plast. 2017;2017:1582182.
15. Dudoit T, Labeyrie PE, Deryckere S, Emery E, Gaberel T. Is systematic post-operative CT scan indicated after chronic subdural hematoma surgery? A case-control study. Acta Neurochir (Wien). 2016;158:1241–6.
16. Farhat Neto J, Araujo JL, Ferraz VR, Haddad L, Veiga JC. Chronic subdural hematoma: epidemiological and prognostic analysis of 176 cases. Rev Col Bras Cir. 2015;42(5):283–7.
17. Feghali J, Yang W, Huang J. Updates in chronic subdural hematoma: epidemiology, etiology, pathogenesis, treatment, and outcome. World Neurosurg. 2020;141:339–45.
18. Flores G, Vicenty JC, Pastrana EA. Post-operative seizures after burr hole evacuation of chronic subdural hematomas: is prophylactic anti-epileptic medication needed? Acta Neurochir (Wien). 2017;159(11):2033–6.
19. Fornebo I, Sjåvik K, Alibeck M, et al. Role of antithrombotic therapy in the risk of hematoma recurrence and thromboembolism after chronic subdural hematoma evacuation: a population-based consecutive cohort study. Acta Neurochir (Wien). 2017;159(11):2045–52.
20. Glancz LJ, Poon MTC, Coulter IC, et al. Does drain position and duration influence outcomes in patients undergoing Burr-Hole evacuation of chronic subdural hematoma? Lessons from a UK multicenter prospective cohort study. Neurosurgery. 2019;85(4):486–93.
21. Gill M, Maheshwari V, Narang A, Lingaraju TS. Impact on cognitive improvement following Burr-Hole evacuation of chronic subdural hematoma: a prospective observational study. J Neurosci Rural Pract. 2018;9(4):457–60.
22. Guha D, Coyne S, Macdonald RL. Timing of the resumption of antithrombotic agents following surgical evacuation of chronic subdural hematomas: a retrospective cohort study. J Neurosurg. 2016;124(3):750–9.
23. Hanak BW, Walcott BP, Nahed BV, et al. Postoperative intensive care unit requirements after elective craniotomy. World Neurosurg. 2014;81(1):165–72.
24. Henaux PL, Le Reste PJ, Laviolle B, Morandi X. Steroids in chronic subdural hematomas (SUCRE trial): study protocol for a randomized controlled trial. Trials. 2017;18(1):252.
25. Huang J, Gao C, Dong J, Zhang J, Jiang R. Drug treatment of chronic subdural hematoma. Expert Opin Pharmacother. 2020;21(4):435–44.
26. Iliescu IA. Current diagnosis and treatment of chronic subdural hematomas. J Med Life. 2015;8(3):278–84.
27. Ishfaq A, Ahmed I, Bhatti SH. Effect of head positioning on outcome after burr hole craniostomy for chronic subdural haematoma. J Coll Physicians Surg Pak. 2009;19(8):492–5.
28. Janowski M, Kunert P. Intravenous fluid administration may improve post-operative course of patients with chronic subdural hematoma: a retrospective study. PLoS One. 2012;7(4):e35634.
29. Kale A, Öz İİ, Gün EG, Kalaycı M, Gül Ş. Is the recurrence rate of chronic subdural hematomas dependent on the duration of drainage? Neurol Res. 2017;39(5):399–402.
30. Kamenova M, Lutz K, Schaedelin S, Fandino J, Mariani L, Soleman J. Does early resumption of low-dose aspirin after evacuation of chronic subdural hematoma with burr-hole drainage Lead to higher recurrence rates? Neurosurgery. 2016;79(5):715–21.
31. Kurabe S, Ozawa T, Watanabe T, Aiba T. Efficacy and safety of postoperative early mobilization for chronic subdural hematoma in elderly patients. Acta Neurochir. 2010;152:1171–4.
32. Liu H, Luo Z, Liu Z, Yang J, Kan S. Atorvastatin may attenuate recurrence of chronic subdural hematoma. Front Neurosci. 2016;10:303.
33. Lutz K, Kamenova M, Schaedelin S, et al. Time to and possible risk factors for recurrence after burr-hole drainage of chronic subdural hematoma: a subanalysis of the cSDH-drain randomized controlled trial. World Neurosurg. 2019;132:e283–9.
34. Matsumoto K, Akagi K, Abekura M, et al. Recurrence factors for chronic subdural hematomas after burr-hole craniostomy and closed system drainage. Neurol Res. 1999;21(3):277–80.
35. Mehta V, Harward SC, Sankey EW, Nayar G, Codd PJ. Evidence based diagnosis and management of chronic subdural hematoma: a review of the literature. J Clin Neurosci.

2018;50:7–15.
36. Merrill SA, Khan D, Richards AE, Kalani MA, Patel NP, Neal MT. Functional recovery following surgery for chronic subdural hematoma. Surg Neurol Int. 2020;11:450.
37. Miah IP, Herklots M, Roks G, et al. Dexamethasone therapy in symptomatic chronic subdural hematoma (DECSA-R): a retrospective evaluation of initial corticosteroid therapy versus primary surgery. J Neurotrauma. 2020;37(2):366–72.
38. Montano N, Stifano V, Skrap B, Mazzucchi E. Management of residual subdural hematoma after burr-hole evacuation. The role of fluid therapy and review of the literature. J Clin Neurosci. 2017;46:26–9.
39. Mulligan P, Raore B, Liu S, Olson JJ. Neurological and functional outcomes of subdural hematoma evacuation in patients over 70 years of age. J Neurosci Rural Pract. 2013;4(3):250–6.
40. Nakaguchi H, Tanishima T, Yoshimasu N. Relationship between drainage catheter location and postoperative recurrence of chronic subdural hematoma after burr-hole irrigation and closed-system drainage. J Neurosurg. 2000;93(5):791–5.
41. Nakaguchi H, Tanishima T, Yoshimasu N. Factors in the natural history of chronic subdural hematomas that influence their postoperative recurrence. J Neurosurg. 2001;95(2):256–62.
42. Nakajima H, Yasui T, Nishikawa M, Kishi H, Kan M. The role of postoperative patient posture in the recurrence of chronic subdural hematoma: a prospective randomized trial. Surg Neurol. 2002;58:385.
43. Nassiri F, Hachem LD, Wang JZ. Reinitiation of anticoagulation after surgical evacuation of subdural hematomas. World Neurosurg. 2020;135:e616–22.
44. Ng HY, Ng WH, King NK. Value of routine early post-operative computed tomography in determining short-term functional outcome after drainage of chronic subdural hematoma: an evaluation of residual volume. Surg Neurol Int. 2014;5:136.
45. Oh HJ, Lee KS, Shim JJ, Yoon SM, Yun IG, Bae HG. Postoperative course and recurrence of chronic subdural hematoma. J Korean Neurosurg Soc. 2010;48(6):518–23.
46. Pedersen CB, Sundbye F, Poulsen FR. No value of routine Brain Computed Tomography 6 weeks after evacuation of chronic subdural hematoma. Surg J (N Y). 2017;3(4):e174–6.
47. Phan K, Abi-Hanna D, Kerferd J, et al. Resumption of antithrombotic agents in chronic subdural hematoma: a systematic review and meta-analysis. World Neurosurg. 2018;109:e792–9.
48. Prud'homme M, Mathieu F, Marcotte N, Cottin S. A pilot placebo controlled randomized controlled trial of Dexamethasone for Chronic Subdural Haematoma. Can J Neurol Sci. 2016;43(2):284–90.
49. Qian Z, Yang D, Sun F, Sun Z. Risk factors for recurrence of chronic subdural hematoma after burr-hole surgery: potential protective role of dexamethasone. Br J Neurosurg. 2017;31(1):84–8.
50. Ragland JT, Lee K. Chronic subdural hematoma ICU management. Neurosurg Clin N Am. 2017;28(2):239–46.
51. Ratilal BO, Pappamikail L, Costa J, Sampaio C. Anticonvulsants for preventing seizures in patients with chronic subdural haematoma. Cochrane Database Syst Rev. 2013;2013(6):CD004893.
52. Rauhala M, Helén P, Huhtala H, et al. Chronic subdural hematoma-incidence, complications, and financial impact. Acta Neurochir (Wien). 2020;162(9):2033–43.
53. Ro HW, Park SK, Jang DK, Yoon WS, Jang KS, Han YM. Preoperative predictive factors for surgical and functional outcomes in chronic subdural hematoma. Acta Neurochir (Wien). 2016;158(1):135–9.
54. Roh D, Reznik M, Claassen J. Chronic subdural medical management. Neurosurg Clin N Am. 2017;28(2):211–7.
55. Sakakibara F, Tsuzuki N, Uozumi Y, Nawashiro H, Shima K. Chronic subdural hematoma—recurrence and prevention. Brain Nerve. 2011;63(1):69–74.
56. Santafé Colomina M, Arikan Abelló F, Sánchez Corral A, Ferrer Roca R. Optimization of the neurosurgical patient in Intensive Care. Med Intensiva. 2019;43(8):489–96.
57. Santarius T, Kirkpatrick PJ, Ganesan D, et al. Use of drains versus no drains after burr-hole evacuation of chronic subdural haematoma: a randomised controlled trial. Lancet. 2009;374(9695):1067–73.
58. Santarius T, Kirkpatrick PJ, Kolias AG, Hutchinson PJ. Working toward rational and evidence-based treatment of chronic subdural hematoma. Clin Neurosurg. 2010;57:112–22.
59. Santarius T, Lawton R, Kirkpatrick PJ, Hutchinson PJ. The management of primary chronic subdural hematoma: a questionnaire survey of practice in the United Kingdom and the Republic of Ireland. Br J Neurosurg. 2008;22:529–234.

60. Scerrati A, Germanò A, Trevisi G, et al. Timing of low-dose aspirin discontinuation and the influence on clinical outcome of patients undergoing surgery for chronic subdural hematoma. World Neurosurg. 2019;129:e695–9.
61. Schucht P, Fischer U, Fung C, et al. Follow-up computed tomography after evacuation of chronic subdural hematoma. N Engl J Med. 2019;380(12):1186–7.
62. Sholapurkar TU, Mahantashetti SS, Shenoy RY, Ghorpade RS, Maste PS. Chronic subdural hematoma: influence of head position (head low/supine) postoperatively on recurrence rate after burr hole craniotomy. J Sci Soc. 2014;41(3):173.
63. Sindou M, Ibrahim I, Maarrawi J. Chronic subdural hematomas: twist drill craniostomy with a closed system of drainage, for 48 hours only, is a valuable surgical treatment. Acta Neurochir. 2010;152(3):545–6.
64. Singh AK, Suryanarayanan B, Choudhary A, Prasad A, Singh S, Gupta LN. A prospective randomized study of use of drain versus no drain after burr-hole evacuation of chronic subdural hematoma. Neurol India. 2014;62(2):169–74.
65. Soleman J, Kamenov M, Lutz K, Guzman R, Fandino J, Mariani L. Drain insertion in chronic subdural hematoma: an international survey of practice. World Neurosurg. 2017;104:528–36.
66. Tanweer O, Frisoli FA, Bravate C, et al. Tranexamic acid for treatment of residual subdural hematoma after bedside twist-drill evacuation. World Neurosurg. 2016;91:29–33.
67. Thotakura AK, Marabathina NR. The role of medical treatment in chronic subdural hematoma. Asian J Neurosurg. 2018;13(4):976–83.
68. Wang H, Zhang M, Zheng H, et al. The effects of antithrombotic drugs on the recurrence and mortality in patients with chronic subdural hematoma: a meta-analysis. Medicine (Baltimore). 2019;98(1):e13972.
69. Won SY, Dubinski D, Sautter L, et al. Seizure and status epilepticus in chronic subdural hematoma. Acta Neurol Scand. 2019;140(3):194–203.
70. Wu L, Ou Y, Liu W. Benefit of postoperative computed tomography in chronic subdural hematoma. J Neurosurg. 2019;131(6):1992–3.
71. Xu M, Chen P, Zhu X, Wang C, Shi X, Yu B. Effects of atorvastatin on conservative and surgical treatments of chronic subdural hematoma in patients. World Neurosurg. 2016;91:23–8.
72. Yasunaga H. Effect of Japanese herbal Kampo medicine Goreisan on reoperation rates after burr-hole surgery for chronic subdural hematoma: analysis of a National Inpatient Database. Evid Based Complement Alternat Med. 2015;2015:817616.
73. Ye HH, Kim JH, Kim YS, Cho CW, Kim DJ. Cognitive impairment in the elderly with chronic subdural hematoma. J Korean Neurotraumatol Soc. 2008;4(2):66–9.
74. Yu GJ, Han CZ, Zhang M, Zhuang HT, Jiang YG. Prolonged drainage reduces the recurrence of chronic subdural hematoma. Br J Neurosurg. 2009;23(6):606–11.
75. Zhang Y, Chen S, Xiao Y, Tang W. Effects of Dexamethasone in the treatment of Recurrent Chronic Subdural Hematoma. World Neurosurg. 2017;105:115–21.

第35章 慢性硬膜下血肿的皮质类固醇治疗

Timothy Beutler 和 Satish Krishnamurthy

译者：吴量

35.1 引言

慢性硬膜下血肿（CSDH）是最常见的神经外科疾病之一，但其病情演变的病理生理及最佳治疗方法仍存在争议。手术治疗包括多种选择，从传统的开颅术到床边微创穿刺针钻孔术。尽管患者接受了最佳的手术治疗方式，但据报道慢性硬膜下血肿的复发率仍高达26%[10]。除了复发的风险外，手术还有引发其他并发症的风险，包括急性出血、感染、气颅和卒中的风险。对于合并多种基础疾病的老年患者，高复发率和再次手术可能会增加发生并发症的风险。

慢性硬膜下血肿的治疗理论建立在该病可能的病理生理学基础上。涉及多种机制，包括创伤、血管生成、感染、反复微出血、降解产物以及局部凝血功能障碍[4, 9]。目前已知皮质类固醇具有抗炎和抗血管生成作用，因此皮质类固醇类药物因其在治疗慢性硬膜下血肿中的潜在作用，而受到临床关注。皮质类固醇不仅作为治疗慢性硬膜下血肿的单一疗法被研究，而且作为手术干预的辅助手段也被研究。皮质激素治疗慢性硬膜下血肿的有效性一直存在争议，因为大多数临床数据主要来自小样本量的回顾研究。皮质类固醇的使用也存在相关副作用，包括高血糖、感染和精神状态障碍，如精神病。

本章综述了CSDH和皮质类固醇激素的相关病理生理学，以及皮质激素作为慢性硬膜下血肿单一治疗和辅助治疗有效性的证据。

35.2 病理生理

慢性硬膜下血肿是一种层状包裹的血液、血液降解产物和蛛网膜与硬脑膜之间液体的集合。关于CSDH形成的最早理论之一是，它们是由大脑的桥静脉流入硬脑膜静脉窦段遭到撕裂引起的。这一理论一直存在争议，因为创伤后CSDH需要一个漫长的过程才能发展并出现症状。慢性硬膜下血肿通常在创伤后平均4～8周出现症状，即使是缓慢的静脉出血，也会在几小时到几天内积聚大量的血肿块，从而出现症状[4]。随时间推移，慢性硬膜下血肿的缓慢扩大表明出血并不是这些积液扩大的唯一机制。

长期以来，炎症一直被怀疑在慢性硬膜下血肿的发展中起到作用。1857年，Virchow最早报告了描述关于慢性硬膜下血肿的炎症及其在发病机制中的作用。他将这种情况称为"内硬脑膜炎出血"，并认为是感染驱动的慢性炎症反应，导致纤维蛋白渗出和血管新生[22]。从那时起，我们对炎症的理解发生了很大变化。现在我们知道，炎症不仅是对感染的反应，也是对任何细胞或创伤性损伤的反应。

随后在1946年，Inglis发现了硬脑膜中一种特殊的修饰结缔组织细胞层，对慢性硬膜下血肿发病机制中炎症的作用提供了理论支持[12]。这些细胞现在被称为硬脑膜边界细胞，参与血液及其降解产物的吞噬和膜的形成[6, 17]。人们认为，持续的炎症导致细胞增殖形成新膜，并释放促血管生成因子，促进新生血管形成[4, 9]。这些新生血管被认为是"通透性增加的"，会导致微出血和液体渗出到新形成的膜结合间隙中。

皮质类固醇与慢性硬膜下血肿形成的许多机制有关（图35.1）。已知它们通过改变基因表达以及细胞因子和炎症蛋白的转录介导抗炎作用[16]；参与介导免疫细胞的细胞分化，并与膜的形成有关[4]。最后，皮质类固醇被猜测会影响与慢性硬膜下血肿相关的血管内皮和"渗漏"血管。众所周知，"渗漏"的内皮释放组织型纤溶酶原激活剂，皮质类固醇已

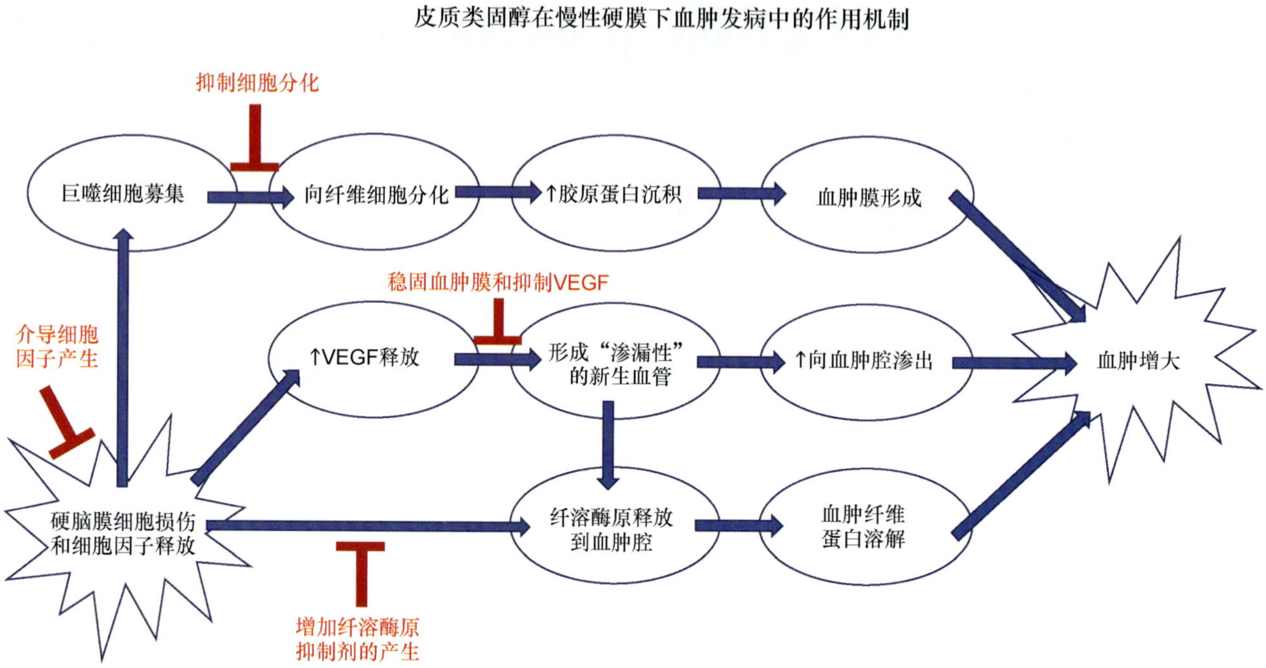

皮质类固醇在慢性硬膜下血肿发病中的作用机制

图 35.1 CSDH 的病理生理过程被推测涉及炎症和血管新生的几种途径。皮质类固醇通过介导细胞因子的产生、抑制细胞分化、促进血肿膜稳定和防止血凝块溶解等多种机制影响 CSDH 的发病机制

被证明通过增加纤溶酶原抑制物介导这种作用[4]。皮质类固醇还通过减轻血管内皮生长因子（VEGF）的作用来降低"渗漏"血管的通透性。据认为，皮质类固醇既可以抑制 VEGF 的产生，又可以直接减轻 VEGF 对血管内皮的影响，降低通透性和液体积聚[18]。

长期以来，皮质类固醇一直被用作 CSDH 的潜在治疗选择。Glover 和 Labadie 在 1976 年的一项早期观察报告称，接受皮质类固醇治疗的患者出现了明显更小、更轻、缺乏膜的血肿腔[8]。这些观察结果很重要，因为它们支持了皮质类固醇在 CSDH 发病中的作用机制。

35.3 皮质类固醇剂量

在慢性硬膜下血肿的治疗中，皮质类固醇已被用作单一疗法和手术的辅助疗法。已使用的最常见的皮质类固醇是地塞米松；然而，少数研究使用了甲泼尼龙。典型的起始日剂量为 12～24 mg，每隔 6～8 h 分次给药，典型的减量疗程为 2～4 周。当用作辅助治疗时，皮质类固醇已在手术前和手术后开始使用。有一些微弱的证据表明，术前皮质类固醇的使用时间与降低慢性硬膜下血肿复发的风险之间存在相关性[1]。

35.4 皮质类固醇作为单一疗法

皮质类固醇已被研究作为治疗慢性硬膜下血肿患者的单一疗法。这种治疗方式对一些患者和医生很有吸引力，因为它是一种潜在的非手术治疗选择。虽然将皮质类固醇治疗与手术或安慰剂进行比较的 1 类随机试验还未完成，但已经完成的一些回顾性综述，在试图解决皮质类固醇作为单一疗法的作用。由于这些研究是回顾性的，因此存在选择偏倚的风险。许多接受皮质类固醇单一治疗的患者要么拒绝接受治疗，要么被认为风险太高而不能进行手术干预。

Sun 等率先完成了一项研究，研究中大量患者接受了皮质类固醇单一疗法治疗慢性硬膜下血肿[19]。他们设定了一组 26 例接受皮质类固醇单药治疗的患者，并将其结果与接受观察、单独手术和手术加辅助类固醇治疗的患者进行了比较。他们发现，年龄较大、有严重合并症和拒绝手术干预的患者通常采用单一疗法。单独接受皮质类固醇治疗的队列与接受手术和辅助皮质类固醇治疗的患者结果相似。与单独观察或手术治疗的患者相比，皮质类固醇单药治疗组的预后也有改善的趋势。

2009 年，Delgado-López 等报道了一项大型回顾性研究，对患者入院时的神经系统检查结果进行了分层[3]。症状轻微的患者最初使用类固醇治疗，症状严重的患者则接受最初的手术治疗，无症状患者未接受治疗。最初分配给类固醇治疗的患者在 48～72 h 后进行评估，如果症状没有改善，则给予手术干预。他们用皮质类固醇单一疗法治疗了近 100 名患者，并报告了与手术治疗的患者相当的结果，甚至在影像上中线移位的患者中也是如此。

虽然有报道称皮质类固醇作为 CSDH 的单药治疗有效，但也有报道称患者预后更差。Fountas 等报道了一系列 CSDH 患者，其中接受皮质类固醇单药治疗的患者复发率（30%）明显高于单独采用钻孔开颅术（7.3%）或手术与皮质类固醇联合治疗（4%）的患者[5]。尽管文献显示皮质类固醇单一疗法的疗效程度不同，但对于拒绝接受手术或有手术干预禁忌证的患者来说，它仍然是一个很好的治疗选择。

35.5　皮质类固醇作为外科手术的辅助治疗

除了作为单一疗法外，皮质类固醇还被研究作为手术的潜在辅助疗法。皮质类固醇作为辅助治疗的目的是降低慢性硬膜下血肿的复发率，以避免额外的手术，而不会显著增加发病率或死亡率。除了几个病例报告外，已经完成了两项将皮质类固醇作为辅助治疗的随机试验。

Berghauser Pont 等研究了术前使用皮质类固醇的情况[1]。他们回顾了近 500 名接受慢性硬膜下血肿治疗的患者。他们发现术前使用皮质类固醇治疗的患者复发的可能性较低，并且发现术前治疗时间与复发风险呈负相关。

Qian 等[15]研究了术后使用皮质类固醇的情况。他们发现高龄、中线移位和混合密度血肿是慢性硬膜下血肿复发的重要危险因素。他们发现，术后接受皮质类固醇治疗的高危患者的复发风险低于单纯接受手术治疗的患者。Fountas 等的回顾性研究也发现，与单纯手术治疗相比，使用皮质类固醇辅助治疗的患者复发率更低[5]。

但是，关于皮质类固醇作为辅助治疗的有效性的文献是混杂的。在为数不多的已完成的随机前瞻性研究中，Chan 等发现，与单纯手术治疗相比，辅助皮质类固醇治疗患者的复发率和再手术率没有显著差异[2]。

最近，Hutchinson 等发表了 680 例症状性 CSDH 患者的多中心随机试验结果，比较了地塞米松与安慰剂的使用[11]。试验的设计允许手术干预，根据临床指征 94% 的患者接受了手术。由于手术干预率高，接受皮质类固醇作为单一治疗的患者数量少，本研究主要考察皮质类固醇作为辅助治疗的使用效果。虽然他们发现地塞米松组的复发率和再手术率较低，但他们发现皮质类固醇也与较高的不良后果发生率相关，包括感染、高血糖和精神状态改变。

总体来说，所有这些研究的数据表明，辅助皮质类固醇治疗的结果可能降低复发和再手术的风险，但可能与并发症发生的高风险相关。无论是术前还是术后，使用类固醇的最佳时机尚不清楚，但均已有报道取得了良好的结果。

35.6　正在进行及未来的研究

不幸的是，很少有随机对照试验研究皮质类固醇对慢性硬膜下血肿的疗效，大多数可用的临床证据来自回顾性观察性研究。虽然这些研究提供了一些有价值的信息，但它们受到非随机分配的潜在偏差的影响，需要更多精心设计的随机试验来比较皮质类固醇激素与安慰剂、皮质类固醇激素与手术、手术单一治疗以及辅助使用皮质类固醇激素的手术。考虑到皮质类固醇可能增加并发症的风险，还需要进一步的研究来确定哪些患者更有可能出现不良后果。

35.7　皮质类固醇使用的积极预后因素

关于皮质类固醇治疗慢性硬膜下血肿的有效性的研究，目前已经从治疗受益的患者中取得了一些结果。已确定的一些变量包括年龄、性别、神经系统检查结果、血肿大小和密度（表 35.1）[21]。

表 35.1　使用皮质类固醇的有利因素

年龄 > 70 岁
女性患者
精神状态没有改变
没有明显的神经功能障碍
轻微症状（如头痛）
CT 显示血肿呈低密度
CT 显示中线没有移位

年龄是 CSDH 的独立危险因素，因为与年龄相关的脑萎缩可以在没有症状的情况下积累更多的血液和液体。年龄大于 70 岁且有脑萎缩迹象且缺乏颅内压升高相关症状的患者被认为是潜在保守治疗的良好候选者[13]。

性别也被认为是一个重要的预后因素。与男性相比，女性 CSDH 的总体发病率和流行率较低。Thotakurta 和 Marabathina 报道了皮质类固醇治疗的女性效果优于男性[20]。这一观察结果被认为与激素因素有关。慢性硬膜下血肿膜的组织学研究表明，男性中雌激素和孕激素受体的含量较高[7]。研究认为雌激素对新生血管膜的局部作用导致组织型纤溶酶原激活物增加和局部纤维蛋白溶解增加。

若慢性硬膜下血肿没有出现中线移位、CT 影像上密度较低，则对皮质类固醇治疗的反应也较好[21]。这些结果也可能与临床症状较轻有关，同时较少的样本量往往出现较少的症状。

对于使用皮质类固醇进行单药治疗，最重要的因素是患者的临床状态。由于类固醇的初始疗效产生可能需要 3 天到 1 周的时间，临床检查状态较差的患者通常被紧急送往手术。精神状态改变和明显神经功能障碍的患者不适合皮质类固醇单药治疗。有轻微症状的患者，如头痛，已被发现对保守治疗的反应良好。

35.8 相关并发症

皮质类固醇的使用与许多并发症有关，包括高血糖、感染和精神状态障碍。高血糖是最常见的并发症，发生率为 6.7%～14.8%[10]；1.5%～12.5%的患者报告感染[10]。最常见的感染报告是浅表伤口感染，然而严重的感染如硬膜下脓肿也有报道[2]。有明显基础疾病（如糖尿病）的患者发生并发症的风险更高。胃肠出血不是常见的并发症，因为大多数患者使用质子泵抑制剂（如奥美拉唑或泮托拉唑）作为预防治疗。最常见的精神状态障碍是由类固醇引起的精神病。考虑到与皮质类固醇治疗相关的风险，有糖尿病病史、胃肠道出血和免疫功能低下的患者是相对禁忌证。

据报道，使用皮质类固醇治疗的患者死亡率为 0～4%[14]。当与单纯的手术治疗相对比时，使用皮质类固醇治疗的患者的死亡率的数据结果是多样的。最近的一项 meta 分析显示，使用皮质类固醇可降低死亡率[10]；然而，该 meta 分析后发表的一项随机试验显示死亡风险增加[11]。

35.9 结论

有证据表明慢性炎症和新生血管在慢性硬膜下血肿的发病机制中起重要作用。由于炎症反应与慢性硬膜下血肿的形成有关，皮质类固醇长期以来一直被用作慢性硬膜下血肿的药物治疗选择，它们已被研究作为单一替代疗法和手术的辅助疗法。

最常用的皮质类固醇是地塞米松。典型的治疗方案为首日剂量范围为 12～24 mg，每 6～8 h 分次给药，减药过程为 2～4 周。在慢性硬膜下血肿中使用皮质类固醇的患者通常耐受性良好，常见的并发症包括感染、高血糖和精神状态障碍。

最近的一项 meta 分析研究了皮质类固醇治疗作为单一疗法和辅助疗法，发现与标准手术治疗相比，治疗方式和神经系统预后没有显著差异[10]。无论采用何种主要治疗方式，高达 90% 的患者报告 GOS 评分为 4～5 的良好结果。然而，接受手术和辅助皮质类固醇治疗的患者再次干预的次数明显减少，死亡率也较低。

有证据表明，在慢性硬膜下血肿的治疗中使用皮质类固醇是安全的，可以单独使用，也可以与手术联合使用作为辅助治疗。根据临床表现使用皮质类固醇可以整合到慢性硬膜下血肿的治疗方案中（图 35.2）。有糖尿病病史、消化道出血或免疫功能低下的患者使用糖皮质激素时应谨慎。对于症状轻微或积液较少的患者以及不希望手术或有手术禁忌证的患者，皮质类固醇是一种合理的单药治疗选择。对于有严重症状或大量积液的患者，皮质类固醇可作为手术的辅助治疗，并可降低复发率和再手术率。

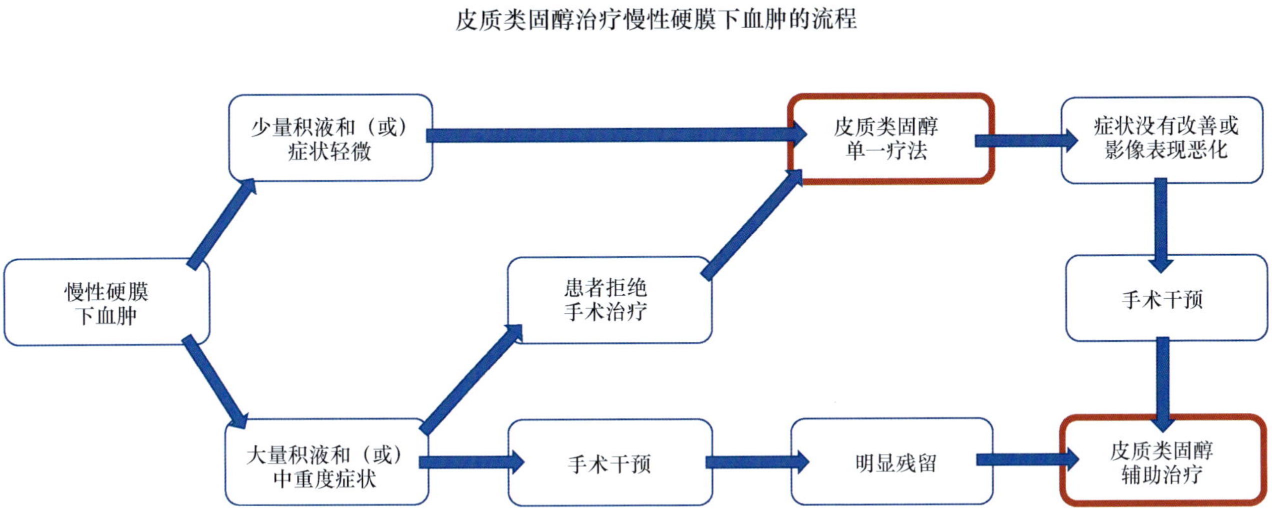

皮质类固醇治疗慢性硬膜下血肿的流程

图 35.2 皮质类固醇作为单一疗法和手术辅助疗法的治疗流程

参考文献

1. Berghauser Pont LM, Dammers R, Schouten JW, Lingsma HF, Dirven CM. Clinical factors associated with outcome in chronic subdural hematoma: a retrospective cohort study of patients on preoperative corticosteroid therapy. Neurosurgery. 2012;70(4):873–80.
2. Chan DYC, Sun TFD, Poon WS. Steroid for chronic subdural hematoma? A prospective phase IIB pilot randomized controlled trial on the use of dexamethasone with surgical drainage for the reduction of recurrence with reoperation. Chin Neurosurg J. 2015;1(1):2.
3. Delgado-López P, Martín-Velasco V, Castilla-Díez J, Rodríguez-Salazar A, Galacho-Harriero A, Fernández-Arconada O. Dexamethasone treatment in chronic subdural haematoma. Neurocirugia. 2009;20(4):346–59.
4. Edlmann E, Giorgi-Coll S, Whitfield PC, Carpenter KL, Hutchinson PJ. Pathophysiology of chronic subdural haematoma: inflammation, angiogenesis and implications for pharmacotherapy. J Neuroinflammation. 2017;14(1):1–13.
5. Fountas K, Kotlia P, Panagiotopoulos V, Fotakopoulos G. The outcome after surgical vs nonsurgical treatment of chronic subdural hematoma with dexamethasone. Interdiscip Neurosurg. 2019;16:70–4.
6. Friede R, Schachenmayr W. The origin of subdural neomembranes. II. Fine structural of neomembranes. Am J Pathol. 1978;92(1):69.
7. Giuffrè R, Palma E, Liccardo G, Sciarra F, Pastore F, Concolino G. Sex steroid-hormones in the pathogenesis of chronic subdural-hematoma. Neurochirurgia. 1992;35(04):103–7.
8. Glover D, Labadie EL. Physiopathogenesis of subdural hematomas: part 2: inhibition of growth of experimental hematomas with dexamethasone. J Neurosurg. 1976;45(4):393–7.
9. Holl DC, Volovici V, Dirven CM, Peul WC, van Kooten F, Jellema K, et al. Pathophysiology and nonsurgical treatment of chronic subdural hematoma: from past to present to future. World Neurosurg. 2018;116:402–11.e2.
10. Holl DC, Volovici V, Dirven CM, van Kooten F, Miah IP, Jellema K, et al. Corticosteroid treatment compared with surgery in chronic subdural hematoma: a systematic review and meta-analysis. Acta Neurochir. 2019;161(6):1231–42.
11. Hutchinson PJ, Edlmann E, Bulters D, Zolnourian A, Holton P, Suttner N, et al. Trial of dexamethasone for chronic subdural hematoma. N Engl J Med. 2020;383(27):2616–27.
12. Inglis K. Subdural haemorrhage, cysts and false membranes: illustrating the influence of intrinsic factors in disease when development of the body is normal. Brain. 1946;69(3):157–94.
13. Parlato C, Guarracino A, Moraci A. Spontaneous resolution of chronic subdural hematoma. Surg Neurol. 2000;53(4):312–7.
14. Pont BL, Dirven C, Dippel D, Verweij B, Dammers R. The role of corticosteroids in the management of chronic subdural hematoma: a systematic review (vol 19, pg 1397, 2012). Eur J Neurol. 2015;22(12):1575.

15. Qian Z, Yang D, Sun F, Sun Z. Risk factors for recurrence of chronic subdural hematoma after burr hole surgery: potential protective role of dexamethasone. Br J Neurosurg. 2017;31(1):84–8.
16. Rhen T, Cidlowski JA. Antiinflammatory action of glucocorticoids—new mechanisms for old drugs. N Engl J Med. 2005;353(16):1711–23.
17. Schachenmayr W, Friede R. The origin of subdural neomembranes. I. Fine structure of the dura-arachnoid interface in man. Am J Pathol. 1978;92(1):53.
18. Stummer W. Mechanisms of tumor-related brain edema. Neurosurg Focus. 2007;22(5):1–7.
19. Sun T, Boet R, Poon W. Non-surgical primary treatment of chronic subdural haematoma: preliminary results of using dexamethasone. Br J Neurosurg. 2005;19(4):327–33.
20. Thotakura AK, Marabathina NR. Nonsurgical treatment of chronic subdural hematoma with steroids. World Neurosurg. 2015;84(6):1968–72.
21. Thotakura AK, Marabathina NR. The role of medical treatment in chronic subdural hematoma. Asian J Neurosurg. 2018;13(4):976.
22. Virchow R. Haematoma durae matris. Verhandl Phys-Med Gesellsch Wurzburg. 1857;7:134–42.

第36章 慢性硬膜下血肿复发的处理

Mohammed Benzagmout

译者：欧云尉

36.1 引言

慢性硬膜下血肿（CSDH）引流术是一种常规手术，通常由住院医师或团队中最初级神经外科医生们来完成。其中钻孔引流是最常用的外科手术方法，术后患者预后通常是良好的[2, 28, 50]。然而，慢性硬膜下血肿的复发是一种严重的并发症，占手术病例的5%～33%[43, 96]，复发可能发生在术后3个月内[45]或更晚[58]。

慢性硬膜下血肿复发是指在初次手术后3个月内，随访时计算机断层成像（CT）发现的导致神经系统症状的同侧血肿。当血肿复发2次及以上时，则被称为难治性慢性硬膜下血肿[47]。若神经功能障碍加重、复发、未改善或出现新的神经症状，则需要再次手术。

一些研究聚焦于慢性硬膜下血肿复发以确定其预测因子，为此研究了众多危险因素，包括患者相关因素（年龄、性别、合并症、临床症状、脑萎缩），血肿特征（偏侧性、厚度、体积、密度、占位效应），和手术相关因素（技术、钻孔数量、引流类型）。虽然已经报道了众多风险因素，但其中某些因素研究结果并不一致，甚至有争议或前后矛盾[13, 18, 22, 53, 55, 77, 80, 84-85]。

值得注意的是，慢性硬膜下血肿复发不仅与一个危险因素有关，而是与它们的组合有关。例如，血肿厚度就与年龄、脑萎缩程度和中线移位密切相关，因为随着年龄增长，脑萎缩发生，老年患者术前血肿量可能更大，导致中线明显移位。此外，老年慢性硬膜下血肿患者具有更多能够影响临床结果的合并症，也意味着术后并发症的进展。

在本章中，我们将总结与慢性硬膜下血肿复发相关的不同风险因素，然后详述其可用的治疗方案及预防措施。

36.2 风险因素

36.2.1 患者相关因素

36.2.1.1 年龄

年龄是慢性硬膜下血肿复发的重要危险因素[59, 84]。部分学者发现，老年患者的复发率明显更高，住院时间更长[68, 84]。然而，其他学者的研究结果并没有发现不同年龄组之间复发率具有统计学差异[39, 59]。

36.2.1.2 性别

一些研究声称，男性是慢性硬膜下血肿复发的独立危险因素，男性比女性会遭受更多的创伤和并发症[59]。然而，其他研究未发现性别与慢性硬膜下血肿复发之间的关系[11, 75]。

36.2.1.3 高血压

动脉性高血压通常与血管动脉硬化性改变相关，是缺血性并发症和出血性并发症的诱因。大量研究表明术前、术中和术后高血压患者出血风险更高[6]。

此外，高血压可能也会影响术后止血。慢性硬脑膜下血肿中脆弱的血管内膜以及外科手术中已受损的头皮血管易再次出血都能解释动脉性高血压导致的更高的复发风险。因此，在围手术期维持正常血压是慢性硬脑膜下血肿管理的基本原则。

36.2.1.4 低颅压

众所周知，低颅压可导致慢性硬脑膜下血肿的形成。这一病因在无颅脑外伤史及血液病史的中青年慢性硬膜下血肿患者中受到广泛关注[99]。同样，低颅压也可促进慢性硬膜下血肿复发[34]。因此，考虑这种可能性并进行治疗以避免血肿复发是必要的。

36.2.1.5 糖尿病

在文献中关于糖尿病这一危险因素的结果也不一致。Pang 等证明糖尿病是慢性硬膜下血肿复发的重要危险因素[60]。相反，Yamamoto 等发现糖尿病可能在降低慢性硬膜下血肿复发率中起作用[100]。他们认为高血糖提高了血液渗透压，激活了血小板聚集，这些可能都有助于降低慢性硬膜下血肿的再出血倾向[100]。

36.2.1.6 癫痫发作史

在 Yamamoto 等的研究中，他们证明癫痫发作史是慢性硬膜下血肿复发的独立预测因子[100]。某些抗惊厥药物引起的凝血功能障碍和肝功能异常也可能同时或独立导致慢性硬膜下血肿的复发[74]。

36.2.1.7 慢性酒精中毒

慢性酒精中毒是慢性硬膜下血肿发生和复发的公认风险因素[32]。慢性硬膜下血肿发生率增加的原因是持续酒精摄入引起的脑萎缩和凝血功能障碍[10]。此外，慢性酒精中毒也会使患者遭受意外头部创伤的风险增加。

36.2.1.8 凝血功能障碍与基础疾病

众所周知，因凝血功能障碍、肝病、慢性肾衰竭或恶性肿瘤而具有出血倾向的患者具有较高的慢性硬膜下血肿复发倾向[32-33, 92]。

Schwarz 等怀疑复发的原因是凝血功能障碍，特别是当没有明确发现其他风险因素时[69]。术前常规血液检查（INR、PTT、血小板、抗凝血酶和纤维蛋白原），维生素 K 拮抗剂的应用似乎对预防手术并发症有一定作用[69]。

36.2.1.9 抗凝/抗血小板治疗

抗凝和抗血小板药物在慢性硬膜下血肿的发生发展中起着重要作用，其发病率为 0.6%～22.5%[10, 42]。这些药物通过抑制血小板聚集、减少天然血小板聚集体的产生或干扰维生素 K 在肝脏的代谢来抑制正常止血机制，显著增加了复发性硬膜下血肿的发生风险[64]。在 Kamenova 等的队列研究中，他们发现 84.2% 的慢性硬膜下血肿复发发生在术后 42 天之内[29]。他们估计，如果早期恢复乙酰水杨酸（ASA）治疗，慢性硬膜下血肿复发的风险会持续增加（每提前 1 周复发风险增加 1%）。然而，在第 42 天之后恢复 ASA 治疗，复发的风险降低。因此，他们主张在术后第 6 周恢复 ASA 治疗。对于需要进行继发性冠状动脉疾病治疗的患者，可能需要在 7～10 天后早期恢复 ASA 治疗，以预防心血管事件的发生[29]。

然而，最近的几项研究表明，抗血小板或抗凝药物的使用与慢性硬膜下血肿复发之间没有关系[29, 42, 60]。

36.2.2 影像学因素

36.2.2.1 中线移位

根据 CT 扫描结果，术前中线移位被认为是慢性硬膜下血肿复发的重要危险因素。中线偏离每增加 1 mm，则复发风险增加 1.18 倍，若中线偏离超过 10 mm，出现手术并发症风险增加 26.93 倍[69]。

Fukuhara 及其同事发现，高龄、脑萎缩、大血肿体积和长时间压迫脑实质会影响脑组织弹性[19]。在这种情况下，大多数患者大脑通常会出现复张不良，导致术后中线移位持续存在[19]，因此术后复发率较高[54]。

另外，巨大慢性硬膜下血肿排空后颅内压突然下降可导致脑实质迅速扩张，随后对周围血管产生压迫，从而增加急性再出血的风险[6]。

36.2.2.2 脑萎缩

在多变量分析中发现，严重的脑实质萎缩是术后血肿体积增加的预测因素。脑萎缩是公认的慢性硬膜下血肿发生和复发的危险因素[100]。这被认为与高龄、脑萎缩和明显的硬膜下腔长期存在导致脑组织弹性增高有关[19, 50]。

脑萎缩导致硬膜下腔扩大。因此，对于脑萎缩程度较大和轴外间隙较大的慢性硬膜下血肿患者，由于压力梯度使得慢性硬膜下血肿引流少于未发生脑萎缩患者，手术治疗效果较差[56]。其次，严重的脑萎缩使硬脑膜和软脑膜之间的间距增加，这导致了更明显的术后气颅。在这两种情况下，脑脊液将积聚并且可能长时间难以吸收，可能增加慢性硬膜下血肿复发的风险。

36.2.2.3 双侧慢性硬膜下血肿

在许多研究中，双侧慢性硬膜下血肿似乎是复发的风险因素[104]。Schwarz 等发现双侧血肿患者再次手术的风险大约是单侧血肿患者的 4 倍[69]。同样，Tsai 等比较了单侧与双侧血肿，并注意到双侧血肿患者年龄较大，使用抗凝药的概率更大，这可能解释了这些患者并发症风险较高的原因[86]。

Tugcu 等发现，双侧血肿更常见于脑萎缩患者，脑萎缩导致术后脑再扩张不良，随后复发概率更高[87]。与单侧慢性硬膜下血肿相比，双侧慢性硬膜下血肿的脑组织再扩张能力较差，可能导致脑实质移位、血管撕裂、术后明显的颅内积气、血肿腔内脑脊液积聚，因此复发率较高[35]。

双侧慢性硬膜下血肿并发症发生率增加的另一种解释可能只是由于统计学上的原因，即一侧血肿的患者再次手术的风险低于两侧血肿的患者[69]。

最后，一些研究表明双侧慢性硬膜下血肿同时双侧减压可降低发生并发症的可能性和慢性硬膜下血肿复发率；然而，其他研究并未证实这一结果[11, 51]。

36.2.2.4 血肿密度

大量研究表明术前血肿密度与慢性硬膜下血肿复发有关，且高密度血肿是复发的独立危险因素[11, 40]。高密度慢性硬膜下血肿中，外膜未成熟毛细血管反复微出血可能解释这种慢性硬膜下血肿类型易复发的现象[40]。

Nakaguchi 等根据血肿密度和内部结构将慢性硬膜下血肿分为四种类型：均质型（均匀密度）、层状型（沿着内膜的薄高密度层）、分离型（不同密度的两种组分）和小梁型（在低密度至等密度背景中具有在内膜和外膜之间延伸的高密度隔膜的非均质内容物）[55]。

根据 Nakaguchi 分类，许多学者已经表明分离型和层状型血肿的复发率较高。在这两种血肿类型中，纤溶强度可能高于凝血强度，导致复发性血肿的形成[55]。至于 Frati 等的研究，显示了炎性细胞因子浓度与复发率之间的相关性，尤其是在层状型中[18]。

36.2.2.5 分隔现象

既往研究发现，慢性硬膜下血肿内存在分隔与高复发风险相关[75, 81, 100]。Jack 等证明，分隔的存在会导致较多的残余血肿量和需要再次引流的慢性硬膜下血肿的复发[27]。Tanikawa 及其同事还证明了存在大量血肿内膜的慢性硬膜下血肿的高复发率[81]。

分隔血肿更难引流，因为必须破坏每个隔室以实现完全引流。破坏血肿内膜并将所有血肿腔室连接在一起以引流血肿液可促进硬膜下液体重吸收，从而防止纤溶及由此导致的再出血[81]。

36.2.2.6 术前血肿体积

通常使用 ABC/2 方法在 CT 扫描上计算血肿体积[76]。术前血肿量的增加是术后残余血肿量增加的重要预测因素。显然，较大的血肿更难以完全引流（特别是通过钻孔引流）。此外，较大的慢性硬膜下血肿具有较低的表面积与体积之比，导致血肿液的吸收减少[17]。总之，引流不完全、血栓形成和再吸收不良可能导致慢性硬膜下血肿复发。

36.2.2.7 术后血肿体积

术后血肿体积被普遍认为是慢性硬膜下血肿复发的最重要的影像学预测因素之一[62]。实际上，Ridwan 等已经证明，当残余血肿体积超过 40 ml 和（或）术前慢性硬膜下血肿体积的 40%（"40/40 原则"）时，复发风险显著增加[62]。

众所周知，慢性硬膜下血肿内存在纤溶亢进和高凝微环境[100]，血肿消退取决于再吸收和微血管渗漏之间的差[25]。因此，术后血肿体积增加与需要二次手术的慢性硬膜下血肿再积聚显著相关。

36.2.2.8 术后颅内积气

颅内积气是慢性硬膜下血肿引流的常见手术并发症[72]。这种并发症是由于颅骨钻孔错位、头部位置不当以及在最终闭合头皮之前用盐水填充血肿腔不充分造成的。

颅内积气会增加慢性硬膜下血肿的复发率[102]。由于患者头部活动所产生的浮动气泡会反复摩擦桥静脉，（译者注：可能导致其破裂出血）所以颅内积气会加重术后血肿腔内的积血[102]。

36.2.3 手术因素

36.2.3.1 手术技术

慢性硬膜下血肿的最佳手术治疗方式仍是一个

有争议的问题。在过去的几十年中已经开发了多种手术技术。然而到目前为止,对于"标准"手术方式还没有共识或指南。钻孔的数量、钻孔的大小、冲洗的有效性以及引流管的位置(无论是硬膜下还是骨膜下)仍存在争议。

许多研究表明,原发性慢性硬膜下血肿钻孔清除术后更低的复发率与使用术后引流相关[36, 41, 50]。这一发现得到了最近发表的随机对照试验结果的支持[66]。两项Meta分析的结论提示,术后引流可以减少慢性硬膜下血肿的并发症和复发率,并推荐常规使用引流[2, 43]。

一些作者推荐使用闭合式非抽吸引流系统,其可显著降低血肿复发率,且不会增加并发症发生率[16]。此外,Smith等回顾了四项不同的研究,比较了每个硬膜下血肿的钻孔次数。作者得出的结论认为,两个钻孔的结果在住院时间和感染率方面优于一个钻孔[73]。

麻花钻钻孔术被证明与传统钻孔术(BHC)一样有效,同时与后者相比在进行硬脑膜下冲洗术后的复发率更低[52]。Almenawer等学者指出,床旁麻花钻引流术在并发症发生率方面略优于传统的钻孔引流术[2]。然而,在另一项前瞻性随机试验中,Gokmen等未发现两种手术技术之间存在任何显著差异[20]。

如今,BHC仍然是慢性硬膜下血肿患者的首选方法[56]。尽管如此,我们认为慢性硬膜下血肿的手术治疗必须根据每位患者的情况进行调整,治疗难点在于确定哪些患者最初应采用更具侵入性的方式进行治疗。

36.2.3.2 引流位置

血肿复发的主要原因被认为是术后脑组织复张不良[50, 55]。术后脑组织复张不良的原因可能是血肿内存在隔膜、血流量减少、引流不充分和脑实质顺应性降低[50]。一些研究评估了手术后脑顺应性与脑组织复张之间的相关性。他们报告称术后硬膜下腔更大时脑组织顺应性更低[19]。Mori和Maeda证明,老年患者、有缺血性损伤既往史的患者、术后硬膜下大量积气的患者和接受抗凝治疗的患者的脑组织复张较少[50]。

关于引流管位置,大量证据表明,引流管放置在额部位置可降低患者术后复发率[55]。

36.2.3.3 引流容量

Shen等报告称,引流量超过100 ml是慢性硬膜下血肿复发的独立风险因素[70]。该结果可能是由于手术期间止血不充分或软脑膜破裂导致脑脊液(CSF)积聚在血肿腔中,即如果脑脊液未能被全部吸收,则导致慢性硬膜下血肿复发。

36.2.3.4 冲洗液容量与温度

Bartley等发现,使用体温(37℃)冲洗液较使用室温(22℃)冲洗液相比,慢性硬膜下血肿复发率显著降低[5]。这一发现可能是由于血肿内的凝血过程的改变以及在体温下进行冲洗时增加慢性硬膜下血肿的溶解度和排空,从而促进积血排空[94, 8]。

此外,还有证据表明术中使用的冲洗液量对复发风险有影响。大致估计,硬膜下腔冲洗液量超过1400 ml与复发风险的降低明显相关[78]。

36.3 复发的治疗

36.3.1 治疗措施

几位学者讨论了皮质激素治疗复发性慢性硬膜下血肿的疗效[53, 83]。Zhang等的结果显示,地塞米松可成功治疗复发性慢性硬膜下血肿,无需再次手术[103]。Drapkin建议在再次手术前,在存在持续或复发症状患者的术后管理中使用皮质激素[15]。

值得注意的是,一些作者主张联合治疗(阿托伐他汀加地塞米松)复发性硬膜下血肿。这种联合的优点是联合抗炎和抗血管生成作用,同时降低了与两种药物相关的并发症的风险[23]。

其他学者主张在治疗复发性硬膜下血肿时使用氨甲环酸作为手术的辅助治疗,特别是在因血栓栓塞风险高而需要持续抗凝治疗的患者中[24]。氨甲环酸可能通过减少血肿周围膜上的小出血、抑制纤溶激肽-激肽释放酶系统和潜在地干扰炎症过程而提高硬膜下血肿的清除率[24]。

36.3.2 外科治疗

36.3.2.1 钻孔引流

对于首次复发患者的治疗,推荐使用相同的手术方式,通常为钻孔颅骨造口术、冲洗和引流,因为这项技术安全性高且围手术期风险更低[47]。通常使用相同的钻孔治疗复发。如果先前存在的钻孔的位置不允许硬膜下腔的完全冲洗，则可以钻取新的钻孔。除了那些经骨孔容易触及的分隔外，不要刻意破坏硬膜下血肿膜的分隔。

可以在钻孔颅骨造口术中联合不同的治疗方法以提高该技术的有效性，特别是调整引流管方向，人工脑脊液灌洗和将纤维蛋白胶注射到血肿腔[54, 1, 93]。

在 Weigel 等的综述中，复发性 CSDH 的报告病例中 85% 病例选择的治疗方法是钻孔引流[95]，其他则采用开颅。如果脑组织体积与颅腔体积有相当大的差异，或者相反由于脑肿胀而导致顽固性高颅内压，则需要进行开颅术或微型开颅术[90]。

36.3.2.2　开颅术

对于机化或难治性慢性硬膜下血肿患者，开颅手术可能是理想的手术选择，血肿清除和血肿膜切除术是非常必要的[63, 90]。文献中描述了几种不同的开颅技术，包括大骨瓣开颅术或小骨瓣开颅术（通常定义为骨瓣直径达 4 cm），以及部分或全膜切除术[65]。

虽然小骨瓣开颅术是一种安全、快速且比大骨瓣开颅术侵入性更小的手术技术，但清除的血肿体积和进行的膜切除术可能不充分[47]。Kim 等报道小骨瓣开颅术的复发率高于大骨瓣开颅术[30]。

许多学者认为机化的慢性硬膜下血肿应该选择大骨瓣颅骨切开术，因为该术式允许足够的暴露范围解决复发性血肿、血肿膜和任何意料之外的棘手出血[30, 63, 65]。

关于血肿膜切除术，是否应部分或全部切除外膜和内膜仍存在争议[88]。一方面，切除外膜和内膜可促进皮质胶质淋巴和硬脑膜淋巴通路对慢性硬膜下血肿内容物排出和重吸收[65]。另一方面，它可以防止外膜的大毛细血管再出血，帮助大脑复张[65]。然而激进的膜切除术，尤其是内膜切除术，可引起皮质静脉损伤。

36.3.2.3　内镜手术

内镜手术最近被建议用于治疗有机化或分隔的慢性硬膜下血肿[46, 79]。在局部麻醉和更好的术中视野下，将柔性内镜穿过钻孔，以便分离在血肿腔内的不同间隔，在血肿内膜上穿孔并清除固体凝块，正确定位引流导管，电凝可能导致血肿复发的新生血管[49, 79]。

虽然内镜手术是治疗慢性硬膜下血肿的微创方法，但与大骨瓣开颅术相比，残留顽固血肿及血肿膜持续残留的可能性大，这反过来可能增加复发率[63, 79]。

36.3.2.4　放置 Ommaya 囊

Sato 等建议使用 Ommaya 囊治疗复发性或难治性慢性硬膜下血肿[67]。Laumer 等主张在第一次钻孔手术后大脑没有充分扩张的患者中植入该装置，此外还在那些患有复发性慢性硬膜下血肿的患者中植入[38]。在全身或局部麻醉下进行植入，通过钻孔将导管穿入硬膜下血肿腔中，之后将导管连接到放置在头皮和颅骨之间的 Ommaya 囊。根据积聚的液体的量，间歇性地穿刺并抽吸囊中液体。

该技术是针对复发性慢性硬膜下血肿的一项新的外科治疗方式，特别是有严重基础疾病或神经系统状态较差不能耐受因多次手术致长期卧床休息的患者[37, 67]。尽管可能会发生一些轻微的并发症（感染、贮器阻塞、出血），但较短的术后卧床期是其主要优点[67]。

36.3.2.5　硬膜下腹腔分流术

使用分流阀对慢性硬膜下血肿进行腹腔引流的第一个成功案例报道于儿童患者[4]。该手术被认为是复发性慢性硬膜下血肿的一种治疗方法，即使是老年人也是如此[61]。所采用的引流系统通常是无阀的。低压阀也已成功使用，主要用于年轻患者中[9]。

该技术治疗复发性慢性硬膜下血肿简单、安全、有效[48]。然而，置入硬膜下腹腔分流需要全身麻醉，并且与一些其他治疗方法相比，手术时间较长，术后感染和腹部并发症的风险相对较高。

在大多数情况下，通常引流约 6 周就足够消除血肿，之后可以移除分流管[48]。有时，硬膜下导管在放置后 3 个月内会与大脑皮质紧密粘连，由于出血等并发症的风险不建议拔除引流管。

36.3.3　血管内治疗

脑膜中动脉（MMA）栓塞术是治疗复发慢性硬膜下血肿最合理、最有效的方法，且手术创伤小[12, 82]。组织学研究表明，脑膜中动脉滋养层外膜可能会增强慢性硬膜下血肿的扩张[80]。脑膜中动脉的栓塞可以破坏外膜的血液供应，从而防止血肿扩大[12, 82]。通过定位出血点，该方法似乎是合理并且有效的。

总体来说，尽管有一些复发病例，但血管栓塞疗法的治疗结局总体良好[12]。在复发的情况下，脑膜中动脉的不充分栓塞或再通被认为是慢性硬膜下血肿复发的原因；二次栓塞或使用钻孔冲洗和引流实现了再发血肿完全治愈[12]。为避免治疗失败，应使用液体栓塞材料，如 2-氰基丙烯酸正丁酯或聚乙烯醇与弹簧圈栓塞[12]。

最后，脑膜中动脉的栓塞可能在一些情况是禁止的或不合适的，如重度肾衰竭患者或脑膜中动脉不通时[47]。

36.4 预防复发

36.4.1 手术技巧

钻孔冲洗和引流已被广泛认为是慢性硬膜下血肿的治疗金标准[66, 99]。防止复发的最好方法之一是充分遵循手术步骤，确保血肿的良好清除。

五项随机试验的 Meta 分析表明，血肿清除后置入引流管可显著降低复发率[2, 66]。已经报道的几种手术技巧和技术存在细微差别，但均可以降低慢性硬膜下血肿复发的风险。在一项随机对照试验中，放置闭式引流或人工脑脊液冲洗与复发率下降相关[1, 99]。术中用大量液体冲洗和术后 3 天静脉注射至少 2000 ml 液体也与复发率降低相关[78]。

使用凝血酶溶液冲洗血肿腔或在冲洗液中加入组织型纤溶酶原激活剂（tPA）也可降低复发率[71, 57]。这种做法增加了血肿清除后排出的液体量，特别是在存在残余固体凝块的情况下。

为了防止血肿复发，Aoki 等通过经皮硬膜下穿刺向血肿腔注满氧气[3]。类似地，Kitakami 等使用 CO_2 气体填充血肿腔，并观察到血肿腔在 CO_2 注射 24 h 内迅速消失，脑重新扩张[31]。此外，Xu 等建议血肿腔内局部应用甲泼尼龙琥珀酸钠联合手术预防复发[97]。

36.4.2 辅助治疗

辅助治疗，如皮质类固醇、血管紧张素转换酶抑制剂、氨甲环酸、阿托伐他汀和中药经常用于预防慢性硬膜下血肿的复发。

在皮质类固醇的辅助治疗方面，术前应用地塞米松可能对预防慢性硬膜下血肿复发有效，尤其是对分层型血肿[53]。据 Berghauser 等报道，术前的地塞米松给药时间越长，术后慢性硬膜下血肿复发率越低[7]。这种现象可以用皮质类固醇抑制血管内皮生长因子（VEGF）来解释[53]。然而，一些学者对复发风险的看法并不相同[77]。

也有报道称，使用血管紧张素转换酶（ACE）抑制剂可降低慢性硬膜下血肿复发风险[96]。这可能与该类别药物的抗血管生成特性有关[96]。血管紧张素转换酶抑制剂被发现可以抑制血肿假膜中的未成熟血管和新生血管的发育[26]。

最近，据报道阿托伐他汀可有效预防慢性硬膜下血肿复发[44, 98]。Wang 等报告了阿托伐他汀治疗的大鼠硬膜下血肿模型，并得出结论低剂量阿托伐他汀可有效诱导血管生成和血管成熟，显著减少硬膜下血肿形成和相关神经功能预后[91]。

在日本，中药如五苓散，由于其副作用发生率低，被广泛用作预防慢性硬膜下血肿复发的辅助治疗[101]。Goto 等证实五苓散可有效预防慢性硬膜下血肿术后复发[21]。作者认为，五苓散可通过抑制慢性硬膜下血肿外膜中水通道蛋白 -4 的表达，从而降低其渗透性来减小血肿体积[89, 101]。

36.5 结论

慢性硬膜下血肿是一种常见的神经外科疾病。手术清除血肿后，慢性硬膜下血肿复发是神经外科临床实践中的一个重要问题，其发生率为 5%～33%，复发性慢性硬膜下血肿的治疗存在广泛争议[43, 95]。因此，全面了解其潜在的危险因素将为改善手术结果和临床结局提供机会。

复发性慢性硬膜下血肿的治疗方法仍有争议。虽然新的外科治疗方法似乎为钻孔引流术提供了合理的替代，但没有一种手术方法已被证明能十分有效地治疗复发性慢性硬膜下血肿。大多数复发性硬膜下血肿需通过钻孔颅骨造瘘术和术后闭式引流术成功治疗。难治性血肿可能需要开颅术和膜切除术、硬膜下-腹腔分流引流术、放置硬膜下导管与持续引流的 Ommaya 囊相连、内窥镜清除、术后持续冲洗和引流，或向脑室腔注入等渗液体以促进脑再扩张[14]。

预计慢性硬膜下血肿的手术量将增加，因此需要使用循证方式优化治疗策略[2]。我们需要更多的调查研究，以明确目前可用的手术方法在复发性慢性硬膜下血肿治疗中的适应证。我们认为，必须根据患者背景、临床状态和影像学结果选择适当的手术技术。

由于大多数可用数据是从对有限数量的具有异质性临床和（或）影像学特征的患者进行的回顾性研究中提取的，从而怀疑存在不同的选择偏倚。因此，需要对大量患者进行大型多中心前瞻性随机对照试验，以确定慢性硬膜下血肿管理中最有效的围手术期策略。

参考文献

1. Adachi A, Higuchi Y, Fujikawa A, Machida T, Sueyoshi S, Harigaya K, et al. Risk factors in chronic subdural hematoma: comparison of irrigation with artificial cerebrospinal fluid and normal saline in a cohort analysis. PLoS One. 2014;9:e103703.
2. Almenawer SA, Farrokhyar F, Hong C, Alhazzani W, Manoranjan B, Yaras-cavitch B, et al. Chronic subdural hematoma management: a systematic review and meta-analysis of 34,829 patients. Ann Surg. 2014;259(3):449–57.
3. Aoki N. A new therapeutic method for chronic subdural hematoma in adults: replacement of the hematoma with oxygen via percutaneous subdural tapping. Surg Neurol. 1992;38:253–6.
4. Aoki N, Mizutani H, Masuzawa H. Unilateral subdural peritoneal shunting for bilateral hematoma in infancy: report of three cases. J Neurosurg. 1985;63:134–7.
5. Bartley A, Jakola AS, Tisell M. The influence of irrigation fluid temperature on recurrence in the evacuation of chronic subdural hematoma. Acta Neurochir. 2020;162(3):485–8.
6. Basali A, Mascha EJ, Kalfas I, Schubert A. Relation between perioperative hypertension and intracranial hemorrhage after craniotomy. Anesthesiology. 2000;93:48–54.
7. Berghauser Pont LM, Dammers R, Schouten JW, Lingsma HF, Dirven CM. Clinical factors associated with outcome in chronic subdural hematoma: a retrospective cohort study of patients on pre-operative corticosteroid therapy. Neurosurgery. 2012;70(4):873–80.
8. Black S, Muller F. On the effect of temperature on aqueous solubility of organic solids. Org Process Res Dev. 2010;14(3):661–5.
9. Cameron MM. Chronic subdural hematoma: a review of 114 cases. J Neurol Neurosurg Psychiatry. 1978;41:834–9.
10. Chen JC, Levy ML. Causes, epidemiology, and risk factors of chronic subdural hematoma. Neurosurg Clin N Am. 2000;11:399–406.
11. Chen FM, Wang K, Xu KL, Wang L, Zhan TX, Cheng F, et al. Predictors of acute intracranial hemorrhage and recurrence of chronic subdural hematoma following burr hole drainage. BMC Neurol. 2020;20(1):92.
12. Chihara H, Imamura H, Ogura T, Adachi H, Imai Y, Sakai N. Recurrence of a refractory chronic subdural hematoma after middle meningeal artery embolization that required craniotomy. NMC Case Rep J. 2014;1:1–5.
13. Chon KH, Lee JM, Koh EJ, Choi HY. Independent predictors for recurrence of chronic subdural hematoma. Acta Neurochir. 2012;154(9):1541–8.
14. Desai VR, Scranton RA, Britz GW. Management of recurrent subdural hematomas. Neurosurg Clin N Am. 2017;28(2):279–86.
15. Drapkin AJ. Chronic subdural hematoma: pathophysiological basis for treatment. Br J Neurosurg. 1991;5:467–73.
16. Ducruet AF, Grobelny BT, Zacharia BE, Hickman ZL, DeRosa PL, Anderson K, et al. The surgical management of chronic subdural hematoma. Neurosurg Rev. 2012;35:155–69.
17. El-Kadi H, Miele VJ, Kaufman HH. Prognosis of chronic subdural hematomas. Neurosurg Clin N Am. 2000;11:553–5567.
18. Frati A, Salvati M, Mainiero F, Ippoliti F, Rocchi G, Raco A, et al. Inflammation markers and risk factors for recurrence in 35 patients with a posttraumatic chronic subdural hematoma: a prospective study. J Neurosurg. 2004;100(1):24–32.
19. Fukuhara T, Gotoh M, Asari S, Ohmoto T, Akioka T. The relationship between brain surface elastance and brain reexpansion after evacuation of chronic subdural hematoma. Surg Neurol. 1996;45:570–4.
20. Gokmen M, Sucu HK, Ergin A, Gokmen A, Bezircio Lu H. Randomized comparative study

of burr-hole craniostomy versus twist drill craniostomy: surgical management of unilateral hemispheric chronic subdural hematomas. Zentralbl Neurochir. 2008;69:129–33.
21. Goto S, Kato K, Yamamoto T, Shimato S, Ohshima T, Nishizawa T. Effectiveness of Goreisan in preventing recurrence of chronic subdural hematoma. Asian J Neurosurg. 2018;13:370–4.
22. Han MH, Ryu JI, Kim CH, Kim JM, Cheong JH, Yi HJ. Predictive factors for recurrence and clinical outcomes in patients with chronic subdural hematoma. J Neurosurg. 2017;127(5):1117–25.
23. Huang J, Li L, Zhang J, Gao C, Quan W, Tian Y, et al. Treatment of relapsed chronic subdural hematoma in four young children with atorvastatin and low-dose dexamethasone. Pharmacotherapy. 2019;39(7):783–9.
24. Iorio-Morin C, Blanchard J, Richer M, Mathieu D. Tranexamic Acid in Chronic Subdural Hematomas (TRACS): study protocol for a randomized controlled trial. Trials. 2016;17(1):235.
25. Ito H, Komai T, Yamamoto S. Fibrinolytic enzyme in the lining walls of chronic subdural hematoma. J Neurosurg. 1978;48:197–200.
26. Ivamoto HS, Lemos HP Jr, Atallah AN. Surgical treatments for chronic subdural hematomas: a comprehensive systematic review. World Neurosurg. 2016;86:399–418.
27. Jack A, O'Kelly C, McDougall C, Findlay JM. Predicting recurrence after chronic subdural hematoma drainage. Can J Neurol Sci. 2015;42(1):34–9.
28. Jang KM, Kwon JT, Hwang SN, Park YS, Nam TK. Comparison of the outcomes and recurrence with three surgical techniques for chronic subdural hematoma: single, double burr hole, and double burr hole drainage with irrigation. Korean J Neurotrauma. 2015;11(2):75–80.
29. Kamenova M, Lutz K, Schaedelin S, Fandino J, Mariani L, Soleman J. Does early resumption of low-dose Aspirin after evacuation of chronic subdural hematoma with burr-hole drainage lead to higher recurrence rates? Neurosurgery. 2016;79(5):715–21.
30. Kim JH, Kang DS, Kim JH, Kong MH, Song KY. Chronic subdural hematoma treated by small or large craniotomy with membranectomy as the initial treatment. J Korean Neurosurg Soc. 2011;50:103–8.
31. Kitakami A, Ogawa A, Hakozaki S, Kidoguchi J, Obonai C, Kubo N. Carbon dioxide gas replacement of chronic subdural hematoma using single burr-hole irrigation. Surg Neurol. 1995;43:574–7.
32. Ko BS, Lee JK, Seo BR, Moon SJ, Kim JH, Kim SH. Clinical analysis of risk factors related to recurrent chronic subdural hematoma. J Korean Neurosurg Soc. 2008;43:11–5.
33. Konig SA, Schick U, Dohnert J, Goldammer A, Vitzthum HE. Coagulopathy and outcome in patients with chronic subdural hematoma. Acta Neurol Scand. 2003;107:110–6.
34. Kristof RA, Grimm JM, Stoffel-Wagner B. Cerebrospinal fluid leakage into the subdural space: possible influence on the pathogenesis and recurrence frequency of chronic subdural hematoma and subdural hygroma. J Neurosurg. 2008;108:275–80.
35. Kung WM, Hung KS, Chiu WT, Tsai SH, Lin JW, Wang YC, et al. Quantitative assessment of impaired post evacuation brain re-expansion in bilateral chronic subdural hematoma: possible mechanism of the higher recurrence rate. Injury. 2012;43(5):598–602.
36. Kutty SA, Johny M. Chronic subdural hematoma: a comparison of recurrence rates following burr-hole craniostomy with and without drains. Turk Neurosurg. 2014;24(4):494–7.
37. Laumer R. Implantation of a reservoir for refractory chronic subdural hematoma. Neurosurgery. 2002;50(3):672.
38. Laumer R, Schramm J, Leykauf K. Implantation of a reservoir for recurrent subdural hematoma drainage. Neurosurgery. 1989;25(6):991–6.
39. Liliang PC, Tsai YD, Liang CL, Lee TC, Chen HJ. Chronic subdural hematoma in young and extremely aged adults: a comparative study of two age groups. Injury. 2002;33:345–8.
40. Lin CC, Lu YM, Chen TH, Wang SP, Hsiao SH, Lin MS. Quantitative assessment of postoperative recurrence of chronic subdural hematoma using mean hematoma density. Brain Inj. 2014;28(8):1082–6.
41. Lind CR, Lind CJ, Mee EW. Reduction in the number of repeated operations for the treatment of subacute and chronic subdural hematomas by placement of subdural drains. J Neurosurg. 2003;99:44–6.
42. Lindvall P, Koskinen LO. Anticoagulants and antiplatelet agents and the risk of development and recurrence of chronic subdural hematomas. J Clin Neurosci. 2009;16:1287–90.
43. Liu W, Bakker NA, Groen RJ. Chronic subdural hematoma: a systematic review and meta-analysis of surgical procedures. J Neurosurg. 2014;121:665–73.
44. Liu H, Luo Z, Liu Z, Yang J, Kan S. Atorvastatin may attenuate recurrence of chronic subdu-

ral hematoma. Front Neurosci. 2016;10:303.
45. Lutz K, Kamenova M, Schaedelin S, Guzman R, Mariani L, Fandino J, Soleman J. Time to and possible risk factors for recurrence after Burr-hole drainage of chronic subdural hematoma: a subanalysis of the cSDH-drain randomized controlled trial. World Neurosurg. 2019;132:e283–9.
46. Majovsky M, Masopust V, Netuka D, Benes V. Flexible endoscope-assisted evacuation of chronic subdural hematomas. Acta Neurochir. 2016;158:1987–92.
47. Matsumoto H, Hanayama H, Okada T, Sakurai Y, Minami H, Masuda A, et al. Which surgical procedure is effective for refractory chronic subdural hematoma? Analysis of our surgical procedures and literature review. J Clin Neurosci. 2018;49:40–7.
48. Misra M, Salazar JL, Bloom DM. Subdural-peritoneal shunt: treatment for bilateral chronic subdural hematoma. Surg Neurol. 1996;46(4):378–83.
49. Mobbs R, Khong P. Endoscopic-assisted evacuation of subdural collections. J Clin Neurosci. 2009;16:701–4.
50. Mori K, Maeda M. Surgical treatment of chronic subdural hematoma in 500 consecutive cases: clinical characteristics, surgical outcome, complications, and recurrence rate. Neurol Med Chir. 2001;41(8):371–81.
51. Motiei-Langroudi R, Thomas AJ, Ascanio L, Alturki A, Papavassiliou E, Kasper EM, et al. Factors predicting the need for surgery of the opposite side after unilateral evacuation of bilateral chronic subdural hematomas. Neurosurgery. 2018;85(5):648–55.
52. Muzii VF, Bistazzoni S, Zalaffi A, Carangelo B, Mariottini A, Palma L. Chronic subdural hematoma: comparison of two surgical techniques. Preliminary results of a prospective randomized study. J Neurosurg Sci. 2005;49:41–6.
53. Nagatani K, Wada K, Takeuchi S, Nawashiro H. Corticosteroid suppression of vascular endothelial growth factor and recurrence of chronic subdural hematoma. Neurosurgery. 2012;70:E1334.
54. Nakaguchi H, Tanishima T, Yoshimasu N. Relationship between drainage catheter location and postoperative recurrence of chronic subdural hematoma after burr-hole irrigation and closed-system drainage. J Neurosurg. 2000;93(5):791–5.
55. Nakaguchi H, Tanishima T, Yoshimasu N. Factors in the natural history of chronic subdural hematomas that influence their postoperative recurrence. J Neurosurg. 2001;95(2):256–62.
56. Neal MT, Hsu W, Urban JE, Angelo NM, Sweasey TA, Branch CL Jr. The subdural evacuation port system: outcomes from a single institution experience and predictors of success. Clin Neurol Neurosurg. 2013;115(6):658–64.
57. Neils DM, Singanallur PS, Wang H, Tracy P, Klopfenstein J, Dinh D, et al. Recurrence-free chronic subdural hematomas: a retrospective analysis of the instillation of tissue plasminogen activator in addition to twist drill or burr-hole drainage in the treatment of chronic subdural hematomas. World Neurosurg. 2012;78:145–9.
58. Oh HJ, Lee KS, Shim JJ, Yoon SM, Yun IG, Bae HG. Postoperative course and recurrence of chronic subdural hematoma. J Korean Neurosurg Soc. 2010;48:518–23.
59. Ou Y, Dong J, Wu L, Xu L, Wang L, Liu B, et al. A comparative study of chronic subdural hematoma in three age ranges: below 40 years, 41-79 years, and 80 years and older. Clin Neurol Neurosurg. 2019;178:63–9.
60. Pang CH, Lee SE, Kim CH, Kim JE, Kang HS, Park CK, et al. Acute intracranial bleeding and recurrence after bur hole craniostomy for chronic subdural hematoma. J Neurosurg. 2015;123(1):65–74.
61. Probst C. Peritoneal drainage of chronic subdural hematomas in older patients. J Neurosurg. 1988;68(6):908–11.
62. Ridwan S, Bohrer AM, Grote A, Simon M. Surgical treatment of chronic subdural hematoma: predicting recurrence and cure. World Neurosurg. 2019;128:e1010–23.
63. Rocchi G, Caroli E, Salvati M, Delfini R. Membranectomy in organized chronic subdural hematomas: indications and technical notes. Surg Neurol. 2007;67:374–80.
64. Rust T, Kiemer N, Erasmus A. Chronic subdural hematomas and anticoagulation or antithrombotic therapy. J Clin Neurosci. 2006;13(8):823–7.
65. Sahyouni R, Mahboubi H, Tran P, Roufail JS, Chen JW. Membranectomy in chronic subdural hematoma: meta-analysis. World Neurosurg. 2017;104:418–29.
66. Santarius T, Kirkpatrick PJ, Ganesan D, Chia HL, Jalloh I, Smielewski P, et al. Use of drains versus no drains after burr-hole evacuation of chronic subdural hematoma: a randomized controlled trial. Lancet. 2009;374:1067–73.
67. Sato M, Iwatsuki K, Akiyama C, Kumura E, Yoshimine T. Implantation of a reservoir for

refractory chronic subdural hematoma. Neurosurgery. 2001;48:1297–301.
68. Schoedel P, Bruendl E, Hochreiter A, Scheitzach J, Bele S, Brawanski A, Schebesch KM. Restoration of functional integrity after evacuation of chronic subdural hematoma-an age-adjusted analysis of 697 patients. World Neurosurg. 2016;94:465–70.
69. Schwarz F, Loos F, Dünisch P, Sakr Y, Safatli DA, Kalff R, Ewald C. Risk factors for reoperation after initial burr hole trephination in chronic subdural hematomas. Clin Neurol Neurosurg. 2015;138:66–71.
70. Shen J, Yuan L, Ge R, Wang Q, Zhou W, Jiang XC, Shao X. Clinical and radiological factors predicting recurrence of chronic subdural hematoma: a retrospective cohort study. Injury. 2019;50(10):1634–40.
71. Shimamura N, Ogasawara Y, Naraoka M, Ohnkuma H. Irrigation with thrombin solution reduces recurrence of chronic subdural hematoma in high-risk patients: preliminary report. J Neurotrauma. 2009;26:1929–33.
72. Shin HS, Lee SH, Ko HC, Koh JS. Extended pneumocephalus after drainage of chronic subdural hematoma associated with intracranial hypotension: case report with pathophysiologic consideration. J Korean Neurosurg Soc. 2016;59(1):69–74.
73. Smith MD, Kishikova L, Norris JM. Surgical management of chronic subdural hematoma: one hole or two? Int J Surg. 2012;10:450–2.
74. So CC, Wong KF. Valproate-associated dysmyelopoiesis in elderly patients. Am J Clin Pathol. 2002;118:225–8.
75. Stanisic M, Lund-Johansen M, Mahesparan R. Treatment of chronic subdural hematoma by burr-hole craniostomy in adults: influence of some factors on postoperative recurrence. Acta Neurochir. 2005;147:1249–57.
76. Sucu HK, Gokmen M, Gelal F. The value of XYZ/2 technique compared with computer-assisted volumetric analysis to estimate the volume of chronic subdural hematoma. Stroke. 2005;36:998–1000.
77. Sun TF, Boet R, Poon WS. Non-surgical primary treatment of chronic subdural haematoma: preliminary results of using dexamethasone. Br J Neurosurg. 2005;19:327–33.
78. Tahsim-Oglou Y, Beseoglu K, Hänggi D, Stummer W, Steiger H-J. Factors predicting recurrence of chronic subdural hematoma: the influence of intraoperative irrigation and low-molecular-weight heparin thromboprophylaxis. Acta Neurochir. 2012;154(6):1063–8.
79. Takahashi S, Yazaki T, Nitori N, Kano T, Yoshida K, Kawase T. Neuroendoscope assisted removal of an organized chronic subdural hematoma in a patient on bevacizumab therapy–case report. Neurol Med Chir. 2011;51:515–8.
80. Tanaka T, Kaimori M. Histological study of vascular structure between the dura mater and the outer membrane in chronic subdural hematoma in an adult. No Shinkei Geka. 1999;27:431–6.
81. Tanikawa M, Mase M, Yamada K, Yamashita N, Matsumoto T, Banno T, Miyati T. Surgical treatment of chronic subdural hematoma based on intrahematomal membrane structure on MRI. Acta Neurochir. 2001;143(6):613–9.
82. Tempaku A, Yamauchi S, Ikeda H, Tsubota N, Furukawa H, Maeda D, et al. Usefulness of interventional embolization of the middle meningeal artery for recurrent chronic subdural hematoma: five cases and a review of the literature. Interv Neuroradiol. 2015;21:366–71.
83. Thotakura AK, Marabathina NR. Nonsurgical treatment of chronic subdural hematoma with steroids. World Neurosurg. 2015;84(6):1968–72.
84. Toi H, Kinoshita K, Hirai S, Takai H, Hara K, Matsushita N, et al. Present epidemiology of chronic subdural hematoma in Japan: analysis of 63,358 cases recorded in a national administrative database. J Neurosurg. 2018;128:222–8.
85. Torihashi K, Sadamasa N, Yoshida K, Narumi O, Chin M, Yamagata S. Independent predictors for recurrence of chronic subdural hematoma: a review of 343 consecutive surgical cases. Neurosurgery. 2008;63(6):1125–9.
86. Tsai TH, Lieu AS, Hwang SL, Huang TY, Hwang YF. A comparative study of the patients with bilateral or unilateral chronic subdural hematoma: precipitating factors and postoperative outcomes. J Trauma. 2010;68:571–5.
87. Tugcu B, Tanriverdi O, Baydin S, Hergunsel B, Gunaldi O, Ofluoglu E, et al. Can recurrence of chronic subdural hematoma be predicted? A retrospective analysis of 292 cases. J Neurol Surg A Cent Eur Neurosurg. 2014;75(1):37–41.
88. Unterhofer C, Freyschlag CF, Thome C, Ortler M. Opening the internal hematoma membrane does not alter the recurrence rate of chronic subdural hematomas: a prospective randomized trial. World Neurosurg. 2016;92:31–6.

89. Utsuki S, Oka H, Kijima C, Inukai M, Abe K, Fujii K. Role of saireito in postoperative chronic subdural hematoma recurrence prevention. J Tradit Med. 2012;29:137–42.
90. Voelker JL, Sambasivan M. The role of craniotomy and trephination in the treatment of chronic subdural hematoma. Neurosurg Clin N Am. 2000;11:535–40.
91. Wang D, Li T, Wei H, Wang Y, Yang G, Tian Y, et al. Atorvastatin enhances angiogenesis to reduce subdural hematoma in a rat model. J Neurol Sci. 2016a;362:91–9.
92. Wang Y, Zhou J, Fan C, Wang D, Jiao F, Liu B, Zhang Q. Influence of antithrombotic agents on the recurrence of chronic subdural hematomas and the quest about the recommencement of antithrombotic agents: a meta-analysis. J Clin Neurosci. 2016b;38:79–83.
93. Watanabe S, Amagasaki K, Shono N, Nakaguchi H. Fibrin glue injection into the hematoma cavity for refractory chronic subdural hematoma: a case report. Surg Neurol Int. 2016;7(Suppl 37):S876–9.
94. Watts DD, Trask A, Soeken K, Perdue P, Dols S, Kaufmann C. Hypothermic coagulopathy in trauma: effect on varying levels of enzyme speed, platelet function and fibrinolytic activity. J Trauma. 1998;44(5):846–54.
95. Weigel R, Schmiedek P, Krauss JK. Outcome of contemporary surgery for chronic subdural hematoma: evidence based review. J Neurol Neurosurg Psychiatry. 2003;74:937–43.
96. Weigel R, Hohenstein A, Schlickum L, Weiss C, Schilling L. Angiotensin converting enzyme inhibition for arterial hypertension reduces the risk of recurrence in patients with chronic subdural hematoma possibly by an antiangiogenic mechanism. Neurosurgery. 2007;61:788–92.
97. Xu XP, Liu C, Liu J, Pang YG, Lu O XD, Fu J, et al. Local application of corticosteroids combined with surgery for the treatment of chronic subdural hematoma. Turk Neurosurg. 2015;25(2):252–5.
98. Xu M, Chen P, Zhu X, Wang C, Shi X, Yu B. Effects of atorvastatin on conservative and surgical treatments of chronic subdural hematoma in patients. World Neurosurg. 2016;91:23–8.
99. Yadav YR, Parihar V, Namdev H, Bajaj J. Chronic subdural hematoma. Asian J Neurosurg. 2016;11(4):330–42.
100. Yamamoto H, Hirashima Y, Hamada H, Hayashi N, Origasa H, Endo S. Independent predictors of recurrence of chronic subdural hematoma: results of multivariate analysis performed using a logistic regression model. J Neurosurg. 2003;98(6):1217–21.
101. Yasunaga H. Effect of japanese herbal Kampo medicine Goreisan on reoperation rates after burr-hole surgery for chronic subdural hematoma: analysis of a National Inpatient Database. Evid Based Complement Alternat Med. 2015;2015:817616.
102. You CG, Zheng XS. Postoperative pneumocephalus increases the recurrence rate of chronic subdural hematoma. Clin Neurol Neurosurg. 2018;166:56–60.
103. Zhang Y, Chen S, Xiao Y, Tang W. Effects of dexamethasone in the treatment of recurrent chronic subdural hematoma. World Neurosurg. 2017;105:115–21.
104. Zumofen D, Regli L, Levivier M, Krayenbuhl N. Chronic subdural hematomas treated by burr hole trepanation and a subperiostal drainage system. Neurosurgery. 2009;64:1116–21.

第 37 章 老年慢性硬膜下血肿的康复治疗

Engin Taştaban 和 Mehmet Turgut

译者：李云飞

37.1 引言

慢性硬膜下血肿（CSDH）是神经外科的常见病，尤其是在老年患者中[12, 18]。这种疾病通常发生在老年人受到轻微外伤后[5]。慢性硬膜下血肿的其他危险因素包括男性性别、慢性酒精中毒史、血液疾病的存在以及抗凝药的使用[28, 37]。人群中慢性硬膜下血肿的发病率为每年每 10 万人中 8.2～14.0 人。

慢性硬膜下血肿的特点是血液和血液分解产物聚集在硬膜下间隙，病程相对缓慢但进展较长[16, 20]。另外，使用计算机断层成像或磁共振成像可快速诊断出慢性硬膜下血肿，影像学结果提示典型的新月形占位性病变[9]。然而，不幸的是，尽管手术治疗对慢性硬膜下血肿患者是有效的，据报道其复发率仍为 6.1%～22%[13]。

慢性硬膜下血肿的临床表现随着症状的出现和持续时间的进展而变化[22, 32]。如果硬膜下间隙内血肿引起的占位效应导致大脑皮质受到压迫，就会出现相应的症状和体征。在临床上，慢性硬膜下血肿患者有多种症状，包括虚弱、头痛、精神状态改变、失语、失用、协调障碍、视觉空间功能障碍、步态改变、跌倒和癫痫[18]。

慢性硬膜下血肿患者临床上多出现偏瘫[2]。偏瘫最初可能是短暂的，然后是持续性的。一般来说，四肢无力一般是轻微的，但有不成比例的嗜睡和神经缺陷症状。神经学上，虽然也有同侧临床症状和体征的病例报告，但临床表现通常是对侧的。步态障碍和跌倒是慢性硬膜下血肿患者常见的表现[31]。反复跌倒被认为是慢性硬膜下血肿发展的主要风险。慢性硬膜下血肿的发展可能会导致复发性跌倒，这可能是由于这些患者的精神状态改变或出现神经缺陷。

37.2 住院康复管理

尽管最近在手术和药物治疗方面取得了进展，但慢性硬膜下血肿仍然是一种使人衰弱的疾病[3]。康复治疗可以减少疾病对身体的影响，减轻关节疼痛，改善生活质量，减少并发症，但慢性硬膜下血肿手术治疗后的理想活动期尚不清楚[19, 29]。人们普遍认为，慢性硬膜下血肿患者术后早期卧床休息可以减少复发率，因为它促进脑组织的复张[21]；但另一方面，早期活动有助于减少各种不活动造成的并发症，特别是静脉血栓栓塞和院内感染[8]。在最近的一项系统综述中，Cunningham 等发现，在 60 岁及以上的慢性硬膜下血肿患者中，有规律的身体活动与死亡率、复发性跌倒、认知能力下降和抑郁发生率的降低有关[11]。

慢性硬膜下血肿患者需要制订医院和门诊康复计划。患者的康复方案需要从重症监护病房开始，然后持续到门诊，康复治疗可以为慢性硬膜下血肿患者提供显著的临床改善[25]。康复团队需要对慢性硬膜下血肿患者的行动能力、自理能力和其他日常生活活动进行训练，采用由个体物理治疗和独立家庭项目相结合的锻炼方案[8]。毫无疑问，为慢性硬膜下血肿患者提供最大限度的运动功能恢复是运动计划的主要目的。从技术上讲，增强患者活动能力是通过锻炼过程获得的，其中柔韧性拉伸的主要目的是增加活动范围和身体功能，必须每周进行 5～7 天运动康复[27]。如果用积极的运动或外部加热方式来刺激肌肉，拉伸会更加有效。

通过运动和阻力练习以及各种矫形器的使用，可以使需要锻炼的关节获得相应的活动范围和力量[6]。早期活动可刺激软组织和关节，预防其挛缩[15]。每天均应进行被动活动范围和主动活动范围的最大拉伸。力量训练应针对负责改善功能的关键肌群，以改善患者运动功能[34]。定期的治疗性运动可提供充足的力量、完整的活动范围和协调性，从而降低心血管并发症和骨质疏松症的风险[4]。最近，Carlisi 等提出辅助康复计划可能有助于改善短期术后平衡和活动状态[8]。

由于长期卧床休息，患者在重症监护病房住院后经常出现虚弱和耐力下降。虚弱的状态可能导致步态的各种异常，行走试验必须从站在床边开始。Weiss 等在之前的研究中发现，早期的物理治疗干预可以促进脑卒中后肌力的恢复[33]。增强活动范围的运动有助于解决软组织挛缩的问题。主动和被动拉伸的治疗目的完全是经验性的，但有证据表明拉伸可以帮助患者减少挛缩的发生[1]，对受影响的肌肉群进行柔韧性活动也是重要的。毫无疑问，当患者承受较大的疼痛时，在被动和主动运动中都需要使用镇痛药物。

37.3 物理治疗方式

越来越多的物理治疗方式，如电疗、热疗、冷热应用等，被广泛用于慢性硬膜下血肿患者的康复，以减轻疼痛，增加肌肉和关节的柔韧性[24]。众所周知，热疗法可以缓解关节和肌肉的僵硬，从而提供拉伸的治疗效果。电疗（即经皮神经电刺激）用于疼痛控制和肌肉刺激。这些方法可以减轻关节和肌肉的疼痛，从而减少对镇痛药物的需求[10]。

37.4 衰弱

衰弱被广泛认为是一种多因素综合征，其特征是存在慢性疾病、体脂量增加和年龄增大。这些患者跌倒的风险增加，导致发病率和死亡率增加[14]。在之前对衰弱治疗的系统综述中，得出的结论是，治疗性运动对于预防严重不良事件非常有效[14]。

37.5 跌倒

有报道称，慢性硬膜下血肿患者经常发生跌倒，跌倒是这些患者发病的主要原因[2]。因此，慢性硬膜下血肿患者应仔细检查，以诊断出跌倒的危险因素，如平衡障碍和（或）肌力不对称。影响平衡和活动的身体功能障碍包括肌肉力量和耐力下降，软组织变化限制关节活动范围，协调能力下降，感觉和知觉过程紊乱以及认知功能障碍，这些都是导致跌倒发生率增加的原因。康复团队必须对存在的风险因素保持警惕。正如预期的那样，与年龄相关的变化和与步态有关的神经功能障碍也是导致跌倒的重要危险因素[35]。

37.6 辅助设备

众所周知，辅助装置是一种辅助患者执行特定任务的外部装置，对于一些慢性硬膜下血肿患者的术后行走可能是必要的[23]。例如，四点式和三点式手杖通过增加手杖底部的着力范围为这些患者提供了足够的稳定性[23]。在这类患者中，使用助行器可以使患者跌倒风险降低，从而增加了患者的稳定性[23]。因此，近年来，辅助装置的益处已被发现，特别是对老年慢性硬膜下血肿患者。

37.7 骨质疏松症

如今，一些学者认为皮质类固醇在慢性硬膜下血肿患者的治疗中是有用的[19]。有研究表明，术前和术后使用皮质类固醇可预防慢性硬膜下血肿的复发[26]。在对有骨质疏松症患者的治疗中，除了运动计划外，还常规使用多种药物，包括补充钙和维生素 D，使用口服抗骨吸收药物，如阿仑膦酸钠或利塞膦酸钠[7]。定期负重或阻力训练可以改善骨量，减少跌倒。慢性硬膜下血肿患者可采用包括步行、重量训练、平衡训练、姿势和柔韧性训练在内的运动方案[17]。有研究表明，脊柱伸展运动和渐进式阻力性背部强化运动有助于减少腰椎前凸的发生[30]。此外，在这些患者出现压缩性骨折时，推荐使用刚性胸腰椎矫形器来提供脊柱的伸展[30]。

37.8 挛缩

"挛缩"是指限制关节在某些特定方向上的运动，从而限制其功能，这意味着肌肉等软组织出现僵硬，是疼痛和皮肤破损的潜在原因[36]。Wong 等认为，长时间的关节制动会导致肌挛缩的发展[36]。众所周知，一些预防措施，如正确的体位、被动和主动的拉伸练习，对于预防关节挛缩是有用的[36]。持续被动牵拉对于维持软组织长度是必要的,一些保护装置如静态和动态夹板通常被应用于此目的[35]。

37.9 门诊康复管理

门诊康复治疗对维持慢性硬膜下血肿患者的运动能力和终身功能具有重要意义。环境的改善可防止患者受到进一步伤害,并对这些患者的生活质量产生积极影响[35]。在慢性硬膜下血肿患者中,使用防滑地毯、改善照明和降低床位高度可能有助于预防跌倒相关的损伤[35]。

37.10 结论

慢性硬膜下血肿患者手术和内科治疗后,受限的活动和功能状态可能会影响正常的日常生活。应在门诊康复计划中提供有关运动重要性的适当教育,以实现终身功能的康复。现如今,众所周知,身体康复训练可以使患者的运动功能更加健全,并提高他们的生活质量。

参考文献

1. Ada L, Dorsch S, Canning CG. Strengthening interventions increase strength and improve activity after stroke: a systematic review. Aust J Physiother. 2006;52:241–8.
2. Adhiyaman V, Asghar M, Ganeshram KN, Bhowmick BK. Chronic subdural haematoma in the elderly. Postgrad Med J. 2002;78:71–5.
3. Almenawer SA, Farrokhyar F, Hong C, Alhazzani W, Manoranjan B, Yarascavitch B, Arjmand P, Baronia B, Reddy K, Murty N, Singh S. Chronic subdural hematoma management: a systematic review and meta-analysis of 34,829 patients. Ann Surg. 2014;259:449–57.
4. American College of Sports Medicine, Chodzko-Zajko WJ, Proctor DN, Fiatarone Singh MA, Minson CT, Nigg CR, Salem GJ, Skinner JS. American College of Sports Medicine position stand. Exercise and physical activity for older adults. Med Sci Sports Exerc. 2009;41:1510–30.
5. Borger V, Vatter H, Oszvald A, Marquardt G, Seifert V, Guresir E. Chronic subdural haematoma in elderly patients: a retrospective analysis of 322 patients between the ages of 65-94 years. Acta Neurochir. 2012;154:1549–54.
6. Cadore EL, Pinto RS, Bottaro M, Izquierdo M. Strength and endurance training prescription in healthy and frail elderly. Aging Dis. 2014;5:183–95.
7. Camacho PM, Petak SM, Binkley N, Diab DL, Eldeiry LS, Farooki A, Harris ST, Hurley DL, Kelly J, Lewiecki EM, Pessah-Pollack R, McClung M, Wimalawansa SJ, Watts NB. American Association of Clinical Endocrinologists/American College of Endocrinology Clinical Practice Guidelines for the diagnosis and treatment of postmenopausal osteoporosis-2020 Update. Endocr Pract. 2020;26:1–46.
8. Carlisi E, Feltroni L, Tinelli C, Verlotta M, Gaetani P, Dalla Toffola E. Postoperative rehabilitation for chronic subdural hematoma in the elderly. An observational study focusing on balance, ambulation and discharge destination. Eur J Phys Rehabil Med. 2017;53:91–7.
9. Carroll JJ, Lavine SD, Meyers PM. Imaging of subdural hematomas. Neurosurg Clin N Am. 2017;28:179–203.
10. Chen N, Wang J, Mucelli A, Zhang X, Wang C. Electro-acupuncture is beneficial for knee osteoarthritis: the evidence from meta-analysis of randomized controlled trials. Am J Chin Med. 2017;45:965–85.
11. Cunningham C, O'Sullivan R, Caserotti P, Tully MA. Consequences of physical inactivity in older adults: a systematic review of reviews and meta-analyses. Scand J Med Sci Sports. 2020;30:816–27.
12. Dumont TM, Rughani AI, Goeckes T, Tranmer BI. Chronic subdural hematoma: a sentinel health event. World Neurosurg. 2013;80:889–92.
13. Edlmann E, Giorgi-Coll S, Whitfield PC, Carpenter KLH, Hutchinson PJ. Pathophysiology of chronic subdural haematoma: inflammation, angiogenesis and implications for pharmacotherapy. J Neuroinflammation. 2017;14:108.
14. Fried LP, Tangen CM, Walston J, Newman AB, Hirsch C, Gottdiener J, Seeman T, Tracy R, Kop WJ, Burke G, McBurnie MA. Frailty in older adults: evidence for a phenotype. J Gerontol A Biol Sci Med Sci. 2001;56:M146–56.
15. Han P, Zhang W, Kang L, Ma Y, Fu L, Jia L, Yu H, Chen X, Hou L, Wang L, Yu X, Kohzuki M,

Guo Q. Clinical evidence of exercise benefits for stroke. Adv Exp Med Biol. 2017;1000:131–51.
16. Holl DC, Volovici V, Dirven CMF, Peul WC, van Kooten F, Jellema K, van der Gaag NA, Miah IP, Kho KH, den Hertog HM, Lingsma HF, Dammers R. Pathophysiology and nonsurgical treatment of chronic subdural hematoma: from past to present to future. World Neurosurg. 2018;116:402–11.
17. Kirazli Y, Atamaz Calis F, El O, Gokce Kutsal Y, Peker O, Sindel D, Tuzun S, Gogas Yavuz D, Durmaz B, Akarirmak U, Bodur H, Hamuryudan V, Inceboz U, Oncel S. Updated approach for the management of osteoporosis in Turkey: a consensus report. Arch Osteoporos. 2020;15:137.
18. Kolias AG, Chari A, Santarius T, Hutchinson PJ. Chronic subdural haematoma: modern management and emerging therapies. Nat Rev Neurol. 2014;10:570–8.
19. Kurabe S, Ozawa T, Watanabe T, Aiba T. Efficacy and safety of postoperative early mobilization for chronic subdural hematoma in elderly patients. Acta Neurochir. 2010;152:1171–4.
20. Kwon CS, Al-Awar O, Richards O, Izu A, Lengvenis G. Predicting prognosis of patients with chronic subdural hematoma: a new scoring system. World Neurosurg. 2018;109:e707–14.
21. Mehta V, Harward SC, Sankey EW, Nayar G, Codd PJ. Evidence based diagnosis and management of chronic subdural hematoma: a review of the literature. J Clin Neurosci. 2018;50:7–15.
22. Merrill SA, Khan D, Richards AE, Kalani MA, Patel NP, Neal MT. Functional recovery following surgery for chronic subdural hematoma. Surg Neurol Int. 2020;11:450.
23. Panel on Prevention of Falls in Older Persons, American Geriatrics Society and British Geriatrics Society. Summary of the Updated American Geriatrics Society/British Geriatrics Society clinical practice guideline for prevention of falls in older persons. J Am Geriatr Soc. 2011;59:148–57.
24. Paolillo FR, Paolillo AR, Joao JP, Frasca D, Duchene M, Joao HA, Bagnato VS. Ultrasound plus low-level laser therapy for knee osteoarthritis rehabilitation: a randomized, placebo-controlled trial. Rheumatol Int. 2018;38:785–93.
25. Ragland JT, Lee K. Chronic subdural hematoma ICU management. Neurosurg Clin N Am. 2017;28:239–46.
26. Roh D, Reznik M, Claassen J. Chronic subdural medical management. Neurosurg Clin N Am. 2017;28:211–7.
27. Sady SP, Wortman M, Blanke D. Flexibility training: ballistic, static or proprioceptive neuromuscular facilitation? Arch Phys Med Rehabil. 1982;63:261–3.
28. Sahyouni R, Goshtasbi K, Mahmoodi A, Tran DK, Chen JW. Chronic subdural hematoma: a historical and clinical perspective. World Neurosurg. 2017;108:948–53.
29. Shapey J, Glancz LJ, Brennan PM. Chronic subdural haematoma in the elderly: is it time for a new paradigm in management? Curr Geriatr Rep. 2016;5:71–7.
30. Sinaki M. Critical appraisal of physical rehabilitation measures after osteoporotic vertebral fracture. Osteoporos Int. 2003;14:773–9.
31. Tabuchi S, Kadowaki M. Chronic subdural hematoma in patients over 90 years old in a super-aged society. J Clin Med Res. 2014;6:379–83.
32. Uno M, Toi H, Hirai S. Chronic subdural hematoma in elderly patients: is this disease benign? Neurol Med Chir. 2017;57:402–9.
33. Weiss A, Suzuki T, Bean J, Fielding RA. High intensity strength training improves strength and functional performance after stroke. Am J Phys Med Rehabil. 2000;79:369–76; quiz 391–64.
34. Williams G, Kahn M, Randall A. Strength training for walking in neurologic rehabilitation is not task specific: a focused review. Am J Phys Med Rehabil. 2014;93:511–22.
35. Winstein CJ, Stein J, Arena R, Bates B, Cherney LR, Cramer SC, Deruyter F, Eng JJ, Fisher B, Harvey RL, Lang CE, MacKay-Lyons M, Ottenbacher KJ, Pugh S, Reeves MJ, Richards LG, Stiers W, Zorowitz RD. Guidelines for adult stroke rehabilitation and recovery: a guideline for healthcare professionals from the American Heart Association/American Stroke Association. Stroke. 2016;47:e98–e169.
36. Wong K, Trudel G, Laneuville O. Noninflammatory joint contractures arising from immobility: animal models to future treatments. Biomed Res Int. 2015;2015:848290.
37. Yang W, Huang J. Chronic subdural hematoma: epidemiology and natural history. Neurosurg Clin N Am. 2017;28:205–10.

第 38 章 慢性硬膜下血肿的转归和预后

Serdar Ercan，Zeki Serdar Ataizi 和 Kemal Yücesoy

译者：欧云尉

38.1 引言

慢性硬膜下血肿（CSDH）是位于硬脑膜和蛛网膜之间存在至少 21 天的血性积液、积血，是成人，尤其是老年患者中最常见的神经外科病理情况。硬脑膜外层增厚是由于硬脑膜胶原蛋白的生成和硬脑膜下出血后硬脑膜内表面成纤维细胞的聚集。随着时间的推移，硬膜下血肿（SDH）液化并形成液性囊肿。在此期间，出血部位的硬脑膜内壁和隔膜可能形成钙化。液性囊肿被认为能引起脑萎缩、神经组织损伤、脱水和颅内压升高。

手术清除是减少血肿的占位效应的可行选择之一。血肿清除可以用许多不同的方法来完成。对于有液化血液、无包膜或钙化血肿的患者，建议单侧或双侧血肿引流[8, 42]。CSDH 的预后一般被认为是良好的。然而，已有许多研究表明 CSDH 可复发甚至导致患者死亡[6, 9]。

38.2 年龄与预后

随着人群中老年人比例的增加，出现硬膜下血肿的患者数量将继续增加。年龄与预后直接相关[9-10, 26, 32, 43]。Gonzales-Vargas 等报道，80 岁以上患者的预后显著更差[17]。这一观点得到了类似研究的支持[16, 43]。但是，尽管高龄是预后不良的原因之一，但这并不影响决定是否需要手术干预。尽管患者年事已高，但仍有许多老年患者在手术干预后得到康复[15, 38, 56]。

虽然高龄是预后不良的一个因素，但各年龄组之间没有观察到显著差异[42]。Gelabert-Gonzales 等在其包含 1000 例患者的队列研究中发现，与年轻患者（21.7%）相比，70 岁以上患者（33.8%）的认知变化更常见，特别是在颅内压升高的患者中[16]。Asghar 报告说，65 岁以上患者最常见的临床症状是精神障碍[2]。

38.3 手术技术与预后

近年来，一些治疗 CSDH 的手术方法如麻花钻开颅术（twist drill，TDC）、钻孔开颅术（burr hole，BHC）、开颅/小骨瓣开颅术等已被提出[11, 49]。手术的目的是清除血肿和降低颅内压。Tabaddor 和 Shulman 在他们的麻花钻闭合引流系统手术研究中显示，在 20% 的硬膜下积液被排空后，颅内压会降至零[47]。他们认为这 20% 的体积减少通常足以引起显著的临床改善[47]。Markwalder 等报道，在钻孔引流术研究中，使用闭合系统引流的 78% 的患者在术后第 10 天仍有硬膜下积液，但不影响愈合。术后 40 天 85% 的患者的硬膜下积液在 CT 上完全吸收，因此他们建议无需积极干预残存积液[31]。

Weigel 等发现这三种手术技术之间的恢复率和死亡率没有显著差异[53]。然而他们报告 TDC 的复发率显著高于 BHC 和开颅术，因此他们得出结论，BHC 的治疗效果与并发症之间比率最佳。相反，Ducruet 表示 BHC 导致的并发症发生率高于 TDC 和开颅术[16]。此外，他们推荐 TDC 作为一线干预措施，同时推荐对于广泛血肿膜形成的患者采用开颅技术（图 38.1）[11]。Almenawer 报道，TDC 和 BHC 在恢复、复发、发病率或死亡率方面没有显著差异，开颅手术引起的并发症发生率较高[1]。

38.4 再出血

在 5% ~ 30% 的患者中可出现 CSDH 的复发。导致复发性出血的危险因素包括高龄、男性性别、脑萎缩和使用抗凝药或抗血小板药物[39]。分隔性 CSDH 是一种特殊类型的血肿，其包含被纤维蛋白分成不同部分的多个腔隙。这些分隔构成了一个完全独立的复发危险因素[7]。由于只有液体形式的 CSDH 可以用钻孔引流术排出，隔膜仍会留在血肿内。虽然在存在厚隔膜的情况下手术并发症发生率较高，仍应

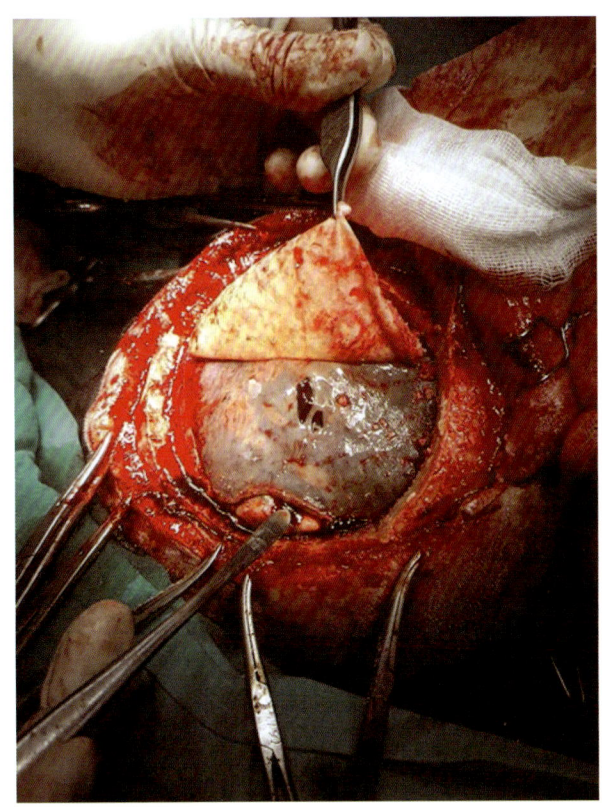

图 38.1　由于广泛的血肿膜形成而对患者采用开颅术

采用开颅术[55]。目前发现与其他钻孔术（BHC）和传统开颅术相比，麻花钻颅骨造口术的复发率更高。此外，钻孔后使用闭合系统引流可降低复发风险。曾有研究指出，与接受引流术的患者相比，未使用引流的患者复发率显著增加[34]。增加再出血的风险因素包括患者年龄超过70岁、既往有脑梗死病史以及正在接受抗凝药或抗血小板治疗。除高龄外，厚包膜下出血和双侧血肿进一步增加了风险。

38.5　大脑复张

影响手术后大脑复张的因素与导致血肿复发的因素相似。脑梗死史，硬膜下腔存在空气导致的张力性气颅，低颅压影响脑顺应性，这些都会阻碍术后脑复张。有报道称，高血压、糖尿病等疾病并不影响大脑皮质的复张[5]。影像学检查可明确显示伴或不伴中线脑结构移位的血肿。血肿宽度大和中线移位提示预后不良。血肿腔内隔膜的存在与较高的复发率有关[24, 33, 36, 43, 52, 54]。术后卧床休息、静脉容量补充或CSDH排空后补液有助于脑的复张。此外，有临床研究表明，在闭合硬脑膜或回纳骨瓣之前，将CO_2或O_2注入手术区域有助于开颅术后大脑复张[16]。

38.6　死亡率和并发症发生率

影响CSDH患者死亡率和并发症发生率的最重要因素之一是患者术前格拉斯哥昏迷评分（GCS）。GCS在3～12，ASA（美国麻醉医师协会）分级为3及以上会增加死亡率和发病率。Rohde等报告总体死亡率为13.3%[42]。此外，存在其他全身和（或）中枢神经系统疾病，如存在感染和静脉血栓栓塞，会使临床表现恶化。并发症发生率介于6%～32%之间[41, 46]。

Weigel及其同事在死亡率研究中比较了麻花钻颅骨造口术（2.7%）、钻孔颅骨造口术（2.9%）和开颅术（4.6%）的死亡率，发现它们之间没有明显差异[21]。在比较手术方式的类似队列研究中，当比较复发率、再手术、住院时间、神经功能恢复和死亡率时，这些手术方式之间没有显著差异[11, 34]。4%的死亡率与之前报道的死亡率相似[4]。

现在认为再出血会影响CSDH的并发症发生率[4, 27]。Brodbelt等将CSDH并发症发生率定义为手术期间或术后发生的除复发以外的任何并发症的发生率。他们发现开颅术（12.3%）的CSDH并发症发生率高于麻花钻开颅术（3%）和钻孔开颅术（3.8%）[5]。因此，开颅术后的二次手术比其他手术方式更常见。然而，神经功能在开颅手术的病例中的改善是最好的[11]。术后感染率各不相同，Borger报道为3.6%，Gelabert报道为1.7%，Rohde报道为2.1%[16, 42]。患者入院时的神经系统状态与其不良预后之间的关系在以前的研究中已有报道[13, 30-31, 43]。Ramachandran发现患者GOS评分与入院时的GCS评分和合并症的存在有关[40]。

38.7　癫痫

CSDH的中枢神经系统并发症可表现为癫痫发作、急性硬膜下和颅内出血、张力性气颅、硬膜下脓肿和伤口感染[32]。在慢性硬膜下血肿中，血肿压迫脑皮质表面，随后产生降解产物刺激皮质而引起癫痫[14]。特别是皮质表面的血红蛋白分解产物，具有高度致痫性[18, 20]。据报道，观察到24%的急性SDH和11%的慢性SDH患者有癫痫发作[19, 22, 50]。

对于慢性 SDH 患者，癫痫发作的危险因素与急性 SDH 不同。一项前瞻性研究报道，酒精中毒是慢性硬膜下血肿患者癫痫发作的危险因素[12]。以往的研究表明，随着年龄的增长，患者功能结局不良的发生率逐渐增加。相比之下，据报道 75 岁以下的患者与更年长的患者相比，这种并发症的发生率没有增加[16, 23, 28]。尽管在 CSDH 患者中报道了 2%～19% 的癫痫发作率，但许多研究对癫痫发作的发生率描述不同。Oshida 等观察到老年患者手术清除血肿后即刻出现 CSDH 下皮质一过性充血[39]。他们认为这一发现可能与急性颅内出血和癫痫发作等并发症有关。类似地，van Havenbergh 等报道称，残留的血肿囊可能导致晚期癫痫[21]。基于这些原因，分析了预防性抗癫痫药对 CSDH 患者的作用，结果表明接受预防性苯妥英钠治疗可以显著降低癫痫的发生发展。

目前，关于 CSDH 患者的预防性抗癫痫治疗仍存在争议。一项针对手术治疗的 CSDH 患者的回顾性研究表明，预防性使用苯妥英可有效减少癫痫发作；然而，预后获益尚未完全确定[28]。另一项研究报告，预防性抗癫痫药治疗可降低 CSDH 的癫痫发生率，但出院后预防性使用抗癫痫药治疗的患者没有从中获益[39]。尽管已建议使用预防性使用抗癫痫药 6 个月，但由于 CSDH 患者癫痫发作的发生率不同，因此目前尚无关于这些患者使用预防性抗癫痫药的共识建议[39, 44-45]。

38.8 抗凝治疗

CSDH 是神经外科临床中最常见的疾病之一，尤其是在轻度头部创伤后的老年人群中。据我们所知，已知的出血危险因素包括高龄、既往颅内出血史、低颅压和创伤前抗凝或抗血小板治疗[3, 25, 29]。据报道，16%～76% 的 CSDH 患者有抗凝治疗史[35, 48, 51]。

术后早期的脑 CT 检查将有助于决定是否开始抗凝治疗。在抗凝治疗中，正确的治疗时机是防止患者再出血或临床恶化的重要因素之一。虽然已知使用阿司匹林有术后颅内出血和慢性硬膜下血肿复发的风险，但对于 CT 上无影像学出血征象的患者，仍建议继续使用阿司匹林[35]。

38.9 结论

年龄与预后直接相关，高龄是预后不良的主要原因之一。然而高龄并不影响治疗决策，因为尽管患者年事已高，但仍有许多老年患者在手术干预后康复。手术的目的是清除血肿和降低颅内压。先前的研究建议将 TDC 作为一线干预，尽管 BHC 比 TDC 和开颅术有更少的血肿复发率，但仍建议对广泛血肿膜形成的患者使用开颅术。尽管建议从确诊时起 6 个月内使用预防性抗癫痫药，但由于 CSDH 患者癫痫发生率不同，目前尚无关于使用预防性抗癫痫药的共识建议。

参考文献

1. Almenawer SA, Farrokhyar F, Hong C, Alhazzani W, Manoranjan B, Yarascavitch B, Arjmand P, Baronia B, Reddy K, Murty N. Chronic subdural hematoma management: a systematic review and meta-analysis of 34829 patients. Ann Surg. 2014;259:449–57.
2. Asghar M, Adhiyaman V, Greenway MW, Bhowmick BK, Bates A. Chronic subdural haematoma in the elderly—a North Wales experience. J R Soc Med. 2002;95:290–2.
3. Aspegren OP, Åstrand R, Lundgren MI, Romner B. Anticoagulation therapy a risk factor for the development of chronic subdural hematoma. Clin Neurol Neurosurg. 2013;115:981–4.
4. Borger V, Vatter H, Oszvald A, Marquardt G, Seifert V, Guresir E. Chronic subdural haematoma in elderly patients: a retrospective analysis of 322 patients between the ages of 65-94 years. Acta Neurochir (Wien). 2012;154:1549–54.
5. Brodbelt A, Warnke P, Weigel R, Krauss JK. Outcome of contemporary surgery for chronic subdural haematoma: evidence based review [3] (multiple letters). J Neurol Neurosurg Psychiatry. 2004;75:1209–10.
6. Bucher B, Maldaner N, Regli L, Sarnthein J, Serra C. Standardized assessment of outcome and complications in chronic subdural hematoma: results from a large case series. Acta Neurochir (Wien). 2019;161:1297–304.
7. Cai Q, Guo Q, Zhang F, Sun D, Zhang W, Ji B, Chen Z, Mao S. Evacuation of chronic and subacute subdural hematoma via transcranial neuroendoscopic approach. Neuropsychiatr Dis Treat. 2019;15:385–90.

8. Cenic A, Bhandari M, Reddy K. Management of chronic subdural hematoma: a national survey and literature review. Can J Neurol Sci. 2005;32:501–6.
9. Cofano F, Pesce A, Vercelli G, Mammi M, Massara A, Minardi M, Palmieri M, D'Andrea G, Fronda C, Lanotte MM, Tartara F, Zenga F, Frati A, Garbossa D. Risk of recurrence of chronic subdural hematomas after surgery: a multicenter observational cohort study. Front Neurol. 2020;11:1–10.
10. Delgado PD, Cogolludo FJ, Mateo O, Cancela P, Garcia R, Carrillo R. Early prognosis in chronic subdural hematomas. Multivariate analysis of 137 cases. Rev Neurol. 2000;30:811–7.
11. Ducruet AF, Grobelny BT, Zacharia BE, Hickman ZL, DeRosa PL, Anderson K, Sussman E, Carpenter A, Connolly ES. The surgical management of chronic subdural hematoma. Neurosurg Rev. 2012;35:155–69.
12. Dudek H, Michno T, Michalski J, Kaczmarek M, Drapało L. Late posttraumatic epilepsy in patients with an alcoholic problem treated surgically for posttraumatic chronic subdural hematomas. Rocz Akad Med Bialymst. 1999;44:119–27.
13. El-Kadi H, Miele VJ, Kaufman HH. Prognosis of chronic subdural hematomas. Neurosurg Clin N Am. 2000;11:553–67.
14. Frey LC. Epidemiology of posttraumatic epilepsy: a critical review. Epilepsia. 2003;44:11–7.
15. Fukui S. Evaluation of surgical treatment for chronic subdural hematoma in extremely aged (over 80 years old) patients (in Japanese). No To Shinkei. 1993;45:449–53.
16. Gelabert-González M, Iglesias-Pais M, García-Allut A, Martínez-Rumbo R. Chronic subdural haematoma: surgical treatment and outcome in 1000 cases. Clin Neurol Neurosurg. 2005;107:223–9.
17. González-Vargas PM, Thenier-Villa JL, Calero Félix L, Galárraga Campoverde RA, Martín-Gallego Á, de la Lama Zaragoza A, Conde Alonso CM. Factors that negatively influence the Glasgow Outcome Scale in patients with chronic subdural hematomas. An analytical and retrospective study in a tertiary center. Interdiscip Neurosurg. 2020;20:100606.
18. Haltiner AM, Temkin NR, Dikmen SS. Risk of seizure recurrence after the first late posttraumatic seizure. Arch Phys Med Rehabil. 1997;78:835–40.
19. Hamasaki T, Yamada K, Kuratsu J. Seizures as a presenting symptom in neurosurgical patients: a retrospective single-institution analysis. Clin Neurol Neurosurg. 2013;115:2336–40.
20. Hammond EJ, Ramsay RE, Villarreal HJ, Wilder BJ. Effects of intracortical injection of blood and blood components on the electrocorticogram. Epilepsia. 1980;21:3–14.
21. van Havenbergh T, van Calenbergh F, Goffin J, Plets C. Outcome of chronic subdural haematoma: analysis of prognostic factors. Br J Neurosurg. 1996;10:35–9.
22. Huang KT, Bi WL, Abd-El-Barr M, Yan SC, Tafel IJ, Dunn IF, Gormley WB. The neurocritical and neurosurgical care of subdural hematomas. Neurocrit Care. 2016;24:294–307.
23. Huang Y-H, Lin W-C, Lu C-H, Chen W-F. Volume of chronic subdural haematoma: is it one of the radiographic factors related to recurrence? Injury. 2014;45:1327–31.
24. Juković MF, Stojanović DB. Midline shift threshold value for hemiparesis in chronic subdural hematoma. Srp Arh Celok Lek. 2015;143:386–90.
25. Kamenova M, Lutz K, Schaedelin S, Fandino J, Mariani L, Soleman J. Does early resumption of low-dose aspirin after evacuation of chronic subdural hematoma with burr-hole drainage lead to higher recurrence rates? Neurosurgery. 2016;79:715–21.
26. Krupp WF, Jans PJ. Treatment of chronic subdural haematoma with burr-hole craniostomy and closed drainage. Br J Neurosurg. 1995;9:619–28.
27. Lee L, Ker J, Ng HY, Munusamy T, King NKK, Kumar D, Ng WH. Outcomes of chronic subdural hematoma drainage in nonagenarians and centenarians: a multicenter study. J Neurosurg. 2016;124:546–51.
28. Leroy H-A, Aboukais R, Reyns N, Bourgeois P, Labreuche J, Duhamel A, Lejeune J-P. Predictors of functional outcomes and recurrence of chronic subdural hematomas. J Clin Neurosci. 2015;22:1895–900.
29. Lindvall P, Koskinen L-OD. Anticoagulants and antiplatelet agents and the risk of development and recurrence of chronic subdural haematomas. J Clin Neurosci. 2009;16:1287–90.
30. Markwalder T-M. Chronic subdural hematomas: a review. J Neurosurg. 1981;54:637–45.
31. Markwalder TM, Steinsiepe KF, Rohner M, Reichenbach W, Markwalder H. The course of chronic subdural hematomas after burr-hole craniostomy and closed-system drainage. J Neurosurg. 1981;55:390–6.
32. Mori K, Maeda M. Surgical treatment of chronic subdural hematoma in 500 consecutive cases: clinical characteristics, surgical outcome, complications, and recurrence rate. Neurol Med Chir (Tokyo). 2001;41:371–81.

33. Motiei-Langroudi R, Alterman RL, Stippler M, Phan K, Alturki AY, Papavassiliou E, Kasper EM, Arle J, Ogilvy CS, Thomas AJ. Factors influencing the presence of hemiparesis in chronic subdural hematoma. J Neurosurg. 2019;131:1926–30.
34. Muzii VF, Bistazzoni S, Zalaffi A, Carangelo B, Mariottini A, Palma L. Chronic subdural hematoma: comparison of two surgical techniques. Preliminary results of a prospective randomized study. J Neurosurg Sci. 2005;49:41–7.
35. Nathan S, Goodarzi Z, Jette N, Gallagher C, Holroyd-Leduc J. Anticoagulant and antiplatelet use in seniors with chronic subdural hematoma: systematic review. Neurology. 2017;88:1889–93.
36. Oh H-J, Lee K-S, Shim J-J, Yoon S-M, Yun I-G, Bae H-G. Postoperative course and recurrence of chronic subdural hematoma. J Korean Neurosurg Soc. 2010;48:518–23.
37. Ohno K, Maehara T, Ichimura K, Suzuki R, Hirakawa K, Monma S. Low incidence of seizures in patients with chronic subdural haematoma. J Neurol Neurosurg Psychiatry. 1993;56:1231–3.
38. Ooba S, Shiomi N, Shigemori M. Clinical features and surgical results of chronic subdural hematoma in the extremely aged patients (in Japanese). No Shinkei Geka. 2006;34:273–8.
39. Oshida S, Akamatsu Y, Matsumoto Y, Ishigame S, Ogasawara Y, Aso K, Kashimura H. A case of chronic subdural hematoma demonstrating the epileptic focus at the area with sulcal hyperintensity on fluid-attenuated inversion recovery image. Radiol Case Rep. 2019;14:1109–12.
40. Ramachandran R, Hegde T. Chronic subdural hematomas-causes of morbidity and mortality. Surg Neurol. 2007;67:367–72.
41. Reponen E, Korja M, Niemi T, Silvasti-Lundell M, Hernesniemi J, Tuominen H. Preoperative identification of neurosurgery patients with a high risk of in-hospital complications: a prospective cohort of 418 consecutive elective craniotomy patients. J Neurosurg. 2015;123:594–604.
42. Rohde V, Graf G, Hassler W. Complications of burr-hole craniostomy and closed-system drainage for chronic subdural hematomas: a retrospective analysis of 376 patients. Neurosurg Rev. 2002;25:89–94.
43. Rovlias A, Theodoropoulos S, Papoutsakis D. Chronic subdural hematoma: surgical management and outcome in 986 cases: a classification and regression tree approach. Surg Neurol Int. 2015;6:127.
44. Rubin G, Rappaport ZH. Epilepsy in chronic subdural haematoma. Acta Neurochir (Wien). 1993;123:39–42.
45. Sabo RA, Hanigan WC, Aldag JC. Chronic subdural hematomas and seizures: the role of prophylactic anticonvulsive medication. Surg Neurol. 1995;43:579–82.
46. Sase T, Furuya Y, Tanaka Y. Hospital discharge arrangements for very elderly patients with chronic subdural hematoma (in Japanese). No Shinkei Geka. 2020;48:1115–20.
47. Schmidek HH, Sweet WH. Surgical management of chronic subdural hematoma in adults. In: Operative neurosurgical techniques. 2012. p. 1573–8.
48. Soleman J, Kamenova M, Guzman R, Mariani L. The management of patients with chronic subdural hematoma treated with low-dose acetylsalicylic acid: an international survey of practice. World Neurosurg. 2017;107:778–88.
49. Tabaddor K, Shulman K. Definitive treatment of chronic subdural hematoma by twist-drill craniostomy and closed-system drainage. J Neurosurg. 1977;46:220–6.
50. Temkin NR, Dikmen SS, Wilensky AJ, Keihm J, Chabal S, Winn HR. A randomized, double-blind study of phenytoin for the prevention of post-traumatic seizures. N Engl J Med. 1990;323:497–502.
51. Wada M, Yamakami I, Higuchi Y, Tanaka M, Suda S, Ono J, Saeki N. Influence of antiplatelet therapy on postoperative recurrence of chronic subdural hematoma: a multicenter retrospective study in 719 patients. Clin Neurol Neurosurg. 2014;120:49–54.
52. Wakuta N, Abe H, Nonaka M, Morishita T, Higashi T, Arima H, Inoue T. Analysis of endoscopic findings in the chronic subdural hematoma cavity: bleeding factors in chronic subdural hematoma natural history and as predictors of recurrence. World Neurosurg. 2019;124:e241–51.
53. Weigel R, Schmiedek P, Krauss JK. Outcome of contemporary surgery for chronic subdural haematoma: evidence based review. J Neurol Neurosurg Psychiatry. 2003;74:937–43.
54. Yan K, Gao H, Wang Q, Xu X, Wu W, Zhou X, Xu W, Ye F. Endoscopic surgery to chronic subdural hematoma with neovessel septation: technical notes and literature review. Neurol Res. 2016;38:467–76.
55. Yan K, Gao H, Zhou X, Wu W, Xu W, Xu Y, Gong K, Xue X, Wang Q, Na H. A retrospective analysis of postoperative recurrence of septated chronic subdural haematoma: endoscopic surgery versus burr hole craniotomy. Neurol Res. 2017;39:803–12.
56. Zingale A, Albanese V, Romano A, Distefano G, Chiaramonte J. Traumatic chronic subdural hematoma over 80 years. A preliminary prospective study. J Neurosurg Sci. 1997;41:169–73.

第 39 章 硬膜下血肿的法医学问题

Mehmet Turgut 和 Erdal Kalkan

译者：欧云尉

39.1 引言

如今，全世界每年有成千上万的人由于机动车事故、跌倒等原因引起的头部损伤而患有硬膜下血肿（SDH）。SDH 的发病率随着年龄的增长而增加，并且因为症状发展缓慢而难以确诊。不幸的是，在这种情况下，误诊或手术过失（医疗事故）会导致进一步的伤害。众所周知，SDH 在老年人、遭受头部创伤的运动员、血友病和镰状细胞病等出血性疾病、服用抗凝药物的患者、酗酒者和早产儿中更为常见[7-8, 13, 26]。因此，全面的查体和神经系统检查是诊断评估的必要部分。

临床中需要注意的是，发展较慢的慢性硬膜下血肿（CSDH）可能会被误认为是其他疾病，如多发性骨髓瘤、脑肿瘤、卒中或痴呆[6, 10, 23]。此外，老年人可能无法记起 SDH 症状发展之前的几周或几个月曾发生的头部外伤史，并且有时创伤非常轻微。外科治疗方面，除了药物治疗，SDH 患者通过在颅骨上钻孔缓解血肿对大脑的压力。然而不幸的是，许多医院和医生可能会对 SDH 的诊断和治疗出现临床错误，导致永久性神经损伤[6, 10]。

在本章中，介绍了有关 SDH 诊疗方面的各种医疗事故，包括漏诊或延误诊断和治疗的情况、对该病危险因素缺乏了解、接受真空或产钳助产的新生早产儿以及"摇晃婴儿综合征"（shaken baby syndrome，SBS）的案例。本章对这些案例进行了详细讨论，并对 SDH 作为医疗事故原因进行了简要的综述。

39.2 硬膜下血肿作为医疗事故的原因

SDH 的特征是在硬脑膜和蛛网膜之间出现血液积聚（图 39.1）。由于大脑和这些脑膜层之间的桥静脉撕裂形成 SDH，可能导致周围脑组织的受压和危及生命的颅内压升高（IICP）。

正如本书前几章详细讨论的那样，考虑到出血发生后的时间，SDH 被分为急性、亚急性和慢性形式。SDH 是由头部创伤引起的，由于各种旋转或线性力作为其发生机制而引起血管破裂出血[12, 26]。通常，血管沿着覆盖大脑凸面的颅骨内侧延伸，被硬脑膜结构如小脑幕和大脑镰限制，因此形状表现为一个"凹"形，与之对应的硬膜外血肿因为无法穿过颅骨线而表现为"双凸"形[10, 29]。

即使仅受到轻微的头部创伤，硬膜下腔扩大的婴儿和脑皮质萎缩的老年酗酒者也可能发生 SDH，这些患者由于桥静脉长度有所增加，因此加大了剪

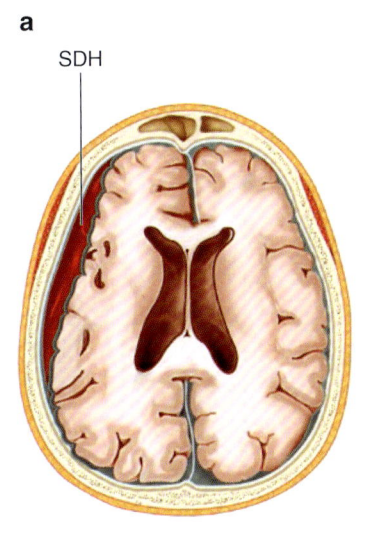
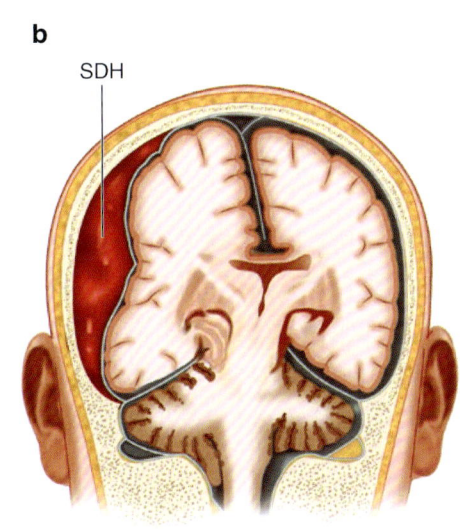

图 39.1 轴向（a）和冠状（b）颅脑示意图显示硬脑膜和蛛网膜之间的血液积聚称为硬膜下血肿（SDH），由医学插画家 Sercan Celebi 创作

切力导致血管撕裂的可能性。另外，SDH 在接受抗血小板或抗凝药物（如华法林和阿司匹林）的患者中也经常出现。此外，青少年年龄组中蛛网膜囊肿和脑脊液（CSF）漏是发生 SDH 的额外危险因素，这是由于 CSF 压力降低使得蛛网膜推离硬脑膜而导致桥静脉破裂[3, 9, 15, 22, 31]。在法医学上，同样重要的是要记住 SDH 可以在 SBS 病例中出现[20]。

在临床中需要特别注意的是，SDH 的症状和体征可能以急性表现在几分钟内进展，也可以慢性形式延迟数月或数年[13, 16, 18, 26]。在临床实践中，患有 SDH 的病例会出现以下症状的任意组合，包括意识丧失、头痛、恶心或呕吐、意识模糊、困倦、嗜睡、头晕、定向障碍、失语、一侧肢体无力、行走困难、失去平衡、记忆丧失、呼吸模式改变、耳鸣、癫痫发作、性格改变、精神症状、视物模糊、易激惹以及婴幼儿头颅增大等[13, 16, 26, 28]。

在影像学上，在完整的神经系统检查后进行计算机断层成像（CT）和（或）磁共振成像（MRI）对诊断 SDH 非常重要。SDH 在 CT 扫描上呈典型的新月形，但也可表现为凸起状，尤其是在出血的早期阶段，导致难以与硬膜外血肿相鉴别[5, 10, 27, 29]。

对 SDH 的治疗取决于血肿的大小和扩大速度。无症状或小的 SDH 可通过密切的临床和影像学监测进行保守治疗，但有症状或大的血肿应通过钻孔或开颅手术置入引流管抽吸或冲洗以清除血肿[13, 25-26]。此外，患者应长期服用抗癫痫药物。急性 SDH 通常比动脉性出血的硬膜外血肿扩张速度更慢，但由于存在严重的相关创伤性损伤，急性 SDH 死亡率较高（50%～90%）。术后并发症包括 IICP、脑水肿、反复出血、感染和癫痫发作[13]。

虽然正常足月分娩的婴儿也可能发生 SDH，但早产儿发生 SDH 的风险最高。在早产儿中，发生 SDH 的危险因素之一是在分娩过程中使用真空助产或产钳助产，导致累及大脑中微小血管损伤。如果婴儿被确诊 SDH，除了输血外可能需要手术干预以防止患儿脑损伤或死亡。从法医学的角度来看，儿科医生漏诊任何谨慎的医生都不难诊断的 SDH 会被认为是一种医疗事故。事实上，在颅脑超声（USG）、CT 和（或）MRI 扫描之后通过神经外科会诊，可以明确某些病例是否具有手术指征[5]。在这些病例中如果能及时正确诊断 SDH，通过小儿神经外科医生的建议，是可能通过适当的外科手术改善预后的。

传统上，在法医学中 SBS 的诊断充满困难与挑战，尽管文献中的相关报道不足，但通过影像学和实验室检查排除其他病因后，合并双侧 SDH、视网膜出血和创伤性脑损伤相应脑病三联征的儿科病例应考虑诊断 SBS[20-21, 24, 30]。最近，Lynøe 等评估了该三联征在识别 SBS 中的诊断价值，他们发现支持性的科学证据并不足（低质量证据）[19]。然而，在这种情况下，重要的是要意识到神经外科医生必须向有关法律当局报告这种疑似虐待儿童的病例，特别是在婴儿出现钙化或骨化的慢性 SDH 并伴有任何形式的身体伤害时[1, 14, 21, 24, 30]。从法律的角度来看，我们认为除了医院保存外，将钙化或骨化的慢性 SDH 患者的医疗文件保存在我们的私人档案中可能是有用的。

如下文详细描述的，常见医疗疏忽包括 SDH 诊治不及时，USG、CT 或 MRI 扫描不及时，或在服用抗凝药物治疗其他健康问题时监测凝血参数如国际标准化比值（INR）存在处置不当。

39.3　硬膜下血肿治疗疏忽导致医疗事故的案例情景

下面描述的是 SDH 诊疗疏忽导致医疗事故的案例，为治疗这些情况的医生做出正确诊断和适当治疗提供了一些有用的指导。

39.3.1　SDH 遗漏或延误诊断与治疗

案例 1：一起 SDH "延误诊断"导致死亡引起的诉讼

一个简单的案例场景可能如下："死者是一个……岁从楼梯上摔下的老年男性……他的格拉斯哥昏迷评分下降……，同时注意到他因……心脏原因服用华法林，他做了一个急诊 CT，放射科医生报告扫描未显示任何颅内出血，未曾尝试停止逆转患者的华法林并增加他的凝血因子。……之后，第二个放射科医生发现了一个……SDH。……这一信息被传达给负责死者的会诊医生……，未能联系值班神经外科医生寻求建议或停用/逆转华法林这一 SDH 的显著出血风险。……死者被转移到……没有人知道死者存在脑损伤并在服用华法林。当天晚些时候，死者出现了严重的神经功能恶化……再次 CT 扫描显示 SDH 进展并导致大脑中线移位，右脑室几乎完全受压。……医生也无能为力……第二天死者去世。"

在这个案例中，未能联系值班的神经外科医生寻求建议或停用/逆转华法林。因此，预计专家将认定未能在 CT 扫描上识别 SDH 的医疗疏忽，这导致未能停用华法林。如果能联系到值班神经外科医生，建议停止华法林，并通过使用适当的药物来逆转其影响，无疑会对患者的预后产生影响。如果没有这些失误，死者本能幸存下来。从法医学角度，这种失误导致了死者的 SDH 再次出血或持续性出血，导致明显的神经功能障碍和死亡。

案例 2：就 SDH "延误诊断" 后患者死亡向医院提出的诉讼

一个简单的案例场景可能如下："患者，……被收住……医院，伴有头痛，视物模糊，……呕吐，……和左眼肿胀眼睑下垂。进行了 CT 扫描并报告正常。她被收入病房观察并等待 MRI 扫描。……等待 MRI 6 天，医院的值班神经科医生没有进行复查。……患者左侧瞳孔散大固定，……对她的头部曾进行了 CT 扫描但报告正常。……复查 CT 扫描显示急性硬膜下血肿，联系另一家医院神经外科团队寻求建议。……到了另一家医院，发现她双侧瞳孔散大固定，……已经出现了不可逆转的脑损伤。进行了脑干测试确定了她的死亡。"

在这个案例中，没有将 SDH 考虑为病因，也没有将此类患者转诊至神经科以获得对症治疗的建议。因此，预计来自影像科医师和专科医师的顾问专家报告将认定对于患者影像检查和临床处置的疏忽，医疗水平低于平均水平。根据 SDH 的标准管理指南，采取积极的诊断策略而非单纯观察患者至关重要，因为引起症状和神经功能缺失的持续扩大的颅内病变可导致灾难性的结果。在这种情况下，研究报告中也存在影像学诊断漏诊，本应确定 SDH 并建议神经外科会诊。无可否认的是，如果这些失误没有发生，患者原本是可能存活的。在法医学上，这些错误明显导致了未能及时进行紧急神经外科干预以止血，导致患者神经功能恶化和死亡。

39.3.2 对危险因素缺乏意识

案例 1：因未能监测血小板计数和（或）给予 SDH 患者新鲜冷冻血浆而导致脑损伤引起的诉讼

一个简单的案例场景可能如下："一位患者表现出……伴有血尿，近期鼻出血病史，腿和胳膊上有瘀点……全血细胞计数（CBC）显示患者的血小板水平无法检出，……联系了血液病医生来评估……患者被诊断为……特发性血小板减少性紫癜（ITP）……血液科医生没有申请任何血小板……患者没有做进一步的血液检测来检查他的血小板。之后，患者出现了头痛……并急剧加重……导致呕吐，患者变得昏睡。CT 扫描显示新发 SDH……神经外科被紧急呼叫……清除血肿。……手术恢复后，他被转到康复医院……现在他存在视力问题和言语障碍。"

在这个案例中，由于未能给 SDH 患者补充血小板导致脑损伤。因此，由于患者血小板在入院时未能检测到，预计来自血液学顾问的专家报告将认定在脑出血前未能给予新鲜冷冻血浆和血小板替代品是对于患者的治疗疏忽。当患者实际上有脑出血时，血液科医生应适当地为患有 ITP 的患者输注新鲜冷冻血浆和血小板。

39.3.3 接受真空抽吸或产钳辅助分娩的新生早产儿

案例 1：因未行 CT 和脑电图（EEG）而做出正确诊断和适当治疗引发的诉讼

一个简单的案例场景可能如下："一个孕期 36 周在真空吸引器辅助下经阴道娩出的婴儿……真空杯压力在 500 mmHg……5 分钟时 Apgar 评分为 9 分。5 h 时婴儿呼吸窘迫加重……呼吸停止，行气管内插管，并被转移到我们的三级医疗机构……，入院时，婴儿的血红蛋白从 15.7 g/dl 降到 9.4 g/dl，血小板值下降到 69 000，提示消耗性凝血病……不幸的是，没有对凝血功能障碍进行进一步检查。之后，婴儿被送往三级医院；CT 显示双侧 SDH，EEG 显示癫痫病灶并继续使用苯巴比妥。……婴儿在出生后第 12 天拔管并复查 CT……。"

在这个案例中，对分娩过程中使用真空吸引或产钳的新生儿，未能使用 USG、CT 和 EEG 正确排除 SDH 的可能性。因此，预计专家将认定治疗婴儿的儿科医生存在疏忽，未能将凝血功能障碍确定为 SDH 的原因而导致了癫痫发作。法医学上，医师有责任正确调查凝血功能障碍的原因；未能及时诊断和进行适当的治疗可能会影响婴儿的预后。如果在这种情况下及时获得神经外科会诊，通过适当的外科手术改善预后是可能的。

39.3.4 "摇晃婴儿综合征"作为双侧 SDH 的原因

案例 1：因医生未能调查虐待的可能性而引发的诉讼

一个简单的案例场景可能如下："2019 年 1 月，一名两个半月大的婴儿因发热和癫痫发作被送往社区医院……婴儿情况稳定并被送回家，但在婴儿前臂上发现了几处香烟灼伤痕迹。然而 1 周后，婴儿因进行性偏瘫被救护车送往三级医院接受进一步治疗……。除了存在视网膜出血外，CT 扫描显示双侧 CSDH，……导致不可逆的脑损伤，报告指出 SBS 的可能性很高……经过进一步调查，婴儿被从父母身边带走，孩子的父亲被指控虐待儿童。"

在这个案例中，未能在婴儿治疗期间正确调查虐待的可能性。因此，预计专家将认定医生的疏忽，因为他们未能通过 CT 扫描查明 SDH，从而导致了不可逆的脑损伤。毫无疑问，如果没有这种疏忽，婴儿就不会遭受脑损伤。法医学上，这一疏忽很明显导致了婴儿的 CSDH，造成了严重的神经功能障碍。如果没有发现外部伤害的迹象，医生有责任彻底调查这种情况下受伤的原因，以防止未来发生类似悲剧。毫无疑问，未能及时诊断和采取适当的治疗措施会严重影响婴儿的预后，就像上述这个婴儿一样。

39.4 对案例场景的评价

如上文给出的病例情景所示，与 SDH 治疗疏忽相关的医疗事故包括漏诊或延误诊断、错误的神经科治疗、延误治疗和神经外科治疗不当。不幸的是这些情况对患者的后果可能是灾难性的，相关医生因此失业会造成严重的经济压力。

世界医学协会（WMA）将医疗事故定义为"由于医生在治疗过程中没有执行标准和最新的治疗方案、缺乏相应技术或没有给予患者治疗而造成的损害"[2, 4, 11, 17]。在法医学上，代理人（医师）在按照代理人（医师）合同的授权履行其治疗受试者的义务时，对未能达到其所期望的结果不负责任，但对因其为达到这一结果而做出的尝试、处理、行动和行为不够认真而造成的损害负有责任[17]。重要的是，代理人（医生）必须谨慎行事，即使是最轻微的过失也要负责[17]。因此，医生在执业范围内的一切失误，哪怕是轻微的失误，都应被认为存在一部分责任[17]。更重要的是，医生有义务对引起临床决策犹豫的情况开展研究工作，即使这种不确定程度很低，也应消除这种不确定，同时采取保护措施[17]。在选择不同治疗方法时，应考虑患者及其疾病的特点，避免使患者处于危险中的态度和行为，并选择最安全的方法[17]。事实上，客户（患者）有权期望代理人（医生）作为一名专业医生，在治疗的各个阶段表现出一丝不苟的照顾和关注。

在上述 4 个病例场景中，揭示了诸如延误诊断、影像学和临床治疗水平不足、由于未能正确评估实验室结果而未对血小板减少采取预防措施、未能预测新生儿凝血病相关 SDH 的发展，以及对 SBS 诊断错误和延迟等原因。代理人（医生）的职责并不是要保证患者完全康复，但也有义务照顾好她/他的患者。

39.5 结论

因为诊疗错误的发生率很高，即使在今天，SDH 也可能被误诊为其他临床疾病，从而导致潜在的永久性重大损伤。因此，经常会遇到有关 SDH 治疗的医疗事故案例，包括漏诊或延误诊断和治疗、危险因素治疗失败、接受真空或产钳辅助分娩的早产儿以及 SBS 病例。从法医学的角度来看，重要的是要能够认识到，作为患者的代理人，每一位医生都应该记住，在 SDH 管理中任何阶段的任何疏忽、粗心和不细致都将导致严重的医疗事故。

参考文献

1. Al Wohaibi M, Russell N, Al Ferayan A. A baby with armoured brain. CMAJ. 2003;169:46–7.
2. Arıkan M, Kalkan E, Erdi F, Deniz M, İzci E. The distinction between cases and malpractice-complications in medical law: the perspectives of the senior students of the faculty of medicine and the faculty of law, problems and suggestions for solution (in Turkish). Türk Nöroşir. 2016;26:40–8.
3. Beck J, Gralla J, Fung C, Ulrich CT, Schucht P, Fichtner J, Andereggen L, Gosau M, Hattingen E, Gutbrod K, Z'Graggen WJ, Reinert M, Hüsler J, Ozdoba C, Raabe A. Spinal cerebrospinal fluid leak as the cause of chronic subdural hematomas in nongeriatric patients. J Neurosurg. 2014;121:1380–7.
4. Birtek F. Complication-malpractice distinction in terms of medical interventions (in Turkish). İstanbul Barosu Dergisi. 2007;81:1997–2007.
5. Carroll JJ, Lavine SD, Meyers PM. Imaging of subdural hematomas. Neurosurg Clin N Am. 2017;28:179–203.
6. Catana D, Koziarz A, Cenic A, Nath S, Singh S, Almenawer SA, Kachur E. Subdural hematoma mimickers: a systematic review. World Neurosurg. 2016;93:73–80.
7. Dobran M, Iacoangeli M, Scortichini AR, Mancini F, Benigni R, Nasi D, Gladi M, Scerrati M. Spontaneous chronic subdural hematoma in young adult: the role of missing coagulation facto. G Chir. 2017;38:66–70.
8. Ellis GL. Subdural hematoma in the elderly. Emerg Med Clin North Am. 1990;8:281–94.
9. Gregori F, Colistra D, Mancarella C, Chiarella V, Marotta N, Domenicucci M. Arachnoid cyst in young soccer players complicated by chronic subdural hematoma: personal experience and review of the literature. Acta Neurol Belg. 2020;120:235–46.
10. Grelat M, Madkouri R, Bousquet O. Acute isodense subdural hematoma on computed tomography scan-diagnostic and therapeutic trap: a case report. J Med Case Rep. 2016;10:43.
11. Hakeri H. Distiction between malpractice and complication in medical law (in Turkish). Toraks Cerrahisi Bülteni. 2014;1:23–8.
12. Holl DC, Volovici V, Dirven CMF, Peul WC, van Kooten F, Jellema K, van der Gaag NA, Miah IP, Kho KH, den Hertog HM, Lingsma HF, Dammers R, Dutch Chronic Subdural Hematoma Research Group (DSHR). Pathophysiology and nonsurgical treatment of chronic subdural hematoma: from past to present to future. World Neurosurg. 2018;116:402–411.e2.
13. Iliescu IA. Current diagnosis and treatment of chronic subdural haematomas. J Med Life. 2015;8:278–84.
14. Ingraham FD, Matson DD. Subdural hematoma in infancy. J Pediatr. 1944;25:1–37.
15. Johnson R, Amine A, Farhat H. Spontaneous acute subdural hematoma associated with arachnoid cyst and intra-cystic hemorrhage. Cureus. 2018;10:e3383.
16. Kar SK, Kumar D, Singh P, Upadhyay PK. Psychiatric manifestation of chronic subdural hematoma: the unfolding of mystery in a homeless patient. Indian J Psychol Med. 2015;37:239–42.
17. Kök N. Malpractice and complication distinction. In: Kalkan E, Serel TA, Yılmaz EN, editors. Legal guide for physicians (in Turkish). Ankara: Turkish Neurosurgery Academy Publications No: 1, Sage Publishing; 2018. p. 109–39.
18. Kushner D. Mild traumatic brain injury: toward understanding manifestations and treatment. Arch Intern Med. 1998;158:1617–24.
19. Lynøe N, Elinder G, Hallberg B, Rosén M, Sundgren P, Eriksson A. Insufficient evidence for 'shaken baby syndrome'—a systematic review. Acta Paediatr. 2017;106:1021–7.
20. Martin HA, Woodson A, Christian CW, Helfaer MA, Raghupathi R, Huh JW. Shaken baby syndrome. Crit Care Nurs Clin North Am. 2006;18:279–86.
21. Mian M, Shah J, Dalpiaz A, Schwamb R, Miao Y, Warren K, Khan S. Shaken baby syndrome: a review. Fetal Pediatr Pathol. 2015;34:169–75.
22. Mori K, Yamamoto T, Horinaka N, Maeda M. Arachnoid cyst is a risk factor for chronic subdural hematoma in juveniles: twelve cases of chronic subdural hematoma associated with arachnoid cyst. J Neurotrauma. 2002;19:1017–27.
23. Prajsnar-Borak A, Balak N, Von Pein H, Glaser M, Boor S, Stadie A. Intracranial multiple myeloma may imitate subdural hemorrhage: how to overcome diagnostic limitations and avoid errors in treatment. Neurol Neurochir Pol. 2017;51:252–8.
24. Richards PG, Bertocci GE, Bonshek RE, Giangrande PL, Gregson RM, Jaspan T, Jenny C, Klein N, Lawler W, Peters M, Rorke-Adams LB, Vyas H, Wade A. Shaken baby syndrome. Arch Dis Child. 2006;91:205–6.

25. Santarius T, Kirkpatrick PJ, Ganesan D, Chia HL, Jalloh I, Smielewski P, Richards HK, Marcus H, Parker RA, Price SJ, Kirollos RW, Pickard JD, Hutchinson PJ. Use of drains versus no drains after burr-hole evacuation of chronic subdural haematoma: a randomised controlled trial. Lancet. 2009;374:1067–73.
26. Schmidt L, Gørtz S, Wohlfahrt J, Melbye M, Munch TN. Recurrence of subdural haematoma in a population-based cohort—risks and predictive factors. PLoS One. 2015;10:e0140450.
27. Sieswerda-Hoogendoorn T, Postema FAM, Verbaan D, Majoie CB, van Rijn RR. Age determination of subdural hematomas with CT and MRI: a systematic review. Eur J Radiol. 2014;83:1257–68.
28. Stone JL, Rifai MH, Sugar O, Lang RG, Oldershaw JB, Moody RA. Subdural hematomas. I. Acute subdural hematoma: progress in definition, clinical pathology, and therapy. Surg Neurol. 1983;19:216–31.
29. Tans JT. Computed tomography of extracerebral hematoma. Clin Neurol Neurosurg. 1977;79:296–306.
30. Vinchon M. Shaken baby syndrome: what certainty do we have? Childs Nerv Syst. 2017;33:1727–33.
31. Wu X, Li G, Zhao J, Zhu X, Zhang Y, Hou K. Arachnoid cyst-associated chronic subdural hematoma: report of 14 cases and a systematic literature review. World Neurosurg. 2018;109:e118–30.

第 40 章　脊柱硬膜下血肿

Arsal Acarbaş，Alican Tahta 和 Mehmet Turgut

译者：吴量

40.1　引言

脊柱硬膜下血肿（spinal subdural hematoma，SDH）是一种罕见情况，血肿块位于脊柱硬膜下腔。本病可压迫脊髓、马尾或脊神经根而导致永久性或暂时性神经功能缺损[25]。因此，如未及时诊断和治疗脊柱 SDH，可能会发生灾难性后果。脊柱 SDH 由 Duverney 于 1682 年首次报道[24]，占所有脊柱血肿的 4.1%。影像学方法的进步提高了脊柱 SDH 的检出率[25]。尤其对于存在进行性神经功能缺损的患者，应通过适当的影像学方法快速诊断并开始正确的治疗。

在本章中，我们将详细回顾脊柱 SDH 的流行病学、病因、发病机制、临床表现、影像学特征和治疗。

40.2　流行病学

脊柱 SDH 是一种罕见疾病，比脊柱硬膜外血肿更为罕见。在一项包含 600 多例脊柱血肿的 meta 分析中，只有 4% 的病例为脊柱 SDH[13]。脊柱 SDH 通常由创伤、脊柱手术或腰椎穿刺引起[4, 8, 23]。由于这是一种罕见的情况且文献中报道的患者多为病例报告，其发病率尚不清楚。

值得注意的是，自发性脊柱 SDH 在女性中略高发（1.25/1）[20]。脊柱 SDH 在不同年龄阶段有两个发病高峰：第一个高峰在 10～20 岁，第二个高峰在 60 岁[20, 22]。第一个高峰与血液疾病引起的出血有关，而第二个高峰与血管性疾病和抗凝治疗有关[20, 22]。

尽管在 46～60 岁和 61～75 岁的患者中主要好发于下胸椎和腰椎，但在 15 岁以下的儿童患者中脊柱 SDH 通常发生在颈椎和颈胸交界区，而 16～30 岁患者则略高发于颈椎和颈胸交界区[13]。Wang 等发表的文献综述也发现，胸段是特发性脊柱 SDH 最常见的部位（9/21，42.9%）[24]。

40.3　病因

脊柱 SDH 通常由创伤、脊柱手术或腰椎穿刺引起，但也可能与脊椎按摩治疗有关[2, 9, 17]。在各种血液疾病、脊髓病变、肿瘤或血管畸形患者中也会发生[6, 9, 23]。自发性脊柱 SDH 主要与凝血功能障碍、血管畸形和医源性原因有关[20]。

异常出血通常是止血机制受损的结果，如典型血友病、严重血小板减少症、急性白血病、真性红细胞增多症和出血倾向[4, 22]。除妊娠和子痫外，文献报道许多风湿性疾病，包括强直性脊柱炎、类风湿关节炎、系统性红斑狼疮以及先天性结缔组织和肾脏疾病如纤维肌肉发育不良、囊性纤维化和多囊肾等都是脊柱 SDH 的危险因素[5-6, 22]。绝大多数自发性脊柱 SDH 病例中均可以确定潜在的血液学或医源性病因[7, 9, 25]。然而，特发性脊柱 SDH 的多数患者没有明确的病因；因此，在这些病例中需要进一步调查以确定正确的诊断[7, 9, 25]。有报道称位于胸段的脊柱 SDH 累及多个脊柱节段[20]。各种血液疾病、凝血功能障碍以及抗凝治疗是近一半脊柱 SDH 患者的病因[22, 25]。

40.4　发病机制

解剖上，与颅内相比，脊髓硬膜下腔没有桥静脉[3]。脊柱 SDH 的发病机制尚不清楚，因为椎管内缺乏桥静脉，而桥静脉通常与颅内 SDH 的发生有关[22]。有研究认为，脊柱 SDH 的出血可能是由 Valsalva 动作引起的蛛网膜下腔内血管破裂造成的，这与腹内和胸内压力的增加有关[8]。根据他们的经验，一些作者注意到脑脊液压力等于硬膜外静脉丛压力，这提示鞘内压力的升高与硬膜外静脉丛的高压力存在密切关联[1, 9, 13, 19-20, 22]。

重要的是要认识到，蛛网膜下腔内血管的任何出血都会被脑脊液稀释，从而防止椎管内实性血肿的发展[22]。有趣的是，文献中有少数脊髓蛛网膜下腔出血合并脊柱 SDH 的病例报道[18, 22]。在这些病例中，普遍认为蛛网膜下腔内的任何出血都可能在出血量较大的情况下穿透进入硬膜下腔[22]。此外，脊柱 SDH 的出血可能与硬膜表面的细小血管破裂有关[11]。因此，在累及蛛网膜下腔或硬膜下腔的脊柱 SDH 病例中，确定出血的来源并不容易[22]。其他理论，包括血肿从幕上或斜坡区在硬膜内迁移到脊柱下部，也得到了广泛的研究[3, 16]。此外，文献中也有由于强烈的背部按摩和椎旁针灸而发生脊柱 SDH 的病例报道[9, 17]。

一般来说，大多数脊柱 SDH 的病因是多因素的，但其中 29.7% 的病例无法确定出血的确切原因，这些被称为特发性脊柱 SDH[13]。此外，脊柱 SDH 可能与抗凝治疗、任何先天性血管畸形以及硬膜外麻醉操作有关[4, 13, 15, 23]。人们普遍认为，自发性脊柱 SDH 的发生是由于在椎静脉丛内压力升高和（或）口服抗凝治疗的同时存在"最薄弱位点"[13]。因此，在接受抗凝药物治疗的病例中，应严格把握脊髓麻醉操作的适应证，并对这些患者进行密切随访[13]。在这些病例中为防止脊柱 SDH 的发生应考虑以下预防措施：（a）谨慎选择患者；（b）非创伤性腰椎穿刺；（c）脊髓麻醉与肝素化方案之间的间隔至少 1 h；（d）对血液凝血参数进行复查[13]。

40.5　临床表现

根据文献回顾，63% 的脊柱 SDH 患者最常见的初始症状是背部和肩胛间的疼痛，但在这类病例中，以头痛为首发症状的情况很少见[1, 3, 13]。脊柱 SDH 患者在出血部位表现为剧烈的刺痛感，可能持续时间较短，但随后会进行性发展为受累脊柱水平以下的肢体瘫痪。有趣的是，如果伴有蛛网膜下腔出血，也可能出现脑膜炎症状、意识丧失和癫痫，从而导致误诊为脑内血肿[13]。

脊柱 SDH 可表现为快速进展的神经系统症状[6]。在临床上，脊柱 SDH 患者的症状可能与脊髓损伤、脊髓受压或马尾综合征相似[22]。脊柱 SDH 最初通常表现为背痛和（或）神经根痛[22]。一般来说，根据脊柱 SDH 的位置不同，神经系统症状可能不同[14, 23]。同样，从最初症状到出现严重神经功能障碍的时间间隔也可能不同，从几小时到 3 周不等[14]。另外，神经功能缺失（运动、感觉或括约肌功能障碍）的程度可能从轻度单瘫到四肢瘫不等[14]。尽管目前有着多种影像学成像技术，但在无症状的脊柱 SDH 患者中，依然存在着漏诊的可能[18]。

40.6　影像学表现

在解剖学上，脊柱硬膜外血肿通常位于椎管后部，并且绝大多数发生在脊柱的颈胸段和胸腰段，这是由于硬膜外静脉丛的脆弱部分也位于相同的椎管部位[16, 21]。脊柱 SDH 发生在硬膜囊内，因此与硬膜外血肿不同，硬膜外脂肪依然存在并且硬膜也不会向内移位[21]。它被成对地置于侧方的齿状韧带处，由背隔包围，在轴位像上形成倒立的梅赛德斯–奔驰征（奔驰征）[12, 21]。因此，SDH 会压迫神经根，但不延伸到神经孔或与骨直接沟通。较小的血肿不会扩大潜在的硬膜下腔，因此它们不会表现为倒立的奔驰征[16, 21]。

40.7　计算机断层成像

计算机断层成像（CT）是急诊医学的主要影像学手段，通常在磁共振成像（MRI）之前用于急诊。然而在紧急情况下脊柱 SDH 很容易被遗漏，特别是当血肿较小的时候。在 MRI 上确定脊柱 SDH 后，回顾 CT 检查并使用窄窗来识别血肿是很好的尝试。此外，回顾 CT 检查有时也有助于明确诊断，可能会观察到新月形高密度影聚集于硬膜内侧，与低密度的硬膜外脂肪相区分[21]。

40.8　磁共振成像

MRI 是诊断脊髓损伤，包括脊柱 SDH 和其他脊髓病变的最佳成像方式。MRI 是鉴别和体现脊柱 SDH 的标准方法[10, 19, 21]。信号特征因血肿的不同时期而有所差异，可按时间顺序加以识别：超急性期 SDH 在 T1 加权像上呈等 / 低信号，在 T2 加权像上呈高信号；急性期 SDH 在 T1 加权像上呈轻度低 / 等信号，在 T2 加权像上呈低信号。亚急性早期 SDH 在 T1 加权像上呈高信号，T2 加权像上呈低信号,而亚急性晚期 SDH 在 T1、T2 加权像上均呈高信号。慢性 SDH 通常在 T1 和 T2 加权像上呈低信号[16, 25]。先前描述的"Y"型征(倒奔驰征)是血肿包裹于蛛网膜内线样结构周围的结果,以此可诊断硬膜外血肿而非硬膜下血肿[16, 21]。在轴位像上确认病灶位于硬膜下后,矢状位可用于检测其累及范围。通常情况下,如果在 MRI 矢状位上发现蛛网膜受压的征象(双凸圆盘样),特别是位于腰 5-骶 1 的区域,则应考虑为液体性出血性病变[16, 21]。然而,硬膜下淋巴瘤通常也可表现为类似的梭状或香肠状,但也可能呈现任何形状[16, 18, 21]。

40.9 治疗

通常,患者的神经系统检查对于治疗方案的选择非常重要[1]。目前对于脊柱 SDH 尚没有明确的治疗指南[8, 22-23]。一些报道建议在动态复查磁共振成像的基础上保守治疗,但也有人主张对脊柱 SDH 患者进行手术减压,包括去除椎板,但某些病例在手术减压后并没有取得临床改善[18-19, 23, 25]。

脊柱 SDH 的治疗方法除了腰椎穿刺外,还包括手术和非手术治疗[1]。一些作者报道了位于斜坡的较大 SDH 延伸至脊柱的患者进行保守治疗取得成功的病例[1, 22, 25]。但总体而言,许多作者建议,对于因脊柱 SDH 压迫伴有神经功能进行性恶化的患者,必须立即进行手术减压,包括椎板切除和血肿清除[2, 13, 24]。发病时的神经功能是预后的最强预测因素[13, 23]。根据我们的实践,手术干预是逆转脊柱 SDH 患者神经功能缺失的最佳选择。

手术的主要目的是通过减轻疼痛和恢复神经功能以改善生活质量。应行去椎板减压术,于后正中开放硬膜并清除 SDH[13]。对位于后方且无凝血功能障碍的 SDH,经皮穿刺引流可能是一种替代治疗方法[14, 22]。针对手术时机,一些作者建议应即刻进行手术,而另一些作者推荐待术前凝血指标正常或至少有所改善后再行手术治疗[8, 13, 18]。

40.10 典型病例

一位 29 岁的孕妇因先兆子痫在脊髓麻醉下接受了紧急剖宫产手术。1 天后患者因头痛、左臂麻木、颈部僵硬行颅脑 CT 检查发现中脑周围 SAH。CT 检查 20 min 后患者头痛加重并出现腿部麻木,因此紧急安排了头颅及颈胸椎 MRI 检查。当患者在进行扫描时,由于突发急性截瘫,MRI 不得不终止。颈椎和胸椎 MRI 显示从斜坡延伸至胸 10 水平的巨大 SDH,以及颈 6~7 水平脊髓前方硬膜下巢样病灶(动静脉畸形?),患者被紧急送入手术室(图 40.1)并进行了颈 6 和颈 7 的全椎板切除术。切开硬膜时,发现 SDH 包绕整个脊髓。位于颈 6~7 水平脊髓前方的致密血肿被清除,但未发现血管性病灶。术后对患者进行神经系统检查,除左肱三头肌肌力为 3/5 级外未见其他异常。术后 1 个月随访时,患者神经系统检查恢复正常。

40.11 结论

脊柱 SDH 是一种罕见的神经外科疾病,因此

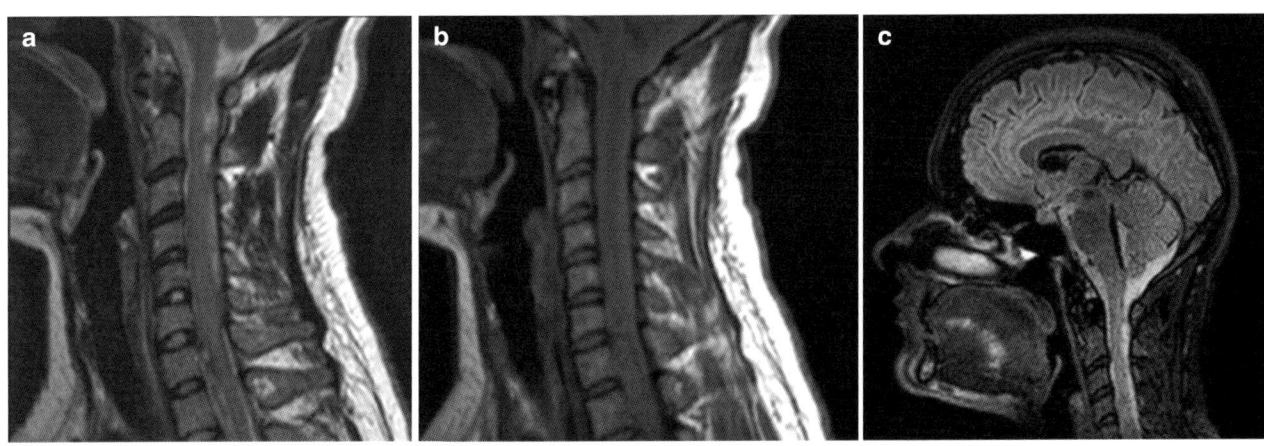

图 40.1 (a) T2 像显示位于脊髓背侧的高信号病变聚集。(b) 在 T1 像,硬膜下血肿使整个硬膜下腔的信号升高。(c) Flair 像显示自斜坡及枕大池向下延伸至椎管的硬膜下腔信号明显增强

选择合适的治疗方法具有挑战性。特别是在没有明确病因的情况下,自发性脊柱 SDH 更是一种极其罕见的情况。即使在今天,人们对脊柱 SDH 仍然知之甚少。如果怀疑脊柱 SDH,首选的影像学检查方法应是 MRI。即使存在一些其他治疗方法,手术减压应是首选治疗方式。特别是如果患者的神经功能进行性恶化,外科医生必须考虑进行减压手术。

参考文献

1. Ahn ES, Smith ER. Acute clival and spinal subdural hematoma with spontaneous resolution: clinical and radiographic correlation in support of a proposed pathophysiological mechanism: case report. J Neurosurg. 2005;103:175–9.
2. Benyaich Z, Laghmari M, Lmejjati M, Aniba K, Ghannane H, Benali SA. Acute lumbar spinal subdural hematoma inducing paraplegia after lumbar spinal manipulation: case report and literature review. World Neurosurg. 2019;128:182–5.
3. Bortolotti C, Wang H, Fraser K, Lanzino G. Subacute spinal subdural hematoma after spontaneous resolution of cranial subdural hematoma: causal relationship or coincidence?: case report. J Neurosurg Spine. 2004;100:372–4.
4. Cha Y-H, Chi JH, Barbaro NM. Spontaneous spinal subdural hematoma associated with low-molecular-weight heparin: case report. J Neurosurg Spine. 2005;2:612–3.
5. Esfahani DR, Shah HP, Behbahani M, Arnone GD, Mehta AI. Spinal subdural hematoma and ankylosing spondylitis: case report and review of literature. Spinal Cord Ser Cases. 2018;4:1–5.
6. Gabl M, Kostron H. Acute spinal subdural haematoma. Neurochirurgia. 1988;31:99–100.
7. Hsieh JK, Colby S, Nichols D, Kondylis E, Liu JK. Delayed development of spinal subdural hematoma following cranial trauma: a case report and review of the literature. World Neurosurg. 2020;141:44–51.
8. Hung K-S, Lui C-C, Wang C-H, Wang C-J, Howng S-L. Traumatic spinal subdural hematoma with spontaneous resolution. Spine. 2002;27:E534–8.
9. Ji GY, Oh CH, Choi W-S, Lee J-B. Three cases of hemiplegia after cervical paraspinal muscle needling. Spine J. 2015;15:e9–e13.
10. Johnson P, Hahn F, McConnell J, Graham E, Leibrock L. The importance of MRI findings for the diagnosis of nontraumatic lumbar subacute subdural haematomas. Acta Neurochir (Wien). 1991;113:186–8.
11. Kakitsubata Y, Theodorou SJ, Theodorou DJ, Miyata Y, Ito Y, Yuki Y, Honbu K, Maehara T. Spontaneous spinal subarachnoid hemorrhage associated with subdural hematoma at different spinal levels. Emerg Radiol. 2010;17:69–72.
12. Kasliwal MK, Shannon LR, O'Toole JE, Byrne RW. Inverted Mercedes Benz sign in lumbar spinal subdural hematoma. J Emerg Med. 2014;47:692–3.
13. Kreppel D, Antoniadis G, Seeling W. Spinal hematoma: a literature survey with meta-analysis of 613 patients. Neurosurg Rev. 2003;26:1–49.
14. Kyriakides AE, Lalam RK, El Masry WS. Acute spontaneous spinal subdural hematoma presenting as paraplegia: a rare case. Spine. 2007;32:E619–22.
15. Maddali P, Walker B, Fisahn C, Page J, Diaz V, Zwillman ME, Oskouian RJ, Tubbs RS, Moisi M. Subdural thoracolumbar spine hematoma after spinal anesthesia: a rare occurrence and literature review of spinal hematomas after spinal anesthesia. Cureus. 2017;9:e1032.
16. Manish K, Chandrakant S, Abhay M. Spinal subdural haematoma. J Orthop Case Rep. 2015;5:72–4.
17. Maste P, Paik S-H, Oh J-K, Kim Y-C, Park M-S, Kim T-H, Kwak Y-H, Jung J-K, Lee H-W, Kim SW. Acute spinal subdural hematoma after vigorous back massage: a case report and review of literature. Spine. 2014;39:E1545–8.
18. Mavroudakis N, Levivier M, Rodesch G. Central cord syndrome due to a spontaneously regressive spinal subdural hematoma. Neurology. 1990;40:1306.
19. Park YJ, Kim SW, Ju CI, Wang HS. Spontaneous resolution of non-traumatic cervical spinal subdural hematoma presenting acute hemiparesis: a case report. Korean J Spine. 2012;9:257.
20. Pereira BJA, de Almeida AN, Muio VMF, de Oliveira JG, de Holanda CVM, Fonseca NC. Predictors of outcome in nontraumatic spontaneous acute spinal subdural hematoma: case report and literature review. World Neurosurg. 2016;89:574–7.
21. Pierce JL, Donahue JH, Nacey NC, Quirk CR, Perry MT, Faulconer N, Falkowski GA,

Maldonado MD, Shaeffer CA, Shen FH. Spinal hematomas: what a radiologist needs to know. Radiographics. 2018;38:1516–35.
22. Rettenmaier LA, Holland MT, Abel TJ. Acute, nontraumatic spontaneous spinal subdural hematoma: a case report and systematic review of the literature. Case Rep Neurol Med. 2017;2017:2431041.
23. Thiex R, Thron A, Gilsbach JM, Rohde V. Functional outcome after surgical treatment of spontaneous and nonspontaneous spinal subdural hematomas. J Neurosurg Spine. 2005;3:12–6.
24. Wang Y, Zheng H, Ji Y, Lu Q, Li X, Jiang X. Idiopathic spinal subdural hematoma: case report and review of the literature. World Neurosurg. 2018;116:378–82.
25. Yokota K, Kawano O, Kaneyama H, Maeda T, Nakashima Y. Acute spinal subdural hematoma: a case report of spontaneous recovery from paraplegia. Medicine. 2020;99:e20032.

结 语

除了位于脊柱的硬脊膜下血肿外，硬脑膜下血肿（SDH）是一种常见的神经外科疾病，由于医学的不断发展和新外科治疗方法的出现，其标准治疗方式仍然存在争议。由于老年患者的预期寿命增加和抗凝治疗的广泛应用，SDH 的发病率正在全球范围内增加。考虑到 SDH 存在急性、亚急性和慢性等多种表现形式，这些不同形式具有不同的临床表现，并影响采用的治疗方式。SDH 患者的临床症状将决定进行何种神经影像学检查，无论是计算机断层成像还是磁共振成像，都将更好地帮助医生判断血肿的位置、范围，以及可能的发病原因。患者的临床病史有时可以提供有价值的信息，以解释 SDH 的发生发展原因，例如在电疗、腰椎穿刺、脑脊液分流术、自发性低颅内压、抗凝治疗、头部创伤或与运动有关的损伤的情况下。

SDH 的治疗方法主要是外科手术清除血肿，手术的目的是减轻颅内或椎管内的占位效应以及对大脑或脊髓的压力。由于现代医学的不断发展，新的治疗方法，如内窥镜血肿探查清除或脑膜中动脉栓塞在内的微创技术，也已广泛应用于临床。同样，通过使用皮质类固醇、阿托伐他汀和氨甲环酸，SDH 的保守治疗也取得了进展。即使医疗水平不断提高，但并发症的出现和血肿的复发，仍可能会导致需要再次手术。由于老年人易复发 SDH，其术后康复治疗也是患者术后恢复的重要组成部分。医学法律关注的焦点集中于成人 SDH 的诊断和治疗过失，以及儿童的非意外创伤。

Aydın, Turkey	Mehmet Turgut, MD, PhD
Marrakech, Morocco	Ali Akhaddar, MD, IFAANS
Syracuse, NY, USA	Walter A. Hall, MD, MBA
Ankara, Turkey	Ahmet T. Turgut, MD